Mosby's

Comprehensive Review

for

VETERINARY TECHNICIANS

Mosby's Comprehensive Review for

VETERINARY TECHNICIANS

Second Edition

Edited by

Monica M. Tighe, RVT, BA
Professor, Veterinary Technician Program
St. Clair College of Applied Arts and Technology
Windsor, Ontario

Marg Brown, RVT, BEd AD ED
Professor, Veterinary Technician Program
Seneca College, King Campus
King City, Ontario

ONTARIO ASSOCIATION VETERINARY TECHNICIANS

With 125 illustrations

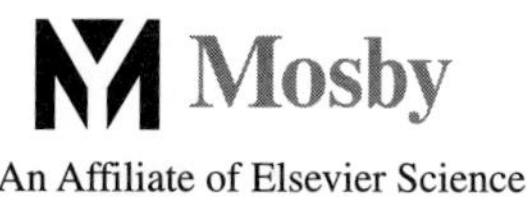

An Affiliate of Elsevier Science

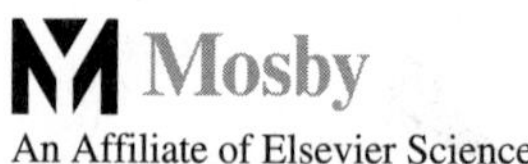
An Affiliate of Elsevier Science

11830 Westline Industrial Drive
St. Louis, Missouri 63146

MOSBY'S COMPREHENSIVE REVIEW FOR VETERINARY TECHNICIANS

0-323-01934-X

Second edition

NOTICE

Pharmacology is an ever-changing field. Standard safety precautions must be followed, but as new research and clinical experience broaden our knowledge, changes in treatment and drug therapy may become necessary or appropriate. Readers are advised to check the most current product information provided by the manufacturer of each drug to be administered to verify the recommended dose, the method and duration of administration, and contraindications. It is the responsibility of the licensed prescriber, relying on experience and knowledge of the patient, to determine dosages and the best treatment for each individual patient. Neither the publisher nor the authors assume any liability for any injury and/or damage to persons or property arising from this publication.

Library of Congress Cataloging-in-Publication Data
Mosby's comprehensive review for veterinary technicians / edited by Monica M. Tighe, Marg Brown.–2nd ed.
p. cm.
Includes bibliographical references.
ISBN 0-323-01934-X (alk. paper)
1. Animal health technicians–Examinations, questions, etc. 2. Animal health technology–Examinations, questions, etc. I. Title: Comprehensive review for veterinary technicians. II. Tighe, Monica M. III. Brown, Marg. IV. Mosby, Inc.

SF774.4 .M67 2002
636.089′06953′076–dc21

2002037896

Managing Editor: Teri Merchant
Publishing Services Manager: John Rogers
Senior Project Manager: Beth Hayes
Designer: Kathi Gosche
Cover Designer: Jennifer Brockett

KI/MVB
Printed in the United States of America

Last digit is the print number: 9 8 7 6 5 4 3 2 1

To my "new" husband John E. Treacy
MMT

To Phil, Jacquie, and Tucker
MB

Contributors

Kathleen Alston, AHT, RVT, LVT
Level II Technician, Anesthesia Department
Cornell University Hospital for Animals
Ithaca, New York

Karen Anderson, AHT
Immediate Past Vice President/Ombudsman
Alberta Association of Animal Health Technologists
Minburn, Alberta

Rebecca M. Atkinson, BSc, RVT
Guelph, Ontario

Patricia L. Bell, BSc, RVT
Instructor, Veterinary Technology/Biotechnology Programs
Saskatchewan Institute of Applied Sciences and Technologies
Saskatoon, Saskatchewan

Patricia Bonnot, AHT
Laboratory Technician, Animal Health Department
Vanier College
Montreal, Quebec

Marg Brown, RVT, BEd AD ED
Professor, Veterinary Technician Program
Seneca College, King Campus
King City, Ontario

Frances Federbush-Cheslo, AHT, RVT
Marketing Services Team Leader
Hill's Pet Nutrition Canada, Inc.
Mississauga, Ontario

Sue Cornwell, RVT
Large Animal Clinic
Ontario Veterinary College
University of Guelph
Guelph, Ontario

Carlene A. Decker, BS, CVT
Associate Professor
Parkland College Veterinary Technology Program
Paxton, Illinois

Barbara Donaldson, BA, BEd, MEd, RVT, VDT
Professor, Veterinary Technology Program
Coordinator, Veterinary Assistant Program
St. Lawrence College
Kingston, Ontario

Melanie K. Gramling, AS, CVT, VTS (ECC)
ICU Nursing Supervisor
Florida Veterinary Specialists
Tampa, Florida

Joanne Hamel, VT, RT, BA
Professor, Coordinator, Veterinary Technology
Veterinary Hospital Managers Programs
St. Lawrence College
Kingston, Ontario

Kim Healey, BA, RVT
Registered Veterinary Technician
Mohawk Equine Services
Mississauga, Ontario

Mary Lake, RVT
Teaching/Research Technician
Department of Pathobiology
Ontario Veterinary College
University of Guelph
Guelph, Ontario

Mary Martini, RVT, RLAT
Manager, Central Animal Facility
Ontario Veterinary College
University of Guelph
Guelph, Ontario

Sandra McCampbell, CAHT
Homestead, Florida

Pierry McLean, RVT
Radiology Department
University of Guelph
Guelph, Ontario

A. Patrick Navarre, BS, RVT
School of Veterinary Medicine
Purdue University
West Lafayette, Indiana

Julie Ovington, RVT
Past President, Ontario Association of Veterinary Technicians
Mississauga, Ontario

Elisa Petrollini, CVT, VTS (ECC)
Emergency Service Nursing
Veterinary Hospital of the University of Pennsylvania
Philadelphia, Pennsylvania

Sally Powell, CVT, VTS (ECC)
Supervisor of Nursing, Emergency Service
University of Pennsylvania Veterinary Hospital
Philadelphia, Pennsylvania

Penny Rivait, RVT, BA, RLAT
Professor, Veterinary Technician Program
St. Clair College of Applied Arts and Technology
Windsor, Ontario

Shirley Sandoval, RVT, AAS
Scientific Instructional Technician II
Washington State University
Veterinary Clinical Sciences
Veterinary Teaching Hospital
Pullman, Washington

Margi Sirois, EdD, MS, RVT
Program Director Thomson Education Direct
Veterinary Technician Program
Holiday, Florida

Teresa Sonsthagen, BS, LVT
Research Specialist II
North Dakota State University
Veterinary Technology Program
Fargo, North Dakota

Monica M. Tighe, RVT, BA
Professor, Veterinary Technician Program
St. Clair College of Applied Arts and Technology
Windsor, Ontario

James A. Topel, CVT
Instructor, Veterinary Technology
Colorado Mountain College
Glenwood Springs, Colorado

William L. Wade, LVT, LATG
Manager, Compliance and Training
Center for Comparative Medicine
Northwestern University
Chicago, Illinois

Dan Walsh, LVT, MPS
Department of Veterinary Science
State University of New York
Delhi, New York

Elizabeth Warren, RVT
Austin Community College
Austin, Texas

Kisha L. White-Farrar, BSc, RVT
Lead Nurse, Hullen Hills Animal Hospital
Fort Worth, Texas

Preface

The new and improved second edition of *Mosby's Comprehensive Review for Veterinary Technicians* builds on the strengths of the first edition while making further enhancements. As with the first publication, this comprehensive review was written collectively by Canadian and American veterinary technicians for veterinary technician students and graduates. This version is also written in outline format for an easy review of the material. Each chapter includes learning outcomes, multiple-choice questions, and a list of current references for further study. Each chapter has been revamped by either its original author or new authors. The chapters have been reorganized and divided into logical sections.

This text cannot possibly cover all areas of veterinary technology; however, it is an excellent primary, overall review guide that can be used in conjunction with textbooks for specific areas.

At the end of the text there is a 300-question comprehensive test. The test is an overview of each topic presented and, as with the book, is not meant to simulate the content or percentage of each topic that might be on a credentialing examination.

The appendixes have been expanded to contain Internet websites for various associations and further resources. Addresses and contacts of provincial and state associations have also been updated and are current at the time of writing. The appendixes also include abbreviations and symbols, species information, normal references, and metric equivalents. We hope you enjoy this study guide/resource text.

Monica M. Tighe
Marg Brown

Acknowledgments

Our thanks to Teri Merchant, Jody McBride, and Mary Schierbaum at Elsevier Science Publishing for helping us maintain quality and focus.

A heartfelt thanks is again extended to the contributors who wrote these chapters and to their families and employers for their support.

Finally, to all technicians who continue to encourage the development of knowledge and professionalism in the field of veterinary technology, may you never stop learning and growing.

Monica M. Tighe
Marg Brown

Contents

Appendixes

Mosby's Comprehensive Review for VETERINARY TECHNICIANS

PART I

Basic and Clinical Sciences

CHAPTER 1

Animal Anatomy and Physiology

Penny Rivait

OUTLINE

LEARNING OUTCOMES

After reading this chapter you should be able to:

1. Explain the various processes that enable substances to move in and out of cells.
2. List the structural and functional characteristics of the four primary body tissues and their subtypes.
3. Define and be able to use all directional terms.
4. Classify and identify basic bones and joints.
5. List the three types of muscle and state the distinct characteristics of each.
6. Describe the divisions of the nervous system and state how they relate to each other.
7. List the parts of the brain and state their functions.
8. List the parts of the cardiovascular system and state their functions.
9. Explain the cardiac cycle and identify its components on a typical electrocardiographic tracing.
10. Compare and contrast the structure and function of arteries and veins.
11. Explain the process of digestion.
12. Name the parts of the ruminant stomach and state their functions.
13. Describe the structure of lymph vessels, lymph nodes, and lymphatic organs and their functions.
14. Name the parts of the respiratory system and state their functions.
15. Describe the three basic processes of respiration.
16. Define *tidal volume, residual volume, dead space, apnea, eupnea,* and *dyspnea.*
17. Explain the anatomy and functions of the excretory system.
18. Explain the anatomy and physiology of the male and female reproductive systems.
19. Explain the estrous cycle.
20. Describe the process of parturition and lactation.
21. List the endocrine glands; state the hormones they release and their functions.
22. Describe the structure and function of all sense organs.

Anatomy and physiology are the essential foundations of veterinary technology. Many clinical procedures such as positioning of a patient for a radiograph, preparing for a surgical procedure, or simply placing a catheter involve a working knowledge of anatomy and physiology. Understanding the unique interrelationships of the animal's body systems is critical in assisting with the management of disease.

DEFINITIONS

I. Anatomy: the science of the structure of the body and the relation of its parts

II. Physiology: the science of how the body functions

CELL STRUCTURE AND PHYSIOLOGY

Cells are the basic unit of life. Cells are either prokaryotes or eukaryotes.

Prokaryote: "Before Nucleus"

I. A cell that lacks a true membrane-bound nucleus

II. All bacteria are prokaryotes

Eukaryote: "True Nucleus"

I. A cell that has a membrane-bound nucleus and contains many different membrane-bound organelles

II. All multicellular organisms are composed of eukaryotic cells

III. Composition of eukaryotic cells

Three major parts: cell membrane, cytoplasm, and nucleus

A. Cell membrane (plasma membrane)

Separates the cell from its external environment

1. Consists of a double phospholipid layer with interspersed proteins (fluid-mosaic model), also contains carbohydrate chains and cholesterol
2. Semipermeable; therefore allows various substances to move in and out of the cell
3. Some cells have surface modifications such as hairlike projections (cilia) that are used for surface movement or a single, longer projection (a flagellum) that is used for cellular movement, or microvilli to increase surface area (especially in absorptive cells)

B. Cytoplasm

Encompasses everything within the cell except the nucleus. Organelles within the cytoplasm have very specialized functions

1. Ribosomes
   - a. Float freely or are attached to the endoplasmic reticulum
   - b. Composed of protein and ribosomal ribonucleic acid (RNA)
   - c. Site of protein synthesis
2. Mitochondria
   - a. "Powerhouse" of the cell
   - b. Contains mitochondrial deoxyribonucleic acid (DNA) and protein
   - c. Double membrane with the inner membrane extending into folds called cristae
   - d. Cristae increase surface area for production of adenosine triphosphate (ATP)
   - e. ATP is produced through the process of cellular respiration (Krebs cycle, citric acid cycle, tricarboxylic acid cycle)
   - f. Cells that use large amounts of energy (e.g., skeletal muscle) have large numbers of mitochondria
3. Endoplasmic reticulum (ER)
   - a. Rough endoplasmic reticulum (RER)
     - (1) Hollow system of flattened membranous channels with attached ribosomes
     - (2) Acts as transportation network for proteins
   - b. Smooth endoplasmic reticulum (SER)
     - (1) Hollow system of flattened membranous channels without attached ribosomes
     - (2) Not involved in protein synthesis
     - (3) Important in synthesizing cholesterol, steroid-based hormones and lipids; also important in detoxification of drugs, breakdown of glycogen, and transportation of fats
     - (4) Liver cells, intestinal cells, and interstitial cells of the testes have large amounts of SER
4. Golgi complex (Golgi apparatus)
   - a. Stacked, saucer-shaped membranes that function as a receiving, packaging, and distribution center
   - b. Modifies and packages substances received from the ER: exports them from the cell or releases them into the cytoplasm for internal use
   - c. Produces lysosomes
5. Lysosomes
   - a. Contain digestive enzymes that digest intracellular bacteria, break down nonfunctional organelles, and are the principal organelles in digestion of nutrients
   - b. Autolysis (i.e., self-digestion of the cell) occurs if the lysosome enzymes are released into cytoplasm
   - c. Large numbers found in phagocytic cells
6. Peroxisomes
   - a. Membrane-bound organelles that contain strong oxidase and catalase enzymes

   b. Use oxygen to detoxify toxic substances, especially alcohol and formaldehyde
   c. Very important in converting free radicals (normal byproducts of cellular metabolism but harmful to biological molecules if left to accumulate) into hydrogen peroxide, which is converted to water by catalase enzymes
   d. Large amounts found in liver and kidney cells
7. Cytoskeleton
   a. Consists of microtubules, microfilaments, and intermediate filaments that are made of proteins
   b. Provides an elaborate internal framework that gives the cell form, structure, and support; anchors organelles; and enables movement
8. Centrioles
   a. Microtubules arranged to form a hollow tube
   b. Important in organizing the mitotic spindle
   c. Form the base of cilia and flagella

C. Nucleus
1. Control center of the cell
2. Contains DNA (deoxyribonucleic acid), which governs heredity and protein synthesis
3. DNA is in the form of chromatin in the nondividing cell and in the form of chromosomes in the dividing cell
4. Has a double, semipermeable nuclear membrane or envelope
5. Contains one or more nucleoli, which manufacture the ribosomal units

MOVEMENT IN AND OUT OF CELLS

I. Definitions
   A. Solute: a substance that can be dissolved
   B. Solvent: a substance that does the dissolving
   C. Solution: when the solute has dissolved and is no longer distinguishable from the solvent (a uniform mixture)
   D. Intracellular: within a cell
   E. Extracellular: outside of a cell
   F. Intercellular: (interstitial) between cells

II. Passive processes: no energy is expended by the cell
   A. Diffusion
      1. Movement of molecules (e.g., water and ions) from a high concentration to a low concentration
      2. Oxygen passes into a cell while carbon dioxide passes out of cells by simple diffusion through the lipid layer of the cell membrane
   B. Facilitated diffusion
      1. Diffusion with the aid of carrier proteins
      2. Glucose enters the cell by this method
   C. Osmosis
      1. Movement of water through a semipermeable membrane from a region of low solute (high solvent) to a region of high solute (low solvent)
      2. Water constantly moves in and out of the cell by osmosis
      3. Osmotic pressure is the amount of pressure necessary to stop the flow of water across the membrane
   D. Filtration
      1. Substances are forced through a membrane by hydrostatic pressure; small solutes will pass through; larger molecules will not
      2. Important in kidney function

III. Active processes: energy is expended by the cell
   A. Endocytosis: taking into the cell
      1. Phagocytosis ("cell eating"): cell membrane extends around solid particles
         a. Some white blood cells and macrophages are phagocytic
      2. Pinocytosis (bulk-phase) ("cell drinking"): cell membrane extends around fluid droplets
         a. Important in absorptive cells in small intestine
      3. Receptor mediated: specialized membrane receptors bind to substances entering the cell
         a. Enzymes, insulin, hormones, iron, and cholesterol enter the cell by this method
   B. Exocytosis: materials are expelled by a cell
      1. Waste products are excreted and useful products are secreted into the extracellular space
      2. Hormones, neurotransmitter chemicals, and mucus are released from the cell by this method
   C. Active transport
      1. Movement of molecules from a low concentration to a high concentration with the aid of carrier proteins
      2. Sodium-potassium pump is an active transport pump within cell membranes, most ions and amino acids move into the cells by this method

IV. Hypotonic, hypertonic, and isotonic
   A. Hypotonic (extracellular fluid is less concentrated than the intracellular fluid)
      1. Red blood cells placed in a hypotonic solution due to osmosis will gain water and burst (hemolysis)

B. Hypertonic (extracellular fluid is more concentrated than the intracellular fluid)
  1. Red blood cells placed in a hypertonic solution due to osmosis will lose water and *crenate* (shrivel)
C. Isotonic (concentrations of the extracellular and intracellular fluids are equal)
  1. Red blood cells placed in an isotonic solution will remain unchanged due to equal osmotic pressures

TISSUES

I. Tissue: groups of similar cells with related functions
II. Histology or microanatomy: the study of tissues
III. Four primary types of tissue
  A. Epithelial
  B. Connective
  C. Muscle
  D. Nervous

Epithelial Tissue

I. Covers body surface, lines body cavities, and forms the active part of glands
  A. Functions are protection, secretion, excretion, filtration, absorption of nutrients, and receipt of sensory information
II. May form simple (one cell layer) or stratified (more than one cell layer) tissue
III. Subtypes
  A. Squamous epithelium
    1. Flat, thin, platelike cells
    2. Simple squamous epithelial tissue lines blood vessels (endothelium), alveoli of lungs, thoracic and abdominal cavities
    3. Stratified squamous epithelial tissue is found in areas of wear: nonkeratinized tissue lines the mouth, esophagus, vagina, and rectum; keratinized tissue makes up the epidermis
  B. Cuboidal epithelium
    1. Cube-shaped cells
    2. Simple cuboidal epithelial tissue is important in absorption and secretion; forms the active part of glands and small ducts, ovary surface, and kidney tubules
    3. Stratified cuboidal epithelial tissue is fairly rare but lines the ducts of sweat, salivary, and mammary glands
  C. Columnar epithelium
    1. Tall, rectangular-shaped cells
      a. Simple columnar epithelial tissue lines the digestive tract from stomach to rectum and is important for absorption and secretion; these cells also have a surface modification known as microvilli and are associated with mucus-secreting cells known as goblet cells
      b. Simple columnar epithelial tissue with cilia lines bronchi, uterine tubes, and uterus
      c. Stratified columnar epithelial tissue is relatively rare but is found in mammary ducts and portions of the male's urethra
  D. Pseudostratified columnar epithelium
    1. Appears to be more than one layer, but all cells touch the basal membrane
    2. Usually ciliated and often associated with goblet cells; found in the respiratory tract
  E. Transitional epithelium
    1. May resemble both cuboidal and squamous shapes depending on the thickness of the organ but is found in areas where a great degree of distention is needed, such as the urinary bladder, ureters, and part of the urethra (cuboidal when bladder is empty and squamous when bladder is full)
  F. Glandular epithelium
    1. Highly specialized epithelial cells with the ability to secrete various products
    2. Classified as endocrine or exocrine
      a. Endocrine: ductless, secrete hormones directly into the bloodstream (e.g., ovaries [estrogen])
      b. Exocrine: have ducts and secrete onto an epithelial surface (e.g., sweat glands)
        (1) Exocrine glands are very numerous and classified in many different ways, especially by their structure, method of secretion, and type of secretion

Connective Tissue

I. Widely distributed throughout the body and composed of three different elements: cells, fibers, and matrix (ground substance)
II. A variety of functions depending on tissue type (connects and supports, protects, insulates, transports fluids, stores energy, defends)
III. Fiber types
  A. Collagen fibers (white fibers): long, straight, very strong white fibers composed of collagen protein
  B. Elastic fibers (yellow fibers): long, thin, branching stretchable yellow fibers composed of elastin protein
  C. Reticular fibers: fine, collagen fibers in a complex network
IV. Cell types
  A. Many different cell types depending on the type of tissue; immature and active cells have the suffix *blast-* and mature cells have the suffix *cyte-*

Table 1-1 Connective tissue

Category	Type	Subtype	Examples and composition
Connective tissue proper	Loose	Aerolar	Most widely distributed supports organs, protective and provide flexibility for all three fiber types, fibroblasts, macrophages, mast cells, white blood cells
		Adipose	Insulates, protects, cushions, reserve energy composed of fat cells (adipocytes)
		Reticular	Supportive tissue Found in spleen, liver, lymph nodes, and bone marrow Network of fine reticular fibers, macrophages, and fibroblasts
	Dense	Regular	Tendons (bone to muscle), ligaments (bone to bone), and aponeuroses (muscle to muscle) Collagen fibers arranged in a parallel pattern and fibroblasts provide strong attachments
		Irregular	Dermis of the skin, organ capsules, joint capsules Collagen fibers arranged in an irregular pattern, elastic fibers, fibroblasts provide strength and support to areas experiencing tension from all directions
		Elastic	Ligaments which contain more elastic fibers than collagen nuchal ligament in horses necks
Specialized	Cartilage	Hyaline	Nose, trachea, larynx, embryonic skeleton, costal cartilage, articular cartilage Collagen fibers and chondrocytes support with some flexibility
		Elastic	Pinna, auditory canal, epiglottis, elastic fibers Provides shape and great flexibility
		Fibrocartilage	Intervertebral discs, pubic symphysis, disk in stifle thick collagen fibers and chondrocytes provide strong support
	Bone (osseous)	Compact (dense)	Bones, collagen fibers, osteocytes, and calcified matrix Supports, protects, houses blood-producing tissue, stores calcium and other minerals
		Spongy (cancellous)	Lattice-like bone structure
	Blood		Erythrocytes, leukocytes, thrombocytes, plasma

V. Connective tissue types are divided into two categories: connective tissue proper and specialized connective tissue and their subtypes (Table 1-1)

Muscle Tissue

I. Skeletal (striated)
   A. Under voluntary control
   B. Long, parallel striated fibers with multiple nuclei located on the periphery
   C. Attach to and move skeletal muscles

II. Smooth
   A. Involuntary control
   B. Spindle-shaped smooth cells with a centrally located nucleus
   C. Found in walls of hollow organs (e.g., digestive tract blood vessels)

III. Cardiac
   A. Involuntary control
   B. Long, striated cells that join together at points known as intercalated discs; single, centrally located nucleus
   C. Found only in the heart (myocardium)

Nervous Tissue

I. Specialized for conducting electrical impulses
II. Major locations are brain, spinal cord, and nerves
III. Two major cell types: neurons, which conduct impulses, and neuroglial (glial) cells, which are supporting cells and do not conduct impulses

DIRECTIONAL TERMINOLOGY

I. Cranial: toward the head (e.g., the thoracic vertebrae are cranial to the sacral vertebrae)
II. Caudal: toward the tail (e.g., the lumbar vertebrae are caudal to the cervical vertebrae)
III. Dorsal: toward the backbone (e.g., the thoracic vertebrae are dorsal to the sternum)
IV. Ventral: away from the backbone (e.g., the umbilicus is on the ventral surface of the cat)
V. Medial: closest to the median plane (e.g., the tibia is medial to the fibula)
VI. Lateral: farthest from the medial plane (e.g., the ribs are lateral to the sternum)
VII. Proximal: the point closest to the backbone, used especially in reference to limbs (e.g., the greater trochanter is on the proximal end of the femur)

VIII. Distal: the point farthest away from the backbone, used especially in reference to limbs (e.g., the fabellae are located at the distal end of the femur)
IX. Anterior: toward the head, used especially in reference to limbs (e.g., the patella is on the anterior aspect of the rear leg)
X. Posterior: toward the tail, used especially in reference to limbs (e.g., the Achilles tendon is on the posterior aspect of the rear leg)
XI. Palmar: bottom of the front foot
XII. Plantar: bottom of the rear foot

BODY SYSTEMS

Skeletal System

I. Osteology: study of the bones
II. Skeletal divisions
  A. Axial skeleton
    1. Bones found on the midline or attached to it (excludes the limbs)
    2. Examples include the ribs, skull, vertebral column, and sternum
  B. Appendicular skeleton
    1. All bones that compose the limbs (e.g., femur, humerus)
III. Function of bones
  A. Support soft tissues of the body
  B. Protect vital organs (e.g., heart)
  C. Act as levers for muscle attachment
  D. Store minerals
  E. Produce blood cells
IV. Types of bone
  A. Compact (dense) bone
    1. Has very few spaces, appears solid, provides strength and support
    2. Made of haversian systems (osteons); each system is composed of the following
      a. Central haversian canal: houses blood vessels and nerves
      b. Canaliculi: very small canals that radiate out, connecting all lacunae to each other and to the central haversian canal
      c. Lamellae: concentric rings of bone
      d. Lacunae: small spaces that house osteocytes (mature bone cells)
  B. Spongy (cancellous) bone
    1. No haversian systems
    2. Large spaces between lattice-like pieces of bone known as trabeculae
    3. Spaces are filled with marrow
V. Bone cells
  A. Osteoblast: immature bone cell that produces bone matrix known as osteoid
  B. Osteocyte: mature bone cell; each cell occupies a lacunae in bone
  C. Osteoclast: very large multinucleated cells that are capable of dissolving bone matrix and releasing minerals, a process known as osteolysis, or resorption
    1. It is important for the body to maintain a balance between osteoblast and osteoclast activity
VI. Classification of bones
  A. Long bones
    1. Consist of long cylindrical shaft (diaphysis), two ends (epiphyses), and a marrow cavity (e.g., radius, femur)
    2. Main supporting bones of the body
    3. Parts of a long bone (Figure 1-1)
      a. Diaphysis: shaft
      b. Epiphysis: proximal or distal end of the bone
      c. Articular cartilage: hyaline cartilage that covers the ends of the bones
      d. Periosteum: fibrous membrane covering outside of bone; rich in blood, nerves, and lymphatic vessels
      e. Endosteum: lines the marrow cavity
      f. Medullary (marrow) cavity: space within the bone center that contains marrow (red or yellow); red marrow is hemopoietic tissue that produces blood cells, yellow marrow is primarily fat
      g. Epiphyseal cartilage: region between diaphysis and epiphysis where bone grows in length; often referred to as the "growth plate"; becomes epiphyseal line in mature animals
  B. Short bones
    1. Small, cube-shaped bones
    2. Two thin layers of compact bone with spongy bone between the layers
    3. Function as shock absorbers (e.g., carpus, tarsus)
  C. Flat bones
    1. Thin, flat bones
    2. Two layers of compact bone with spongy bone between the layers; resembles a sandwich
    3. Protective function (e.g., pelvis, scapula, ribs, and many bones of the skull)
  D. Pneumatic bones
    1. Contain sinuses (e.g., frontal)
  E. Irregular bones
    1. Unpaired bones with complicated shapes that do not fit any other category (e.g., vertebra, some skull bones) (Table 1-2)
  F. Sesamoid bones
    1. Small short bones attached to tendons
    2. Reduce friction along a joint (e.g., patella)

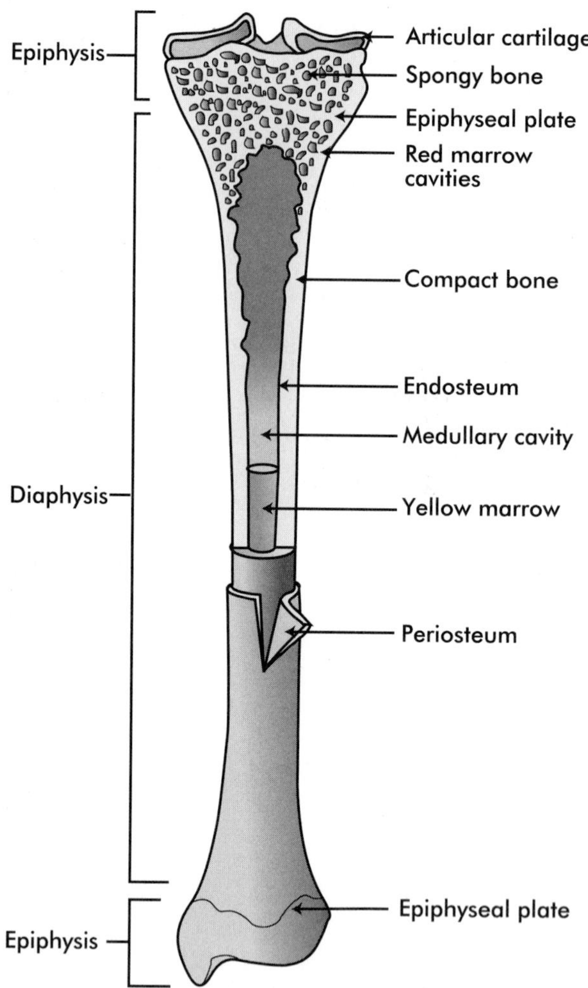

Figure 1-1 Parts of a long bone. (From Colville T, Bassert JM: *Clinical anatomy and physiology for veterinary technicians,* St Louis, 2002, Mosby.)

Table 1-2 Vertebral formulas

Species	No. of cervical vertebra	No. of thoracic vertebra	No. of lumbar vertebra	No. of sacral vertebra	No. of caudal or coccygeal vertebra
Dog, cat	7	13	7	3	21-23
Horse	7	18	6	5	15-20
Cow	7	13	6	5	18-20
Pig	7	14-15	6-7	4	20-23
Sheep	7	13	6-7	4	16-18
Human	7	12	5	5	4

VII. Osteogenesis (ossification): formation of bone (Figure 1-2)
  A. Types
    1. Endochondral
      a. Bones formed from cartilage bars laid down in the embryo
      b. Majority of bones in the body are formed by this method
    2. Intramembranous
      a. Bones formed from fibrous membranes laid down in the embryo
      b. Most flat bones are formed by this method
      c. Osteoblasts produce new bone and become mature osteocytes

VIII. Skeletal species differences (see Table 1-2 for species variations)

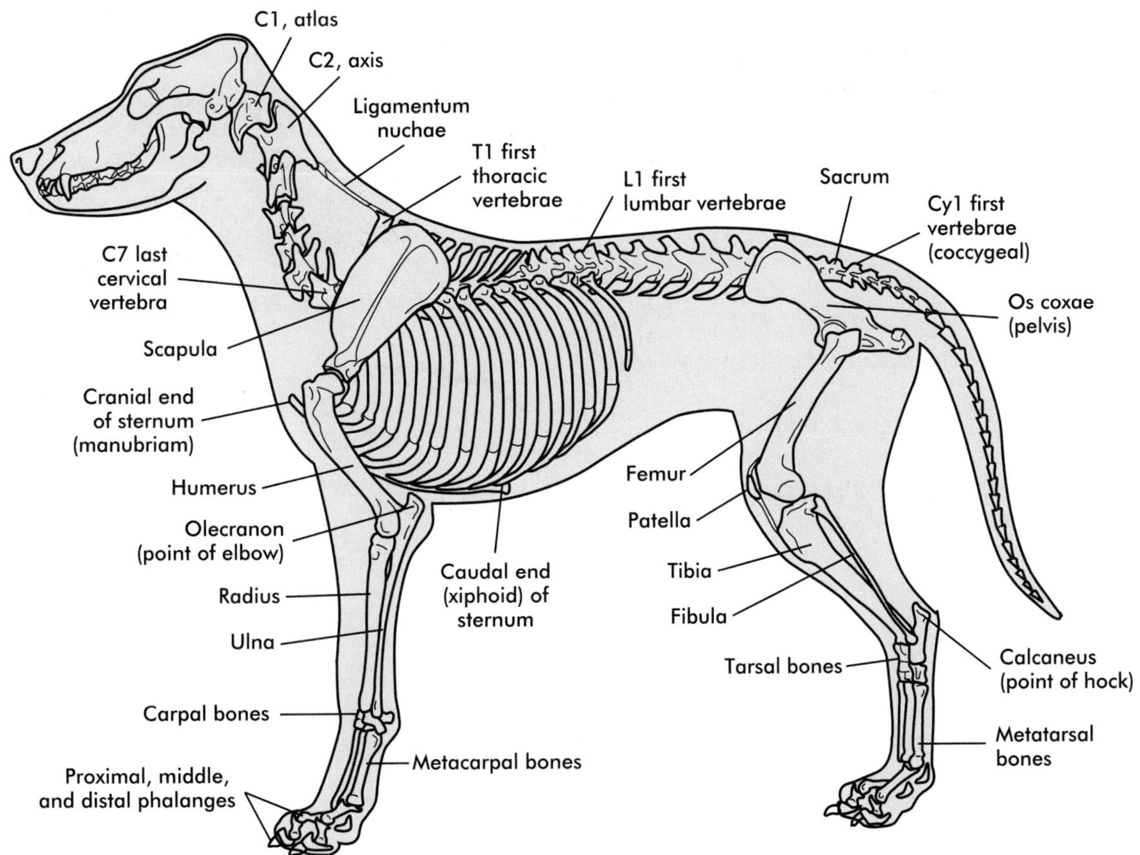

Figure 1-2 Canine skeleton. (From Colville T, Bassert JM: *Clinical anatomy and physiology for veterinary technicians,* St Louis, 2002, Mosby.)

Table 1-3 Types of synovial joints

Synovial joint	Structure	Location	Movement
Ball and socket (spheroid)	Ball-shaped head articulates with cup-shaped depression	Shoulder, hip	Flexion, extension, abduction, adduction, rotation, circumduction
Arthrodial (condyloid)	Oval articulating surfaces	Radial-carpal joints	Flexion, extension
Trochoid (pivot)	Rounded end of one bone articulates with a ring of bone	Atlantoaxial	Rotation
Hinge (ginglymus)	Cylindrical bone fits into depression	Stifle, elbow	Flexion, extension
Gliding	Flat, articulating surfaces	Radioulnar, intervertebral	Flexion, extension
Saddle	Concave surface articulates with a convex bone	Carpometacarpal in primates only	Flexion, extension, abduction, adduction, rotation, circumduction

A. Cat has a clavicle; dog does not
B. Male dogs have a nonarticulating bone (os penis) in the penis

IX. Articulations (joints)
A. Formed when two or more bones are united by fibrous, elastic, or cartilaginous tissue
B. Classification by function
1. Synarthrosis: immovable joint (e.g., skull sutures)
2. Amphiarthrosis: slightly moveable joint (e.g., pubic symphysis)
3. Diarthrosis: freely moveable joint (e.g., stifle)
C. Classification by structure
1. Fibrous: united by fibrous tissue, no joint cavity, synarthroses (e.g., skull sutures)
2. Cartilaginous: united by cartilage, no joint cavity, amphiarthroses (e.g., intervertebral discs, pubic symphysis)
3. Synovial: joint cavity filled with synovial fluid, synovial membrane, joint capsule, diarthroses (e.g., all joints of the limbs)

a. Majority of the joints in the body are synovial
b. They are classified into several different types (Table 1-3)

Muscular System

I. Function
  A. Produces movement of entire body or parts
  B. Maintains posture
  C. Produces heat

II. Types
  There are three types of muscle: skeletal, smooth, and cardiac
  A. Skeletal muscle (striated, voluntary)
    1. Skeletal muscle cells are long, striated fibers that run parallel to each other
    2. Cells are multinucleated with the nuclei on the periphery
    3. Functional unit is a sarcomere
    4. Each muscle fiber is a muscle cell consisting of many myofibrils
    5. Myofibrils are composed of myofilaments (i.e., actin and myosin)
  B. Smooth muscle (visceral, unstriated, involuntary)
    1. Smooth muscle cells are spindle shaped with one centrally located nucleus and no striations
    2. Responsible for involuntary movement (e.g., digestion)
    3. Two types of smooth muscle: single unit or visceral smooth muscle and multiunit smooth muscle
    4. Single-unit smooth muscle is found in sheets and forms the walls of many hollow organs (e.g., intestines); contraction occurs in waves
    5. Multiunit smooth muscle is found as individual fibers and the fibers are activated by the autonomic nervous system (e.g., arrector pili muscle, eye muscles)
  C. Cardiac muscle (myocardium)
    1. Involuntary, striated cells that branch together to form a network
    2. Cells are joined by intercalated discs, which aid in conduction of the nervous impulse to coordinate contraction
  D. Contraction of skeletal muscle
    1. Contraction occurs by means of the sliding-filament theory
    2. A nerve impulse travels down a motor nerve axon
    3. Acetylcholine is released into the synaptic cleft, transmitting the impulse to the sarcolemma
    4. Impulse is conducted into the T-tubules and to the sarcoplasmic reticulum

Nervous System

ORGANIZATION

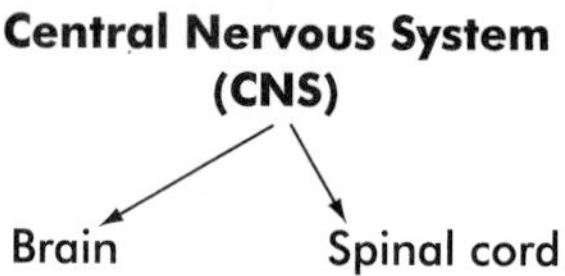

Peripheral Nervous System (PNS)

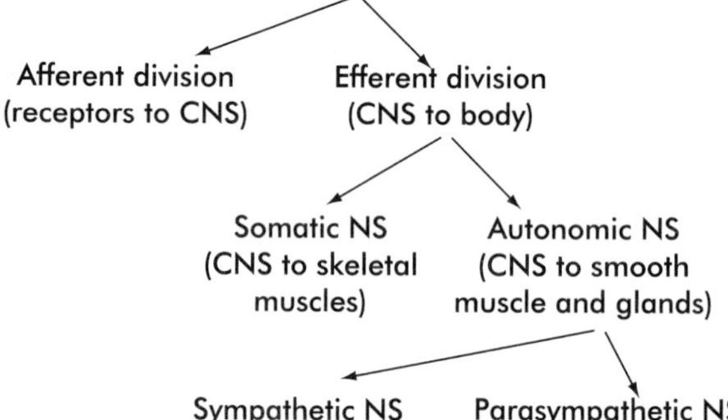

    5. Calcium is released, causing ATP to be split and providing the energy required for contraction
    6. Myosin and actin form cross-bridges during muscle contraction
    7. When the nerve impulse stops, muscle relaxes; energy is also required for relaxation
    8. All-or-none principle states that muscle fibers contract to their fullest or not at all
  E. Skeletal muscle actions
    1. Flexor: usually decreases the angle of a joint
    2. Extensor: usually increases the angle of a joint
    3. Abductor: moves a bone away from the midline
    4. Adductor: moves a bone toward the midline
    5. Levator: produces a dorsally directed movement
    6. Depressor: produces a ventrally directed movement
    7. Sphincter: decreases the size of an opening

Nervous System

The central nervous system (CNS) consists of the brain and spinal cord.

I. Brain
  A. Cerebrum
    1. Site of motor control, interpretation of sensory impulses, and areas of association
    2. Surface area increased by gyri (elevations) and sulci (fissures)
  B. Diencephalon
    1. Region of thalamus and hypothalamus
    2. Thalamus acts as a relay station for sensory impulses and interprets some sensations such as temperature and pain

3. Hypothalamus controls body temperature, fluid balance, sexual drives and influences the pituitary

C. Brain stem
1. Consists of midbrain, pons, and medulla oblongata
2. Midbrain serves as a connecting link
3. Pons contains important respiratory centers
4. In the medulla oblongata, nerve fibers cross from left to right, and vice versa
5. Medulla also influences respiratory rate, heart rate, vomiting, coughing, and sneezing
6. Throughout the brain stem is the reticular activating system (RAS), which is responsible for sleep/wake cycles

D. Cerebellum
1. Responsible for coordination and balance

II. Spinal cord
A. Runs through the vertebral foramen
B. Contains ascending and descending nerve tracts
C. Major function is to convey sensory (afferent) nerve impulses from the periphery to the brain and to conduct motor (efferent) nerve impulses from the brain to the periphery
D. Brain and spinal cord are protected by bone and meninges

III. Meninges
A. Dura mater: dense fibrous connective tissue
B. Arachnoid (arachnoidea mater): middle layer, very delicate and elastic connective tissue
C. Pia mater: transparent delicate connective tissue that contains tiny blood vessels and adheres to the surface of the brain and spinal cord
D. Epidural space between bone and dura mater contains loose connective tissue, blood vessels, and fat; injection of anesthetic agents into this region causes temporary nerve paralysis
E. Subarachnoid space contains cerebrospinal fluid (CSF) and large blood vessels

IV. Cerebrospinal fluid
A. Colorless fluid of watery consistency; contains protein, glucose, ions, and other substances
B. pH and pressure are particularly important
C. Functions to cushion and nourish the brain
D. A lumbar or CSF tap is used for CSF sampling

V. Blood-brain barrier
A. A protective barrier in the brain; separates blood from nerve cells
B. Consists of selectively permeable capillaries that are tightly connected, forming an effective barrier
C. Substances such as oxygen, glucose, and fat-soluble substances enter the brain easily; many waste products and drugs are blocked by the barrier

VI. Peripheral nervous system
A. Consists of all nerve processes connecting to the CNS; includes all cranial and spinal nerves
B. Divided into major divisions: afferent (sensory) and efferent (motor)
C. Afferent or sensory nerves carry impulses that arise from receptors to the CNS for interpretation
D. Efferent or motor nerves carry impulses from the CNS to skeletal muscle as part of the somatic division and to smooth muscle, glands, and heart as part of the autonomic system
E. All voluntary movements are part of the somatic division
F. Autonomic division serves all the involuntary functions and is further divided into sympathetic and parasympathetic
1. Sympathetic nerve fibers act to elicit the fight-or-flight response in emergencies or stressful situations (e.g., increased heart rate, respiratory rate, and blood flow)
2. Parasympathetic nerve fibers are responsible for quiet activities (e.g., digestion, heart rate) and return the body to normal levels after the sympathetic response

VII. Principal cells of the nervous system
A. Neuron (nerve cell)
1. Composed of dendrites, cell body, and axon
2. Dendrites receive the impulse and conducts it to the cell body, which in turn conducts it to the axon, which leads the impulse away to a synapse
3. Nerve impulses are generated of action potentials
4. An action potential is depolarization followed by repolarization; the electrical charge of the cell is reversed and then returned to normal
5. Impulses travel in one direction
6. Nerve cell bodies cannot regenerate if damaged
7. Some nerve cells have an insulative covering known as myelin; myelin is interrupted at the nodes of Ranvier—impulses jump from node to node, making transmission along myelinated nerve fibers faster than along nonmyelinated nerve fibers

B. Neuroglial cells (glial)
1. Connective tissue cells of CNS; are supportive and protective only, do not transmit impulses
a. Astrocytes: most numerous, form blood-brain barrier
b. Oligodendrocyte: smaller, wrap around axons to form myelin in CNS

c. Microglia: smallest, phagocytic
d. Schwann cells: wrap around axons to form myelin on peripheral nerves

C. Reflex
1. Automatic response to a stimulus
a. Reflex arc involves a stimulus that is picked up by the receptor
b. Transmits the impulse along a sensory neuron to the spinal cord, where it synapses with an interneuron (three-head neuron reflex) or directly with a motor neuron (two-head neuron reflex)
c. Impulse hits the effector organ, causing a response
d. Some typical reflexes are the stretch reflex (knee-jerk reflex), withdrawal reflex, corneal reflex, and papillary light reflex

Cardiovascular System

Deals with the heart *(cardio)* and blood vessels *(vascular).*

I. Function
A. Heart provides the force to circulate blood to all parts of the body

II. Structure (Figure 1-3)
A. Myocardium is the heart (cardiac) muscle
B. Cardiac muscle cells are striated and are connected by intercalated discs
C. Intercalated discs have a low electrical resistance; therefore, the impulse spreads very quickly and all cells seem to function as one

III. Protective layers
A. Pericardium: a double-walled membranous sac covering the myocardium
1. Outer layer, enveloping the heart, is a tough fibrous connective tissue known as fibrous pericardium; deep to this layer is an inner, more delicate, serous layer known as serous pericardium
2. Serous pericardium has two layers: the parietal layer adheres to the fibrous pericardium and the visceral layer adheres to the myocardium
3. Space between the two layers of serous pericardium is the pericardial cavity, filled with pericardial fluid that reduces friction when the heart beats

B. Endocardium: a serous membrane lining the inner chambers of the heart

IV. Pulmonary circulation
A. Consists of the precava (cranial vena cava or superior vena cava) and postcava (caudal vena cava or inferior vena cava)
B. Precava and postcava empty into the right atrium, through the tricuspid valve into the

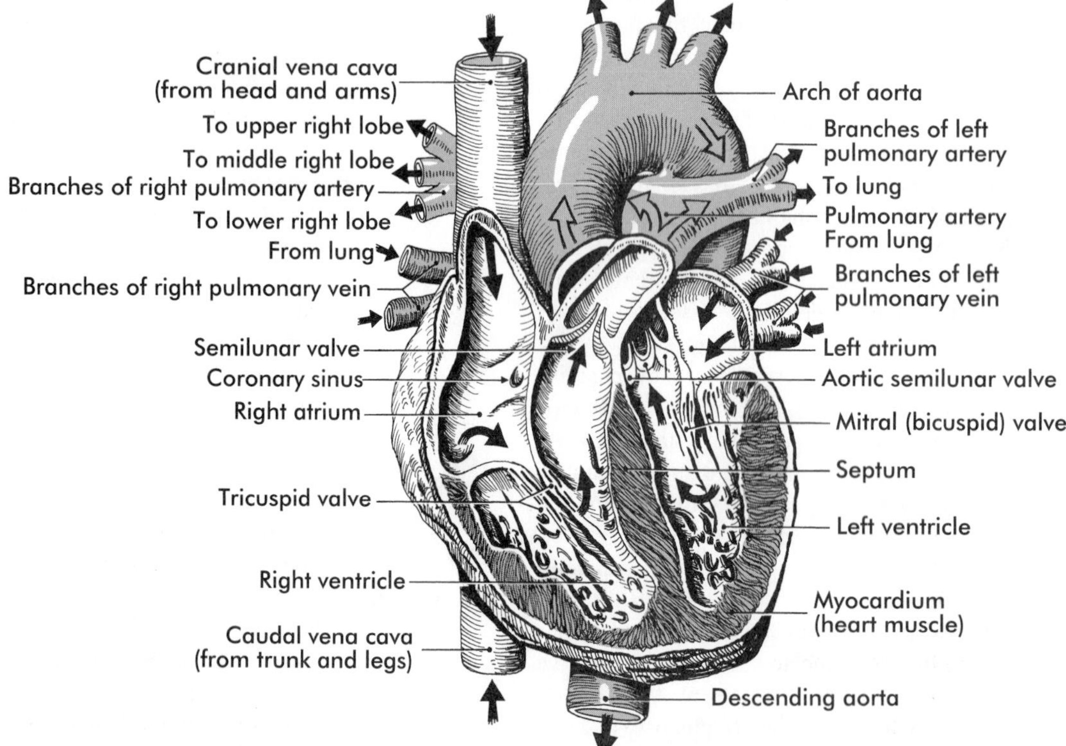

Figure 1-3 Anatomy of the heart. (From McBride DF: *Learning veterinary terminology,* ed 2, St Louis, 2002, Mosby.)

right ventricle, and through the pulmonary artery (passes pulmonary semilunar valve) to the lungs, where the blood is oxygenated and returned to the heart via pulmonary veins

V. Systemic circulation (somatic circulation)
   A. Oxygenated blood in the left atrium flows through the bicuspid (mitral) valve to the left ventricle and out of the aorta (passes aortic semilunar valve) to all parts of the body
   B. Two branches come off of the aortic arch in dogs and cats
      1. Innominate artery (brachiocephalic), which branches into the right subclavian artery and right and left common carotid arteries
      2. Left subclavian artery

VI. Coronary circulation
   A. Coronary arteries provide nutrients and oxygen to the myocardium; coronary veins drain waste and carbon dioxide from the myocardium

VII. Cardiac cycle
   A. One complete cycle: as atria contract (systole), the ventricles relax (diastole), and as ventricles contract, the atria relax
   B. Atrial diastole: atria are at rest
      1. Right atrium is receiving blood from the precava and postcava while the left atrium is receiving blood from the pulmonary veins
   C. Atrial systole: atria are contracting
      1. Sinoatrial (SA) node fires, causing contraction of the atria; blood is pushed through the tricuspid and bicuspid valves into the right and left ventricles
   D. Ventricular diastole
      1. Ventricles receive blood from the atria
   E. Ventricular systole
      1. Impulse from the SA node has been conducted to the atrioventricular (AV) node, which conducts the impulse down the bundle of HIS (AV bundle) to the Purkinje fibers
      2. Ventricles are now stimulated to contract; blood is forced through the semilunar valves into the pulmonary artery to the lungs and out of the aorta to all parts of the body

VIII. Heart sounds
   A. Auscultation (listening to heart sounds)
      1. Lubb, dupp, pause
         a. Lubb is the first sound; it is a long sound made when the AV valves close
         b. Dupp is the second sound; it is a short, sharp sound made when the semilunar valves close

IX. Heart rate
   A. Animal heart rates vary with age, size, breed, health, and fitness
   B. Dog: 70 to 160 beats per minute
   C. Cat: 150 to 210 beats per minute
   D. Heart rate may also be affected by chemicals, hormones, temperature, behavior, and respiratory rate

X. Electrocardiography (ECG [or EKG])
   A. Electrocardiogram records the electrical activity of the heart
   B. First wave is the P wave, which represents the electrical events during atrial systole (depolarization)
   C. Large QRS complex represents the electrical events of ventricular systole (depolarization)
   D. T wave represents the electrical events during ventricular diastole (repolarization)
   E. Atrial diastole occurs during ventricular systole; therefore, it is masked by the QRS complex

Central Vascular System

I. Blood vessels
   A. Arteries
      1. Carry blood away from the heart
      2. Carry oxygenated blood (except for pulmonary artery)
      3. Thicker and stronger than veins
      4. Pressure within is greater than in veins
   B. Arterioles
      1. Small arteries
      2. Lead to capillaries and regulate the blood flow into them
   C. Capillaries
      1. Consist of one layer of endothelium
      2. Microscopic in size
      3. Exchange of oxygen and carbon dioxide takes place here
   D. Venules
      1. Emerge from capillaries and enlarge into veins
   E. Veins
      1. Larger than arteries and thinner walled
      2. Low blood pressure; therefore have valves to prevent the backflow of blood
      3. Carry blood back to the heart

II. Fetal circulation
   A. Lungs, kidneys, and digestive tract are nonfunctional in fetus but must be nourished with oxygen
   B. Exchange of nutrients and waste takes place within the placenta
   C. Oxygenated blood enters the fetus via one umbilical vein

D. Vein ascends toward the fetal liver and divides into two: one branch joins the hepatic portal vein and enters the liver while the majority of blood flows into the ductus venosus, which connects to the postcava
E. Postcava enters the right atrium; precava from the head enters the right atrium as well
F. Most of the blood goes directly through the foramen ovale to the left atrium into the left ventricle and out of the aorta to all parts of the fetus
G. Blood that goes into the right ventricle passes into the pulmonary artery; most is diverted through the ductus arteriosus into the aorta (a small amount goes to the lungs)
H. Blood in the descending aorta branches into the iliac arteries; the two umbilical arteries branch off and return deoxygenated blood to the placenta

Digestive System

The digestive system functions to break down foodstuffs into absorbable nutrients to fuel the body. There are anatomical variations among different species depending on their diet.

I. Process
  A. Digestive system uses five basic processes to prepare the food for utilization by the body
    1. Ingestion of food
    2. Peristalsis: moving food through the digestive tract
    3. Mechanical and chemical digestion
    4. Absorption
    5. Defecation
II. Types of diet
  A. Herbivore: plant-eating animal (e.g., rabbit, cow, horse, sheep)
  B. Carnivore: meat-eating animal (e.g., cat, dog, tiger)
  C. Omnivore: plant- and meat-eating animal (e.g., rats, pigs, humans)
III. Histological layers
  A. Walls of gastrointestinal tract or alimentary canal can be divided into four layers
    1. Mucosa closest to the lumen; three sublayers
      a. Epithelium: stratified squamous and simple columnar
      b. Lamina propria: connective tissue
      c. Muscularis mucosa: smooth muscle
    2. Submucosa: loose connective tissue
    3. Muscularis externa: two or three layers of smooth muscle depending on location
      a. Oblique muscle: stomach only
      b. Circular muscle
      c. Longitudinal muscle
    4. Serosa: loose connective tissue
IV. Structures
  A. Mouth
    1. Receives food and mixes food with saliva during mastication
    2. Bolus is formed
  B. Pharynx
    1. Common passageway for digestive and respiratory systems
  C. Esophagus
    1. Muscular tube running from the pharynx to the cardia (opening to stomach)
    2. Food moves through the esophagus via peristalsis
  D. Stomach
    1. Simple stomach: monogastric animals
      a. Found in humans, pigs, horses, and dogs
      b. Four regions: esophageal, cardiac, fundic, pyloric
        (1) Esophageal region is nonglandular
        (2) Cardiac region produces mucus
        (3) Fundic region is the true body of the stomach and contains true gastric glands, which have four distinct cell types
          (a) Mucous neck cells, which secrete mucus
          (b) Chief cells, which produce the enzyme pepsinogen
          (c) Parietal cells, which produce hydrochloric acid
          (d) Endocrine cells, which produce the hormone gastrin
        (4) Pyloric region produces mucus
      c. Inner folds known as rugae
      d. Food is mixed in the stomach with secretions from the digestive glands until it is reduced to a liquid known as chyme
      e. pH of stomach is acidic
    2. Ruminant stomach
      a. Found in cattle, sheep, goats, and llamas
      b. All ruminants are herbivores, but not all herbivores are ruminants
      c. Animal regurgitates food (bolus), remasticates (rechews), and swallows (deglutition) it again
      d. Composed of four compartments: rumen, reticulum, omasum, and abomasum
        (1) Rumen: called "fermentation vat"
          (a) Largest compartment
          (b) Food is mixed and churned in a favorable environment (i.e., proper pH, temperature, bacteria, and anaerobic conditions)

(2) Reticulum: called "hardware compartment"
   (a) Most cranial compartment that is not completely separate from the rumen
   (b) Also called the "honeycomb"
   (c) Acts as a passageway for food, paces the contraction of the rumen, and is the usual site for ingested foreign objects
(3) Omasum
   (a) Grinds up the food and absorbs water and bicarbonate
   (b) Composed of many layers of laminae, which resemble leaves
(4) Abomasum
   (a) True glandular stomach
   (b) Mixes the food with enzymes, initiating chemical digestion

E. Small intestine
   1. Divided into three regions: duodenum, jejunum, ileum
   2. Major site of digestion and absorption
   3. Three specialized structures increase the surface area of the small intestine
      a. Circular folds: deep, mucosal folds
      b. Intestinal villi: long slender projections
      c. Microvilli: columnar epithelial cells have microvilli
   4. Produces digestive enzymes (proteases, amylases, and lipase)

F. Large intestine
   1. Cecum found at the ileocecocolic junction
   2. Colon (ascending, transverse, descending)
   3. Has no villi, no circular folds, and no enzymes secreted; large number of goblet cells secrete mucus
   4. Absorbs water, produces vitamins B and K, and propels waste toward the rectum

G. Rectum
   1. End portion of the large intestine that secretes mucus

H. Anus
   1. Terminal ending of gastrointestinal tract
   2. Has two sphincters: one internal involuntary sphincter and one external voluntary sphincter

I. Other organs that are involved
   1. Pancreas: releases sodium bicarbonate to neutralize acidic chyme and digestive enzymes into the duodenum
      a. Trypsin: to digest proteins
      b. Lipase: to digest fat
      c. Amylase: to digest starch
   2. Liver: produces bile, which emulsifies fats
   3. Gallbladder: stores bile and releases it into the duodenum when fats are present
      a. Under the influence of cholecystokinin (CCK)
      b. Rat and horse do not have a gallbladder

V. Digestive process (simple stomach)
   A. Food enters the mouth and is mixed with salivary amylase (from salivary glands: parotid, sublingual, mandibular, and zygomatic)
   B. Amylase begins to break down starch
   C. Food entering the stomach is mixed with gastric juice composed of protein-digesting enzymes, hydrochloric acid, and mucus
   D. Rennin (chymosin) is also present in the young to coagulate milk
   E. In the small intestine, the chyme is acted on by pancreatic enzymes
      1. Pancreatic amylase: to act on starch
      2. Trypsin: to act on proteins
      3. Chymotrypsin: to act on proteins
      4. Elastase: to act on elastin
      5. Peptidases: to act on large peptides (proteins)
      6. Lipase: to act on fats
      7. Nucleases: to act on nucleic acids
   F. Pancreatic enzymes are delivered in an alkaline fluid to help neutralize the acidic chyme
   G. Small intestine also secretes enzymes
      1. Trypsin: to act on dipeptides
      2. Maltase, sucrase, and lactase: to act on disaccharides
      3. Nuclease: to act on nucleic acids
      4. Chyme is mixed with enzymes through segmentation and moves via peristalsis
      5. Monosaccharides and amino acids are absorbed through the intestinal capillaries, and fats are absorbed through the lacteals of the intestinal villi
   H. Large intestine moves solid waste to the rectum for defecation, water is absorbed here, and vitamins B and K are produced
   I. Defecation of undigested waste occurs through the anus

Lymphatic System

I. Function
   A. Absorbs protein-containing tissue fluid that escapes from capillaries and returns it to the venous system
   B. Transports fats from digestive tract to blood
   C. Produces lymphocytes
   D. Develops immunity

II. Structure
   A. Lymph vessels
   1. Blind end tubes running parallel to venous system, which eventually empty into precava

2. Resemble veins but have thinner walls and more valves; lymph fluid is filtered through the lymph nodes

B. Lymph nodes (glands)
   1. Oval-shaped structures
   2. Filter lymph fluid
   3. Produce lymphocytes

C. Lymph organs
   1. Tonsils
      a. Mass of lymphoid tissue embedded in mucous membrane
      b. Supplied with reticuloendothelial cells
   2. Spleen
      a. Largest mass of lymphoid tissue
      b. Phagocytic function
      c. Produces lymphocytes
      d. Stores and releases blood as needed
   3. Thymus
      a. Important in developing immune response in the young
      b. Eventually replaced by fat in the adult, depending on the species

Respiratory System

I. Structures

A. Nostrils (nares)
   1. External openings

B. Nasal cavity
   1. Lined with mucous membrane
   2. Houses turbinate bones
   3. Air is warmed by capillaries, moistened, and filtered

C. Pharynx
   1. Nasopharynx: from posterior nares to the soft palate
   2. Oropharynx: from soft palate to the hyoid bone
   3. Laryngopharynx: from hyoid bone to the larynx
   4. Eustachian tube: from the middle ear to the nasopharynx

D. Larynx (voice box)
   1. Consists of cartilage (e.g., thyroid, cricoid, arytenoid, and epiglottis)
   2. Epiglottis covers the glottis during swallowing
   3. Vocal folds attach to arytenoid cartilage

E. Trachea
   1. Consists of noncollapsible, C-shaped, cartilaginous rings
   2. Lined with ciliated columnar cells
   3. Divides into bronchi at the tracheal bifurcation

F. Bronchi
   1. Right and left cartilaginous bronchi enter the lungs
   2. Passageways become progressively smaller, and the amount of cartilage diminishes

G. Bronchiole
   1. Consists of smooth muscle, no cartilage
   2. Lead to the alveoli

H. Lungs
   1. Varying number of lobes, depending on species
   2. Covered with visceral pleura
   3. House microscopic air sacs known as alveoli, where exchange of oxygen and carbon dioxide takes place

II. Physiology

A. Respiration of mammals: three basic processes
   1. Ventilation: movement of air between the atmosphere and the lungs
   2. External respiration: exchange of gases between the atmosphere and the blood
   3. Internal respiration: exchange of gases between the blood and the cells

B. Ventilation
   1. Inspiration (inhalation)
      a. Nervous impulse from the brain causes the diaphragm and external intercostal muscles to contract
      b. Diaphragm moves caudally and the chest moves ventrally; therefore the size of the thoracic cavity is increased, causing a decrease in intrathoracic pressure and a decrease in intraalveolar pressure
      c. Because intraalveolar pressure is now less than atmospheric pressure, air moves into the lungs
   2. Expiration (exhalation)
      a. Diaphragm and external intercostal muscles relax
      b. Diaphragm moves cranially and the chest moves dorsally; this decreases the size of the thoracic cavity, thereby causing an increase in intrathoracic pressure and an increase in intraalveolar pressure
      c. Because intraalveolar pressure is now greater than atmospheric pressure, air moves out of the lungs

III. Lung volumes

A. Tidal volume: the volume of air exchanged during normal breathing

B. Inspiratory reserve volume: the amount of air inspired over the tidal volume

C. Expiratory reserve volume: the amount of air expired over the tidal volume

D. Residual volume: air remaining in the lungs after a forced expiration

E. Dead space: air in the pathways of the respiratory system

IV. Respiratory rate
  A. Dog: 10 to 30 breaths per minute
  B. Cat: 24 to 42 breaths per minute
  C. Horse: 8 to 16 breaths per minute
V. Control of respiration
  A. Medullary rhythmicity center in the medulla oblongata, a region that has inspiratory and expiratory neurons
  B. Apneustic area in the pons, which prolongs inspiration
  C. Pneumotaxic area in the pons, which inhibits the apneustic area and causes expiration
  D. Hering-Breuer reflex: stretch receptors in the lungs that prevent the lungs from overinflating
  E. Carbon dioxide: an increase causes an increase in respiratory rate
  F. Other factors may affect the rate of respiration (e.g., pain, cold, blood pressure, pH, oxygen, stress)
VI. Terminology
  A. Pneumothorax: air in the thoracic cavity
  B. Atelectasis: collapsed lungs
  C. Pleuritis (pleurisy): inflammation of the pleural membranes
  D. Pneumonia: inflammation of the lungs caused primarily by bacteria, viruses, or chemical irritants
  E. Eupnea: normal, quiet respiration
  F. Dyspnea: difficult breathing
  G. Apnea: no breathing

Excretory System

I. Anatomy
  A. Kidneys
    1. Extract and remove metabolic waste from the blood; blood pressure provides the force
    2. Size and shape vary according to the species; majority are bean shaped
    3. Right kidney is more firmly attached and cranial to the left kidney
    4. Microscopic unit is the nephron
    5. Outer cortex: contains the glomerulus, Bowman's capsule, proximal convoluted tubules (PCTs), and distal convoluted tubules (DCTs)
    6. Medulla: contains the loop of Henle and most of collecting tubules
    7. Medulla is arranged into various numbers of pyramids
    8. Apex of the pyramid is the papilla, which opens into the minor calyx, major calyx, and renal pelvis
  B. Ureters
    1. Consist of smooth muscle
    2. Capable of peristalsis to move urine to the urinary bladder
  C. Urinary bladder
    1. Consists of smooth muscle
    2. Lined with transitional cell epithelium
  D. Urethra
    1. Tube of smooth muscle to transport urine from the urinary bladder to the exterior
II. Physiology: three phases to urine production
  A. Filtration
    1. Blood enters glomerulus by the afferent arteriole
    2. Due to various pressures, water, salt, and small molecules move out of the glomerulus into Bowman's capsule
      a. It is now called the glomerular filtrate; rate at which it was formed is called the glomerular filtration rate (GFR)
  B. Reabsorption
    1. Occurs in the PCTs and loop of Henle; substances needed by the body are reabsorbed from the glomerular filtrate into the peritubular capillaries
  C. Secretion
    1. Substances are selectively secreted from the peritubular capillaries into the DCT
III. Urination (micturition)
  A. To void urine
  B. Filtrate flows into collecting ducts, renal pelvis, ureter, urinary bladder, and urethra and is voided as urine
  C. Urine is water plus waste products (e.g., urea, excess ions)
IV. Hormonal influence
  A. Antidiuretic hormone (ADH [vasopressin])
    1. Increase in ADH increases the reabsorption of water within the kidney
  B. Aldosterone
    1. Stimulates sodium (Na) reabsorption in the kidney

Reproductive System: Male

I. Male anatomy
  A. Testicles
    1. Two oval-shaped glands in a skin-covered scrotum
    2. Seminiferous tubules produce sperm
    3. Cells of Leydig produce testosterone
    4. Epididymis adheres to the side of the testicle; it connects the seminiferous tubules to the vas deferens and provides storage for sperm and a place for maturation
    5. Testicles develop inside the abdomen but descend into the scrotum (after birth in dogs

and cats), where the body temperature is more favorable for sperm development

B. Vas deferens (ductus deferens)
   1. Connects from the epididymis to the urethra
   2. Is a part of the spermatic cord along with blood vessels and nerves
   3. Spermatic cord passes through the inguinal ring; at this point, the vas deferens separates and joins the urethra

C. Accessory sex glands
   1. These glands produce semen
   2. Semen provides a transport medium for sperm, protects the sperm against the acidity in the female genital tract, and provides a source of nutrition
   3. Glands vary with the species
   4. Dogs have a prostate only
   5. Cats have a prostate and bulbourethral (or Cowper's) glands
   6. Stallions have seminal vesicles (vesicular glands), prostate, bulbourethral glands, and ampulla

D. Penis
   1. Houses the urethra, which transports sperm into the female genital tract
   2. Consists of a shaft and the tip known as the glans penis
   3. Erectile tissue surrounds the urethra; with sexual excitement the tissue becomes engorged with blood, leading to an erection, followed by the release of sperm during ejaculation
      a. Penis of the dog and stallion is composed of almost all erectile tissue and a small amount of connective tissue
      b. Penis of the bull, ram, and boar is composed of almost all connective tissue and very little erectile tissue
         (1) These animals achieve erection by the straightening of the sigmoid flexure (S-shaped)
   4. Dog penis is unique in that it has a very long glans penis and a bone (os penis)
   5. Cat penis is retracted and covered with spiny epithelial projections

II. Male physiology

A. Follicle-stimulating hormone (FSH) is secreted from the pituitary, causing spermatogenesis to begin

B. Spermatogonia in the testicle undergo meiosis; each cell will give rise to four mature sperm with the haploid number

C. Interstitial cell–stimulating hormone (ICSH) is secreted from the pituitary, causing the cells of Leydig to produce testosterone

Reproductive System: Female

I. Female anatomy

A. Ovaries
   1. Paired oval organs found in the abdomen
   2. Produce ova and hormones

B. Oviduct
   1. Conducts ova from ovary to uterine horn or uterus (depending on the species)

C. Uterus
   1. Consists of uterine horns, body, and a cervix
   2. Presence or absence of uterine horns varies with the species
   3. In dogs and cats, young develop within the uterine horns
   4. In monotocous or uniparous (giving birth to one offspring at a time) animals, young develop in the body of the uterus
   5. In polytocous or multiparous (giving birth to more than one offspring at a time) animals, young develop in uterine horns
   6. Opening to the uterus is the cervix; some species may have a double cervix
   7. Uterine horns and uterus have three layers
      a. Endometrium: epithelial cells and mucous membrane
         (1) Varies in thickness with the cycle
         (2) Is reabsorbed in animals with an estrous cycle and sloughed in animals with a menstrual cycle (primates)
      b. Myometrium: smooth muscle
      c. Perimetrium: serous covering, which is continuous with peritoneum

D. Vagina (birth canal)
   1. Muscular tube from the cervix to the urethral orifice

E. Vulva
   1. Internally from the urethral opening to the external genitalia
   2. Many female animals have a common urogenital pathway

II. Female physiology

A. Estrous cycle
   1. Monestrous: usually one cycle per year, usually seasonal breeders (e.g., mink)
   2. Diestrous: cycle in spring and fall (e.g., dog)
   3. Polyestrous: more than one cycle per year (continuous) (e.g., swine)
   4. Seasonally polyestrous: cycle continuously in specific seasons (e.g., cat, horse, sheep)
   5. Reflex or induced ovulators: ovulate after being bred (e.g., cat, rabbit, mink, ferret)
   6. Spontaneous ovulator: ovulation occurs naturally regardless of coitus (e.g., humans)

III. Estrous cycle
   A. Proestrus
      1. Period of preparation
      2. Under influence of FSH from the pituitary
      3. New ovarian follicles grow and release estrogen, which builds up the uterus and uterine horns
   B. Estrus ("standing heat"): period of sexual receptivity
      1. Female is sexually receptive to the male
      2. Uterus and uterine horns are ready to receive an embryo
      3. Release of luteinizing hormone (LH) from the pituitary causes ovulation in dogs
      4. Cats and rabbits are nonspontaneous ovulators or induced ovulators and ovulate when bred; they have a longer estrus if not bred
      5. Dogs may have a bloody discharge; cats exhibit behavioral changes (e.g., rubbing, lordosis, vocalization)
   C. Metestrus
      1. Short postovulatory phase
      2. Each ruptured follicle develops into a corpus luteum
      3. Corpus luteum produces progesterone, which puts final maturation on uterine horns and/or uterus and inhibits development of new follicles
   D. Diestrus
      1. Corpus luteum continues to secrete hormones
      2. If pregnancy does not occur, the corpus luteum degenerates
      3. If pregnancy occurs, the corpus luteum is maintained and continues to secrete hormones: in some species for the entire pregnancy, and in others only until the placenta is developed
      4. Some animals remain in this stage and appear pregnant; this is known as pseudopregnancy
   E. Anestrus
      1. Long period of inactivity in seasonally polyestrus animals

IV. Fertilization and pregnancy
   A. Copulation or coitus is the act of mating or sexual intercourse
   B. Male will mount the female, followed by intromission of the penis; ejaculation causes the deposition of semen into the vagina
   C. Fertilization begins with the union of sperm and egg within the oviduct
   D. Zygote undergoes mitotic divisions as it is propelled through the uterine tubes and then implants in the uterine horns or uterus, depending on the species
   E. Placenta forms to allow the exchange of nutrients and waste products between mother and fetus (fetal and maternal blood do not mix)
   F. Fetal membranes form around the developing embryo for protection
   G. As the embryo grows, it develops a placenta and attaches to the endometrial lining of the uterus
   H. After implantation until parturition, the developing organism is called a fetus
   I. Protective fetal membranes
      1. Amnion: forms a fluid-filled sac closest to the fetus; this is filled with amniotic fluid
      2. Allantois: a two-layered membrane: one layer adheres to the amnion, the other layer to the chorion; fluid fills this cavity
      3. Chorion: outermost layer, which attaches to the endometrium
         a. Different species have various types of fetal attachment

V. Parturition: act of giving birth
   A. Labor
      1. Under the influence of oxytocin from the pituitary, the uterus and/or uterine horns begin to contract
      2. Delivery of fetus: fetus is pushed through the cervix and vagina
      3. Delivery of placenta: placenta (afterbirth) is delivered after the birth of each fetus

VI. Gestation periods: length of time from fertilization to birth
   A. Cat and dog: average 63 days
   B. Horse: average 336 days
   C. Cow: average 285 days

VII. Dystocia: difficult birth
   A. May result in a cesarean section

VIII. Lactation: milk production
   A. First milk is colostrum; contains antibodies, proteins, and vitamins and is important for the neonate
   B. Milk production is under the influence of prolactin from the pituitary

Endocrine System

Endocrine glands (Table 1-4) are ductless and produce chemical substances (hormones) that have a specific effect on a target area. The hormones are secreted directly into the bloodstream.

I. Characteristics
   A. Hormones may
      1. Change the permeability of a cell
      2. Change the permeability of an organelle
      3. Activate or inactivate an enzyme system
      4. Change the rate of enzyme production

Table 1-4 Endocrine glands

Gland	Hormone/Steroid-Hormone	Action
Thyroid	Thyroxin	Accelerates metabolism
	Calcitonin	Regulates calcium levels
Parathyroid	Parathormone	Regulates calcium and phosphorus levels
Adrenal cortex	Glucocorticoids, mineralocorticoids, gonadocorticoids	Protein and carbohydrate metabolism, stress resistance, anti-inflammatory, regulates sodium and potassium levels, male and female sex hormones
Adrenal medulla	Epinephrine, norepinephrine	Stimulate sympathetic nervous system; "fight or flight"
Pituitary (master gland)	Growth hormone	Stimulates growth
	Thyroid-stimulating (thyrotropic)	Stimulates thyroid gland
	Adrenocorticotropic (corticotropin)	Stimulates adrenal cortex
	Follicle-stimulating	Growth of ovarian follicle
	Luteinizing, (interstitial cell–stimulating)	Causes ovulation, stimulates testosterone production
	Prolactin	Stimulates lactation
	Oxytocin	Causes uterine contractions
	Antidiuretic (vasopressin)	Causes water reabsorption
Pancreas	Insulin	Decreases blood glucose
	Glucagon	Increases blood glucose
Ovary	Estrogen	Female sex characteristics
	Progesterone	Prepare uterus and uterine horns
Testes	Testosterone	Male sex characteristics

II. Control
   A. Hormone secretion is regulated through a feedback system; as the hormone levels rise, their secretion is inhibited
   B. Only the adrenal medulla is under neural control

Integumentary System

Anatomy

I. Skin: consists of two layers
   A. Epidermis
      1. Superficial layer is the stratum corneum; this is a nonvascular, cornified layer
      2. Constantly being shed and replaced
      3. Deep to this is the actively growing stratum germinativum
      4. Melanocytes (pigment cells) produce melanin, giving skin its color, and are found in this region
   B. Dermis (corium)
      1. Deep to the epidermis
      2. Contains arteries, veins, capillaries, lymphatics, and nerve fibers
   C. Hypodermis
      1. Deep to the dermis is the subcutaneous layer consisting of connective and adipose tissue

Function

I. Protective barrier, sense organ, site for vitamin D synthesis
II. Contains many glands and nerve receptors (e.g., Meissner's corpuscle [touch receptor], sweat glands, Ruffini endings [heat], Pacini's corpuscles [pressure], sebaceous glands)

Hair

I. Hair contains an inner medulla, which is covered by the thicker cortex, followed by a keratinized layer called the cuticle
II. Hair is produced within a follicle with growth originating in the bulb region
III. Hair below the skin is known as the root; the region above the skin is the shaft
IV. Number of hairs per follicle varies
V. Each hair follicle is supplied with sebaceous glands and an arrector pili muscle
VI. Contraction of this muscle is responsible for the hair raising seen in frightened cats
VII. Types
   A. Normal guard or cover hair: usually accompanied by shorter wool hair in the same follicle
   B. Wool hair: shorter, wavy, no medulla (e.g., sheep)
   C. Tactile hairs (sinus hairs) (e.g., whiskers): used as feelers; very sensitive to movement

Specialized Integument

I. Horns, claws, hooves grow from a specialized dermis and consist of cornified epidermal cells

Senses

Vision

I. Anatomy: eye
   A. Sclera: outermost fibrous coat (white of the eye)
   B. Choroid: vascular coat between the sclera and retina
   C. Retina: nervous coat housing photoreceptors (e.g., rods and cones)

D. Vitreous humor: clear, watery fluid filling the vitreous body
E. Lens: focuses light onto the retina
F. Iris: colored, contractile membrane between the lens and the cornea; regulates amount of light passing through the pupil
G. Pupil: opening in the center of the iris
H. Aqueous humor: clear, watery fluid filling the anterior and posterior chambers
I. Cornea: transparent covering on the eye
J. Conjunctiva: mucous membrane that lines the eyelids
K. Nictitating membrane: third eyelid

II. Lacrimal apparatus
A. Tears from the lacrimal gland located in the upper eyelids flow onto the eyeball to flush debris from the eye, moisten, and lubricate
B. Tears drain out a lacrimal duct located in the medial canthi of the upper and lower lids into the nasal cavity via the nasolacrimal duct

III. Physiology
A. Light passes through the pupil, is refracted by the lens, and hits the photoreceptors (i.e., rods and cones of the retina)
B. Rods respond to dim light and occur in greater numbers in nocturnal animals
C. Cones respond to bright light and color
D. Nervous impulse is passed via the optic nerve to the brain

Hearing

I. Anatomy: ear (consists of three regions)
A. Outer ear
1. From the pinna up to and including the tympanic membrane
2. Air filled
B. Middle ear
1. Houses three ossicles: malleus (hammer), incus (anvil), stapes (stirrup)
2. Air filled, communicates with the nasopharynx by way of the eustachian tube
C. Inner ear
1. Houses the cochlea and semicircular canals
2. Fluid filled
3. Cochlea houses the organ of Corti (hearing receptors)
4. Semicircular canals contain nerve receptors that respond to balance

II. Physiology
A. Sound waves are transmitted through the outer ear and strike the tympanic membrane
B. Sound is concentrated and conducted through the three ossicles to the round window of the cochlea
C. Cochlea houses the organ of Corti, which when stimulated conducts a nervous impulse along the auditory nerve to the brain

III. Deafness
A. Nerve deafness
1. Results from malfunction of receptors or auditory nerve
2. Most common in white blue-eyed cats, Sealyham terriers, Scotch terriers, Border collies, and fox terriers
B. Transmission deafness
1. Results from malfunction in transmission of sound waves from outer to inner ear

Smell

I. Associated with the olfactory bulb
II. Receptors lie in the mucous membranes of the nasal cavity
III. Odor is dissolved in receptors and transmitted to the brain

Taste

I. Taste receptors are enclosed in papillae on the tongue
II. Four types of papillae: fungiform, foliate, filiform, and vallate
A. Fungiform papillae resemble fungus and contain taste buds in all animals
B. Foliate papillae resemble leaves of a plant and are found in the horse, pig, and dog
1. They contain taste buds and serous glands
2. Mucous glands are also found in the foliate papillae of the horse and dog
C. Filiform papillae are hair-like in appearance
1. These papillae are shorter and softer in the horse; hence the velvet-like tongue
D. Vallate (circumvallate) papillae are large, circular projections surrounded by a deep groove
1. Contain taste buds and serous glands in all domestic animals
2. Contain mucous glands in the horse

Glossary

anatomy The study of the form and structure of the body
apnea No breathing
articulation Where two or more bones meet; also called a joint
canthi (singular, canthus) The junction of the upper and lower eyelids at either corner of the eyes
carnivore Meat-eating animal
conjunctiva Mucous membrane that lines the eyelids
cornea Transparent covering on the eye
coronary circulation Blood circulation that nourishes the myocardium
dead space Air in the respiratory passageways
dyspnea Difficult breathing
dystocia Difficult birth
endocrine glands Secrete hormones directly into the bloodstream
estrous cycle Interval from the beginning of one heat period to the beginning of the next heat period

estrus Time of the female's cycle when she is receptive to a male
eupnea Normal respiration
exocrine glands Secretions are through ducts, usually onto an epithelial surface
extracellular Outside of a cell
herbivore Plant-eating animal
hormone Chemical substance that has a specific effect on target area
hypertonic Having a higher osmotic pressure than another solution
hypotonic Having a lower osmotic pressure than another solution
intercellular Between the cells
intracellular Within a cell
isotonic Having equal osmotic pressures
lacrimal apparatus Lacrimal duct conducts tears from the medial corners to the nasal cavity
lactation Milk production
laminae (singular, lamina) Thin, flat layer or membrane
meninges Protective coverings of the brain and spinal cord
monestrous One estrous cycle per year
monotocous Producing one offspring at birth
myocardium Heart muscle
nonspontaneous ovulator Ovulation occurs only when bred
omnivore Animal that eats meat and plants
osmotic pressure Amount of pressure necessary to stop the flow of water across a membrane
osteology Study of bones
parturition Act of giving birth
physiology Study of body functions
polyestrous More than one estrous cycle per year
polytocous Giving birth to several offspring at one time
residual volume Air remaining in the lungs after a forced expiration
ruminant Animal with a four-chambered stomach; animal that commonly chews its cud
spontaneous ovulator Ovulation occurs naturally within the cycle
tidal volume Volume of air exchanged during eupnea

Review Questions

1 The process by which bone is formed from cartilage bars is known as
a. Intramembranous ossification
b. Endochondral ossification
c. Heteroplastic osteogenesis
d. Chondrabar osteogenesis

2 Skeletal muscle is composed of
a. Parallel, multinucleated fibers
b. Interconnected, uninucleated fibers
c. Spindle-shaped, uninucleated fibers
d. Parallel, uninucleated fibers

3 The scientific discipline that studies the functions of living things is
a. Anatomy
b. Systemic anatomy
c. Physomy
d. Physiology

4 The canine foreleg is composed of the following bones
a. Tibia, radius, ulna
b. Humerus, radius, ulna
c. Humerus, radius, fibula
d. Femur, tibia, fibula

5 A dog that has had a major hemorrhage accidentally receives a large transfusion of distilled water into the cephalic vein. This would probably have
a. No result as long as the water was sterile
b. Serious, perhaps fatal, results because the red blood cells would shrink
c. No effect because the dog was dehydrated
d. Serious, perhaps fatal, results because the red blood cells would burst

6 In the digestive tract, the three histological layers of the mucosa are
a. Stratified squamous, simple columnar, stratified squamous
b. Epithelium, lamina propria, muscularis mucosa
c. Submucosa, muscularis externa, serosa
d. Muscularis mucosa, lamina propria, columnar epithelium

7 In the dog, the SA node is located in the
a. Left auricle
b. Right atrium
c. Left ventricle
d. Right ventricle

8 Which one of the following hormones is not secreted by the pituitary?
a. FSH
b. ACTH
c. Cortisone
d. Growth hormone

9 All of the following are major sites of lymphatic tissue except
a. Tonsils
b. Thymus
c. Spleen
d. Kidneys

10 Which of the following statements about the middle ear is false?
a. It contains three ossicles
b. Infection in the middle ear is called otitis media
c. It communicates with the nasopharynx by means of the eustachian tube
d. The cochlea is located here

BIBLIOGRAPHY

Colville T, Bassert J: *Clinical anatomy and physiology for veterinary technicians,* St Louis, 2002, Mosby.

Frandson RD: *Anatomy and physiology of farm animals,* ed 5, Philadelphia, 1992, Lea & Febiger.

Marieb E: *Human anatomy and physiology,* ed 5, San Francisco, Calif, 2001, Benjamin Cummings.

Martini F: *Fundamentals of anatomy and physiology,* ed 5, Upper Saddle River, NJ, 2001, Prentice Hall.

McBride DF: *Learning veterinary terminology,* ed 2, St Louis, 2002, Mosby.

Romich JA: *An illustrated guide to veterinary terminology,* Albany, NY, 2000, Delmar Thomson Learning.

Ruckebusch Y, Phaneuf L-P, Dunlop R: *Physiology of small & large animals,* St Louis, 1991, Mosby.

CHAPTER 2

Urinalysis and Hematology

William L. Wade *Dan Walsh*

OUTLINE

LEARNING OUTCOMES

After reading this chapter you should be able to:

1. Demonstrate proper collection and analysis of urine.
2. Recommend the important concepts with blood collection.
3. Explain the hematological examinations that are commonly performed on blood samples.
4. Understand how hematological tests are used to evaluate organ function.

Veterinarians depend on accurate laboratory test results to offer the best patient care. Consistent, high-quality results provided by the veterinary technician are an essential component of this care. Many tests are routinely performed in-house rather than forwarded to a reference laboratory. (Values given in parentheses are SI units.)

URINALYSIS

A complete urinalysis provides information on the state of the kidneys and the animal's ability to normally filter and excrete metabolites. When an endocrine or a metabolic disturbance occurs, a complete analysis of the urine is indicated to demonstrate any abnormalities in chemical or structural components. These tests are easily performed in most veterinary settings using a minimal amount of diagnostic equipment, time, and expense.

Specimen Collection

I. Containers
   A. Collect the specimen in a clean, opaque container to prevent contamination and degradation of light-sensitive components (e.g., bilirubin and urobilinogen)
   B. Sterile containers should be used for urine samples for bacterial cultures collected through cystocentesis or catheterization
II. Free flow, clean catch, or voiding
   A. Simple, noninvasive procedure but unsatisfactory for bacterial culture
   B. Preferably, a midstream sample is collected; avoid initial or end portion of the voided urine
   C. Vulva or prepuce should be cleansed before collection
III. Cystocentesis
   A. Performed by inserting a needle through the ventral abdominal wall and into the urinary bladder
   B. Should be performed using aseptic technique
   C. Perform in an animal with a full bladder to avoid possible damage to other abdominal organs
   D. Collection through cystocentesis avoids contaminants from the lower portions of the

urinary tract, making the sample suitable for bacterial culture

IV. Catheterization
   A. Performed by passing a rubber, plastic, or metal catheter through the urethra and into the urinary bladder
   B. Type and size of catheter depend on sex and species of animal
   C. Should be completed as aseptically as possible and with caution to avoid undue trauma and erroneous test results
   D. Sample is easily aspirated into a syringe attached to the exposed end of the catheter

V. Manual expression
   A. As with collection for a voided sample, midstream collection is preferred
   B. Sample is not suitable for bacterial culture
   C. Vulva or prepuce should be cleansed before sample collection
   D. Must be performed with care and patience; avoid excessive pressure to the bladder
   E. Should never be attempted on an animal with a suspected obstruction

VI. Metabolism cage
   A. Usually of value to determine urine volume only
      1. Extended periods of time between collection and testing may cause contamination and sample degradation
         a. Exception is the alarm-sensitive cage that is used in some research facilities

VII. Tabletop
   A. May be adequate for screening if the table is clean and the sample is analyzed in an expedient manner
      1. Sample is not suitable for bacterial culture

VIII. Client-collected samples
   A. Usually, client-collected samples are not satisfactory because of improper collection procedures and extended periods of time between collection and testing, as well as improper container use
   B. Have the client discourage the pet from voiding urine for 2 to 3 hours before the appointment to facilitate collection at the clinic

Evaluation

I. Sample preservation
   A. Samples should be analyzed within 30 minutes for maximum valid information
      1. Degradation of urine components

a. Ammonia	increases
b. Bacteria	increases
c. Bilirubin	decreases
d. Casts	disappear
e. Color	darkens
f. Crystals	change
g. Erythrocytes	hemolyze
h. Glucose	decreases
i. Ketones	decrease
j. Leukocytes	decrease
k. Nitrites	appear
l. Hemolyzed blood	increases
m. Odor	becomes stronger
n. pH	usually increases
o. Protein	increases or decreases
p. Turbidity	develops
q. Urobilinogen	decreases (dipstick tests not reliable in animals)

   B. Refrigerate for an additional 6 to 12 hours if necessary but bring to room temperature before evaluation, especially if evaluating for specific gravity (SG) and crystals
   C. For cytological evaluation, centrifuge immediately
   D. The sample can be preserved by the addition of formalin, toluene, or phenol, but changes may occur with some chemical analyses

II. Gross examination
   A. Volume may be influenced by several factors, including water intake, environmental temperature, physical activity, size, and species
      1. Ideally, a 24-hour urine estimation should be made
   B. Pollakiuria: refers to frequent urination; often confused with polyuria by clients
   C. Polyuria: increase in urine output or production
      1. Associated with nephritis, diabetes mellitus, and polydipsia
   D. Oliguria: decrease in the formation or elimination of urine
      1. Occurs with shock, dehydration, water conservation, or renal failure
   E. Anuria: complete absence of urine formation or elimination
      1. Can occur as a result of renal shutdown; usually associated with obstruction

III. Color
   A. In most species, urine is transparent light-yellow to amber
   B. Yellow is normally due to pigments called urochromes
   C. Color usually correlates with SG
      1. Lighter-colored urine tends to have a lower SG; darker urine generally has a higher SG
      2. Bile pigments are likely contained in yellow-brown to greenish urine that foams when shaken

3. Red or reddish-brown urine indicates hematuria (red blood cells [RBCs]) or hemoglobinuria (hemoglobin [Hb])
4. Brown urine may contain myoglobinuria (myoglobins from muscle cell breakdown)

D. Some species, such as rabbits, normally have darker urine (orange to reddish brown)

IV. Transparency

A. Transparency is described as clear, cloudy, or flocculent

B. Cloudy urine can be associated with the presence of cellular debris such as RBCs, WBCs, epithelial cells, crystals, bacteria, casts, mucus, semen, and lipids

1. Bacteria or crystal formation can cause standing urine to become cloudy

C. Normal freshly voided urine in many species is clear; exceptions include

1. Horse, because of the presence of calcium carbonate crystals and mucus
2. Rabbit, hamster, and guinea pig because of the presence of calcium salts
3. On standing, urine typically becomes more cloudy with the increased numbers of bacteria and possible formation of crystals (e.g., calcium carbonate crystals form in cattle urine)

V. Odor

A. Not highly diagnostic but may be useful in detecting some bacterial growth or excessive ammonia content

B. Strong urine odor is typical in mice, tom cats, goats, and pigs

C. In some cases, a sweet or fruity odor can be indicative of ketones and is commonly associated with diabetes mellitus, pregnancy toxemia in sheep, or acetonemia in cows

D. Ammonia is due to bacterial proliferation, which may also cause an odor in standing urine

VI. Specific gravity is the density of a quantity of liquid compared with that of distilled water. In practical applications, it is used to assess the ability of the renal tubule to concentrate or dilute filtrates from the glomerulus, indicating how well the kidney can maintain water and osmotic balance

A. Refractometer method

1. Approximately measures SG or total solids of urine
2. Place a few drops of urine on the prism cover glass
3. Point refractometer toward bright light and read at the light-dark boundary
4. Ensure that results are read from the SG scale, which differs from the total protein scale
5. If reading is off the scale, dilute the urine 1:1 and adjust result accordingly, for accuracy

B. Urinometer method

1. Requires a larger volume of urine
2. Lower weighted bulb with attached scale into cylinder containing urine sample
3. Read results at bottom of the meniscus
4. Urinometers are calibrated to read samples at room temperature

C. Reagent test strips

1. Made for use in human samples
2. Least reliable method of determining SG, especially if SG is greater than 1.030
3. Place strip in sample to saturate reagent at tip
4. Read results by comparing color changes with color on scale on container

D. Changes in urine SG

1. Average SG values for the following species
   a. Canine 1.025
   b. Feline 1.030
   c. Equine 1.035
   d. Cattle and swine 1.015
   e. Sheep 1.030
2. Range for canine is from 1.001 to 1.060, and that for feline is 1.001 to 1.080
3. Increased SG occurs with dehydration, decreased water intake, acute renal disease, and shock
   a. In these situations, it would be expected that SG would be higer than 1.035 in feline, 1.030 in canine, and 1.025 in large animals
4. Decreased SG occurs with increased fluid intake and renal and other diseases

Chemical Components

I. Urine pH

A. Used to generally assess the body's acid-base balance. pH number expresses the hydrogen ion (H^+) concentration or the acidity of the urine

B. Reagent strips are most commonly used to determine pH. After being dipped into urine sample, the color change is compared with the color on a scale on the container

C. pH is often affected by diet

1. Herbivores commonly have an alkaline pH (7 to 8.5)
2. Carnivores have an acidic pH (feline 6 to 7)
3. Omnivores may have either

D. Loss of CO_2 occurs with samples left open and standing at room temperature, resulting in higher pH readings

E. Standing urine, containing urease-producing bacteria, also increases the reading

F. In highly acidic urine, a false reduction of the pH reading may result because of dripping from the protein pad onto the pH pad

II. Protein
   A. Proteinuria usually describes an abnormal level of proteins or protein metabolites in the urine
   B. Detection of protein levels is commonly made by use of reagent test strips (Multistix, Ames, Petstix)
   C. Color comparison is made and results are recorded in mg/dL
      1. Normal should be none or trace (10 mg/dL)
   D. Results are considered semiquantitative because of variables in chemical reaction and color chart comparison
   E. Errors can occur
      1. False-positive results can occur with alkaline urine
      2. If proteinuria is caused by globulins rather than albumin, false-negative results can occur
      3. Depending on the reader, different values may be obtained
      4. Proteinuria in diluted urine indicates greater protein loss than in concentrated urine
   F. Proteinuria results from several pre and post renal causes; abnormality in the urogenital system is most often suggested
   G. Values must be taken in context with other results such as urine blood and microscopic sediment
      1. Good evaluation of protein loss in the animal can be made by comparing urine protein and urine creatinine values (should be performed at a reference laboratory)
   H. Protein values can also be evaluated with sulfosalicylic acid, which determines urine protein levels through acid precipitation

III. Glucose
   A. Detectable levels of sugar are referred to as glucosuria or glycosuria and depend on glucose levels in the blood
      1. Unless the renal threshold is reached (about 170 to 180 mg/dL [greater than 6.8 mmol/L in dogs]), glucosuria does not usually occur
   B. Testing is usually performed by using any number of reagent strips available; Clinitest (Ames) reagent tablets detect sugars in the urine; reagent strips detect only glucose
      1. If the proteinaceous labile enzymes found in the glucose test pads become inactive, a false-negative result occurs. Check with the manufacturer for details on prolonging the life of unopened, in-date packages by freezing
   C. Hyperglycemia along with glucosuria can be attributed to diabetes mellitus created by insulin deficiency or function
      1. For confirmation of diabetes mellitus, blood glucose level should be evaluated
   D. Other factors such as fear, stress, excitement, intravenous fluids with glucose, and other diseases also cause glucosuria
      1. Fasting is recommended before glucose testing to avoid higher levels after a high-carbohydrate meal
      2. False-positive results can occur after the use of various drugs such as salicylates, ascorbic acid, and penicillin

IV. Ketones
   A. Ketones include acetone, acetoacetic (diacetic) acid, and β-hydroxybutyric acid
      1. Acetone and β-hydroxybutyric acid are derived from acetoacetic acid and result from the catabolism of fatty acids
      2. Ketones are produced during fat metabolism and are important sources of energy
      3. Excessive ketones are toxic, producing central nervous system depression and acidosis
   B. In normal animals, very small amounts are found in the blood
      1. If there is increased fat metabolism, decreased carbohydrate metabolism, or both, excess ketones spill into the urine, causing ketonuria
      2. Ketonemia (ketosis) often causes ketonuria
   C. In large animals, ketosis is associated with hypoglycemia because of insufficient carbohydrate intake, often during lactation or pregnancy
   D. In small animals, ketosis occurs with diabetes mellitus
      1. Lack of insulin prevents carbohydrate utilization
   E. Ketone measurement is accomplished by using one of several reagent test strips or separate reagent tablets (Ketostix, Acetest, Ames)
      1. Color intensity is proportional to ketone concentration
      2. These tests are most sensitive to acetoacetic acid

V. Bile pigments
   A. Commonly detected bile pigments include bilirubin and urobilinogen
      1. Only conjugated bilirubin is found in the urine
      2. Small amount of urobilinogen, from the breakdown of bilirubin by bacteria in the intestines, is excreted into the urine
      3. Positive bilirubin test pads in cats are usually reliable, whereas in dogs there is a significant number of false-negative and false-positive results

a. Urobilinogen test pads in both dogs and cats have not been reliable

B. Bilirubinuria can be seen in several diseases, including biliary obstruction, hepatic infections, toxicity, and hemolytic anemia
   1. Light will oxidize bilirubin if urine is left standing, resulting in a false-negative result
   2. Because the liver and kidneys of dogs and cattle have an enzyme that can conjugate bilirubin, slight bilirubinuria may be present in these species

C. Determination of bile pigments is made with reagent test strips (Bili-labstix, Multistix, Ames). Urobilinogen is not easily detected
   1. More accurate test is the Ictotest (Ames)
   2. Rough determination of the presence of bilirubinuria can be determined if urine is shaken and a yellow foam forms

VI. Blood
   A. Presence of intact RBCs in the urine is referred to as hematuria
      1. Presence of free Hb is referred to as hemoglobinuria
      2. Hematuria is usually seen as red and cloudy urine
      3. Hemoglobinuria and myoglobinuria are a red to brown color
   B. Occult blood may also be present, with no visible changes to the urine
   C. Hematuria is associated with disease of the urogenital tract
      1. Hemoglobinuria indicates some intravascular hemolysis
      2. Myoglobinuria generally indicates a muscle disease
   D. Besides color interpretation, blood or blood components in the urine are detected with reagent strips (Hemastix, Ames), as well as with tablets (Occultest Reagent Tablets)
      1. Because these do not differentiate the cause of blood in urine, microscopic evaluation to determine RBC numbers, as well as animal history and examination, along with other tests, should be included in the evaluation process
   E. Leukocyte test pads usually yield false-positive results for cats and false-negative results for dogs. It is best to evaluate fresh urine samples microscopically for the presence or absence of leukocytes

VII. Nitrites
   A. In humans, nitrite is used as an indirect indication of bacteriuria. It is believed that ascorbic acid normally present in canine and feline urine usually gives false-negative results
   B. Bacterial cultures and microscopic evaluation of fresh urine samples are the best methods for detecting the presence of bacteriuria

Microscopic Evaluation

Examination of the urine sediment is a highly valuable tool used in conjunction with the interpretation of color, SG, turbidity, protein, pH, and occult blood tests. Microscopic evaluation may be considered a form of exfoliate cytology.

I. Sample preparation
   A. Best sample is obtained in the early morning because it is fresh and well concentrated
   B. Refrigerate the sample if it cannot be examined within 30 minutes. Room temperature storage can result in natural chemical breakdown and lysing of cells
   C. Thoroughly mix the specimen, transfer to a conical tip centrifuge tube, and centrifuge sample at 1500 to 2000 rpm for 3 to 5 minutes
      1. A 5-mL sample of fresh urine is usually adequate
   D. Note the volume of sediment; leave about 0.3 mL of the supernatant and resuspend the sediment
      1. Transfer a small drop to a clean microscope slide and examine
   E. Examination can be done with or without stain; staining may be done with 1 drop of 0.5% new methylene blue (NMB) or Sedi-Stain
   F. Reduce illumination, scan entire area under the coverslip under ×10 (low-power field [LPF]) objective, and then identify through ×40 (high-power field [HPF]) objective
   G. Crystals and cast numbers are estimated as the average per LPF
      1. Epithelial cells and blood cells are estimated as the average number per HPF
      2. Bacteria and sperm are noted as few, moderate, or many under HPF
   H. Contaminated or nonrefrigerated "stale" samples should be avoided
      1. Samples that have not been thoroughly resuspended after centrifugation may yield a nonrepresentative sediment
      2. Sediments that were allowed to dry on the microscope slide may make cells unrecognizable

II. Components of sediment (Figure 2-1)
   A. WBCs (leukocytes) are normally found very few in number
      1. Most cells in urine are neutrophils and appear spherical, granular, and larger than RBCs but smaller than epithelial cells
      2. Excessive number of WBCs is referred to as pyuria or leukocyturia

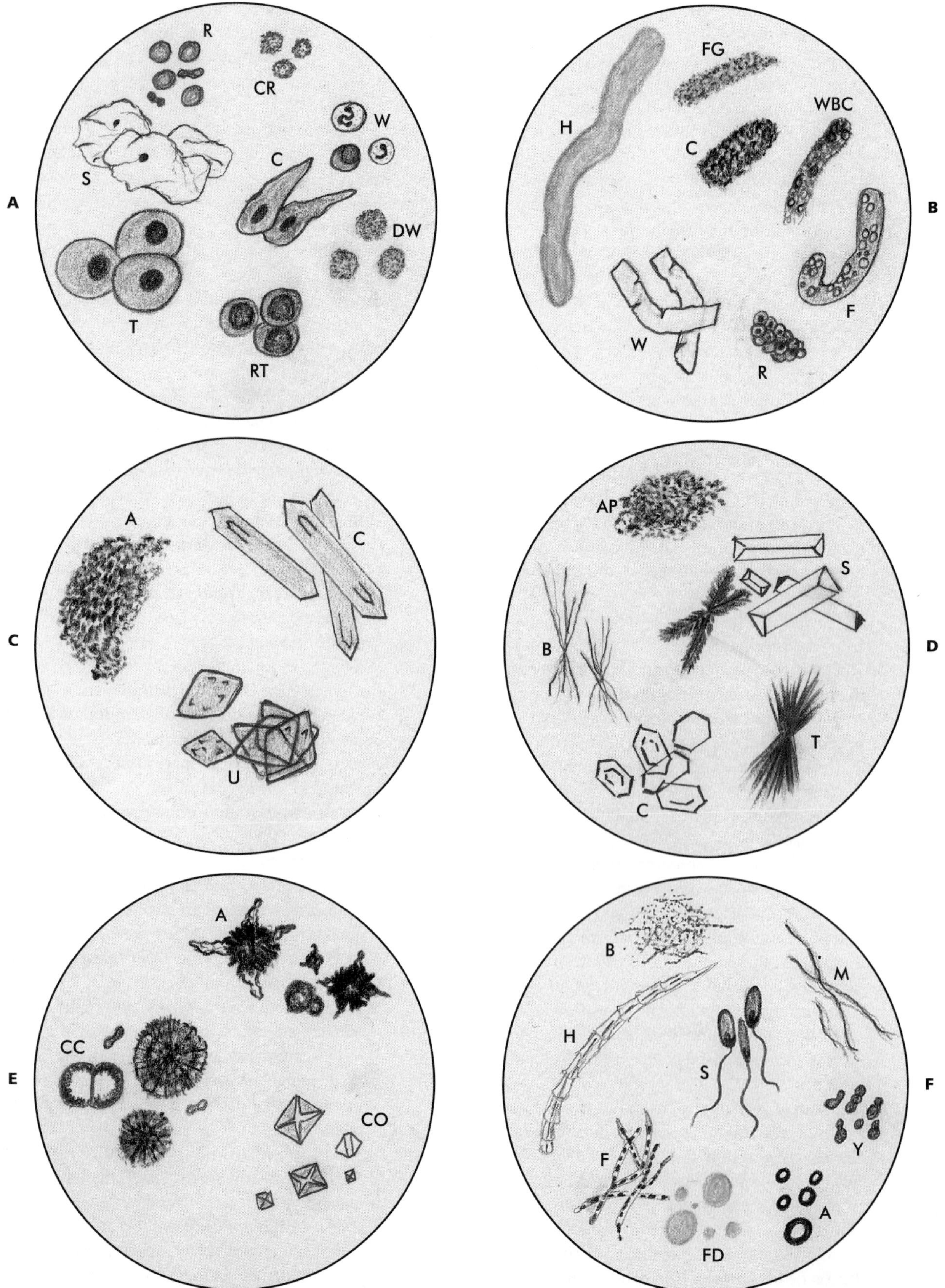

Figure 2-1 For legend see p. 29.

Figure 2-1 Common components of urine sediment. **A,** Caudate cells *(C)*, crenated RBC *(CR)*, degenerated white blood cell *(DW)*, red blood cell *(R)*, renal tubular *(RT)*, squamous *(S)*, transitional *(T)*, white blood cell *(W)*. **B,** Casts. Coarse granular *(C)*, fatty *(F)*, fine granular *(FG)*, hyaline *(H)*, red blood cell *(R)*, waxy *(W)*, white blood cell *(WBC)*. **C,** Amorphous urates *(A)*, calcium oxalate monohydrate *(C)*, uric acid *(U)*. **D,** Amorphous phosphate *(AP)*, bilirubin *(B)*, cytine *(C)*, strubite/triple phosphate *(S)*, tyrosine *(T)*. **E,** Ammonium ruate/"thorn apple" *(A)*, calcium cargonate *(CC)*, calcium oxalate dihydrate/"envelope" *(CO)*. **F,** Air bubbles *(A)*, bacteria *(B)*, fat droplets *(FS)*, fungi *(F)*, hair *(H)*, mucus *(M)*, sperm *(S)*, yeast *(Y)*. (Drawings by Toni D'Amato-Scheck, AAS, LVT, from Walsh D, D'Amato-Scheck T, eds: *Clinical technician lab manual*, State University of New York at Delhi, 2001.)

3. Increased numbers indicate active inflammatory disease along the urinary tract but can also be from the genital tract
4. More than a few (5 to 8 per HPF) should be regarded as abnormal and further investigated
5. Note any evidence of bacteria

B. RBCs (erythrocytes) are also normally very few in number
1. Excessive number of RBCs is referred to as hematuria
2. Hematuria is associated with trauma, calculi, infection, and benign or malignant neoplasia
3. RBCs appear as pale yellow refractive disks, usually uniform in shape and smaller than WBCs
   a. Sample manipulation can create distortion, crenation and hemolysis, and confusion with fat or yeast
      (1) Fat droplets will float in and out of planes of focus; RBCs do not
      (2) If a small amount of 2% acetic acid is added to the slide and the structures disappear, they were RBCs
4. In concentrated urine, RBCs may lose fluid and become crenated (shrunken and spiked)
   a. In dilute urine they may swell or lyse, becoming ghost cells
5. More than a few (5 per HPF) should be noted as abnormal and further investigated

C. Epithelial cells
1. Three types usually found in urine sediment: squamous, transitional, renal
2. Squamous cells are derived from the urethra, vagina, and vulva and are the largest cells found in urine sediment
   a. Appear as flat, irregularly shaped cells with angular borders and small round nuclei
   b. Usually not seen in samples obtained by cystocentesis or catheterization
   c. Their presence is not considered significant
3. Transitional cells come from the bladder, ureters, renal pelvis, and part of the urethra
   a. Wide variation in size; may be round, pear shaped, or caudate, typically with granular cytoplasm
   b. Increased numbers are associated with inflammation such as cystitis or pyelonephritis
4. Renal cells originate from the renal tubules, are found in small numbers, are slightly larger than WBCs, and are sometimes difficult to differentiate from WBCs
   a. Usually round with a large nucleus
   b. Increased numbers indicate renal tubular disease

D. Casts (see Figure 2-1)
1. Found in the distal and collecting tubules of the kidneys
2. Dissolve in alkaline urine; so analyze fresh samples immediately
3. Any structures that are in the tubules at the time the casts are formed embed themselves in the cast
4. Larger numbers of casts help localize pathology to the renal tubules, but numbers do not always indicate the severity of the disease
   a. May be only a few casts in severe chronic nephritis
5. Hyaline casts
   a. A few may be seen in normal urine
   b. Clear, colorless, highly refractile, and composed of mucoprotein
   c. Cylindrical with symmetrical sides and rounded ends
   d. Indicates mildest form of renal irritation
6. Granular casts
   a. Most common type seen in animals
   b. Contain granules from degenerate epithelial cells and WBCs
   c. Seen in greater numbers with acute nephritis; indicates severe kidney disease
7. Epithelial, fatty, and waxy casts
   a. Epithelial casts contain cells from renal epithelium
      (1) Seen in acute nephritis and renal tubule degeneration
   b. Fatty casts contain small fat droplets that are refractile
      (1) Seen in cats with renal disease and dogs with diabetes mellitus
   c. Waxy casts are wide and square ended and have a dull appearance
      (1) More opaque than hyaline casts and indicate chronic to severe tubular degeneration

E. Crystals (see Figure 2-1)

1. May be normal or abnormal; term "crystalline" may or may not be of clinical significance
2. Crystal formation is influenced by pH, temperature, concentration, and medication
3. Triple phosphates appear as classic "coffin lids:" three- to six-sided colorless prisms normally found in alkaline urine
   a. May be associated with urease-producing bacteria of lower urinary tract disease, often in association with uroliths
   b. Can be found in slightly acidic urine
4. Amorphous phosphate/urates
   a. Phosphates found in alkaline urine appear as granular precipitate
   b. Urates are similar but are found in acidic urine
   c. Ammonium biurate crystals are round and brownish, with long spicules
      (1) Seen in liver disease or portal caval shunts
5. Calcium carbonate crystals are often found in normal horses and cattle
   a. Resemble colorless dumbbells
6. Calcium oxalate are small, colorless envelopes, sometimes dumbbell or ring formed, usually with a characteristic X form in the center
   a. Generally in acidic urine but can be seen in neutral or alkaline urine
   b. Dihydrate calcium oxalate crystals are found in normal urine
      (1) Monohydrate calcium oxalate crystals seen in animals with ethylene glycol toxicity or large animals that ingested oxalates
         (a) Also associated with calcium oxalate urolithiasis
7. Leucine/cystine/tyrosine crystals may indicate hepatic disease
   a. Leucine crystals are small and round, with sectioned centers
   b. Tyrosine crystals appear spiculated and spindle shaped
   c. Cystine crystals are flat and hexagon shaped (six sided)
      (1) Their presence may indicate metabolic defect of cysteine metabolism
      (2) Possible association with uroliths
   d. All three are found in acidic urine
8. Uric acid crystals are in alkaline urine and associated with metabolic defect
   a. Common in Dalmatians and animals with uroliths
   b. Bilirubin crystals often found if there is bilirubinuria
      (1) Presence is not significant
9. Some drugs, such as sulfonamides, may precipitate and form crystals

F. Other cells may be found in urine sediment
   1. Spermatozoa can be seen in the urine of an intact male, but they are clinically insignificant
   2. Parasite ova in the urine sediment may be fecal contamination or urine parasites
   3. Fat droplets are highly refractile and spherical and of various shapes, thus often difficult to differentiate from other cells; however, they can be stained with Sudan stain
   4. Bacteria may not be detected in the sediment until their numbers approach 10,000+ per mL
      a. When stains are used, be careful to avoid precipitated or bacterial contaminated stains, because both may be falsely identified as sediment bacteria
      b. Cultures and antimicrobial sensitivity testing should be used for identification of bacteria and selection of the antimicrobial agent

G. Uroliths
   1. Most common type of canine uroliths (urinary stones) are triphosphate (struvite) concretions, whereas most feline uroliths are calcium oxalate
   2. Although there are in-house chemical methods for the determination of the composition of the stones, quantitative mineral analysis at reference laboratories tends to provide the most accurate determinations

HEMATOLOGY

The most commonly performed hematology procedure is the complete blood count (CBC). It includes determination of total RBC and WBC numbers, packed cell volume (PCV), total plasma protein, Hb, RBC indices, and blood film evaluation. Normal values can be found in the tables at the end of the chapter. It should be understood that actual values vary with the laboratory performing the tests and population of animals tested. Abnormal patients may fall within the reference value range, while normal patients may be outside of the range. Reference value ranges for the species tend to be wide while individual normal ranges are narrower.

Erythrocyte Evaluation

I. Erythrocyte PCV
   A. Also termed hematocrit (HCT)
   B. Determines percentage of RBCs in the circulating blood volume
   C. Most easily measured by filling a microcapillary or hematocrit tube with fresh, anticoagulated blood
   D. Tubes are sealed and generally centrifuged at high speed for 5 minutes
      1. Actual time is dependent on the speed and centrifugation angle
      2. Hematocrit centrifuges are often preset for speed
      3. For manual setting, 1500 rpm for 5 minutes is recommended

4. Goat and sheep blood should be centrifuged for 10 to 20 minutes
   a. The small RBCs (<4 to 5 μm) mean increased cell numbers and subsequent packing time

E. Results are determined by use of a scale on the centrifuge, hand-held card or mechanical reader
F. Results are reported as percentage (%) in conventional units (or as liter per liter [L/L] in SI units)
G. Color and clarity of plasma, as well as screening for microfilaria and total plasma protein (TPP), can be evaluated from the plasma fraction of the PCV (hematocrit) tube

II. Erythrocyte total numbers
   A. Determined by using an automated or a manual cell counting device
   B. Automated counters require calibration for cell size, depending on species
   C. Manual counts are made with a hemacytometer and are usually not as accurate
   D. Both methods require that the sample be greatly diluted before counting
   E. Total erythrocyte count usually has no advantage over the PCV except to determine the RBC indices
   F. Total RBC numbers are reported as millions per microliter ($n \times 10^6/\mu L$ or $n \times 10^{12}/L$ in SI units)

III. Hemoglobin
   A. Part of the RBCs responsible for carrying oxygen and carbon dioxide
   B. Assists in acid-base regulation by eliminating carbon dioxide
   C. Can be measured by photometric methods or automated cell counters
   D. Used for determining erythrocytic indices
   E. Measured in g/dL (g/L)
   F. For a quick qualitative analysis, the normal animal Hb is about one third of the PCV

IV. Erythrocyte indices
   A. Determined by use of the total RBC numbers, Hb content, and PCV. Many electronic units automatically include these values
      1. Used to assist in classifying some anemias
   B. Mean corpuscular volume (MCV) is the mean volume of a group of erythrocytes (their size)
      1. MCV is calculated by dividing the PCV (%) by the total RBC count and multiplying by 10
      2. MCV is recorded in femtoliters (fL); normal ranges vary among species
      3. For SI units, divide the PCV (L/L) by the RBC count and multiply by 1000
   C. Mean corpuscular Hb (MCH) is the mean weight of Hb contained in the average RBC
      1. MCH is calculated by dividing the Hb concentration by the total RBC count and multiplying by 10
      2. Results are recorded in picograms (pg)
      3. Considered least accurate of the indices because Hb and RBC counts are less accurate than the PCV
   D. Mean corpuscular hemoglobin concentration (MCHC) is the concentration of Hb in the average RBC (color of the cell)
      1. MCHC is calculated by dividing the Hb concentration by the PCV (%) and multiplying by 100
      2. Results are reported in g/dL (g/L)
         a. For SI units, divide the Hb concentration (g/L) by the PCV (L/L)
      3. Considered the most accurate of the RBC indices because it does not require the RBC count
   E. Red cell distribution (RDW) is an electronic measurement of anisocytosis
      1. Higher RDWs indicate anisocytosis, whereas normal values indicate normal cell size

V. Reticulocyte count
   A. Expression of the percentage of RBCs that are reticulocytes or immature erythrocytes still containing the ribosomes
   B. Wright's stain causes a polychromatophilic staining or diffuse, blue-gray color
   C. Cats possess two forms: aggregate and punctate
      1. Only the aggregate form should be counted
      2. Similar to other species, this contains large clumps that appear polychromatophilic
   D. A few drops of blood are mixed with an equal amount of NMB stain
      1. This mixture is used to prepare a conventional blood film that shows up as granular precipitate
   E. Percentage of reticulocytes per 1000 RBCs or an absolute count in reticulocytes per milliliter is reported
   F. Useful in assessing the bone marrow response to anemia in all domestic animals, except for horses, because they do not release reticulocytes from the bone marrow

Blood Collection and Sampling

I. General rules
   A. Collect the smallest amount of blood necessary to perform all tests plus an adequate amount for retest or errors
      1. This will usually be approximately two times the initial amount necessary to accomplish the tests

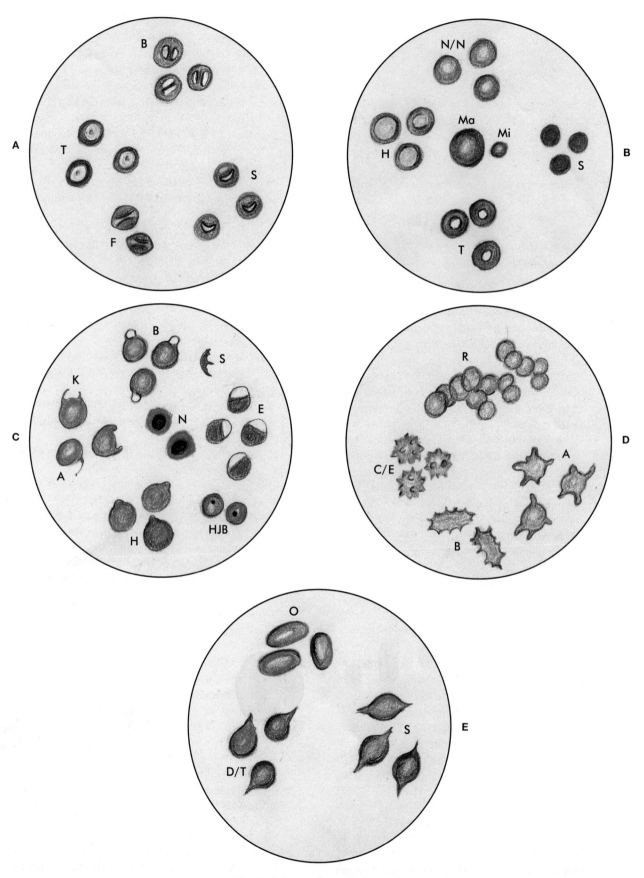

Figure 2-2 For legend see p. 33.

Figure 2-2 Common red blood cell morphological changes and inclusions. **A,** Stomatocytes *(S)* and leptocytes: bar cell *(B)*, folded *(F)*, target cell *(T)*. **B,** Hypochromic *(H)*, macrocyte *(Ma)*, microcyte *(Mi)*, normocyte/normochromic *(N/N)*, spherocyte *(S)*. **C,** Apple stem cell *(A)*, blister cell *(B)*, eccentrocyte *(E)*, Heinz body *(H)*, Howell-Jolly body *(HJB)*, nucleated red blood cell *(N)*, shistocyte *(S)*. **D,** Acanthocyte *(A)*, burr cell *(B)*, crenated echinocyte *(C/E)*, rouleaux *(R)*. **E,** Sacrocyte/teardrop *(D/T)*, ovalocyte *(O)*, spindle cell *(S)*. (Drawings by Toni D'Amato-Scheck, AAS, LVT, from Walsh D, D'Amato-Scheck T, eds: *Clinical technician lab manual*, State University of New York at Delhi, 2001.)

2. Use syringes and vacuum collection devices proportional to the size of the patient and volume needed

B. Ethylenediaminetetraacetic acid (EDTA) is the best anticoagulant

1. When used in the proper ratio of anticoagulant to blood, will cause the least changes in cell morphology

C. When using anticoagulants, fill the tube to at least 90% of the capacity of the tube to maintain the proper anticoagulant-to-blood ratio

1. Do not put in more than the volume that a vacuum tube will collect
2. Inadequate sample amount will cause crenation of the erythrocytes and reactive changes in the leukocytes

D. Be cautious when aspirating with a syringe, or a vacuum collection device that is too large

1. Excessive vacuum may cause cell destruction and injury to the patient

E. When transferring blood from a syringe to a vacuum container, either

1. Remove the stopper from the tube and needle from the syringe
   a. Gently push on the plunger to evacuate the blood from the syringe
2. Carefully pass the needle through the stopper and allow the vacuum to pull the blood from the syringe
3. Simultaneously pushing the plunger on the syringe along with the vacuum from the tube, will cause excessive pressure and damage cells

F. Avoid repeated collection from the same site in close proximity of time

1. May cause localized increases in the number of leukocytes and platelets, trauma, pain, and increased chances for hematomas

G. Samples collected immediately postprandial may be lipemic

H. Fear, excitement, struggling, stress, and restraint may cause relative changes in the patient's values because of redistribution of cells from and to the marginal and circulating pools of blood

I. Medications and fluids may have biological or dilution effects on the sample or may influence the test procedure

J. Patient history, such as recent vaccinations or surgery, may influence results

K. Time of collection to time of testing is critical

1. Sample degradation starts immediately after collection
2. EDTA prevents coagulation but does not preserve the sample

Erythrocyte Film Evaluation (Figure 2-2)

I. Erythrocyte size, shape, appearance, and color can vary among species of animals

A. These parameters can also be affected by environment, handling, technique, and other factors

II. Size of mature erythrocyte can range from 3 to 7 μm, depending on the species, and may be characterized as follows

A. Macrocytosis: an increased number of larger-than-normal, usually immature, polychromatic RBCs

B. Microcytosis: an increased number of RBCs smaller in diameter than normal, decreased MCV

C. Normocytic: refers to normal-size mature erythrocytes

D. Anisocytosis: variation in the size of RBCs

1. Normal amount varies with species
2. Can be due to large and/or small cells
3. Graded as mild, moderate, or marked

III. Color

A. Normochromic: a mature cell that stains pink in color with an area of central pallor (mammals); nucleated in reptiles, birds, and amphibians

B. Polychromasia: cells that have a bluish tint, because of remaining organelles in the cytoplasm

1. Are referred to as reticulocytes if stained with NMB

C. Hypochromic: lack of or decrease in staining intensity, because of decrease in cellular Hb

1. Iron deficiency most common cause
2. Because of large diameter, macrocytic erythrocytes may appear hypochromic
3. True hypochromia is usually concurrent with microcytosis and determined by MCV

IV. Shape

A. Acanthocyte: cells with irregularly shaped margins/projections from the cell wall; also known as spur cells

1. Can be due to faulty technique or disease in which cholesterol concentration changes occur at the membrane

B. Crenation: cells with spiny projections around the margin
   1. Often associated with slow drying of the blood film
C. Echinocyte (burr cells): have regular spinelike projections from all surfaces of the cell
   1. Echinocytes are usually more round
   2. Burr cells are more elongated and are seen with renal disease
   3. Observed in blood of horses after exercising or with renal disease and lymphosarcoma in dogs
   4. Can be due to faulty technique (crenation)
   5. Appear as dark red spots when seen on top of the cell
D. Target cells: "Mexican hat" cells
   1. Contain a central, round portion of Hb inside the area of central pallor
   2. Form of leptocyte; may be called codocyte
   3. Bar cells found in similar conditions and have barlike protrusions of the cell membrane
E. Leptocyte: large, thin RBC that is folded or misshapen because of increased membrane or decreased volume
   1. Common finding with regenerative anemias
F. Stomatocyte: also a type of leptocyte
   1. Large, thin cell that warps when passing through small blood vessels
   2. Seen in dogs with rare inherited disorders
G. Spherocytes: smaller, dense, and dark staining; lack central pallor
   1. Suggestive of immune-mediated hemolytic anemia
      a. Because of loss of surface membrane (partial erythrophagocytosis)
H. Schistocytes: fragmented erythrocytes, also known as helmet cells
   1. Suggestive of mechanical damage or vascular occlusion (disseminated intravascular coagulation)
I. Poikilocytosis: a general presence of a variation in cell shape
J. Rouleaux: erythrocytes appearing as stacks of coins or rows
   1. Can indicate inflammatory changes or alteration of plasma protein
   2. Normal finding in equine species (marked)
K. Agglutination: an amorphous clumping of erythrocytes, typically associated with immune disease
   1. May be visibly seen: a grainy appearance on the slide
   2. If seen, do not use automated RBC counting or sizing
L. Anisocytosis: variation in size of RBCs
   1. Normal amount varies with species
   2. Can be due to large and/or small cells
   3. Graded as mild, moderate, or marked
M. Ovalocytes (elliptocytes): a membrane defect causing the cell to be oval with an oval central pallor
N. Blister cell: an oxidative defect associated with iron deficiency anemia, causing a blister-like protrusion on the cell membrane surface
   1. Keratocyte: a rupturing of the blister causing a hornlike protrusion
   2. Apple stem cell: a rupturing of the blister causing a singular protrusion
O. Ghost cell: pale remnants of RBC membranes caused by intravascular lysis
P. Eccentrocytes: Hb is displaced to one side of the cell, resulting in a half-moon appearance caused by oxidative injury to the RBC
Q. Torocyte: a spreading artifact resulting in an abrupt change between the outer ring of Hb and the central pallor, causing a "Life-Saver"- or "Cheerio"-like punched-out appearance
   1. Must be distinguished from the gradual change seen in hypochromic cells

V. Inclusions
   A. Howell-Jolly bodies: erythrocytes that retain small, round nuclear fragments, dark staining, intracellular bodies
      1. Noted in regenerative anemias and splenic disorders
      2. Nonrefractile when out of focus
      3. In 1% of feline and equine RBCs
   B. Heinz bodies: small, round areas of denatured Hb attached to the cell membrane
      1. Appear transparent with Wright's or Diff-Quick stain; stain blue with NMB (1 to 2 mL)
      2. Associated with oxidant drugs, lymphosarcoma, hyperthyroidism, and diabetes mellitus in cats
      3. Common in cats
   C. Basophilic stippling: small, blue-staining granules (RNA) within the erythrocyte
      1. Seen in very responsive anemias in cattle, sheep, and cats
      2. Suggestive of lead toxicity
   D. Nucleated RBC (NRBC): slightly larger than mature RBC, darker-staining cytoplasm, retained nucleus
      1. Immature cell, not normally seen in circulation, released in response to anemia (see Table 2-1 for list of precursors)
      2. Mature RBCs are normally oval and nucleated in non-mammalian species (i.e., bird, reptiles, fish and amphibians)

VI. Blood parasites
   A. *Hemobartonella felis:* small cocci or rod-shaped, dark purple–stained structures (with Wright's stain) at the margin of feline RBCs

Table 2-1 Precursor blood cells in order of least immature to most mature cells

Erythrocyte precursors	Granulocyte precursors	Platelet precursors
Rubriblast	Myeloblast	Megakaryoblast
Prorubricyte	Progranulocyte	Promegakaryocyte
Rubricyte	Myelocyte	Megakaryocyte
Metarubricyte	Metamyelocyte	Platelet
Polychromatic erythrocyte	Band	

B. *Hemobartonella canis:* long, dark purple–staining chains on the surface of the canine RBC
   1. Rare and usually apparent in immunocompromised or splenectomized dogs
   2. Similar to *Eperythrozoon* in swine, cattle, and llamas
C. *Babesia* spp.: protozoa
   1. *Babesia canis* in dogs; *Babesia caballi* in horses
   2. Appear as fairly large, paired, teardrop-shaped organisms in the RBC
   3. More noticeable in cells along feathered edge
   4. Affected cells tend to accumulate below buffy coat
   5. Can lyse cells and stain with Giemsa or diagnose through serology
   6. Transmitted by *Ixodes* ticks
D. *Cytauxzoon felis:* very rare organism found in RBCs, lymphocytes, and macrophages of cats
   1. Small, dark-staining ring forms in the cells
E. *Anaplasma marginale:* intracellular parasite of the RBC in cattle and wild ruminants
   1. Small, dark-staining cocci at the cell margin
   2. Must be differentiated from similar-sized Howell-Jolly bodies
F. *Dirofilaria immitis:* heartworm of dogs, may be seen on blood films
   1. Unless present in large numbers, may be missed; best to use buffy coat
   2. Modified Knott's and filter technique increase the chance of finding microfilaria, but are still considered screening tests
      a. Not detect afilarial cases or cases with low microfilaria concentrations
   3. Enzyme-linked immunosorbent assays (ELISAs) and other immunological techniques tend to have an increased level of sensitivity over techniques used to detect the presence of microfilaria
      a. ELISA techniques detect the antigen of the gravid female *D. immitis* or antibodies that develop by the patient
   4. Must differentiate the nonpathogenic *Dipetalonema* spp. by morphology

Leukocyte (White Blood Cell) Evaluation

I. Total leukocyte counts may be made manually or with automated cell counters
   A. Both methods require blood sample dilution and lysis of the RBCs before counting
   B. Neubauer hemacytometer method: sample preparation using the Unopette system (Becton, Dickinson & Co.) is a common method
      1. Calibrated blood sample (20 μL) is diluted 1:100 in acetic acid diluent
      2. Sample is mixed, left for at least 10 minutes to hemolyze the RBCs, and then placed on the hemacytometer chamber
      3. Cells are counted in the nine primary squares at ×10 objective magnification
   C. Calculating total WBCs with a hemacytometer
      1. Total cells counted from both chambers is averaged
      2. Add 10% of cells counted to this number and multiply by 100 (the dilution factor)
         a. Example: 75 cells counted, 75 + 7.5 (10%) = 82.5 × 100 = 8250/μL
         b. Value is then 8.250×10^3/μL conventional units (8.25×10^9/L SI units)
      3. Automated counters use an electronic impulse to sense and count cells as they pass through the aperture; some calibration may be necessary
      4. Corrected WBC count for automated and manual counts if NRBCs present due to inflation of count
         a. Corrected with use of the blood film evaluation and NRBC count
         b. Practical method is to include the NRBC in the differential count and calculate using absolute numbers
            (1) Example: total WBC is 9000/μL (n × 10^9/L) with 10% NRBCs or 900 absolute
               (a) 9000 – 900 = 8100 as the corrected total
      5. Avian and reptilian leukocyte count
         a. Birds and reptiles have NRBCs, which makes determining a WBC count difficult with the normal methods
            (1) Eosinophil unopette is used: the anticoagulated blood is added to the unopette and allowed to sit for 5 minutes
               (a) If it rests much longer, the cells will take up all the stain and errors will result
               (b) Hemacytometer is filled with eosinophils and heterophils, which are the nonmammalian equivalent of neutrophils
               (c) All nine squares are counted

(d) Microscope condenser should be kept up to decrease contrast
(e) WBC count is calculated using the formula: Cells Counted on Hemacytometer × 32 × (100/heterophils + eosinophils) = WBCs/μL

6. Increased WBC count is leukocytosis
7. Decreased WBC count is leukopenia

II. Leukocyte evaluation and differentiation
A. WBC evaluation and differentiation is performed by examining the stained blood film
1. Traditional stains include Wright's, Wright-Giemsa, and Diff-Quick (American Scientific Products)
2. Techniques vary; follow manufacturer directions
B. Cells should be examined and counted in an area of the film where distribution and staining properties are best
1. Monolayer of cells is preferable; examination is completed under ×40 or ×100 oil immersion magnification
2. Avoid the feathered edge because of increased amounts of artifacts
3. If a coverslip is put on immersion oil, there is more definition of cells
C. Leukocyte differential numbers should always be reported as absolutes
1. Percentage of each cell type is multiplied by the total WBC counts
2. Example: 60% neutrophils × 10,000 WBC/μL total = 6000 absolute neutrophils
D. Leukocyte morphology
1. Neutrophils: most common peripheral WBCs in companion animals
a. Irregular, segmented nucleus with coarse clumped chromatin staining dark purple
b. Horse neutrophils show more segmentation than dog neutrophils
c. Cytoplasm is pale pink with faint granulation
d. Phagocytic and bactericidal properties, with an average life span of 10 hours
e. Inflammation is usually indicated by neutrophilia with increased bands
f. Increase may also be due to stress, exercise, glucocorticoid use, or leukemia
g. Neutropenia may be due to decreased survival of cells, reduced or ineffective production, or sequestration
(1) Will likely produce a degenerative left shift (more immature than mature neutrophils)
h. Avian neutrophil is called a heterophil
2. Neutrophilic bands: immature neutrophil stage
a. Horseshoe shaped, symmetrical nucleus with rounded ends
(1) Increased numbers denote left shift
3. Toxic neutrophils: changes with toxicity
a. Döhle bodies: appear as small, gray-blue cytoplasmic inclusions, indicative of mild toxemia
b. Basophilia or blue cytoplasm and vacuoles are slightly more severe signs of toxicity
c. Nuclear hypersegmentation implies older neutrophils
d. More evident in many feline illnesses
e. Other species with toxic neutrophils are often indicative of bacterial disease
4. Lymphocytes: small and large forms are recognized
a. High nuclear-to-cytoplasm ratio
b. Coarse, clumped (often round), dark-staining chromatin
c. Slight sky blue cytoplasm surrounding nucleus of small forms with more cytoplasm in large lymphocytes
d. Cytoplasm may contain pink-purple granules (azurophilic)
e. Cattle tend to have more lymphocytes than neutrophils
(1) May be large and have indented nuclei and increased cytoplasm, and granules
(2) Difficult to separate from neoplastic lymphoid cells
f. Reactive lymphocytes, a sign of antigenic stimulation, are shown by a pale perinuclear zone surrounded by basophilic cytoplasm and possible azurophilic granules
5. Monocytes: largest of the peripheral WBCs
a. Variable nuclear shape (kidney bean shape, elongated, lobulated) with diffuse chromatin, not as intensely stained
b. Blue-gray cytoplasm, possibly with vacuoles and fine pink granules
c. May be difficult to distinguish from band neutrophils or metamyelocytes
d. Circulate briefly in blood before entering tissues as macrophages
6. Eosinophils: nuclear structure similar to neutrophils but not as coarsely clumped chromatin
a. Distinctive red- to purple-staining cytoplasmic granules that vary in size and shape among species
(1) Dog: size and shape vary
(2) Cat: eosinophil granules tend to be rod shaped, small, and numerous
(3) Horse: intense orange-red and large granules

(4) Cattle, sheep, and pig: stain intense pink and are round

b. Increase is noted in allergic or hypersensitive reactions

(1) Mast cells often present

7. Basophils: a rare finding in peripheral blood

a. Cytoplasmic granules stain blue to blue-black (lavender in cat) and may be few in number (in dog) or more numerous (in horse and cow)

b. Gray-blue cytoplasm often with small vacuoles

c. As with mast cells, involved with hypersensitivity reactions

III. Inclusions

A. *Ehrlichia canis:* an intracellular parasite of monocytes and neutrophils

1. Tropical pancytopenia; transmitted by ticks
2. Appear as small lightly stained clusters in the cytoplasm (called morulae)
3. Diagnosis through buffy coat smear or serology (best)
4. Signs include leukopenia, anemia, thrombocytopenia, increased TPP, and lymphocytosis

Thrombocyte (Platelet) Evaluation

I. General information

A. Anuclear cytoplasmic fragments from bone marrow megakaryocytes

B. Vary in size, shape, and color

1. Usually small pale blue to pink-purple in color

C. May be found in clumps (especially in cat)

D. Thrombocytes (platelets) are an important component of hemostasis

E. Adequate numbers are estimated to be 8 to 10 per oil immersion field

1. Average number of platelets on 10 fields, per ×100 oil immersion field, in an area where RBCs are overlapping, is multiplied by 15,000 for a rough estimate
2. With decreased estimates, platelet aggregation on the blood film or tube of blood must be ruled out before thrombocytopenia is confirmed

F. Actual counts can be done manually with the hemacytometer or an automated cell counter

Total Protein

I. Combination of various proteins produced mostly by the liver

II. Abnormalities indicate diseases in tissues responsible for protein synthesis, catabolism, and loss

III. Total plasma or serum protein measured by total solids refractometer or chemical analysis in g/dL (g/L)

Nonmanual Instrumentation

I. Quantitative buffy coat analysis (QBC)

A. Specialized equipment and capillary tubes used for measurements of PCV, total WBC count, platelet count, and limited differential

B. Buffy coat band lengths are converted to numerical readings

1. Various types and degrees of fluorescence, depending on the layers, are also observed

C. It is essential that a differential also be performed to ensure accuracy

D. Layers of cells from uppermost to lowest are platelets, mononuclear cells (monocytes and lymphocytes), eosinophils, granulocytes, reticulocytes, NRBCs, and RBCs

II. Electronic cell counters

A. Various instruments ranging in costs are available

B. Many now available that automatically change instrument settings for multiple species application

C. Speed, accuracy, and reproducibility are major advantages

D. Depending on unit, will calibrate WBC and RBC count, Hb, PCV (indirectly), erythrocytic indices, and platelets

1. Some will give RBC distribution width (RDW), which is an indication of the variation in RBC size

a. The greater the variation, the higher the RDW

E. Sample must be diluted, but some machines do so automatically

F. Good quality control is essential

G. Impedance and laser technologies are used in the counting process

1. Size of the particle determines the threshold setting that most instruments will detect

a. If the machine is calibrated for human use, may not accurately count RBCs of cat, horse, cow, pig, and goat because the cells are smaller and the mean cell volumes fall below 55 fL

b. WBCs of dog are smaller; WBCs of cat are larger, and the cat's platelets tend to clump, which will create false elevations of the WBC count

c. Important to do an actual differential inspection to make sure results are accurate

Table 2-2 Hematologic reference values for domestic animals* in SI units

	Ox	Sheep	Goat	Pig	Horse	Dog	Cat
Hemoglobin (g/L)	80-150	90-150	80-120	100-160	110-190	120-180	80-150
Hemogram (μmol/L)	5.0-9.3	5.6-9.3	5.0-7.4	6.2-9.9	6.8-11.8	7.4-11.2	5.0-9.3
PCV (L/L)	0.24-0.46	0.27-0.45	0.22-0.38	0.32-0.50	0.32-0.53	0.37-0.55	0.24-0.45
RBC ($\times 10^{12}$/L)	5-10	9-15	8-18	5-8	7-13	6-9	5-10
MCV (fl)	40-60	28-40	16-25	50-68	37-58	60-77	39-55
MCH (pg)	11-17	8-12	5-8	17-21	12-20	20-25	13-18
MCHC (g/L)	300-360	310-340	300-360	300-340	310-390	320-360	300-360
Reticulocytes ($\times 10^9$/L)	0	0	0	0-80	0	0-128	0-0.5[†]
WBC ($\times 10^9$/L)	4.0-12.0	4.0-12.0	4.0-13.0	11.0-22.0	5.4-14.3	6.0-17.0	5.5-19.5
Neutrophils (mature) ($\times 10^9$/L)	0.6-4.0	0.7-6.0	1.2-7.2	3.1-10.5	2.3-8.6	3.0-11.5	2.5-12.5
Neutrophils (bands) ($\times 10^9$/L)	0-0.1	Rare	Rare	0-0.9	0-0.1	0-0.3	0-0.3
Lymphocytes ($\times 10^9$/L)	2.5-7.5	2.0-9.0	2.0-9.0	4.3-13.6	1.5-7.7	1.0-4.8	1.5-7.0
Monocytes ($\times 10^9$/L)	0-0.8	0-0.8	0-0.6	0.2-2.2	0-1.0	0.2-1.4	0-0.9
Eosinophils ($\times 10^9$/L)	0-2.4	0-1.0	0.1-0.7	0.1-2.4	0-1.0	0.1-1.3	0-1.5
Basophils ($\times 10^9$/L)	0-0.2	0-0.3	0-0.1	0-0.4	0-0.3	Rare	Rare
Platelets ($\times 10^9$/L)	100-800	250-750	300-600	320-720	100-350	200-500	300-800
Plasma proteins (g/L)	60-85	60-75	60-75	60-80	58-87	60-80	60-80
Fibrinogen (g/L)	3-7	1-5	1-4	1-5	1-4	1-5	0.5-3.0

*Reference values may be influenced by the method of measurement and by the animal's breed, sex, age, and environment; hence, these values are guidelines only.
†Aggregate reticulocytes derived from Fan LC, Dorner JL, Hoffman WE: *J Am Anim Hosp Assoc,* 14: 219, 1978.
Updated by BW Parry from first edition.
From Blood DC, Studdert VP: *Saunders, comprehensive veterinary dictionary,* ed 2, Philadelphia, 1999, WB Saunders, p 1252.

Table 2-3 Hematologic reference values for domestic animals in conventional units

	Dog	Cat	Horse	Cattle	Sheep	Pig
PCV (%)	37-55 (45)	24-45 (37)	32-52 (42)	24-46 (35)	24-50 (38)	32-50 (42)
Hemoglobin (g/dl)	12-18 (15)	8-15 (12)	11-19 (15)	8-15 (12)	8-16 (12)	10-16 (13)
RBC (×10⁶)/μl	5.5-8.5 (6.8)	5-10 (7.5)	6.5-12.5 (9.5)	5-10 (7)	8-16 (12)	5-8 (6.5)
Total protein (g/dl)	6.0-7.5	6.0-7.5	6.0-8.0	6.0-8.0	6-7.5	6-7
WBC (×10³)/μl	6.0-17.0 (11.5)	5.5-19.5 (12.5)	5.5-12.5 (9.0)	4.0-12.0 (8.0)	4-12 (8)	11-22 (16)
Differential, absolute						
Segmented	60%-77%; 3000-11,500 (7000)	35%-75%; 2500-12,500 (7500)	30%-65%; 2700-6700 (4700)	15%-45%; 600-4000 (7000)	10%-50%; 700-6000 (2400)	28%-47%; 3000-10,500
Bands	0%-3%; 0-300 (70)	0%-3%; 0-300 (100)	0%-2%; 0-100 (2.0)	0%-2%; 0-120 (20)	Rare	0%-2%
Lymphocytes	12%-30%; 1000-4800 (2800)	20%-55%; 1500-7000 (4000)	27-70; 1500-5500 (3500)	45%-75%; 2500-7500 (4500)	40%-75%; 2000-9000 (5000)	39%-62%; 4300-13,700
Monocytes	3%-10%; 150-1350 (750)	1%-4%; 0-850 (350)	0.5%-7%; 0-800 (400)	2%-7%; 25-840 (400)	0.6%; 0-750 (200)	2%-30%; 220-2200
Eosinophils	2%-10%; 100-1250 (550)	2%-12%; 0-1500 (650)	0%-11%; 0-925 (375)	2%-20%; 0-2400 (700)	0.1%; 0-1000 (400)	0.5%-11%; 0-2500
Basophils	Rare	Rare	0%-3%; 0-170 (50)	0%-2%; 0-200 (50)	0-3%; 0-300 (50)	0%-2%; 0-400
Platelets (×10⁵)	2.0-9.0	3-7 (4.5)	1-6 (3.3)	1-8 (5)	2.5-7.5 (4.0)	3.25-7.15 (5.2)
MCV (fl)	60-77 (70)	39-55 (45)	34-58 (46)	40-60 (52)	23-48 (52)	50-68 (63)
MCH (pg)	19-23	13-17	15.2-18.6	14.4-18.6	9-13	16.6-22
MCHC (g/dl)	32.0-36.0 (34.0)	30-36 (33.2)	31-37 (35)	30-36 (32.7)	31-38 (33.5)	30-34 (32)

PCV, Packed cell volume; *RBC*, red blood cell(s); *WBC*, White blood cell(s); *MCV*, mean corpuscular volume; *MCH*, mean corpuscular hemoglobin; *MCHC*, mean corpuscular hemoglobin concentration.
Values given as range (mean).
From Pratt PW: *Principles and practice of veterinary technology*, St Louis, 1998, Mosby, pp 146-147.

Table 2-4 Conversions factors for hematology data

Analyte	Conventional unit	Multiplication factor	SI unit	Multiplication factor	Conventional unit
Hemoglobin	g/dL	10	g/L	0.10	g/dL
Hemoglobin	g/dL	0.6206	mmol/L	1.6113	g/dL
PCV	%	0.01	L/L	100	%
RBC	×10⁶/μL	1	×10¹²/L	1	×10⁶/μL
MCHC	g/dL	10	g/L	0.10	g/dL
Leukocytes (all types)	×10³/μL	0.001	×10⁹/L	1000	×10³/μ/L
Plasma proteins	g/dL	10	g/L	0.10	g/dL
Fibrinogen	mg/dL	0.01	g/L	100	mg/dL

PCV, Packed cell volume; *RBC*, red blood cell(s); *MCHC*, mean corpuscular hemoglobin concentration.
From Blood DC, Studdert VP: *Saunders' comprehensive veterinary dictionary*, ed 2, Philadelphia, 1999, WB Saunders, p 1253.

Glossary

absolute count Calculation of absolute cell numbers based on percentage of type multiplied by the total cell count
acanthocyte Erythrocyte with irregularly shaped margins
agglutination Aggregate of particles that have clumped together
agranulocyte WBCs such as monocyte and lymphocyte that do not have obvious cytoplasmic granules when viewed under a light microscope
anemia Below normal values in PCV, RBC count, or Hb
anisocytosis Variation in cell size
anuria Complete absence of urine formation or elimination
azurophilic granules Large homogeneous and dense granules that stain blue with Romanowsky stains
basophilia Increased number of basophils
basophilic stippling Presence of small, blue-staining granules in the erythrocyte
bilirubinuria Detectable conjugated bile pigments in the urine
buffy coat Layer of WBCs, platelets, and nucleated RBCs in sedimented or centrifuged blood
codocyte Form of leptocyte or target cell
crenation Erythrocytes with spiny projections on the margin of the cell
eosinopenia Decreased number of eosinophils
eosinophilia Increased number of eosinophils
erythrophagocytosis Engulfing, or phagocytosis, of the erythrocyte
erythropoiesis Production of RBCs
exfoliative cytology Study of cells shed from body surfaces such as tissues, lesions, and fluids
exudate Fluid escaped from blood vessels with a high content of protein and cellular debris
glucosuria Detectable levels of glucose in the urine (glycosuria)
granulocyte Cell containing granules
granulomatous Composed of a tumorlike mass or nodule of granulation tissue
hematuria Presence of intact erythrocytes in the urine
hemoglobinuria Free Hb in the urine
hemolysis Destruction of RBCs
heterophil Avian neutrophil
hypersegmented Neutrophil with more than five lobes in the nucleus
hypertonic Greater than isotonic concentration
hypochromic Erythrocyte with lack or decrease in staining intensity, low cellular Hb
hypotonic Less than isotonic concentration
isotonic Of similar osmolality to normal plasma
ketonuria Excessive ketones (e.g., acetone) in the urine
left shift Presence of an increased number of immature (nonsegmented) neutrophils in the circulation
leptocyte Thin, flattened hypochromic erythrocyte that has a normal diameter and a decreased mean corpuscular volume
leukemia Neoplastic disease in which a significant number of immature blast cells are found in the bone marrow and blood
leukocytosis Increase in circulating WBC numbers
leukopenia Decrease in circulating WBC numbers
lymphocytosis Increased number of circulating lymphocytes
macrocyte RBC that has a diameter that is larger than normal
macrocytic Increased number of large RBCs
mast cell Tissue cell having granules that contain histamine and heparin
microcyte RBC with a diameter that is smaller than normal
microcytic Increased number of small RBCs
monocytopenia Decreased number of monocytes
monocytosis Increased number of monocytes
neutropenia Decreased number of neutrophils
neutrophilia Increased number of neutrophils
NMB New methylene blue, a basic dye used to stain cell nuclei and granules
normochromic Normal, pink-staining erythrocyte
normocytic Adjective used to describe an RBC of normal size (volume)
NRBC Nucleated RBC, an immature erythrocyte
oliguria Decrease in urine formation
pancytopenia Decrease in the RBC, WBC, and platelet lines
PCV Packed cell volume, or hematocrit
plasma Fluid portion of the blood in which cells are suspended
poikilocytosis Variation in general cell shape
pollakiuria Frequent urination
polychromasia Erythrocytes that have a bluish tint when stained with regular blood stains and are reticulocytes (granular precipitates) with NMB
polyuria Increased urine production
postprandial Immediately after eating
proteinuria Abnormal level of proteins in the urine
RBC Red blood cell, or erythrocyte
right shift Presence of an increased number of hypersegmented neutrophils in circulation
rouleaux Erythrocytes formed in stacks or columns
schistocyte Fragmented erythrocyte, "helmet cell"
sedimentation rate Rate at which RBCs settle in their own plasma in a given amount of time
smudge cell Nucleated cell that has ruptured during smearing due to mechanical damage or increased fragility of the cell
spherocyte Small, dense, dark-staining erythrocyte
supravital staining Use of a stain that has a low toxicity so that vital and functional processes can be studied in live cells
thrombocytopenia Decreased number of platelets (thrombocytes)
thrombocytosis Increased number of platelets (thrombocytes)
toxic neutrophils Neutrophil showing certain morphological changes such as vacuolation, toxic granules, increased basophilia, or nuclear changes
WBC White blood cell, or leukocyte

Review Questions

1 Of the following collection methods, which is primarily of use for urine volume only?
a. Cystocentesis
b. Metabolism cage
c. Client-collected samples
d. Catheterization

2 Urine samples should be analyzed within ________ for maximum valid information.
   a. 1 hour
   b. 2 minutes
   c. 30 minutes
   d. 12 hours
3 Normal freshly voided urine of many species is clear. Exceptions include which of the following species?
   a. Rabbit
   b. Horse
   c. Hamster
   d. All of the above
4 It is recommended that urine sample size be standardized. An adequate sample of fresh urine is considered to be
   a. 1 mL
   b. 5 mL
   c. 10 mL
   d. 20 mL
5 The fluid portion of the blood from which fibrinogen has been removed is termed
   a. Serum
   b. Plasma
   c. Buffy coat
   d. Packed cells
6 If used in the proper ratio to blood, which anticoagulant is most recommended to cause the least changes in cell morphology?
   a. Heparin
   b. EDTA
   c. Potassium chloride
   d. Acid-citrate-dextrose (ACD)
7 To maintain proper anticoagulant to blood ratio, sample tubes should be filled to at least what capacity?
   a. 90%
   b. 50%
   c. 75%
   d. 60%
8 Blood samples collected immediately postprandial will be
   a. Icteric
   b. High in TPP
   c. Lipemic
   d. Low in RBCs
9 Which of the following urine collection methods should be utilized for bacterial culture?
   a. Manual expression
   b. Cystocentesis
   c. Midstream
   d. Litterpan pour off
10 Pollakiuria is defined as
   a. Complete absence of urine formation
   b. Increased urine production
   c. Frequent urination
   d. Decreased urine formation

BIBLIOGRAPHY

Baker P: Lecture notes, Seneca College, King City, Ontario 2002.

Campbell TW: *Avian hematology and cytology,* Ames, 1995, Iowa State University Press.

Cowell RL, Tyler RD, Meinkoth JH: *Diagnostic cytology and hematology of the dog and cat,* St Louis, 1999, Mosby.

Free HM, ed: *Modern urine chemistry,* Elkhart, IN, 1991, Miles Diagnostic Division.

Fudge AM: *Laboratory medicine: avian and exotic pets,* Philadelphia, 2000, WB Saunders.

Harvey JW: *Atlas of veterinary hematology: blood and bone marrow of domestic animals,* Philadelphia, 2001, WB Saunders.

Hendrix CM: *Laboratory procedures for veterinary technicians,* ed 4, St Louis, 2002, Mosby.

Joseph SL: *Urinalysis: the picture of health,* Proceedings of EXPO for veterinary technicians, Washington, DC, 1987.

McCurnin DM: *Clinical textbook for veterinary technicians,* ed 5, St Louis, 2002, WB Saunders.

Osborne CA, Stevens JB: *Handbook of canine & feline urinalysis,* ed 1, St Louis, 1981, Ralston Purina Co.

Raskin RE, Meyer DJ: *Atlas of canine and feline cytology,* Philadelphia, 2001, WB Saunders.

Reagan WJ, Saunders TG, DeNicola DB: *Veterinary hematology: atlas of common domestic species,* Ames, 1998, Iowa State University Press.

Rich LJ: *The morphology of canine & feline blood cells,* ed 2, St Louis, 1976, Ralston Purina Co.

Walsh DJ, Wade WL: The differential film: errors and normal variations, *Vet Tech* 17:7, 1996.

CHAPTER 3

Cytology

Margi Sirois

OUTLINE

LEARNING OUTCOMES

After reading this chapter, you should be able to:

1. Describe a variety of sample collection and processing techniques for cytology samples.
2. Identify common normal cells found in cytology samples.
3. Identify common abnormal cells in cytology samples.
4. Describe methods for differentiation of inflammatory and neoplastic cytology samples.

Microscopic examination of cells, primarily those exfoliated from tissues, lesions, and internal organs, has become an increasingly valuable tool in veterinary diagnostics. Fluid aspirates also provide valuable diagnostic information to the clinician. Sample collection can be easily performed, and in most cases no special equipment is required.

INDICATIONS

I. Purpose
   A. Differentiation between inflammatory processes and neoplastic diseases
   B. Identification of cell types present to aid in diagnosis and treatment
II. Advantages
   A. Can be collected quickly and easily
   B. No specialized equipment is required
   C. Inexpensive
III. Disadvantages
   A. Quality control concerns
      1. Improper specimen collection can damage cells
      2. Staining techniques are variable and subject to greater error than standard staining methods
      3. Formalin fumes near specimen collection or processing areas cause cells to become partially fixed and therefore unusable for cytological evaluation

SPECIMEN COLLECTION

I. Fine needle aspiration
   A. Used to collect samples from the skin, lymph nodes, and internal organs
   B. Recommended needle sizes range from 22 to 25 gauge, attached to a 3- to 12-mL syringe
   C. Softer masses require smaller syringes and smaller-gauge needles; firmer masses require larger-bore syringes and larger-gauge needles
   D. Samples should be collected from several areas and depths within the tissue by releasing the pressure on the syringe and redirecting the needle into another location
   E. Samples are collected and pushed onto clean microscope slides for staining
II. Fluid aspiration

A. Includes thoracocentesis, cystocentesis, arthrocentesis, cerebrospinal fluid (CSF) taps, and abdominocentesis
B. Collection site must be cleaned. If samples are being submitted for microbiology testing, a surgical scrub should be performed
   1. Surgical preparation also for CSF and joint taps
C. Usually performed with animal in standing position
   1. For cystocentesis, dorsal or lateral recumbency may be used
   2. CSF is usually completed in lateral recumbency
D. Fluids may be centrifuged for sediment examination or submitted for bacterial culture

III. Solid mass imprinting and scraping
A. For collection and preparation of cytologic specimens in situ
B. Can also be performed on surgically removed tissues
C. Fresh edge is cut to expose the center of the mass, and the specimen is blotted to remove excess fluid and blood
D. Several small imprints are made onto a clean slide
E. Scrapings are made on a freshly cut surface with a clean scalpel blade; the film is spread across a clean slide and stained

IV. Swab technique
A. Used as an aid in determining stage of estrous cycle and evaluating uterine and vaginal disease and in collecting samples from ears
B. Also useful for evaluation of fistulated lesions
C. For vaginal cytology, vulva and surrounding area are washed clean, and a vaginal speculum is carefully introduced
D. Sample of the vaginal mucosa is taken with a sterile swab moistened with sterile saline
E. Swabs of fistulated lesions should be taken before and immediately after cleaning of the site
F. Samples are rolled onto clean slides for staining

V. Transtracheal and bronchial washes
A. Evaluation of mucus secretions from the trachea, bronchi, and bronchioles and in differential diagnosis of inflammation, neoplasia, mycosis, bacterial, and protozoal diseases
B. Two techniques
   1. Percutaneous technique provides samples with the least amount of contamination
      a. Requires placement of a jugular catheter within the tracheal lumen through the cricothyroid ligament
      b. Saline is infused through the catheter at a maximum dose of 1 to 2 mL/10 lb (4.5 kg)
      c. When the animal coughs or the entire dose has been given, a small amount of fluid is aspirated and the catheter is removed
   2. Endotracheal tube technique requires that the patient be lightly anesthetized
      a. Sterile endotracheal tube is inserted
      b. Large-bore indwelling catheter is then placed down the endotracheal tube so that the catheter extends just beyond the end of the endotracheal tube
      c. Saline is infused at a dose of 1 to 2 mL/10 lb (4.5 kg), and then a small amount of aspirate is collected

CONCENTRATION TECHNIQUES

I. May be needed if cellularity of sample is low
II. Place anticoagulated fluid in a standard clinical centrifuge
III. Spin for 5 minutes at 1000 to 2000 rpm (165 to 400 *g*)
IV. Pour off supernatant. Leave a few drops in the tube and then gently resuspend sediment
V. Prepare multiple smears using several different smearing techniques

CHARACTERISTICS OF FLUID SAMPLES

I. Before preparation of any fluid sample, the gross characteristics of the sample, such as color, turbidity, and odor, should be determined
A. Total nucleated cell count (TNCC) and total protein should also be determined

II. Usually sample can then be characterized as a transudate, exudate, or modified transudate (Figure 3-1)
A. Transudate samples are clear or colorless, with TNCC less than 500/mL and total protein less than 3 g/dL
   1. Transudates are more commonly found in ascites and are usually colorless
B. Modified transudates are moderately cellular and have total protein concentrations between 2.5 and 7.5 g/dL
C. They are often amber or pink and turbid in appearance

III. Exudates are characterized by increased cellularity and total protein greater than 3.0 g/dL
A. This higher cell count and protein value are usually indicative of inflammation

SLIDE PREPARATION

I. Squash prep method (Figure 3-2)
A. Small amount of aspirate is placed in the center of a clean slide
B. Second slide is placed over the sample at a 90 degree angle and is carefully slid apart from the bottom slide
C. Excessive pressure can distort and rupture cells

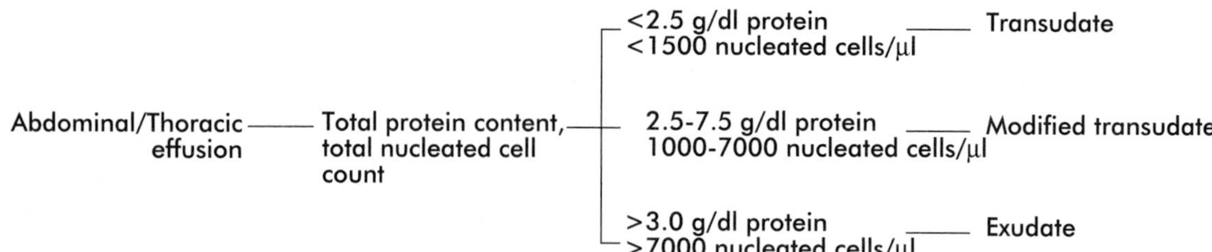

Figure 3-1 An algorithm to classify effusions as transudates, modified transudates, or exudates, based on total protein content and total nucleated cell count. (From Cowell RL, Tyler RD, Meinkoth JH: *Diagnostic cytology and hematology of the dog and cat,* ed 2, St Louis, 1999, Mosby.)

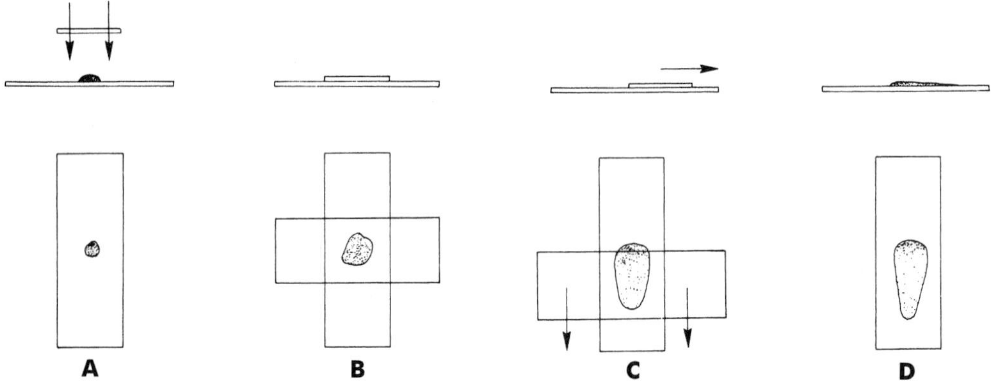

Figure 3-2 Squash preparation. **A,** A portion of the aspirate is expelled onto a glass microscope slide, and another slide is placed over the sample. **B,** This spreads the sample. If the sample does not spread well, gentle digital pressure can be applied to the top slide. Care must be taken not to place excessive pressure on the slide, causing the cells to rupture. **C,** The slides are smoothly slid apart. **D,** This usually produces well-spread smears but may result in excessive cell rupture. (From Cowell RL, Tyler RD, Meinkoth JH: *Diagnostic cytology and hematology of the dog and cat,* ed 2, St Louis, 1999, Mosby.)

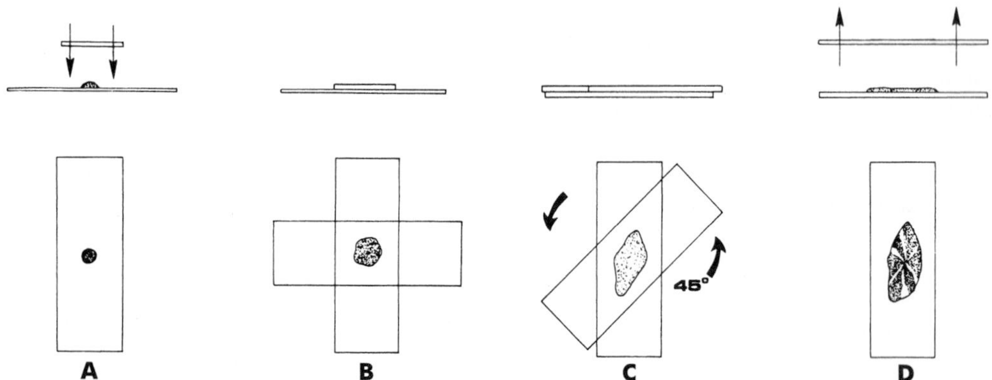

Figure 3-3 A modification of the squash preparation. **A,** A portion of the aspirate is expelled onto a glass microscope slide, and another slide is placed over the sample. **B,** This causes the sample to spread. If necessary, gentle digital pressure can be applied to the top slide to spread the sample more. Care must be taken not to use excessive pressure and cause cell rupture. **C,** The top slide is rotated about 45 degrees and lifted directly upward, producing a spread preparation with subtle ridges and valleys of cells **(D).** (From Cowell RL, Tyler RD, Meinkoth JH: *Diagnostic cytology and hematology of the dog and cat,* ed 2, St Louis, 1999, Mosby.)

II. Modified squash preparation (Figure 3-3)
   A. Combination method especially useful when cells are unusually fragile or for thin samples
   B. Small amount of aspirate is placed in the center of a clean slide

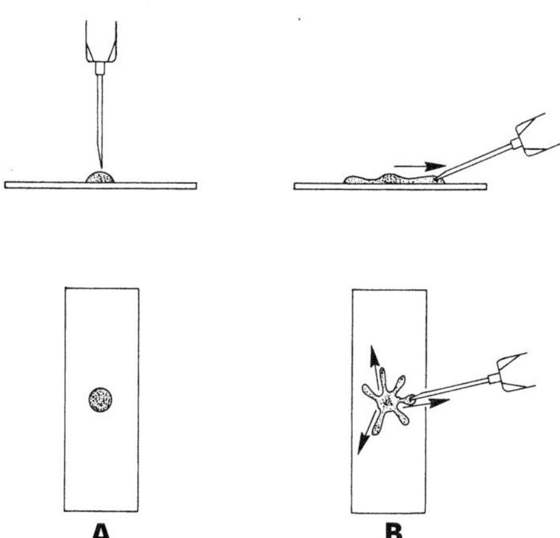

Figure 3-4 Needle spread, or "starfish" preparation. **A,** A portion of the aspirate is expelled onto a glass microscope slide. **B,** The tip of a needle is placed in the aspirate and moved peripherally, pulling a trail of the sample with it. This procedure is repeated in several directions, resulting in a preparation with multiple projections. (From Cowell RL, Tyler RD, Meinkoth JH: *Diagnostic cytology and hematology of the dog and cat,* ed 2, St Louis, 1999, Mosby.)

   C. Second slide is placed on top at a 90 degree angle
   D. Second slide is rotated 45 degrees and then lifted straight off

III. Starfish method (Figure 3-4)
   A. Most useful for highly viscous samples
   B. Small amount of aspirate is placed in the center of a clean slide
   C. Tip of the needle is then used to pull the sample out into several projections: a starfish appearance is formed

IV. Line smear (Figure 3-5)
   A. Used when fluid samples cannot be concentrated or when the amount of sediment is very small
   B. Small drop of the sample is placed near the end of a clean glass slide, and a second slide is used to spread the specimen in a manner similar to that used for preparation of a peripheral blood film
   C. When the smear covers approximately three fourths of the slide, the second slide is abruptly lifted off the first
   D. This produces a smear with a thick edge that contains a line of concentrated sediment from the sample
   E. Smear should be dried quickly; using a hairdryer is one method

V. Wedge smear

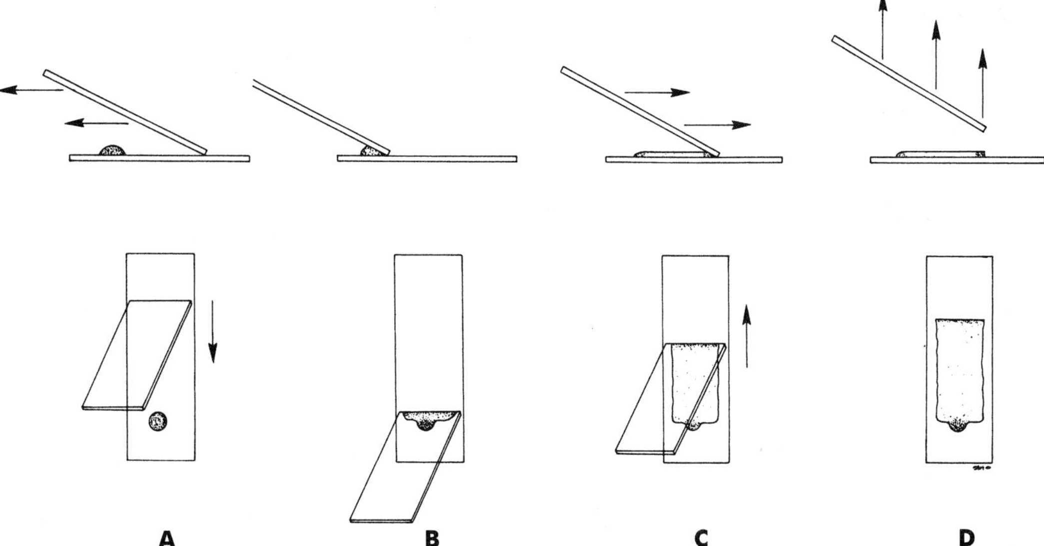

Figure 3-5 Line smear concentration technique. **A,** A drop of fluid sample is placed onto a glass microscope slide close to one end, and another slide is slid backward to contact the front of the drop. **B,** When the drop is contacted, it rapidly spreads along the juncture between the two slides. **C,** The spreader slide is then smoothly and rapidly slid forward. **D,** After the spreader slide has been advanced about two thirds to three fourths the distance required to make a smear with a feathered edge, the spreader slide is raised directly upward. This produces a smear with a line of concentrated cells at its end, instead of a feathered edge. (From Cowell RL, Tyler RD, Meinkoth JH: *Diagnostic cytology and hematology of the dog and cat,* ed 2, St Louis, 1999, Mosby.)

A. Small amount of aspirate is placed on one end of a clean slide
B. Second slide is then used to smoothly pull the sample toward the other end
C. This technique produces a film similar to that used for a whole blood differential count

STAINING TECHNIQUES

I. Stains should be applied according to the recommendations of the manufacturer
II. Denser, thicker preparations tend to require longer amounts of time to stain structures correctly
III. Types of stains
A. Romanowsky-type stains
1. Include Wright's, Giemsa, and Diff-Quik
2. Provide satisfactory staining of cytological specimens
3. Some variation in staining quality is evident: consistent use of one type is recommended
B. New methylene blue
1. Will stain nuclei, mast cell granules, and most infectious agents
2. Can be applied directly to an air-dried slide
3. Selected uses include presence of nucleated cells, bacteria, fungi, and mast cells
C. Gram staining
1. For classification of bacterial agents
2. Gram-negative bacteria and cells stain pink; gram-positive organisms stain purple
D. Other stains
1. Hematoxylin/eosin stain: normally used for histological evaluations
2. Papanicolaou stains
a. Commonly used in human gynecological examinations
b. Multiple steps required in staining technique
(1) Excellent for accentuating nuclear detail

EVALUATION AND INTERPRETATION

I. Initial examination
A. Low power (×100) to evaluate overall cellularity, quality of preparation
1. Scan for large objects such as parasites, fungal hyphae, crystals, etc.
B. High power (×430) to determine predominant cell types
C. Oil immersion (×1000) to describe cellular characteristics
D. Algorithm such as the one in Figure 3-6 should be used to assist with differentiation
II. Cells commonly found in exfoliative cytology
A. Neutrophils
1. May resemble those in blood, be degenerative, or have undergone morphological changes
a. Hypersegmentation: more than five lobes
b. Pyknosis: condensed nucleus
c. Karyolysis: loss of nuclear membrane
d. Karyorrhexis: fragmented nucleus
B. Lymphocytes: usually appear the same as in peripheral blood
C. Plasma cells
1. Represent activated lymphocytes
a. Appear as oval cell with eccentric nucleus, basophilic cytoplasm, and a perinuclear clear zone
D. Eosinophils: usually appear the same as in peripheral blood
E. Macrophages: large cells derived from the monocyte found in peripheral blood
1. Oval to pleomorphic nucleus with lacy to condensed chromatin
2. Abundant blue cytoplasm with vacuoles that may contain phagocytized cells or debris
3. May be multinucleated or giant cells (nuclei uniform in size and shape)
F. Mesothelial cells
1. Cells that line the pleural, peritoneal, and visceral surfaces
2. Round, usually with one round to oval nucleus, but may be multinucleated
3. May have nucleoli, corona (a fringe), or be seen singularly or in clusters
4. Nuclear chromatin is finely reticulated
5. Cytoplasm is slightly basophilic and may contain phagocytic debris
a. Difficult to distinguish from macrophages once they are activated
G. Mast cells
1. Round to oval with round to oval nuclei
2. Numerous blue to purple cytoplasmic granules
H. Erythrocytes: may be free in sample or seen inside phagocytic cells, particularly macrophages
III. Cytology of inflammation
A. Inflammation is a normal physiological response
1. Chemotactic factors released from damaged tissue attract neutrophils and macrophages to inflammatory site
B. Eosinophils and basophils may also be evident
IV. Classifications: inflammation can be classified as purulent, pyogranulomatous, granulomatous, or eosinophilic
A. Purulent (suppurative) inflammation
1. May also be referred to as acute inflammation
2. Most common type of inflammation, with the majority being caused by bacteria

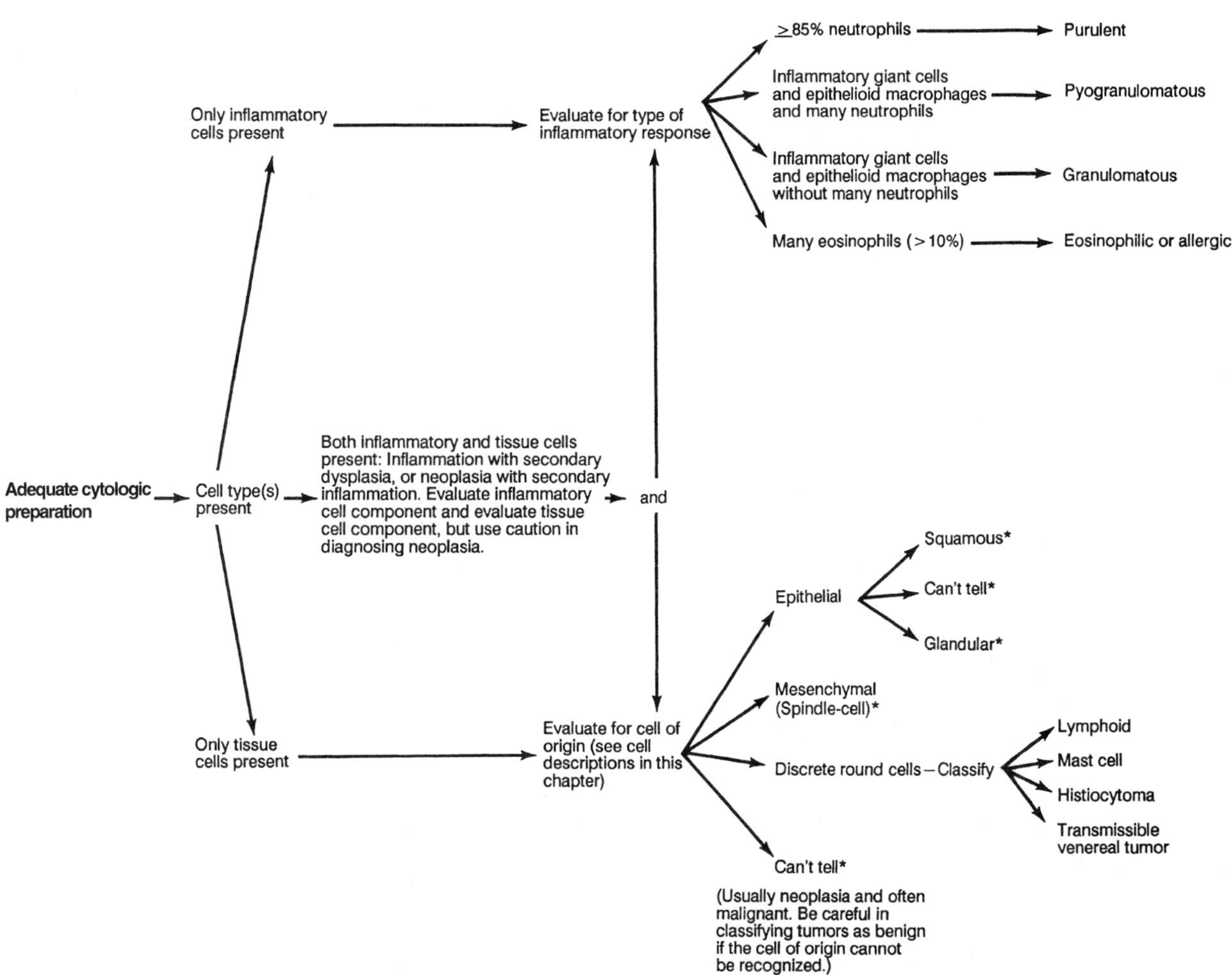

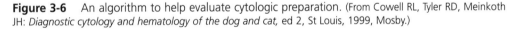

Figure 3-6 An algorithm to help evaluate cytologic preparation. (From Cowell RL, Tyler RD, Meinkoth JH: *Diagnostic cytology and hematology of the dog and cat,* ed 2, St Louis, 1999, Mosby.)

3. Samples usually characterized by greater than 70% neutrophils
4. Small numbers of macrophages and lymphocytes may also be present

B. Pyogranulomatous inflammation
   1. May also be referred to as chronic/active
   2. Consists of macrophages and 50% to 75% neutrophils

C. Granulomatous inflammation
   1. May also be referred to as chronic inflammation
   2. Greater than 70% of cells mononuclear (monocytes, macrophages, giant cells) with few neutrophils

D. Eosinophilic
   1. Consists of greater than 10% eosinophils
   2. Often a few mast cells, plasma cells, and lymphocytes

NONINFLAMMATORY, NON-NEOPLASTIC LESIONS

Include cysts such as epidermal inclusion cysts (sebaceous cysts), hyperplasia, dysplasia, hematoma, seroma, adipocytes, and salivary mucocele.

Neoplasia and Lesions

I. Best indication is presence of homogeneous population of cells, which may or may not be pleomorphic, in a location where they should not be found

II. May be benign or malignant and may have associated inflammation

III. Benign neoplasia is characterized by homogeneous populations of the same cell type with no evidence of malignant characteristics within cells

IV. Malignant neoplasia is characterized by morphological changes in cytoplasm and nuclei
V. A minimum of three criteria should be met before determining malignancy in a cytological sample
   A. Five criteria are more diagnostic
VI. Not as indicative of neoplasia if inflammation is also present or changes are only in cytoplasm
VII. Criteria of malignancy (Table 3-1)
   A. General criteria of malignancy
      1. Anisocytosis and macrocytosis
      2. Hypercellularity
      3. Pleomorphism (except lymphoid tissue)
   B. Cellular changes
      1. Anisocytosis: abnormal variation in cell size of same type
      2. Pleomorphism: variability in the size, shape, and appearance of same cell type
      3. Hypercellularity: increased cell exfoliation
   C. Nuclear changes: most important criteria for determining malignancy
      1. Anisokaryosis: any unusual variation in overall nuclear size
      2. High or variable "N:C ratio:" specifically, an increased ratio of nucleus to cytoplasm
      3. Increased mitotic activity: mitosis is rare in normal tissue, and cells usually divide evenly in two. Any increase in the presence of mitotic figures or cells that are not dividing equally is considered a malignant criterion
      4. Coarse chromatin pattern: chromatin pattern is coarser than normal and may appear ropy or cordlike
      5. Nuclear molding: deformation of nuclei by other nuclei within the same cell or adjacent cells
      6. Multinucleation: multiple nuclei within a cell
      7. Nucleoli that vary in size, shape, and number
         a. Anisonucleolosis
         b. Angular nucleoli
         c. Multiple nucleoli
         d. Very large nucleoli
   D. Cytoplasmic changes
      1. Extreme basophilia of cytoplasm
      2. Vacuolation
      3. Boundaries may be irregular and indistinct
VIII. Tissue origin
   A. Malignant neoplasia should be further characterized by origin of tissue cells present
   B. Common neoplastic tissue cells include epithelial, mesenchymal, and discrete round cell
      1. Epithelial cell tumors
         a. Also referred to as carcinoma or adenocarcinoma
         b. Samples tend to be highly cellular, and often exfoliate in clumps or sheets
         c. Cells tend to be large to very large
            (1) Show marked variation
            (2) Nuclei are round with smooth to slightly coarse chromatin pattern that increases with increased malignancy
            (3) Nuclei contains one or more notable nucleoli
            (4) Cytoplasm is moderate to abundant
         d. Increased N:C ratio with nuclear molding evident
      2. Mesenchymal cell tumors or spindle cell tumors
         a. Also referred to as sarcoma and are usually less cellular
         b. Tend to exfoliate singly or as wispy spindles
            (1) Cytoplasm tails away from nucleus: fusiform shape
            (2) Generally small to medium sized
            (3) Moderate degree of light to medium blue cytoplasm
            (4) Round to oval nucleus with smooth fine chromatin that is lacy
            (5) Nucleoli more evident as malignancy increases
               (a) Also change in shape, chromatin pattern, and N:C ratio
      3. Discrete round cell tumors
         a. Exfoliate very well but are usually not in clumps or clusters
         b. Individual round cells that are small to medium sized
         c. Round cell tumors include histiocytoma, lymphoma, mast cell tumors, plasma cell tumors, transmissible venereal tumors, and melanoma
            (1) Histiocytoma and transmissible venereal tumor appear similar except that histiocytoma is not usually highly cellular
               (a) Histiocytoma cells have poorly defined boundaries, contain a few vacuoles, and have a moderate amount of pale blue cytoplasm
               (b) Boundaries of transmissible venereal tumors appear distinct; there are usually many definite vacuoles with a light smoky to medium blue cytoplasm
            (2) Lymphosarcomas can be recognized by the presence of large numbers of cells with a prominent perinuclear\ clear zone

Table 3-1 Easily recognized general and nuclear criteria of malignancy

Criteria	Description	Schematic representation
GENERAL CRITERIA		
Anisocytosis and macrocytosis	Variation in cell size, with some cells ≥1.5 times larger than normal.	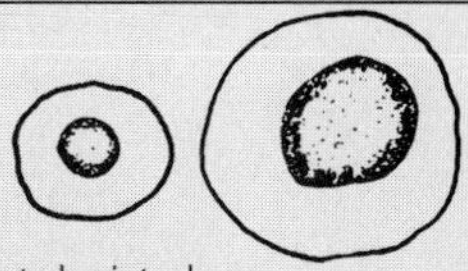
Hypercellularity	Increased cell exfoliation due to decreased cell adherence.	Not depicted
Pleomorphism (except in lymphoid tissue)	Variable size and shape in cells of the same type.	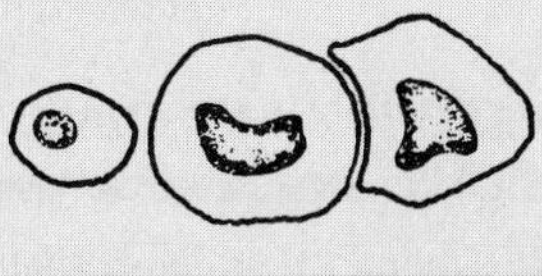
NUCLEAR CRITERIA		
Macrokaryosis	Increased nuclear size. Cells with nuclei larger than 10 μm in diameter suggest malignancy.	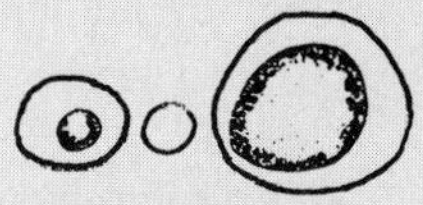 RBC
Increased nucleus-to-cytoplasm (N:C) ratio	Normal nonlymphoid cells usually have an N:C ratio of 1:3 to 1:8, depending on the tissue. Increased ratios (1:2, 1:1, etc.) suggest malignancy.	See "Macrokaryosis"
Anisokaryosis	Variation in nuclear size. This is especially important if the nuclei of multinucleated cells vary in size.	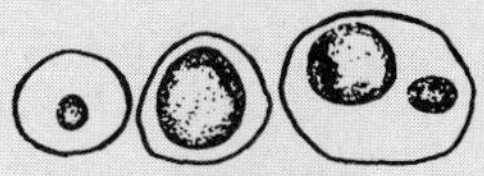
Multinucleation	Multiple nucleation in a cell. This is especially important if the nuclei vary in size.	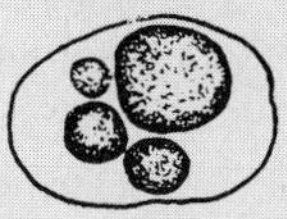
Increased mitotic figures	Mitosis is rare in normal tissue.	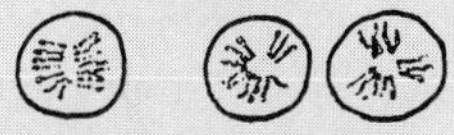 normal abnormal
Abnormal mitosis	Improper alignment of chromosomes.	See "Increased mitotic figures"
Coarse chromatin pattern	The chromatin pattern is coarser than normal. It may appear ropy or cordlike.	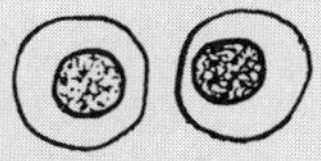
Nuclear molding	Deformation of nuclei by other nuclei within the same cell or adjacent cells.	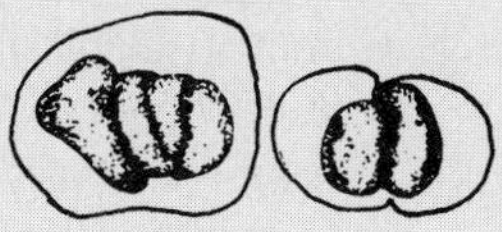
Macronucleoli	Nucleoli are increased in size. Nucleoli of ≥5 μm strongly suggest malignancy. For reference, RBCs are 5-6 μm in the cat and 7-8 μm in the dog.	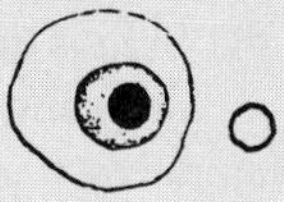 RBC
Angular nucleoli	Nucleoli are fusiform or have other angular shapes, instead of their normal round to slightly oval shape.	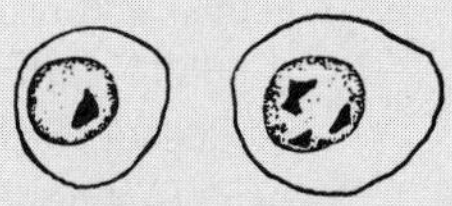
Anisonucleoliosis	Variation in nucleolar shape or size (especially important if the variation is within the same nucleus).	See "Angular nucleoli"

RBC, Red blood cell.

(a) Cells are round; size and characteristics depend on the type of lymphosarcoma
(3) Mast cells can be recognized by their prominent purple/black granules
(a) Granules not as dark in cats
(b) Few to many cells with moderate amount of cytoplasm
(c) Round nuclei stain pale
(4) Melanoma is generally characterized by cells with prominent dark black granules

COLLECTION AND EVALUATION OF COMMON LESIONS

I. Cutaneous and subcutaneous tissues
A. Collection is usually made by swabbing, scraping, imprint, or fine needle aspiration
B. Collect sample before and after cleaning of the lesion
C. If scabs are present, remove them before sample collection
D. Scraping should be performed at several levels within the lesion
E. Common inflammatory lesions include bacterial, fungal, and parasitic infections
1. Infectious agents are often visible within phagocytic cells
a. Gram-positive cocci (*Staphylococcus* sp., *Streptococcus* sp.)
b. Gram-negative bacilli (*Nocardia* sp., *Actinomycetes* sp., *Pseudomonas* sp.)
c. Fungi (*Microsporum* sp.)
d. Parasites (*Leishmania* sp.)
2. Noninfectious inflammation may result from injection site reactions, trauma, insect bites, snakebites, etc.
F. Common neoplastic lesions are numerous and include lipomas, mast cell tumors, histiocytomas, squamous cell carcinomas, fibromas, and hemangiosarcomas
1. Skin is the most common site for neoplasia in dogs and cats
II. Respiratory system
A. Tracheal and bronchial samples
1. Usually collected with transtracheal wash or endoscopically
2. Aids in determining cause of chronic coughing
3. Presence of mucus makes actual cell counts difficult
a. Estimate of increased or normal numbers on stained sediment smears may be useful
(1) Inflammatory conditions will increase mucus production
b. Mucus will appear as twisted or whorled blue to pink amorphous sheets
(1) Increased cellularity often accompanies a granular appearance
4. Normal cell types
a. Columnar and cuboidal epithelia can be ciliated or nonciliated
(1) Columnar cells are elongated or cone shaped with a generally round to oval nucleus showing a finely granular chromatin pattern at one end of the cell
(2) Cuboidal cells are similar except they are more square in shape
b. Neutrophils are similar to those found in peripheral blood with greater toxic changes
(1) Increase in neutrophils indicates inflammation
c. Alveolar macrophages will generally have an eccentrically placed, round to bean-shaped nucleus
(1) Cytoplasm is abundant, blue-gray, and granular
d. If oral contamination occurs, superficial squamous cells may be common
(1) Large epithelial cells with small nucleus and abundant angular cytoplasm
5. Increase in macrophages and neutrophils is not normal
6. Eosinophils are commonly seen in allergic disease
7. Mast cells may also be present and have little diagnostic significance unless found in high numbers
a. Red-purple intracytoplasmic granules are characteristic
8. Bacterial and fungal diseases are routinely identified by transtracheal wash
B. Lung tissue
1. Fine needle aspiration is used to collect samples from masses identified radiographically
a. Complications include pneumothorax and hemorrhage
2. Tissues removed during biopsy are prepared by scraping and/or impression
3. Normal cell types found are similar to those obtained from transtracheal wash
4. Common neoplasias of lung tissue include carcinoma and adenocarcinoma
a. Inflammation may be the result of bacterial (*Mycobacterium* sp.), fungal (*Cryptococcus* sp., *Blastomyces* sp.), parasitic (*Toxoplasma* sp., *Pneumocystis* sp.), and viral diseases
5. Nasal exudates and masses
a. Usually collected by aspiration of nasal flushing
b. Bacterial and fungal organisms may be present

c. Trauma or foreign body inflammation is common
d. Neoplasia of nasal cavities is uncommon but usually malignant

III. Oral cavity
A. Usually collected by imprint or scraping
B. Normal flora includes the bacterium *Simonsiella* sp.
C. Neoplasia may occur on lips, cheeks, palate, gingiva, tonsils, or tongue
1. Watch carefully for oral melanomas
2. Epuli are commonly seen

IV. Sensory organs
A. Specimens are usually collected from eyelids using scraping or fine needle aspiration
1. Sebaceous gland tumors are common
B. Samples for evaluation of the conjunctiva are usually collected by scraping with a flat round-tip spatula
1. May help identify the cause of chronic conjunctivitis
C. Samples for evaluation of corneal lesions are collected by applying topical anesthetic and scraping the lesion
D. Secretions from ear canals are collected with cotton swabs
1. Bacterial and fungal (*Malassezia* spp.) infections are common
2. Parasites (*Otobius* sp., *Otodectes* sp.) may also be present
3. Neoplasia is uncommon and usually benign

V. Glandular tissues
A. Samples from mammary, parathyroid, thyroid, and salivary glands are usually collected by fine needle aspiration
B. Common inflammatory and benign neoplastic conditions include mastitis, cysts, sialoceles, and lymphocytic thyroiditis
C. Mammary tumors are common in female dogs and cats and are usually malignant. These are often histologically "mixed" (contain a variety of cell types)
D. Malignant neoplastic conditions of salivary, thyroid, and parathyroid tissues are extremely rare

VI. Lymph nodes
A. Lymph node tissue: complex cytology evaluations
1. Normal lymph nodes
a. Consist of 75% to 95% small lymphocytes
(1) Smaller than a neutrophil and has scant, pale-blue cytoplasm
(2) Round nuclei is about the size of a red blood cell (RBC) with dense aggregated chromatin
b. Only a few plasma cells, medium and large lymphocytes, and macrophages
c. Reticular and endothelial cells are common, but because of aspiration techniques, the large swollen nuclei often appear without any cytoplasm
d. Small numbers of neutrophils, eosinophils, and mast cells are occasionally present
e. Cytoplasmic fragments referred to as lymphoglandular bodies are round, homogeneous, basophilic structures about the size of platelets
f. Free nuclei that are pink and amorphous result from the aspiration pressure forcing fragile lymphocytes to rupture and release the nuclei
2. Wide variety of diseases can manifest with changes in lymph node cytology
3. Inflammation (lymphadenitis)
a. Will have an increase in inflammatory cells: neutrophils, eosinophils, and macrophages
(1) Likely have more than 5% neutrophils or 3% eosinophils
4. Hyperplasia (benign neoplasia)
a. Cytologically not that different from a normal lymph node
5. Mixed (both inflammatory and neoplastic cells present)
6. Neoplasia (lymph node cells with abnormal nuclear features)
7. Metastasis (neoplastic cells from other body tissues that spread to lymph nodes)

VII. Hepatobiliary tissues
A. Samples for cytological evaluation of the hepatobiliary system may be collected by fine needle aspiration or biopsy
B. Normal findings in hepatobiliary cytology include hepatocytes and blood cells
C. Hepatocytes commonly contain bile pigments and hemosiderin
D. Abnormal findings usually involve changes in the morphology of the hepatocytes (vacuoles, excessive or unusual granulation, or unstained areas within the cytoplasm)
E. Common non-neoplastic disorders include feline hepatic lipidosis
F. Inflammatory disorders include amyloidosis, hepatitis, and cholangiohepatitis
G. Often blood chemistry and physical examination assist in identifying the cause of any inflammatory or non-neoplastic condition
H. Common neoplastic disorders include epithelial cell tumors, lymphosarcoma, and hemangiosarcoma

I. Metastasis from other body tissues is a common finding

VIII. Fluid aspirates: may involve removal and evaluation of abnormal fluid accumulation (i.e., abdominocentesis, thoracocentesis) or removal and evaluation of body fluids normally found (i.e., arthrocentesis, spinal tap)

A. Abdominal and thoracic fluid

1. Accumulations of thoracic or abdominal fluid indicate pathology in other body systems
2. Sample collection is accomplished by fine needle aspiration into a sterile ethylenediaminetetraacetic acid (EDTA) collection tube
    a. If cultures or biochemical testing are required, additional samples should be collected in a transport media container and a plain sterile blood collection tube
3. Samples are initially evaluated for volume, total nucleated cell count, total protein, color, and clarity
4. Abdominal and thoracic fluids should be classified as to type of effusion (transudate, exudate, modified transudate) using the classification system described earlier
5. Techniques for preparation of slides depend on the character of the sample
    a. Samples with low cellularity should be concentrated before preparation or prepared as line smears
    b. Turbid samples usually have high cellularity and can be prepared with direct smears
6. Cells seen in most thoracic effusions include neutrophils, mesothelial cells, macrophages, lymphocytes, and other peripheral blood cells
    a. Predominance of neutrophils indicates an inflammatory process
        (1) Neutrophils should be evaluated for degenerative characteristics, toxic granulation, presence of phagocytized material, etc.
    b. Common inflammatory conditions include infectious peritonitis, infectious pleuritis, and feline infectious peritonitis
    c. Macrophages and mesothelial cells look similar in effusions
        (1) They may appear atypical, but this is an expected response to the presence of abnormal fluid around the cells and should not be confused with neoplasia
    d. Increased number of lymphocytes usually indicates neoplasia, particularly lymphosarcoma
    e. Chylous effusions often have a predominance of mature lymphocytes
    f. Reactive lymphocytes are present in inflammatory conditions and can be differentiated from neoplastic cells by evaluating the cytoplasm
        (1) Reactive lymphocytes are larger than small lymphocytes and usually have scant to moderate deep blue cytoplasm
        (2) Neoplastic lymphocytes usually have moderate clear to light blue cytoplasm
            (a) Nuclei shape is variable and contains finely stippled nuclear chromatin and nucleoli
            (b) They are larger than neutrophils
    g. Increased number of mast cells indicates a mast cell tumor
    h. Other neoplastic conditions that may be identified cytologically include carcinoma, sarcoma, and mesothelioma
    i. Some tumors do not exfoliate well into effusions. The absence of neoplastic cells does not rule out neoplasia

B. Synovial fluid

1. Evaluation of synovial fluid may aid in differential diagnosis of lameness
2. Collection method: arthrocentesis usually involves fine needle aspiration from the flexed joint space, but techniques vary depending on the joint of interest
3. Normal synovial fluid contains a variety of proteins, electrolytes, and other substances (i.e., glucose) similar to blood plasma
4. Synovial fluid does not clot unless the sample is contaminated with blood or intraarticular hemorrhage is present
    a. If needed, heparin is the anticoagulant of choice
5. Samples should be evaluated for volume, total nucleated cell counts, color, turbidity, viscosity, total protein, and mucin concentration
6. Abnormal cytological findings include increased RBCs, vacuolization of large mononuclear cells (macrophages and/or clasmatocytes), and other degenerative characteristics (karyorrhexis, pyknosis)
7. Infectious disorders are uncommon but usually bacterial in origin

a. Phagocytized bacteria normally would be evident
8. Variety of degenerative joint diseases can occur (e.g., arthritis, systemic lupus erythematosus) and are usually immune mediated
a. Radiography is often used for confirmation

C. Cerebrospinal fluid
1. Evaluation of cerebrospinal fluid (CSF) can aid in diagnosis of neurological disorders
2. Sample collection is by fine needle aspiration on the anesthetized patient
3. Site of collection depends on suspected neuropathy; lumbar puncture and atlantooccipital space are the most common collection sites
4. CSF should be examined for total cellularity, color, turbidity, total protein, and total RBC count. Biochemical testing may also be needed
5. CSF fluid generally needs to be concentrated before performing cytological evaluation
6. In normal CSF tap, most cells are small lymphocytes, with a few monocytes and macrophages (look like monocytes with phagocytic vacuoles)
a. Neutrophils are not normally found unless the tap was traumatic
7. Increases in total nucleated cells or alterations in the relative proportions of the various cell types indicate a pathological condition
8. Variety of inflammatory disorders can occur, including bacterial meningitis, feline infectious peritonitis, and toxoplasmosis
9. Neoplastic cells are a rare finding in CSF

IX. Urogenital system
A. Kidney tissue
1. Samples are usually collected by fine needle aspiration or biopsy
2. Renal tubular epithelial cells and peripheral blood cells are common findings
a. Large polygonal to round, found singly or in clusters
(1) Abundant light-blue cytoplasm with round, centrally located nucleus
3. Abnormal findings include lymphoid cells, lymphoblasts, and plasma cells
4. Inflammation is a common finding and may be septic (pyelonephritis) or nonseptic. Benign cysts also occur
5. Renal lymphosarcoma is common in cat; carcinoma is common in dog
6. Majority of renal tumors in dog and cat are malignant

B. Urinary tract
1. Cytological evaluation of the urinary tract may aid in differentiation of urinary tract masses
2. Samples can be collected with routine urine collection methods or by fine needle aspiration of radiographically identified masses
3. Infectious cystitis is characterized by the presence of large numbers of neutrophils. Infectious agents may also be present either free or within phagocytic cells
4. Neoplasia of the urinary tract usually involves bladder epithelial cells
5. Prostatic enlargement usually requires cytological evaluation
a. Samples are collected by fine needle aspiration
b. Prostatitis is common and characterized by large numbers of neutrophils that may also be septic
c. Benign hyperplasia is common in older animals
d. Prostatic carcinoma may also occur

C. Vaginal cytology
1. Indicated to assist in timing mating programs such as artificial insemination in small animals or to evaluate infectious or neoplastic processes
2. History and clinical signs are important for proper interpretation of cytology specimen
3. Samples with very large numbers of degenerate neutrophils may indicate vaginitis, pyometra, or metritis
4. Transitional cell carcinoma or squamous cell carcinoma may also be identified cytologically
5. Cells commonly found vary depending on the stage during the cycle
a. Basal cells are small with small amount of cytoplasm
b. Parabasal cells are generally uniform in shape and small and round with a small amount of cytoplasm
c. Intermediate cells are twice the size of parabasal cells
(1) As they increase, the cytoplasmbecomes more irregular, folded, and angular
d. Superficial cells are the largest cells seen
(1) With age the nuclei become pyknotic, fade, and occasionally disappear
(2) Cytoplasm is abundant, angular, and folded
(3) Commonly referred to as cornified cells
6. Identification of cell populations during the estrous cycle is easily accomplished through cytologic examination
a. Anestrus
(1) Predominantly noncornified squamous epithelial cells
(2) Smaller cells, basophilic cytoplasm, and large, round nucleus

(a) Cells are intermediate or parabasal
(3) Some neutrophils but no RBCs
b. Proestrus
(1) In early to mid-proestrus, there is a mixture of parabasal, intermediate, and superficial cells
(a) Neutrophils and RBCs are present
(2) By late proestrus, there is a decrease in neutrophil numbers
(a) Mostly large intermediate and superficial cells
(b) RBCs may or may not be present
(c) Bacteria often present
c. Estrus
(1) All superficial cells
(2) Many appear to be anuclear or have small pyknotic nuclei
(3) RBCs may be present, but no neutrophils
(4) Bacteria often present
d. Metestrus
(1) Parabasal and intermediate cells replace superficial cells
(2) Neutrophil numbers increase
(3) RBCs generally absent but may be present
(4) Cytologically, late estrus to early metestrus resembles early or mid-proestrus

D. Testes
1. Sample collection by fine needle aspiration can aid in differentiation of testicular enlargement
2. Inflammatory conditions (orchitis and epididymitis) appear similar to other inflammatory processes
3. Common neoplastic conditions include Sertoli cell tumors and interstitial cell tumors
4. Transmissible venereal tumor may be present on external genitalia
a. May also be found in the oral and nasal cavities

X. Miscellaneous
A. Musculoskeletal system
1. Muscle tissue samples can be collected in a manner similar to that used for cutaneous and subcutaneous lesions
a. Bone tissue samples are collected by fine needle aspiration or biopsy
2. Primary muscle tissue tumors are extremely rare
3. Inflammatory disorders of bone tissue (osteomyelitis) can be caused by a variety of infectious agents such as fungi and bacteria
4. Neoplastic disorders of bone are common
a. Osteosarcoma is characterized by highly cellular samples and pleomorphic cell types
b. Chondrosarcoma is characterized by the presence of a diffuse cartilaginous matrix with imbedded cells
c. Fibrosarcoma and hemangiosarcoma may also occur in bone tissue

B. Spleen
1. Samples for analysis of the spleen can be collected by fine needle aspiration or biopsy
2. Care must be taken when collecting samples by fine needle aspiration to avoid fracturing delicate splenic tissues
3. Cytology evaluation is combined with clinical signs (e.g., degree of splenic enlargement) when determining diagnosis
4. Hyperplasia can result from a variety of infectious or immune-mediated conditions, including parasites and fungi
5. Splenic enlargement can also occur as a result of extramedullary hematopoiesis involving the spleen
6. Neoplastic disorders of the spleen include hemangiosarcoma and fibrosarcoma, as well as a number of other tumor types

C. Rectal mucosa
1. Presence of mucus or blood in fecal samples may indicate the need for rectal mucosal scraping
2. Normal cells in rectal scrapings include columnar epithelial cells and bacteria
3. Infections with *Histoplasma* or *Balantidium* organisms may be identified with rectal scraping
4. Lymphosarcoma may be identified with rectal scraping. Most other intestinal masses require fine needle aspiration for evaluation

ACKNOWLEDGMENT

The author recognizes and appreciates the original work of Marg Brown and Bill Wade on which this chapter is based.

Glossary

abdominocentesis Removal of fluid from the abdominal cavity
adenocarcinoma Tumors of epithelial cell origin that tend to be highly cellular and often exfoliate in clumps or sheets
adenoma Benign epithelial tumor
adipocytes Fat storage cell
amyloidosis Deposition of an almost insoluble protein in various tissues
anisocytosis Abnormal variation in size of cell
anisokaryosis Abnormal variation in size of nucleus
anisonucleoliosis Abnormal variation in size of nucleoli

benign Neoplasia that is characterized by homogeneous populations of cells that are not malignant, including lipoma, fibroma, papilloma, and adenoma

carcinoma Tumors of epithelial cell origin that tend to be highly cellular and often exfoliate in clumps or sheets

chemotactic Molecules such as phagocytes that attract and guide the movement of cells

cholangiohepatitis Inflammation of the biliary and liver parenchyma

chondrosarcoma Malignant tumor of the cartilage cells or their precursors

chylous effusion A milky-appearing liquid that contains a high concentration of lymph fluid

clasmatocyte Synovial fluid monocytic leukocytes other than lymphocytes, monocytes, and macrophages

cystocentesis Aspiration of fluid from the urinary bladder

effusion Fluid in a body cavity that is abnormally increased in volume

epulis Benign tumor of mixed cells found in the oral cavity

erythrocytophagia Phagocytosis of erythrocytes

exfoliative cytology Study of cells from body surfaces

exudate Effusion characterized by greater than 3.0 g/dL of protein and greater than 7000 nucleated cells/µL

fibroma A tumor of the fibrous or well-developed connective tissue

fibrosarcoma Sarcoma found in fibrous connective tissue

fistula Abnormal passage between two internal organs or from an internal organ to the body surface

granulomatous Inflammatory condition characterized by greater than 70% of mononuclear cells (monocytes, macrophages, giant cells) with few neutrophils

hemangiosarcoma Malignant neoplasia consisting of epithelial cells and fibroblasts

hemosiderin Insoluble form of intracellular iron storage

hepatocytes Liver cells

histiocytoma Tumor of discrete round cell origin that tends to exfoliate singly and have high cellularity

hypercellularity Abnormal increase in number of cells present

hyperplasia Abnormal increase in overall cell numbers as a result of an external stimulus

hypersegmentation Excessive division into segments or lobes

in situ Within the body

karyolysis Loss of nuclear membrane

karyorrhexis Fragmentation of the cell nucleus

lymphadenitis Inflammation of the lymph nodes

lymphoblast Immature, nucleated precursor of the mature lymphocyte; also called large lymphocyte

macrocytosis Increase in number of abnormally large erythrocytes

macrophage Tissue phagocyte derived from the peripheral blood monocyte

malignant Neoplasia that displays multiple abnormal nuclear criteria

mast cell Tissue cell containing dark-staining granules of histamine and heparin

melanoma Tumor arising from cells that contain melanin

mesenchyma Muscular, connective tissue and vessels that are derived from the embryonic connective tissue in the mesoderm

mesoderm Middle of the three primary germ layers of the embryo

mesothelial Cells that line pleural, peritoneal, and visceral surfaces

mesothelioma Rare malignant tumor derived from mesothelial cells

metastasis Neoplasia that is present in an area other than where it initially developed

modified transudate Effusion characterized by moderate cellularity and total protein

mucocele Accumulated mucous secretion in a cavity

neoplasia Any new or abnormal growth, especially if it is uncontrolled and progressive; a tumor

osteomyelitis Inflammation of the bone

osteosarcoma Malignant tumor of the bone

papilloma Common wart

percutaneous Performed through the skin

perinuclear Space between the inner and outer nuclear membranes

plasma cell Activated lymphocyte characterized by basophilic cytoplasm and a perinuclear clear zone

pleomorphic Abnormal variation in size and/or shape of cells of the same type

pleuritis Inflammation of the pleura

pnuemothorax Air in the pleural cavity that causes lung collapse

purulent Inflammation containing greater than 85% neutrophils

pyknosis Condensed nucleus

pyogranulomatous Inflammatory process consisting of macrophages and 50% to 75% neutrophils

sarcoma Malignant tumor derived from connective tissue cells

sialocele Common non-neoplastic condition of salivary gland characterized by fluid-filled cavities composed primarily of epithelial cells

suppurative Purulent inflammation containing greater than 85% neutrophils

thoracocentesis Removal of fluid from the thoracic cavity

transudate Effusion with less than 2.5 g/dL protein and fewer than 1500 cells/µL

Review Questions

1 The preferred sample preparation technique when cellularity is low is
   a. Wedge smear
   b. Starfish smear
   c. Line smear
   d. Squash prep

2 The preferred preparation technique for highly viscous samples is
   a. Wedge smear
   b. Starfish smear
   c. Line smear
   d. Squash prep

3 A chylous effusion appears
   a. Milky
   b. Pink
   c. Amber
   d. Colorless

4 The presence of predominantly anuclear cornified epithelial cells indicates
a. Proestrus
b. Anestrus
c. Diestrus
d. Estrus

5 Cells that line the pleural, peritoneal, and visceral surfaces are
a. Plasma cells
b. Mast cells
c. Mesothelial cells
d. Macrophages

6 Cells that contain a perinuclear clear zone are
a. Plasma cells
b. Mast cells
c. Mesothelial cells
d. Macrophages

7 The most common site for neoplasia in dog and cat is
a. Bone
b. Skin
c. Liver
d. Kidney

8 A nuclear criterion of malignancy that involves variability in the size and shape of same cell type is referred to as
a. Anisocytosis
b. Anisokaryosis
c. Pleomorphism
d. Nuclear molding

9 The presence of imbedded cells in a diffuse cartilaginous matrix is characteristic of
a. Osteosarcoma
b. Chondrosarcoma
c. Osteomyelitis
d. Chondromyelitis

10 A deformation of nuclei by other nuclei within the same cell or adjacent cells is referred to as
a. Nuclear molding
b. Angular nuclei
c. Anisonucleosis
d. Multinucleation

BIBLIOGRAPHY

Baker R, Lumsden J: *Color atlas of cytology of the dog and cat,* St Louis, 2000, Mosby.

Cowell R, Tyler R, Meinkoth J: *Diagnostic cytology and hematology of the dog and cat,* ed 2, St Louis, 1999, Mosby.

Meyer DJ: The management of cytology specimens, *Comp Cont Educ Pract Vet* 9:1, 1987.

Perman V: *Cytology of the dog and cat,* 1979, American Animal Hospital Association.

Rebar A: *Handbook of veterinary cytology,* St Louis, 1980, Ralston Purina Co.

CHAPTER 4

Parasitology

Mary Lake

OUTLINE

LEARNING OUTCOMES

After reading this chapter, you should be able to:

1. List the scientific and common names of parasites.
2. Define and describe the life cycles of various parasites.
3. Describe clinical signs associated with each parasite.
4. Describe how to identify a parasite infestation.
5. Define treatment and control of parasite infestations.
6. Define various basic laboratory techniques for the identification of parasites.

The parasite/host relationship is unique. A parasite is an organism that in its natural habitat feeds and lives on or in another organism. The parasite may cause clinical signs in the host, but its goal is to use the host to live and reproduce without causing death. However, a parasite infection of sufficient numbers can overwhelm the host and cause death. Familiarity with life cycles helps us to control parasites. For example, heartworm in dogs can be controlled with preventives. In other cases, such as flea infestation, the environment and the host need to be treated. Proper identification of parasites or ova allows the veterinarian to determine which treatment regimen is appropriate. This chapter describes common parasites by host, beginning with the domestic dog and cat and moving on to horses, food animals, and some common laboratory animals.

Ten tables at the end of the chapter list diagnosis and treatment options for common parasites.

FECES EXAMINATION

Gross Examination of Feces

I. Gross characteristics of feces should be recorded and reported to the veterinarian

II. Characteristics noted include consistency, color, and presence of blood, mucus, or adult parasites, including tapeworm segments

Standard Vial Gravitation Flotation Technique

I. Based on specific gravity of parasitic material and fecal debris
   - A. Specific gravity of most parasite eggs is between 1.100 and 1.200
   - B. Specific gravity of water is 1.000
   - C. Flotation solution must have a higher specific gravity than that of the parasitic material to facilitate flotation of parasite eggs, oocysts, etc.

II. A simple, inexpensive technique but of poor efficiency

A. Materials
 1. Vial (approximately 2 inches deep by 1 inch in diameter)
 2. Two paper cups
 3. Wire strainer
 4. Tongue depressor
 5. Glass slide and coverslip
 6. Solution of sodium nitrate with specific gravity of 1.340
  a. Other common flotation solutions
   (1) Sugar solution: inexpensive, does not crystallize or distort eggs, specific gravity of 1.330
   (2) Zinc sulfate solution: for *Giardia* cysts, specific gravity of 1.180
   (3) Saturated sodium chloride solution: specific gravity of 1.200

B. Fill a paper cup with approximately 60 mL of sodium nitrate solution
C. Using a tongue depressor, add approximately 2 to 4 g (0.5 to 1 teaspoon) of feces
D. Mix feces well with sodium nitrate solution
E. Strain, using wire strainer, into a second cup. Remove as much fluid as possible from the fecal material in the strainer
F. Discard feces on the strainer and wash strainer with hot water for reuse
G. Swirl strained fecal suspension in the cup to randomly disperse eggs and pour mixture into vial until fluid projects above rim of the vial, creating a positive meniscus
H. Place a coverslip on top of the fluid and allow eggs to float upward
I. After a minimum of 10 to 15 minutes, remove coverslip (straight up), trying not to tilt fluid back into vial, and place it on a glass slide
J. Using ×10 objective, systematically examine entire area under the coverslip, noting type and number of parasites seen
 1. Sample should also be examined using ×40 for small protozoa
K. Although the procedure cannot be classified as quantitative, results are reported as follows
 1. 1 to 100 eggs seen: graded as one plus (+)
 2. 101 to 300 eggs seen: graded as two plus (++)
 3. 301 or more eggs seen: graded as three plus (+++)

Quantitative Fecal Examination

I. Quantitative procedures are used to determine the number of eggs present per gram of feces
 A. Examples include the Wisconsin double centrifugation technique and the McMaster technique
 B. Other quantitative procedures can be found in the reference books listed at the end of this chapter

Commercial Flotation Kits

I. Common examples
 A. Ovassay (Synbiotics, San Diego, CA)
 B. Fecalyzer (EVSCO Pharmaceuticals, Buena, NJ)
 C. Ovatector (BGS Medical Products, Venice, FL)
II. Kits are easy to use but expensive and have low sensitivity
III. A kit generally comes with a vial, which may or may not have a cap; an insert (or funnel or filter), to collect or pick up feces; and possibly flotation solution
IV. Follow insert instructions

Direct Smear

I. Direct smear is used to
 A. Detect protozoa in feces
 B. Quickly estimate the number of parasites
II. Materials
 A. Microscope slides and coverslip
 B. Applicator sticks or tongue depressors
 C. Lugol's iodine or new methylene blue stain (optional)
III. Procedure
 A. Place a drop of saline or water on a slide with an equal amount of feces. A drop of stain may be added at this time
 B. Mix feces and saline with applicator stick
 C. Make a very thin smear on the slide
 D. Remove large pieces of feces on slide for easier viewing
 E. Examine smear using ×10 objective for parasite eggs and larvae and ×40 objective for protozoal organisms

OVC Puddle Technique for (*Cryptosporidium* Oocysts)

I. Materials
 A. Microscope slide and coverslip
 B. Applicator stick
 C. Saturated sugar solution (e.g., corn syrup)
II. Procedure
 A. Place a drop of sugar solution on a glass slide
 B. Add a small amount of feces to slide and mix
 C. Add a coverslip and examine under ×40 objective
  1. Oocysts of *Cryptosporidium* are up to 5 μm in diameter and have a slight pinkish color
  2. There may be fungal spores present similar in size and shape to an oocyst; however, spores usually will bud if observed for a period of time

PRESERVATION OF PARASITIC SAMPLES

I. Fresh specimens should be packaged in leak-proof containers, sealed, and labeled
   A. Label should include the following information: date, location from which the specimen was obtained, owner's name, animal's species, animal's name or identification number, referring veterinarian, clinic address, and telephone number
II. Feces can be sent fresh or mixed at a ratio of 1:3 with 10% formalin
III. Whole parasites or segments can be preserved in alcohol or formalin

Examples of ova are illustrated at the end of the chapter.

BLOOD PARASITE EXAMINATION (*DIROFILARIA IMMITIS* AND *DIPETALONEMA RECONDITUM*)

Modified Knott's Technique

I. Materials
   A. 15 mL centrifuge tube and centrifuge
   B. 2% Formalin
   C. Methylene blue stain
   D. Pasteur pipettes and bulbs
   E. Slides and coverslips
II. Procedure
   A. Place 1 mL of EDTA blood in a 15 mL conical centrifuge tube
   B. Add 9 mL of 2% formalin (or water)
   C. Mix by inversion and shake to lyse the red blood cells
   D. Spin in centrifuge for 5 minutes at 1000 rpm or let stand for 1 hour
   E. Decant supernatant by inverting tube once and letting it drain
   F. Add 2 drops of methylene blue stain to the sediment and mix with a pipette by gently aspirating the mixture
   G. Place a drop of the mixture on a slide, add coverslip, and examine under ×10 objective
   H. Examine entire slide for microfilariae

Commercial Filter Technique

I. Common example of a commercial kit
   A. Di-Fil (EVSCO, Buena, NJ)
II. These kits come with filters, lysing solution, stain, and directions
III. Most kits require 1 mL of whole blood to test for heartworms
IV. Mix blood with 10 to 12 mL of lysing solution
V. Place a new filter in the filter holder, inject the fluid into the filter holder, and rinse with 10 mL of water
VI. Place the filter on a slide, and add a drop of stain
VII. Add a coverslip to the slide, and examine slide

Buffy Coat Method

I. A concentration method using a small amount of blood
II. Quick and can be performed after evaluation of a packed cell volume (PCV) and before total protein evaluation
III. Materials
   A. Microhematocrit tubes and sealer
   B. Centrifuge
   C. Microscope slides and coverslips
   D. Saline
   E. Methylene blue stain
   F. Small file or glass cutter
IV. Procedure
   A. Centrifuge blood-filled microhematocrit tube for 3 minutes
   B. Read PCV
   C. Examine surface of buffy coat (white blood cells) layer of the blood under microscope
      1. When a blood-filled microhematocrit tube is spun in the centrifuge, the blood separates into three layers
         a. Plasma
         b. White blood cell layer (buffy coat)
         c. Red blood cell layer
   D. Use a file to scratch tube at level of the buffy coat. Snap tube and gently tap tube to place buffy coat on slide
   E. Add a drop of saline and a drop of methylene blue stain to the buffy coat. Add coverslip, and examine for microfilariae
   F. Use remaining plasma from the hematocrit tube to evaluate total protein

ENZYME-LINKED IMMUNOSORBENT ASSAY

I. Enzyme-linked immunosorbent assay (ELISA) kits do not detect microfilariae. Only the host's response to parasites or antigens present in the blood is detected
II. This type of test can be used to identify
   A. Occult heartworm
   B. *Dirofilaria immitis*
III. Common examples
   A. Dirochek (Synbiotics, San Diego, CA)
   B. PetChek/Snap (Idexx)
   C. Witness (Binax)
IV. ELISA antigen detection system
   A. Monoclonal antibody is bound to the walls of a well in a test tray, to a membrane, or to a plastic wand
   B. If the specific antigen is present in the sample, it will bind to this antibody and to the second enzyme-labeled antibody that is added
   C. When a color-producing agent is added to the mixture, the agent reacts to develop a specific

color that indicates presence of the antigen in the sample

D. If the sample contains no antigen, the second antibody is washed away during a rinsing process and no other color reactions take place

V. ELISA tests are easy to perform when following manufacturer directions and take approximately 10 to 15 minutes to complete

EXTERNAL PARASITE IDENTIFICATION

Skin Scraping

I. Materials
   A. No. 10 scalpel blade
   B. Mineral oil in a dropper bottle
   C. Microscope slides
   D. Microscope

II. Procedure
   A. Add mineral oil to a slide and dip scalpel blade in it
   B. Begin scraping by holding skin between thumb and index finger of one hand and scalpel blade in the other hand
   C. While scraping, the blade must be held perpendicular to the skin
      1. Holding the blade at any other angle could result in an incision into the skin
   D. Depth of scraping depends on the suspected parasite
      1. *Sarcoptes* (burrowing mite) and *Demodex* (hair follicle mite): scrape until blood begins to seep from the abrasion
      2. *Chorioptes* (nonburrowing mite) and *Cheyletiella* (walking dandruff): skin is scraped superficially to collect loose scales and crusts
   E. All of the harvest (material scraped from the skin) is placed on a slide with mineral oil
   F. After adding a coverslip, examine entire slide under the ×10 objective
   G. For thorough evaluation, examine at least 10 slides

Skin Digestion Technique

I. Used for scraping samples where there is a large amount of scurf and skin debris

II. Materials
   A. Conical centrifuge tube
   B. 4% NaOH
   C. Hot plate, beaker
   D. Centrifuge

III. Procedure
   A. Place the skin scraping (with scalpel blade if desired) in a 15 mL conical centrifuge tube
   B. Add about 10 mL of 4% NaOH solution
   C. Place the tube in the water bath (glass beaker with water) on the hot plate. Allow the water to boil gently for 5 to 10 minutes
   D. Remove the centrifuge tube, and centrifuge at 1000 rpm (×264) for 5 minutes
   E. Decant supernatant, mix sediment with a pipette, place a drop on a slide, add a coverslip, and examine under the microscope (×10)

Cellophane Tape Method

I. Used for mites and pinworms, that are primarily on skin surface and the hair (e.g., *Cheyletiella* sp., *Oxyuris equi*)

II. Materials
   A. Cellophane tape
   B. Mineral oil
   C. Microscope slides

III. Procedure
   A. Using cellophane tape, lift off epidermal dermis from skin surface
   B. Place a drop of mineral oil on a slide and stick tape on top of the slide
   C. Examine slide using ×10 objective

Baermann Technique

I. This is used for removing lungworm larvae from small amounts of feces

II. Materials
   A. Paper cup
   B. Disposable cellulose tissue (Kimwipe)
   C. Elastic band
   D. Sedimentation jar
   E. Long Pasteur pipette with bulb
   F. Dissecting microscope

III. Procedure
   A. Place the fecal sample in a paper cup
   B. Cover the opening of the cup with a disposable cellulose tissue and secure with an elastic band
   C. Fill a sedimentation jar half-way with warm water
   D. Invert the paper cup with the feces, and punch a small hole in the bottom of the cup
   E. Immerse the tissue end of the cup into the water in the sedimentation jar
   F. Tuck the overhanging tissue into the jar
   G. After 12 to 18 hours, withdraw a sample from the bottom of the sedimentation jar
      1. Gently tilt the paper cup, and insert a long Pasteur pipette down to the bottom of the jar
      2. Refill the pipette three or four times, and place the fluid collected into a small Petri dish
   H. Examine with a dissecting microscope
      1. The larvae should be alive and motile

EXTERNAL AND INTERNAL PARASITE IDENTIFICATION (TABLES 4-1 TO 4-10)

Table 4-1 Diagnostic characteristics of internal parasites of domestic animals

Parasite	Location	Prepatent period	Diagnostic stage	Test	Method of infection	Clinical signs	Control
DOGS							
Toxocara canis	Small intestines	3-5 weeks	Dark brown, thick-walled egg, with a pitted eggshell; single-celled zygote, 90-75 μ	Fecal flotation	Ingestion of infective egg Paratenic host Transplacentally Transmammary Ingestion of larvae in bitch's feces	Poor growth, emaciation, intestinal blockage, vomiting, diarrhea, death	Remove feces from environment
Ancylostoma caninum	Small intestines	2-3 weeks	Clear, smooth, thin-walled hookworm egg; zygote 8- to 16-cell morula; 55-65 × 27-43 μ	Fecal flotation	Skin penetration Ingestion of infective larvae Transmammary Paratenic host Larval 'leak' Transplacentally	Anemia, weakness, melena	Remove feces from environment
Uncinaria stenocephala	Small intestines	2 weeks	Hookworm egg; 63-93 × 32-55 μ	Fecal flotation	Ingestion of infective larvae Skin penetration (not likely)	Usually no obvious clinical signs In heavy infection in dogs, hypoproteinemia, dehydration, weakness	Remove feces from environment
Trichuris vulpis	Large intestines	3 months	Smooth, amber, thick-walled, barrel-shaped egg with bipolar plugs; single-celled zygote; 72-90 × 2-40 μ	Fecal flotation	Ingestion of infective egg	In heavy infection, severe watery diarrhea, hematochezia (frank blood in feces) leading to rapid dehydration and death	Remove from environment
Eucoleus bohmi	Nasal sinuses	Unknown	Smooth, yellow-brown, thick-walled egg with a striated shell and asymmetric bipolar plugs; single-celled zygote	Fecal flotation	Ingestion of infective egg	Upper respiratory signs, sneezing and nasal discharge	
Filaroides spp.	Lungs	5-10 weeks	L1 with S-shaped tail lacking a dorsal spine; esophagus third of length of body; 230-266 μ long	Fecal flotation, Baermann	Paratenic host Ingestion of infective egg	Chronic coughing	
Crenosoma spp.	Lungs	19-21 days	L1 with a straight, pointed tail; esophagus third of length of body; 265-330 μ long	Baermann	Ingestion of infected snails	Coughing	
Spirocerca lupi	Esophagus	5-6 months	Clear, smooth, thick-walled, paperclip-shaped, larvated egg; 30-37 × 11-15 μ	Flotation	Ingestion of intermediate host (dung beetle) Ingestion of paratenic host	Vomit, dysphagia, weight loss, sudden death Most infections not diagnosed until necropsy	In endemic areas, dogs should be prevented from eating dung

Continued

Table 4-1 Diagnostic characteristics of internal parasites of domestic animals—cont'd

Parasite	Location	Prepatent period	Diagnostic stage	Test	Method of infection	Clinical signs	Control
Spirocera lupi—cont'd							beetles, frogs, mice, and lizards, and they should not be fed raw chicken scraps
Dirofilaria immitis	Heart	6-8 months	Microfilaria (L1) lacks an esophagus	Modified Knott's millipore filtration, ELISA, antigen test	Transmission from infective mosquitoe bites Transplacental infection of microfilariae only	Lethargy, exercise intolerance, signs referable to right-sided cardiac enlargement	Use of preventives, reduce exposure to mosquitoes and endemic areas
Dipetalonema reconditum	Subcutaneous	9 weeks	Microfilaria	Modified Knott's tissue millipore filtration	Transmission from infective flea bites Ingestion of fleas	Considered to be nonpathogenic, microfilariae may cause problems in kidney tubules	Control flea population
Dioctophyma renale	Kidney	5 months	Dark brown, thick-walled, barrel-shaped egg with a pitted shell and an operculum at each pole; single-celled zygote; 71-84 × 46-52 μ	Sedimentation of urine	Ingestion of intermediate host (annelid worm) Ingestion of paratenic host (i.e., fish and green frogs)	May be none Vague abdominal pain after kidney rupture Adult worms often found in abdominal cavity at surgery	Surgical removal–nephrectomy if in the kidney
Dracunculus insignis	Subcutaneous tissue	309-410 days	Comma-shaped larva with an esophagus and a straight tail; 500-750 μ long	Direct smear of fluid in blister	Ingestion of paratenic host	Pea-sized blisters on legs, elbow, and axillary area, break open Adult worms coiled in subcutaneous tissue	Surgical removal
				CAT			
Toxocara cati	Small intestines	8 weeks	Dark brown, thick-walled, pitted egg; single-celled zygote; 65-75 μ	Fecal flotation	Ingestion of infective eggs Transmammary Ingestion paratenic host	Usually none, cat may vomit worm or two	Clean up environment
Ancylostoma	Small intestines	3 weeks	Hookworm egg; 55-76 × 34-45 μ	Fecal flotation	Skin penetration Ingestion of infective larvae Transmammary infection	Anemia, emaciation, weakness, melena, death	
Aelurostrongylus abstrusus	Bronchioles alveoli	4-6 weeks	L1 with S-shaped tail and a dorsal spine; 360 μ long; esophagus one-fourth the length of body	Baermann	Ingestion of infected snail Ingestion of paratenic host	Usually asymptomatic, may see chronic coughing	
Platynosomum fastosum	Liver	8-12 weeks	Dark amber, oval, operculated egg containing a miracidium; 34-50 × 20-35 μ	Sedimentation of feces	Ingestion of intermediate host (snail) Ingestion of paratenic host	Severe infections characterized by anorexia, persistent vomiting, diarrhea, jaundice, death	

Toxoplasma gondii	Small intestines	1-3 weeks	Clear, smooth, thin-walled spherical oocyst; single-celled zygote; 8-10 μ	Fecal flotation	Ingestion of cysts in meat Ingestion of sporulated oocysts	Most infections are latent or asymptomatic Young animals signs may include fever, anorexia, cough, dyspnea, diarrhea, jaundice, and central nervous system dysfunction	Cats should not be fed raw meat, remove litter daily before sporulation can occur
DOG AND CAT							
Toxascaris leonina	Small intestines	11 weeks	Clear, smooth, thick-walled eggshell with wavy internal membrane; single-celled zygote and does not completely fill the eggshell; 75 × 85 μ	Fecal flotation	Ingestion of infective eggs Ingestion of paratenic host	Heavy worm burdens may cause weakness, dehydration, poor condition	Clean environment
Ancylostoma braziliense	Small intestines	3 weeks	Hookworm egg; 75-95 × 41-45 μ	Fecal flotation	Ingestion of infective larvae Skin penetration	Anemia, diarrhea, melena, emaciation, weakness	Clean environment
Capillaria aerophilus	Trachea bronchi	6 weeks	Rough, granular, thick-walled, barrel-shaped, straw-colored egg with asymmetric bipolar plugs; single-celled zygote; 58-79 × 29-40 μ	Fecal flotation	Ingestion of infective egg	Light infection—none Heavy infection—signs of bronchitis, bronchi and bronchioles may fill with blood and mucus	
Capillaria plica (dog) *Capillaria feliscati* (cat)	Urinary bladder	60 days	Rough, striated, thick-walled, barrel-shaped, amber-colored egg with asymmetric bipolar plugs; single-celled zygote; 60-68 × 24-30 μ	Sedimentation of urine	Ingestion of intermediate host (earthworm)	Usually none, may be signs of chronic cystitis, frequent urination, painful urination, hematuria	
Strongyloides stercoralis	Small intestines	8-14 days	L1 with a rhabditiform esophagus and a straight pointed tail L3 with a filariform esophagus and a bipartite tail	Baermann Fecal culture	Skin penetration Ingestion of infective larvae Transmammary	Heavy infection—mucoid diarrhea in young animals Emaciation and reduced growth rate	
Physaloptera spp.	Stomach	56-83 days	Smooth, clear, thick-walled, larvated egg; 45-53 × 29-42 μ	Fecal flotation	Ingestion of intermediate host (beetles)	Cause gastritis and duodenitis, often resulting in vomiting, anorexia, and dark feces	
Dipylidium caninum	Small intestines	3 weeks	Proglottid with bilateral genital pores; eggs containing 6-hooked hexacanth embryos in packets; 35-60 μ	ID proglottids fecal flotation	Ingestion of a cysticercoid in intermediate host, (i.e., flea, lice)	Usually none, may see segments in feces May see 'scooting'	Control of intermediate hosts
Taenia spp.	Small intestines	2 months	Dark brown, thick, radially striated eggshell; 6-hooked hexacanth embryo; 32-37 μ; rectangular proglottids with unilateral genital pore	ID proglottid	Ingestion of cysticercous in intermediate host, (i.e., rabbit, rodent)	Usually none, may see segments in feces	Restrict pets from eating wildlife

Continued

Table 4-1 Diagnostic characteristics of internal parasites of domestic animals—cont'd

Parasite	Location	Prepatent period	Diagnostic stage	Test	Method of infection	Clinical signs	Control
Echinococcus spp.	Small intestines	47 days	Similar to *Taenia* eggs	Fecal flotation	Ingestion of hydatid or alveolar hydatid cysts in intermediate host, (i.e., moose, sheep, goats, cattle, horse, deer *[E. granulosis]* or rodents *[E. multilocularis]*)	Usually none	Restrict pets from eating raw meat/viscera and wildlife
Mesocestoides spp.	Small intestines	16-20 days	Smooth, thin egg capsule containing 6-hooked hexacanth embryo; 20-25 µ; globular proglottid with parauterine body	Fecal flotation ID proglottid	Complete life cycle is unknown, arthropods/ mammals/reptiles/birds are suspected intermediate hosts	Usually none	
Spirometra mansonoides	Small intestines	10-30 days	Unembryonated, thin-walled, smooth, amber-colored egg; operculated; 70 × 45 µ	Fecal flotation	Ingestion of intermediate host (crustaceans, water snake)	Vague/none	Control environment
Paragonimus kellicotti	Lung	1 month	Smooth, golden brown, urn-shaped, operculated egg; 75-118 × 42-67 µ	Sedimentation of urine	Ingestion of metacercariae in crayfish	Often none, may be intermittent chronic coughing	Control environment
Nanophyetus salmincola	Small intestines	1 week	Rough, brown, operculated egg; 52-82 × 32-56 µ	Sedimentation of feces	Ingestion of metacercariae in various tissues in fish	None; clinical signs due to salmon poisoning complex caused by rickettsial organism	Control environment
Isospora spp.	Small intestines	4-12 days	Clear, spherical to ellipsoid thin-walled oocyst, size varies with species	Fecal flotation	Ingestion of sporulated oocyst	Persistent diarrhea, may lead to dehydration and death	Clean environment to prevent accumulation and sporulation of oocysts
Sarcocystis spp.	Small intestines	7-33 days	Thin-walled oocyst with 2 sporocysts containing 4 sporozoites each or sporocyst; size varies with species	Fecal flotation	Ingestion of cysts in muscle tissue—various intermediate hosts	None	Restrict pets from eating raw meat offal
				HORSE			
Parascaris equorum	Small intestines	10 weeks	Rough, brown, thick-walled, spherical egg; single-celled zygote; 90-100 µ	Fecal flotation	Ingestion of infective egg	Adult horses—none Foals—may retard growth, may cause colic, (e.g., intussusception, or volvulus of gut)	
Eimerial leukarti	Small intestines	15-33 days	Dark brown, piriform, thick-walled oocyst; 70-90 × 49-69 µ	Fecal flotation	Ingestion of sporulated oocysts	Not pathogenic, no clinical signs	

Cyathostomes (small strongyles)	Large intestines	2-3 months	Smooth, thin-walled, clear strongyle egg; zygote 8- to 16-cell morula; size varies with species	Fecal flotation	Ingestion of infective larvae	Poor growth, decreased performance, profuse diarrhea In acute conditions, large numbers of worms seen grossly in feces	
Strongylus spp. (large strongyles) *Strongylus vulgaris* *Strongylus ledentatus* and *S. equinus*	Large intestines	6-12 months	Strongyle egg	Fecal flotation	Ingestion of infective larvae Larvae not too pathogenic, adults may cause anemia, loss of condition	Colic, fever, diarrhea, weight loss, death	Strategic deworming
Oxyuris equi	Large intestines	5 months	Clear, smooth, thin-walled egg with 1 side flattened; operculated; 90 × 42 μ	Cellophane tape preparation	Ingestion of infective eggs	Pruritus ani, fraying of hairs on tail head May see female worms passed in feces, white egg masses on perianal skin	Removal of egg masses on perianal skin with soap and water, clean stalls and woodwork
Anoplocephala spp.	Small and large intestines	1-2 months	Clear, thick-walled, square eggs with a pear-shaped (piriform) apparatus containing an hexacanth embryo	Fecal flotation	Ingestion of cysticercoid in pasture mite	Most asymptomatic, but *A. perfoliata* causes colic and death due to intestinal accident	
Strongyloides westeri	Small intestines	8-14 days	Smooth, thin-walled, larvated egg; 40-50 × 32-40 μ	Fecal flotation	Transmammary Skin penetration Ingestion of infective larvae	Adult horses—none Foals—diarrhea	
Gasterophilus spp.	Stomach		2.5-cm, robust grub with rows of spines and straight spiracular slits (breathing tubes)	ID 3rd instar at necropsy	Ingestion of larvae	Bots in tongue and gums may cause ulcers on surface of tongue and tooth problems Bots in stomach occasionally cause perforation of stomach wall with with fatal peritonitis	Remove bot eggs from horses legs and shoulder area
CATTLE, SHEEP, GOAT							
Trichostrongyles: *Haemonchus, Ostertagia, Cooperia., Tricho-strongylus*	Abomasum, small intestines	15-28 days	Strongyle egg	Fecal flotation	Ingestion of infective larvae while grazing	Clinical signs depend on age, host resistance and number of worms Acute signs; seen mainly in younger animals, diarrhea, anorexia and loss of condition Chronic signs are more subtle may see poor weight gain and general poor doing animal	Try to prevent pasture contamination by strategic worming\ of animals

Continued

Table 4-1 Diagnostic characteristics of internal parasites of domestic animals—cont'd

Parasite	Location	Prepatent period	Diagnostic stage	Test	Method of infection	Clinical signs	Control
Dictyocaulus spp.	Lungs	3-4 weeks	L1 with dark granular intestines; esophagus one-third the length of larva; straight pointed tail; 550-580 μ long	Baermann	Ingestion of infective larvae	Coughing, dyspnea	
Strongyloides spp.	Small intestines	3-4 weeks	Thin-walled egg with parallel sides; 40-60 × 20-25 μ	Fecal flotation	Ingestion of infective larvae	Rarely a clinical problem	
Oesophagostomum spp.	Large intestines	45 days	Strongyle egg	Fecal flotation	Ingestion of infective larvae	Usually not a clinical problem in cattle and goats in moderate numbers In sheep, large numbers can cause diarrhea and weight loss	
Skrjabinema spp.	Large intestines	25 days	Clear, smooth, thin-walled egg with one side flattened, single-celled zygote	Fecal flotation	Ingestion of infective egg	Typical of pinworms Eggs deposited on perianal skin—possibly pruritus ani Seen in goats, rarely in sheep	
Eimeria spp.	Small and large intestines	10-30 days	Smooth or rough, thin-walled, clear to yellowish brown oocysts; single-celled zygote; size varies with species	Fecal flotation	Ingestion of infective egg	Light infections usually no clinical signs Heavy infections, diarrhea, sometimes bloody, and tenesmus Note: clinical signs are possible before oocysts pass in the feces, repeat fecal examination will eventually reveal oocysts	
Moniezia spp.	Small intestines	6 weeks	Thick-walled, clear, triangular to square egg with a piriform apparatus containing an hexacanth embryo	Fecal flotation	Ingestion of cysticercoid in a free-living pasture mite	Not considered very pathogenic Heavy burdens may affect weight gain	
Thysanosoma actinoides	Bile ducts		Thin-walled egg with hexacanth embryos in packets; 21-45 μ	Fecal flotation			
Fasciola spp.	Liver	10-12 weeks	Dark amber, oval, operculated egg; 130-150 × 63-90 μ	Sedimentation of feces	Ingestion of metacercariae	Devastating disease in sheep, is dependent on the number of metacercariae eaten over a short period of time Produces a distended, painful abdomen, anemia, and sudden death Chronic disease may show signs of anemia, unthriftiness, submandibular edema, and reduced milk secretion	

Bunostomum spp.	Small intestines	2-3 weeks	Strongyle egg	Fecal flotation	Ingestion of infective larvae Skin penetration	Ruminant hookworms Occasionally low worm burdens Heavy infections can cause anemia	Strategic deworming
Chabertia ovina	Large intestines	47-63 days	Strongyle egg	Fecal flotation	Ingestion of infective larvae	Larvae and adults can cause small hemorrhages with edema in the colon: the feces may be coated with mucus when passed	Deworming
Trichuris spp.	Large intestines	2-3 months	Dark, brownish, thick-walled, smooth egg with symmetric bipolar plugs; single-celled zygote; size varies with species	Fecal flotation	Ingestion of infective larvae Skin penetration	Clinical signs are unlikely, heavy worm burdens seldom seen In occasional heavy infections may see dark feces, anemia, and anorexia Trichuris is not transmissible between ruminants and dogs	Deworming
Capillaria spp.	Small intestines		Brownish, thick-walled striated egg with asymmetric bipolar plugs; single-celled zygote; 45-52 × 21-30 μ	Fecal flotation	Ingestion of infective eggs	None	
				CATTLE			
Cryptosporidium muris	Abomasum	4-10 days	Clear, smooth, thin-walled oocyst containing 4 sporozoites; 5 × 7 μ	Fecal flotation	Transmission by the fecal-oral route Oocysts shed in the feces are immediately infective	Usually seen in calves 1-3 weeks old Diarrhea, tenesmus, weight loss, anorexia are usually seen	No treatment Disease is usually self-limiting Supportive therapy is (i.e., fluids)
				SHEEP			
Protostrongylus rufescens	Lungs	30-37 days	L1 with a straight, pointed tail 48-56 μ long without a dorsal spine; 340-400 × 19-20 μ	Baermann	Ingestion of intermediate host (slug or snail)	Chronic eosinophilic granulomatous pneumonia	
Mullerius spp.	Lungs	6 weeks	L1 are 300-320 × 14-15 μ with S-shaped tail bearing a dorsal spine	Baermann	Ingestion of infective larvae in slugs on pasture	More common in goats Coughing	

Continued

Table 4-1 Diagnostic characteristics of internal parasites of domestic animals—cont'd

Parasite	Location	Prepatent period	Diagnostic stage	Test	Method of infection	Clinical signs	Control
				PIG			
Eimeria spp.	Small intestines	4-10 days	Smooth or rough, thin-walled oocyst; single-celled zygote; size varies with species	Fecal flotation	Ingestion of sporulated oocysts	Essentially nonpathogenic May see diarrhea	
Isospora spp.	Small intestines	5 days	Smooth, clear, thin-walled oocyst; single-celled zygote; 17-25 × 16-21 μ	Fecal flotation	Ingestion of sporulated oocysts	Adult pigs usually do not show clinical signs but contaminate the environment Nursing piglets: diarrhea, dehydration, emaciation	
Balantidium coli	Large intestines		Thin-walled, greenish cyst with hyaline cytoplasm; 40-60 μ; 30-150 × 25-120 μ trophozoite with rows of cilia	Fecal flotation Direct smear	Ingestion of cysts	Found commonly in the feces of swine, not considered pathogenic	Not usually treated
Ascaris suum	Small intestines	7-9 weeks	Brownish yellow, thick-walled, mammilated egg; single-celled zygote; 50-80 × 40-60 μ	Fecal flotation	Ingestion of infective egg	Nursing pigs may show dyspnea Growing pigs—reduced weight gains Adult pigs—usually none	
Strongyloides ransomi	Small intestines	3-7 days	Smooth, thin-walled, larvated egg with parallel sides; 45-55 × 26-35 μ	Fecal flotation	Larvae can be transmitted via colostrum Ingestion of larvae	Heavy infections in piglets produce severe diarrhea when 10-14 days of age, with high mortality	
Oesophagostomum spp.	Large intestines	32-42 days	Strongyle egg	Fecal flotation	Ingestion of infective larvae	Reduced weight of gain in grower pigs	
Hyostrongylus rubidus	Stomach	15-21 days	Strongyle egg	Fecal flotation			
Metastrongylus spp.	Lungs	24 days	Rough, clear, thick-walled, larvated egg with a corrugated surface; 45-57 × 38-41 μ	Fecal flotation	Ingestion of infective larvae	Diarrhea, anorexia, decreased weight gain	
Trichuris suis	Large intestines	2-3 months	Brownish yellow, smooth, thick-walled egg with symmetric bipolar plugs; single-celled zygote 50-56 × 21-25 μ	Fecal flotation	Ingestion of the intermediate host (earthworm)	Coughing and predisposition to bacterial and viral respiratory infections	
Trichinella spiralis	Small intestines	2-6 days	L3 encysted in striated muscles; esophagus composed of stichocytes (single cells stacked on top of one another); cysts are 400-600 × 250 μ	Squash preparation of muscle	Ingestion of larvae in muscle, (i.e., carnivorism)	Usually no clinical signs Economic loss at slaughter	

DOG, CAT, CATTLE, HORSE, SHEEP, GOAT, PIG							
Thelazia californiensis	Eye	3-6 weeks	Adult worm in conjunctival sac and tear duct	ID adult	Flies (*Musca* spp., *Fannia* spp.) deposit infective larvae on the eye while feeding on ocular secretions	Excessive tearing, conjunctivitis, corneal opacity and ulceration	Not commonly seen
Giardia duodenalis	Small intestines	7-10 days	Smooth, clear, thin-walled cyst with 2-4 nuclei; 4-10 × 8-16 µ	Fecal flotation	Ingestion of cyst stage	Predominantly diarrhea	
			Piriform, bilaterally symmetric greenish trophozoite with 2 nuclei and 4 pair of flagella; 9-20 × 5-15 µ	Direct smear			
Trichomonads	Digestive tract		Spindle-shaped to piriform trophozoite with 3-5 anterior flagella, an undulating membrane and 1 posterior flagellum	Direct smear	Ingestion of trophozoite	Diarrhea	
Cryptosporidium spp.	Small and large intestines	4-10 days	Clear, thin-walled, spherical oocyst containing 4 sporozoites; 5 × 5 µ	Fecal flotation	Ingestion of oocysts	Diarrhea, dehydration, anorexia	

Table 4-2 Diagnostic characteristics of blood parasites of domestic animals

Parasite	Definitive host	Location	Prepatient period	Diagnostic stage	Diagnostic test
Babesia spp.	Humans, dogs, cattle, horses	Blood (erythrocytes)	10-21 days	Paired piriform (tear-shaped) merozoites in erythrocytes	Romanowsky-stained blood film, indirect fluorescent antibody test
Trypanosoma spp.	Humans, dogs, cats, cattle, sheep, horses	Blood and lymph, heart, striated muscle, reticuloendothelial muscle	Acute and chronic disease	Trypanosome form, spindle-shaped flagellate with undulating membrane, central nucleus and kinetoplast, found in blood Amastigote form, intracellular spherical bodies with single nucleus and rod-shaped kinetoplast, found in myocardium, striated muscle cells, and macrophages	Blood smears; xenodiagnosis (clean vector allowed to feed on suspect patient and organism isolated from the vector), biopsy, animal inoculation, serology
Leishmania donovani	Humans, dogs	Intracellular in cytoplasm of macrophages of reticuloendothelial system	Several months up to 1 year	Amastigote form, oval, single nucleus, with a rod-shaped kinetoplast, in clusters within the cytoplasm of macrophages	Impression smears and biopsy of skin, lymph nodes, and bone marrow

From Johnson EM: Diagnostic parasitology. In Pratt PW: ***Principles and practice of veterinary technology***, St Louis, 1998, Mosby.

Table 4-3 Zoonotic internal parasites

Parasite	Host	Reservoir	Infective stage	Condition
Toxocara spp.	Dogs, cats	Dogs, cats	Egg with L2	Visceral larva migrans
Ancylostoma spp.	Dogs, cats	Dogs, cats	L3	Cutaneous larva migrans
Uncinaria stenocephala	Dogs, cats	Dogs, cats	L3	Cutaneous larva migrans
Toxoplasma gondii	Cats	Cats, raw meat	Sporulated oocyst, bradyzoite, tachyzoite	Toxoplasmosis
Strongyloides stercoralis	Dogs, cats, humans	Humans, dogs, cats	L3	Strongyloidiasis
Dipylidium caninum	Dogs, cats, humans	Flea	Cysticercoid	Cestodiasis
Taenia saginata	Humans	Bovine muscle	Cysticercus	Cestodiasis
Taenia solium	Humans	Porcine muscle	Cysticercus	Cestodiasis
	Humans	Humans	Egg	Cysticercosis
Echinococcus granulosus	Dogs	Dogs	Egg	Hydatidosis
Echinococcus multilocularis	Dogs, cats	Dogs, cats	Egg	Hydatidosis
Spirometra mansonoides	Dogs, cats	Unknown	Procercoid in arthropod	Sparganosis
Sarcocystis spp.	Humans	Cattle, pigs	Sarcocyst in muscle	Sarcocystiasis
	Dogs, cats	Dogs, cats	Oocyst	Sarcosporidiosis
Cryptosporidium parvum	Mammals	Mammals	Oocyst	Cryptosporidiosis
Balantidium coli	Humans, pigs	Humans, pigs	Cyst, trophozoite	Balantidiasis
Ascaris suum	Pigs	Pigs	Egg with L2	Visceral larva migrans
Trichinella spiralis	Mammals	Porcine and bear muscle	Encysted L3	Trichinellosis
Thelazia spp.	Mammals	Fly	L3	Verminous conjunctivitis
Giardia duodenalis	Mammals	Mammals	Cyst	Giardiasis
Babesia microti	Rodents, humans	Hard tick	Sporozoite	Babesiosis
Trypanosoma	Mammals	Reduviids	Trypanosomal form in kissing bug	Chagas' disease
Leishmania donovani	Mammals	Phlebotomine fly	Leptomonad form in sandfly	Leishmaniasis

From Johnson EM: Diagnostic parasitology. In Pratt PW: ***Principles and practice of veterinary technology***, St. Louis 1998, Mosby.

Table 4-4 Common parasites in laboratory animals

Parasite/hosts	Transmission	Clinical signs	Diagnosis
Pinworms			
Syphacia obvelata, mice/hamsters	Ingestion of infective egg Retroinfection	Usually none Heavy infections; impaction, intussusception, rectal prolapse,	Eggs are thin walled Flattened along one side measuring 100-142 × 30-40 μ
Syphacia muris, rats	Eggs hatch in perianal region, and larvae migrate back into the colon	Poor growth rate	Eggs larvate within 6-24 hours *S. muris:* eggs measure 72-82× 25-36 μ
Aspiculuris tetraptera, mouse	Ingestion of infective egg	Often none	Eggs on fecal float are elliptical, thin shelled 89-93 × 36-42 μ
Passalurus ambiguous, rabbit	Ingestion of infective egg	Usually none Large numbers in young animals may cause gastric disturbances	Eggs are slightly flattened, 95-103 × 43 μ
Tapeworms (dwarf)	Ingestion of egg	Heavy infection in mice can cause weight loss, poor growth, intestinal	Eggs are oval with a hexacanth larvae 40-45 × 34-37 μ
Hymenolepis nana, mouse rat hamster	Ingestion of cysticercoid in paratenic host Autoinfection	Heavy infection in hamsters can cause intestinal occlusion and impaction	

Table 4-4 Common parasites in laboratory animals—cont'd

Parasite/hosts	Transmission	Clinical signs	Diagnosis
Hymenolepis diminuta, mouse/rat/hamster	Ingestion of cysticercoid	Usually none	Eggs semispherical 60-66 with dark outer capsule, hexacanth larvae
Cysticerus pisiformis, rabbit	Larval stage of *Taenia pisiformis*	Cysts in peritoneal cavity Heavy infection; abdominal distention	Cysticercus with opaque body at one end with an inverted scolex
Multiceps seralis, rabbit	Larval stage of *Taenia multiceps*	Swelling, puffy skin	Cyst in subcutaneous tissue (may be palpable)
Coccidia			
Eimeria spp., E. separata, rat	Ingestion of sporulated oocysts	Nonpathogenic	Smooth-walled ellipsoidal oocysts 10-19 × 10-17 μ
Eimeria spp., mouse	Ingestion of sporulated oocysts	Nonpathogenic—moderate infections causing diarrhea	Typical oocyst
Eimeria caviae, guinea pig	Ingestion of sporulated oocysts	Usually none Heavy infections; diarrhea, anorexia, lethargy, death	Smooth, oval, light brown oocyst measuring 13-26 × 12-23 μ
Eimeria spp., rabbits	Ingestion of sporulated oocysts	Mild to severe Heavy infection; anorexia, severe diarrhea, distended abdomen, death	Characteristic oocysts
Cryptosporidium sp.	Ingestion of oocyst	Diarrhea	Smooth walled oocyst 7 × 5 μ
Klossiella muris, mouse *Klossiella cobayae* *Klossiella caviae*, guinea pig	Ingestion of sporocyst	None—mild nephritis	Sporocyst passed in the urine
Fleas			
Leptopsylla segnis, mouse		None Intermediate host for *H. dimunita* and *H. nana*	Very small flea 1-3 mm in length
Spilopsyllus cuniculi, rabbit		Adults feed in clumps inside pinna Vector of myxoma virus	1.2-1.5 mm in length Head long and slender
Lice			
Polyplax spinulosa, rat	Direct contact	Large numbers cause irritation and anemia	Three pairs of legs end in clasping claws
Polyplax serrata, mice		Vector for *Haemobartonella muris* (rat) Vector for Eperythrozoon coccoides (mice)	Eggs laid on host cemented firmly to the base of the hair
Gliricola porcelli, guinea pig		General body surface	Broad head, elongated body Eggs have distinctive operculum
Gryopus ovalis, guinea pig		Preference for head and face	Broad head Eggs with operculum
Mites			
Fur dwelling			
Myobia musculi	Direct contact	Mange head and face	First pair of legs modified for gripping hair
Radfordia		Mange shoulders and back	Myobia—one claw on second pair of legs Radfordia—two claws on the second pair of legs
Mycoptes musculins, rat mouse		Mange shoulders and back	
Cheyletiella parasitivorax	Direct contact	Occasional mange shoulders and back	Medium-sized mite, very active, yellowish white body
		None	Short palpi with claw curving inward

Continued

Table 4-4 Common parasites in laboratory animals—cont'd

Parasite/hosts	Transmission	Clinical signs	Diagnosis
Listorphorus gibbus, rabbit			*Listorphorus* sp smaller mite, body laterally compressed, broad head
Chirodiscoides caviae, guinea pig	Direct contact	None	Small mite, twice as long as broad
Surface dwelling			
Psoroptes cuniculi, rabbit	Direct contact	Ear cankers	Macroscopic, moving rapidly inside ear pinnae
Scarcoptes sp. *Notoedres* sp., mice/rats/rabbit	Transfer of larvae and nymphs	Located in epidermal tunnels Causes generalized mange and alopecia	Round, fat mites, Short stubby legs Nonjointed pedicles
Follicle dwelling			
Demodex sp., hamster/ gerbil/rat		Mite found in hair follicles Dry, scaly skin with scabby lesions	Cigar-shaped mite with stumpy limbs placed evenly along the body

Table 4-5 Ectoparasites: general

Parasite/host	Transmission and life cycle	Clinical signs and location	Diagnosis
Melophagus ovinus (sheep ked)	Obligatory parasite; spends entire life on host	Rubbing and scratching causes damage to wool and skin Large numbers can cause anemia	Macroscopic
Hypoderma spp. (cattle grub)	Fly → egg → larva (migrate through host) → pupate on ground	Irritation to cattle, reduced weight gain, milk production, economic loss at slaughter	Macroscopic
Oestrus ovis nasal bot (sheep, goat)	Fly (L1-L3 in host) → pupate on ground	Nasal discharge, sneezing, rubbing nose	Macroscopic
Cuterbra spp. (lagomorph, dog, cat)	Fly → egg on ground, L1 on host migrate to L3 → pupate on ground	Fibrotic cyst in subcutaneous tissue Secondary infection with abcessation	Macroscopic
		LICE	
Anoplura (sucking)		Lice on skin usually in areas that can be protected from being rubbed off Pruritic	Adult, dorsoventrally flattened, head narrower than thorax; nymph,small adult; egg (nit) elongate, operculate, glued to hairs
Haematopinus spp.	Cattle, pig, horse		
Linognathus spp.	Dog, cattle, sheep		
Solenopotes sp.	Cattle		
Pediculus spp.	Humans		
Mallophaga (biting)		Lice on skin and hair; cause rubbing and scratching	Adult, dorsoventrally flattened, head wider than thorax; nymph, small adult; egg elongate operculate, whitish
Damalinia spp.	Horse, cattle, sheep		
Felicola subrostratus	Cat		
Trichodectes canis	Dog		
		FLEAS	
Ctenocephalides spp.	Dog, cat	Adult on skin of host; larvae and pupae in the bedding/ living area of host; can cause flea allergy dermatitis	Adults seen grossly Flea "dirt" (feces) on host

Table 4-5 Ectoparasites: general—cont'd

Parasite/host	Transmission and life cycle	Clinical signs and location	Diagnosis
		TICKS	
Hard		Vectors for Rocky Mountain spotted fever, tularemia, Q fever	Scutum ornate; basis capitulum parallel sided, palps short with festoons
Dermacentor spp.	Dog, cat three-host tick		
Ixodes scapularis	Animals, humans three-host tick	Vector for Lyme disease *(Borrelia burgdorferi)*	Scutum ornate; basis capitulum parallel sided, palps long, without festoons
Rhipicephalus sanguineus	Primarily dog three-host tick	Vector for *Babesia canis* and *Ehrlichia canis*	Scutum ornate; basis capitulum angular, palps short, with festoons
Soft			
Argasid	Birds	Not routinely seen	Soft ticks have a leathery dorsal surface that lacks a hard plate (scutum)
		MITES	
Sarcoptes spp. pig, dog, cat, horse, cattle, humans	Egg → larvae → nymph → adult all takes place on the host Transmission by direct contact	Scratching, chewing, self-excoriation causing crust and scab formation Secondary infections can occur	Round mite with short stubby legs; posterior two pairs not extending beyond margins of the body; long unsegmented pedicles; dorsal spines
Demodex spp. dog, cat, cattle, goat, humans	Adults in hair follicles lay eggs, larvae and nymphs at mouth of follicles Transmission by direct contact	More common in dogs Lesions consist of varying degrees of scaling, alopecia, erythema, hyperpigmentation	Adult, anterior half of mite; eggs elongate; stubbly legs on adults may be seen on fecal float
Cheyletiella spp. dog, cat, rabbit (also called "walking dandruff")	All stages on host, mites feed on epidermal debris Transmission by direct contact	Dorsal seborrhea, generally non-pruritic	Adult, oval, long legs that extend beyond the margins of the body; terminal appendage on each leg is a fine comblike structure
Chorioptes spp. cattle, sheep, goat, horse	Mites live on surface of the skin Transmission by direct contact	Tail mange: cattle Scrotal mange: sheep Leg mange: horse	Adult, oval, long legs that extend beyond the margins of the body; pedicles are short and unsegmented with large suckers
Psoroptes spp. cattle, sheep, goat, horse	Transmission by direct contact or with infested material	Pruritus, alopecia Skin becomes thick and wrinkled Animals may become emaciated and die Not commonly seen	Adults, oval, long legs that extend beyond the margins of the body; pedicles are long and segmented

Table 4-6 Anthelmintics registered in Canada for use in dogs (D) and cats (C)—2002

Compound	Trade name	Manufacturer	*Toxocara* spp.	*Toxascaris leonina*	*Ancylostoma* spp.	*Uncinaria stenocephala*	*Trichuris vulpis*	*Dipylidium caninum*	*Taenia* spp.	*Echinococcus* spp.	*Dirofilaria immitis*	*Ctenocephalides* spp.	*Otodectes cynotis*	*Sarcoptes scabiei*
Piperazine	Once-a-month roundworm treatment for dogs and cats	Beaphar	DC	DC										
Pyrantel pamoate	Pyran	P.V.U. (Merial)	DC	D	DC	D								
	Pyr-a-Pam	Pfizer	DC	D	DC	D								
	Pyr-a-Pam II	Pfizer	DC	D	DC	D								
Pyrantel pamoate + oxantel pamoate	Pyr-a-Pam Plus	Pfizer	D	D	D	D	D							
Ivermectin + pyrantel pamoate	Heartgard-30 Plus	Merial	D	D	D	D					D*			
Milbemycin	Interceptor	Novartis	DC	D	DC		D				DC*			
Lufenuron + milbemycin	Sentinel	Novartis	D	D	D		D				D*	D		
Nitroscanate	Lopatol	Novartis	D	D	D	D		D	D					
Fenbendazole	Panacur	Intervet	D	D	D	D	D		D					
Praziquantel + pyrantel pamoate + febantel	Drontal Plus	Bayer	D	D	D	D	D	D	D	D				
Praziquantel + pyrantel pamoate	Drontal	Bayer	C		C			C	C					
Praziquantel	Droncit	Bayer						DC	DC	D				
	Prazarid	Bimeda-MTC						DC	DC	D				
Epsiprantel	Cestex	Pfizer						DC	DC					
Ivermectin	Heartgard-30	Merial			C						DC*			
(Moxidectin)	(ProHeart 6)	(Ayerst)			D						D*			
Diethylcarbamazine	Decacide	P.V.L.	DC	DC							D*			
Melarsomine	Immiticide	Merial									D			
Lufenuron	Program	Novartis										DC		
Selamectin	Revolution	Pfizer	C		C						DC*	DC	DC	D

Table was produced by Andrew S. Peregrine.
*, Preventive activity; (), not yet licensed.

Table 4-7 Anthelmintics registered in Canada for use in horses—2002

Anthelmintic	Trade name	Manufacturer	*Anoplocephala perfoliata*	*Draschia megastoma*	*Habronema* spp.	*Gasterophilus* spp.	*Trichostrongylus* spp.	*Strongyloides westeri*	*Parascaris equorum*	*Strongylus* spp.	Small strongyles	*Oxyuris equi*	*Onchocerca cervicalis*
Ivermectin	Eqvalan	Merial		1	A+1	O/G	A	A	A+2	A+3	A+4	A+4	7
	Equimectrin	A.P.A		1	A+1	O/G	A	A	A+2	A+3	A+4	A+4	7
	Zimecterin												
Moxidectin	Quest	Ayerst			A	O/G	A		A+4	A+5	A+6	A+4	
Febantel + trichlorfon	Equitron 2	Davis & Lawrence				O/G			A	A	A	A+4	
Oxibendazole	Anthelcide EQ	Pfizer						A	A	A	A	A+4	
Oxfendazole	Benzelmin	Ayerst							A	A+3	A	A+4	
Fenbendazole	Panacur Paste	Intervet							A	A	A	A	
	Safe-Guard Paste	Intervet							A	A	A	A	
	Safe-Guard Suspension	Intervet							A	A	A	A	
Pyrantel tartrate	Strongid-C	Pfizer							A+4	A	A+4	A+4	
Pyrantel pamoate	Strongid-P	Pfizer	A						A	A	A	A	
	Strongid-T	Pfizer	A						A	A	A	A	
Piperazine	Co-op Wormer	IPCO							A		A	A	
	52%	A.P.A							A		A	A	
	Piperazine 52	JAMP							A		A		
	Worazine 53%	Dominion							A		A		
	Piperazine Dihydrochloride	Dominion							A		A		
	Super Pip-Zine 34												

Table was produced by Andrew S. Peregrine.
Activity against: *A*, adult parasites; *O/G*, oral and gastric stages; *1*, cutaneous larvae; *2*, L_4 and L_3; *3*, arterial larval stages of *S. vulgaris; 4*, L_4; *5*, arterial larval stages of *S. vulgaris* + tissue stages of *S. edentatus; 6*, late L_3, L_4 mucosal larvae, and undifferentiated lumen larvae; *7*, microfilariae.

Table 4-8 Antiparasitic compounds registered in Canada for use in cattle—2002

Compound	Trade name	Manufacturer	*Bunostomum* spp.	*Chorioptes*	*Coccidia*	*Cooperia* spp.	*Damalinia bovis*	*Dictyocaulus* spp.	*Fasciola* spp.	*Haematobia irritans*	*Haematopinus*	*Haemonchus* spp.	*Hypoderma* spp.	*Linognathus vituli*	*Moniezia* spp.	*Nematodirus* spp.	*Oesophagostomum* spp.	*Ostertagia* spp.	*Psoroptes*	*Sarcoptes scablei*	*Solenopotes*	*Strongyloides* spp.	*Thelazia* spp.	*Trichostrongylus* spp.	*Trichuris* spp.
Oxfendazole	Synanthic Suspension	Ayerst				A						A					A	A						A	
Morantel	Banminth II	Phibro				A						A				A	A	A						A	
Levamisole	Tramisol Powder	Ayerst	A			A		A				A				A	A	A						A	
Fenbendazole	SafeGuard Suspension	Intervet	A			A		A1				A1				A	A	A1						A1	
	Panacur Suspension	Intervet	A1			A1		A1				A1				A1	A1	A1						A	
	SafeGuard Premix	Intervet	A1			A1		A1				A1				A1	A1	A1						A1	
Albendazole	Valbazen	Pfizer	A			A1		A1	A			A			A	A	A	A2						A	
Ivermectin	Ivomec SR Bolus	Merial	cA			cA		c2			A	cA	IP	A		cA	cA	c2	A	A				cA	A
	Ivomec Pour-On	Merial		A		A	A	A1		A	A	A1	IP	A		L4	A1	A2		A		A	A	A1	A
	Ivomec Injection	Merial				A1		A1			A	A1	IP	A			A1	A2	A	A	A	A	A	A1	

Doramectin	Dectomax Injection	Pfizer	A			A1		A1			A	A1	IP	A		A	A1	A2	A	A	A	A	A	A1	A
	Dectomax Pour-On	Pfizer	A	A		A1	A	A1		A	A	A1	IP	A			A1	A2		A	A		A	A1	A
Moxidectin	Cydectin Injection	Ayerst	A1			A1		A1			A	A1	IP	A		A1	A1	A2	A		A			A1	A
	Cydectin Pour-On	Ayerst	A	A		A	A	A1			A	A1	IP	A		A1	A	A2	A	A	A			A1	
Eprinomectin	Ivomec Eprinex	Merial	A1	A		A2	A	A1		A	A	A1	IP	A		A1	A1	A2		A	A			A1	A
Amprolium	Amprol 9.6% Solution	Merial			T																				
	Amprol 25% FeedMix	Merial			TP																				
Triple S*	Cocci Bol-O-Tab	Intervet			TP																				
Decoquinate	Deccox	Alpharma			P																				
Lasalocid	Bovatec Premix	Alpharma			P																				
Monensin	Rumensin	Elanco			P																				
Sulfametha-zine	Neo-Sulfalyte	Pfizer			T																				
	Boluses	Citadel			P																				
	Sodium Sulfametha-zine 25%; Sulfa 25%	Bimeda-MTC			P																				

Table was produced by Andrew S. Peregrine.
A, Activity against adult parasites; *A1*, activity against adult parasites and L_4; *A2*, activity against adult parasites, L_4 and inhibited L_4; *IP*, activity against internal parasitic stages; *cA*, prevents establishment of newly ingested L_3 for 135 days, and activity against adult parasites; *c2*, prevents establishment of newly ingested L_3 for 135 days, and activity against both adult parasites and hypobiotic stage; *, sulfacetamide, sulfabenzamide, sulfaquinoxaline; *T*, therapeutic activity; *P*, preventive activity; *L4*, activity against L_4.

Table 4-9 Antiparasitic compounds registered in Canada for use in pigs—2002

Compound	Trade name	Manufacturer	*Ascaris* spp.	*Strongyloides ransomi*	*Hyostrongylus rubidus*	*Oesophagostomum* spp.	*Trichuris suis*	*Metastrongylus* spp.	*Haematopinus suis*	*Sarcoptes scabiei*	*Stephanurus dentatus*	*Ascarops strongylina*
Pyrantel	Pro-Banminth Premix	Phibro	⊕									
Hygromycin B	Hygromix 8	Elanco	⊕			⊕						
Piperazine	Co-op Wormer 52%	IPCO	A			A						
	Piperazine 34	A.P.A.	A			A						
	Piperazine 52	A.P.A.	A			A						
	Piperazine Dihydrochloride	Dominion	A			A						
	Super Pip-Zine 34	Dominion	A			A						
	Worazine 53%	JAMP	A			A						
Morantel	Banminth II 20% Premix	Phibro	A+1		A	A + 1						
Dichlorvos	Atgard C	Boehringer	A+1			A+1	A + 1					
Levamisole	Tramisol Soluble Pig Wormer	Ayerst	A	A	A	A		A				
	Tramisol Soluble Powder	Ayerst	A	A	A	A		A				
Fenbendazole	Safe-Guard Premix 20%	Intervet	A + 1		A	A	A+1	A				
Ivermectin	Ivomec Injection for Cattle, Sheep and Swine	Merial	A+1	A+2	A+1	A + 1		A	A	A		
	Ivomec Premix for Swine	Merial	A+1	A+2	A + 1	A+1		A	A	A	A+1	A
Doramectin	Dectomax Injectable Solution	Pfizer	A + 1	A	A+1	A+1		A	A	A	A	

Table was produced by Andrew S. Peregrine.
A, Adult parasites; *1*, L_4; *2*, somatic larvae; ⊕, prevention of registration and establishment.

Table 4-10 Antiparasitic compounds registered in Canada for use in sheep—2002

Compound	Trade name	Manufacturer	*Bunostomum* spp.	*Chabertia* spp.	*Coccidia*	*Cooperia* spp.	*Dictyocaulus* spp.	*Haemonchus* spp.	*Nematodirus* spp.	*Oesophagostomum* spp.	*Oestrus ovis*	*Ostertagia* spp.	*Strongyloides* spp.	*Trichostrongylus* spp.	*Trichuris* spp.
Levamisole	Tramisol Sheep Wormer Oblets	Ayerst	A	A		A	A	A	A	A		A		A	
	Tramisol Soluble Powder	Ayerst	A	A		A	A	A	A	A		A		A	
Ivermectin	Ivomec Injection for Cattle, Sheep and Swine	Merial		A1		A1	A1	A1		A1	L	A1		A1	A
	Ivomec Drench for Sheep	Merial		A		A1	A1	A1	A	A1	L	A1	A	A1	A
Sulfamethazine	Sodium sulfamethazine 25%	Citadel			T										
	Sulfa 25%	Bimeda-MTC			T										
Sulfacetamide/ sulfabenzamide/ sulfaquinoxaline	Cocci Bol-O-Tab	Intervet			TP										
	Cocci Bol-O-Tab Jr.	Intervet			TP										

Table was produced by Andrew S. Peregrine.
A, Activity against adult parasites; *A1,* activity against adult parasites and L_4; *L,* activity against all larval stages; *T,* therapeutic activity; *P,* preventive activity.

Glossary

acariasis Infestion by mites

anthelmintic "Against worms"; therefore a drug used to remove worms

arthropod Invertebrate animals having segmented external coverings and jointed legs (e.g., ticks and mites)

Baermann technique Generally used for removing lungworm larvae from small amounts of feces

cestode Commonly called "tapeworms"; flat, segmented worms

efficacy Effectiveness of a drug

ELISA Enzyme-linked immunosorbent assay

final host Normal host or definitive host; type of animal in which the adult worm is found

hexacanth Infective stage of development in a cestode egg after fertilization takes place

infective Developed to a stage capable of causing infection

intermediate host Any organism in which a parasite lives during its larval or non-reproductive stage

mange Infestation by mites

meniscus Curved upper surface of a liquid on the top of a container

morulated Solid mass of cells clustered together

myiasis Invasion of living tissue by fly maggots

nematode Free-living or parasitic unsegmented worms, usually cylindrical and elongated in shape and tapering at the extremities

non-infective Not yet developed to a stage capable of causing infection

OVC Ontario Veterinary College

paratenic host One in which the parasite does not develop to adult, remains alive for long periods of time, and does not rely on host exclusively to complete its life cycle

PCV Packed cell volume

pediculosis Infestation by lice

prepatent infection Occurs when worms have not yet developed to mature adults; therefore no eggs are being shed and a diagnosis is not possible by fecal examination or other laboratory testing

prepatent period (ppp) Period of time between infection of the host and when eggs or larvae can be recovered by laboratory methods

protozoa A unicellular organism

rpm Rotations per minute

trematode Group of parasites that are hermaphroditic, have two suckers (oral and ventral), and require an intermediate host, commonly called "flukes"

zoonosis Disease that can be transmitted to humans

Review Questions

1 ELISA tests can detect
   a. *Dirofilaria immitis*
   b. *Dirofilaria* antigen
   c. Microfilaria
   d. Only occult heartworm

2 *Eimeria steidae* is associated with
   a. Hepatic coccidiosis in rabbits
   b. Cecal coccidiosis in chickens
   c. Renal coccidiosis in geese
   d. Intestinal coccidiosis in dogs

3 Biting lice have which characteristic?
   a. Head wider than thorax
   b. Feed on blood
   c. Narrower head than thorax
   d. Barely move

4 Cutaneous larval migrans is caused by
   a. *Toxocara cati*
   b. *Trichuris vulpis*
   c. *Ancylostoma caninum*
   d. *Aeleurostrongylus* sp.

5 Visceral larval migrans is caused by ingestion of
   a. *Echinococcus* sp.
   b. *Toxocara* sp.
   c. *Uncinaria* sp.
   d. *Dioctophyma renale*

6 The intermediate host for the bovine tapeworm *Moniezia* sp. is a
   a. Bird
   b. Pasture mite
   c. Snail
   d. Mudworm

7 *Eimeria* spp. when sporulated contain
   a. Four sporocysts with two sporozoites
   b. Two sporocysts with four sporozoites
   c. One sporocyst with three sporozoites
   d. None of the above

8 The term "pediculosis" means
   a. Infestation by mites
   b. Invasion of living tissue by fly maggots
   c. Intense itching and hair loss
   d. Infestation by lice

9 Which of the following is not true about ticks?
   a. Often carry disease-causing organisms
   b. Are generally picked up from wooded areas
   c. Feed on blood
   d. Are microscopic

10 The prepatent period for *Dirofilaria immitis* is
   a. 6.5 weeks
   b. 3 months
   c. 8 months
   d. 6.5 months

BIBLIOGRAPHY

Barta JR: *Principles of disease,* lecture notes from Veterinary Parasitology, Ontario Veterinary College, 2001, Guelph, Ontario, Canada.

Coles EH: *Veterinary clinical pathology,* ed 3, Philadelphia, 1980, WB Saunders.

Flynn RJ: *Parasites of laboratory animals,* Ames, 1973, Iowa State University Press.

Georgi JR: *Parasitology for veterinarians,* ed 3, Philadelphia, 1974, WB Saunders.

Harkness JE, Wagner JE: *The biology and medicine of rabbits and rodents,* ed 3, Philadelphia, 1988, Lea & Febiger.

Hendrix CM: *Laboratory procedures for veterinary technicians,* ed 4, St Louis, 2002, Mosby.

Ivens VR et al: *Principal parasites of domestic animals in the U.S.,* Urbana, IL, 1989, University of Illinois.

Lautenslagerb P: *Notes from veterinary parasitology for animal health technicians,* Centralia, Ontario, Canada, 1982, Centralia College.

Owen DG: *Parasites of laboratory animals, Handbook #12,* London, 1992, Royal Society of Medicine Services Ltd.

Peregrine A: *Anthelmintics registered in Canada, principles of disease in veterinary medicine,* lecture notes from Veterinary Parasitology, Guelph, Ontario, Canada, 2001, Ontario Veterinary College.

Pratt PW: *Principles and practice of veterinary technology,* St Louis, 1998, Mosby.

Sloss MW, Kemp RL: *Veterinary clinical parasitology,* Ames, 1978, Iowa State University Press.

APPENDIX

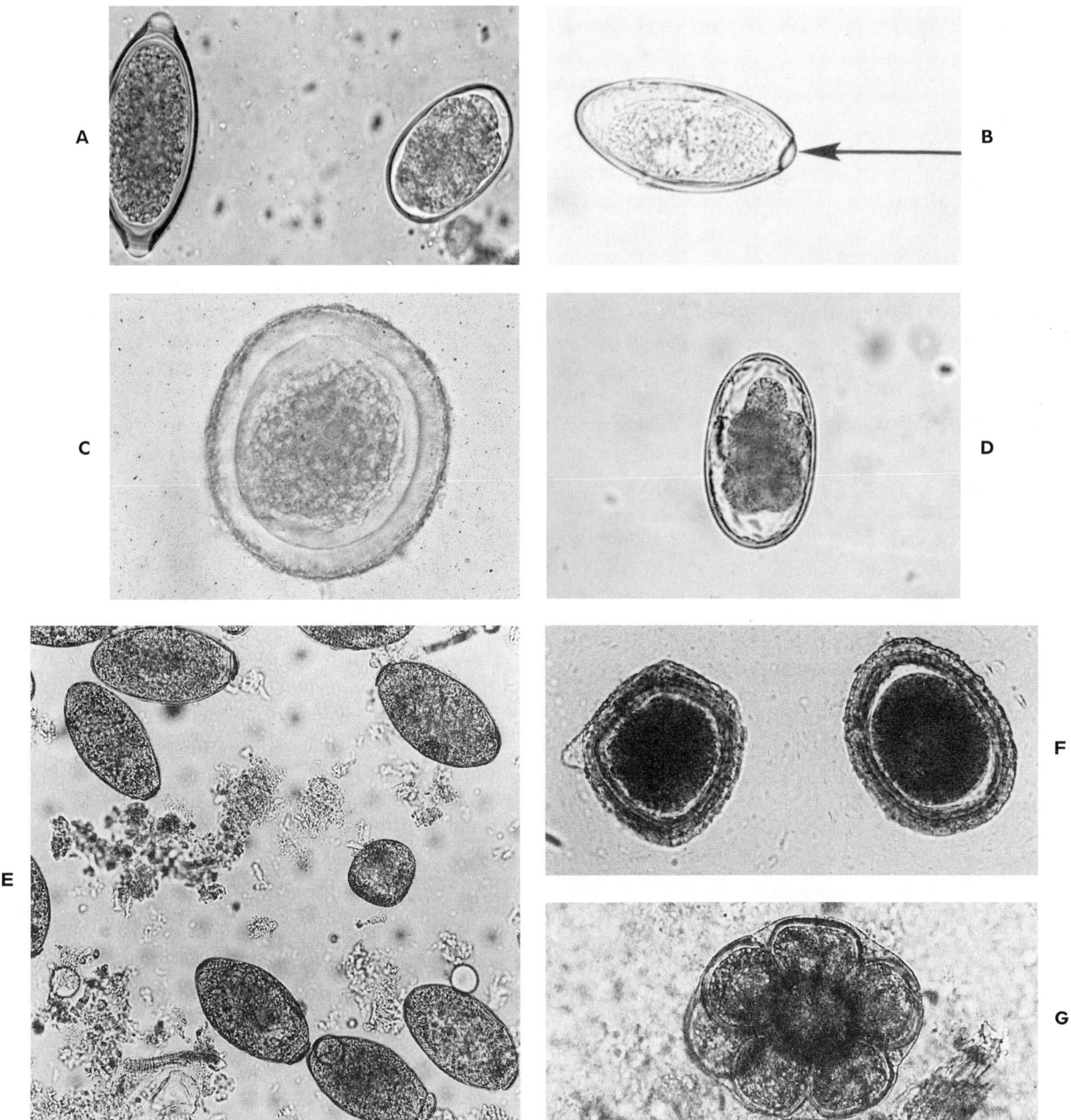

Figure A-1 **A,** *Trichuris vulpis and Ancylostoma caninum.* **B,** *Oxyuris equi.* **C,** *Parascaris equorum.* **D,** Strongyle-type ovum. **E,** *Fasciola hepatica/Moniezia* sp. **F,** *Toxocara canis.* **G,** *Dipylidium caninum.*

CHAPTER 5

Diagnostic Microbiology and Mycology

Sandra McCampbell

OUTLINE

LEARNING OUTCOMES

After reading this chapter you should be able to:

1. List and describe equipment needed to perform diagnostic microbiology.
2. Describe and list the purposes of various bacterial and fungal media.
3. Describe the types of samples that may be obtained from the body for microbiological culture.
4. Describe the collection of specimens.
5. Explain bacterial identification procedures for gram-positive and gram-negative bacteria.
6. Explain fungal identification.
7. Describe how to perform various diagnostic tests to identify specific bacteria and fungi.

Microbiology is the study of microscopic organisms. *Clinical microbiology* is the identification of these organisms, including bacteria, fungi, parasites, and viruses, that cause clinical illness. In this chapter we will explore the fundamental components of a working clinical microbiology laboratory, the most common causes of bacterial and fungal diseases of domestic animals, and how to use this information to assist the veterinarian in the diagnosis and treatment of these diseases.

PURPOSE

The purpose of a veterinary clinical microbiology laboratory is to

I. Assist the veterinarian in the diagnosis and treatment of bacteriological and fungal disease
II. Provide accurate identification of the causes of infections
III. Provide useful information about the organisms cultured (i.e., antibiotic sensitivity)

IV. Maintain cost- and time-effectiveness while presenting all of the above
  A. Many practices send out cultures to commercial laboratories because their low volume of samples makes keeping media impractical
  B. Competent staff must be available to perform microbiological procedures
  C. Clients may benefit from the quick turnaround time of an in-house laboratory

EQUIPMENT

Light Microscope

I. Probably the most expensive piece of equipment needed
II. Parts of a light microscope
  A. Eyepiece(s): one in a monocular microscope; two in a binocular microscope. The eyepiece(s) magnify the viewed field 5, 10, or 15 times (×5, ×10, or ×15; most are ×10). A binocular microscope is more expensive but is preferred because of the ease in viewing and increased clarity
  B. Light source: an attached, internal lightbulb with a variable intensity best illuminates the viewed slide
  C. Light condenser: another means of increasing or decreasing the amount of light on the slide; most good microscopes have two: one directly above the light source and one under the stage
  D. Stage: the platform on which the slide is placed for viewing; most stages are movable by means of two knobs on the side of the microscope: one for horizontal movement and one for vertical movement
  E. Objectives: magnify the specimen
  F. Focus: most microscopes have two types of focus-adjusting knobs: a coarse focus for initially viewing the specimen and a fine focus for sharpening the image
III. Many different models available; for use in a clinical microbiology laboratory, must have at least three objectives
  A. ×10 (dry): used to scan the slide
  B. ×40 (dry): used to identify fungal elements
  C. ×100 (oil immersion): used to differentiate stained bacteria

Incubator

An incubator allows an organism to be grown under controlled conditions. There are many different types of incubators available, but for most clinical microbiology laboratories all that is needed is an incubator that keeps the specimens at 37° C (98.6° F), which is human body temperature, and room air oxygen concentration.

I. Most cultures are grown overnight and held at least 48 hours
II. Most veterinary cultures are grown at 37° C (98.6° F), including reptile and amphibian cultures
  A. Even though reptiles and amphibians are poikilothermic (i.e., their bodies stay at ambient temperature), most organisms present will grow at 37° C (98.6° F)
  B. This temperature is especially critical when performing such standardized tests as the Kirby-Bauer sensitivity

Sterilizing Heat Sources

I. Bunsen burner
  A. Attaches to gas wall outlets
  B. Allows flame to be ignited with a spark striker
  C. Quickly sterilizes the metal loop used for transferring microorganisms to be inoculated into growing media
  D. Also used to heat fix slides for staining procedures
II. Electric heating element
  A. Usually ceramic, an enclosed heater that sterilizes metal loops
  B. Eliminates the need for a natural gas source
  C. Provides more even heating of loop
III. Alcohol lamps
  A. Usually a small glass lamp with a wick that extends into alcohol in the base
  B. Wick must be ignited with another flame source (i.e., matches)
  C. Does not sterilize metal loops as quickly or thoroughly as a Bunsen burner
  D. Less expensive than above options

Media

I. MUST CHOOSE APPROPRIATE TYPE OF MEDIA FOR ISOLATION NEEDS
  A. Nutritive media grow all types of bacteria (and some fungi)
  B. Selective media grow only certain types of bacteria (e.g., gram-negative or gram-positive types) or fungi
  C. Differential media contain elements that differentiate certain types of bacteria (e.g., lactose fermenters [LFs] or hydrogen sulfide [H_2S] producers)
II. All media must be examined for accidental bacterial/fungal contaminants before use
III. All media plates are incubated upside down (media side up) to prevent condensation from dripping onto cultures

Miscellaneous Equipment

I. Metal loop: for transferring bacterial or fungal specimens onto media or slides; many sizes are available
II. Glass microscope slides: for placing a specimen to be examined under the microscope
III. Wooden applicator sticks: disposable; used when performing quick identification tests
IV. Sterile cotton-tipped applicators: many uses, including applying specimens to media or microscope slide
V. Wax or permanent markers: to identify specimens on media or slides
VI. Filter paper: used to perform some identification tests

BACTERIOLOGICAL AND FUNGAL MEDIA

Basic Media

I. Agar: a semisolid media
II. Broth: a liquid media
III. Plate: a flat, round container of agar
IV. Tube: a screw-top container; can contain broth or agar
V. Slant: a tube of agar that has been allowed to gel at an angle
VI. Selective media: contain compounds that inhibit growth of certain types of organisms
VII. Differential media: contain compounds that identify certain characteristics of organisms grown on the media

Specific Types of Media

I. Trypticase Soy Agar with 5% Sheep's Blood (TSA) also referred to as Blood Agar Plate (BAP)
   A. General, nutritive medium for cultivation of fastidious microorganisms
   B. Used for the observation of bacterial hemolytic reactions
II. MacConkey II Agar (MAC)
   A. Selects for gram-negative organisms using crystal violet as a gram-positive bacterial inhibitor
   B. Differentiates between lactose fermenters (LFs) and non–lactose fermenters (NLFs) using a neutral red indicator that colors LF colonies purple
   C. Designed to inhibit the swarming of *Proteus* spp. bacteria
III. Columbia Colistin–Nalidixic Acid Agar (CNA) with 5% Sheep Blood
   A. Selects for gram-positive organisms using colistin and naladixic acid
IV. *Salmonella-Shigella* Agar (SS)
   A. Selects for pathogenic enteric gram-negative bacteria
   B. Differentiates colonies on the basis of lactose fermentation [see MacConkey II Agar (MAC)]
   C. Differentiates H_2S-producing bacteria by use of ferric citrate in the formula, which produce black pigment in their presence
V. Mueller-Hinton Agar (MH)
   A. General-use medium specially formulated to give standardized results during antibiotic sensitivity testing
   B. Can be enriched with blood for more fastidious organisms
VI. *Campylobacter* Agar with 5 Antimicrobics and 10% Sheep Blood (Campy BAP)
   A. Highly selective medium for use in a microaerophilic environment for the growth of *Campylobacter* spp. from fecal specimens
VII. Thioglycollate Broth (THIO) Without Indicator –135C
   A. General-use broth that grows most bacterial organisms, including anaerobes, and some fungi
VIII. Trypticase Soy Broth (TSB)
   A. General-use media that grows most bacteria, particularly fastidious organisms
   B. Used primarily in blood cultures and sterility testing
IX. Gram Negative Broth (GN)
   A. Selective enrichment medium for *Salmonella* and *Shigella* used in fecal culturing
X. Campylobacter Thioglycollate Medium (Campy THIO) with 5 Antimicrobics
   A. Selective broth used in a microaerophilic environment to isolate *Campylobacter* from fecal specimens
XI. Brain Heart Infusion (BHI)
   A. Enriched broth used to bring bacteria to a certain turbidity level when performing diffusion antibiotic sensitivity testing
XII. Bile Esculin agar (BE)
   A. Slanted medium used to identify bacteria that hydrolyse esculin, especially enterococci
   B. Positive reaction is indicated by ferric citrate, which reacts by producing a dark brown color
XIII. Sodium chloride 0.85% (NaCl 0.85%)
   A. Sterile solution used for diluting gram-negative bacteria for API testing
XIV. Motility Test Medium
   A. Semisolid medium used to demonstrate motility of bacteria
XV. Dermatophyte Test Medium (DTM)
   A. Solid tubed medium, supplemented with gentamicin and chlortetracycline; used to isolate pathogenic fungi

B. Differentiation is provided by phenol red, which causes a color change in the presence of acid-producing, rapidly growing pathogenic fungi

XVI. Mycosel Agar
A. Selective fungal medium that contains cyclohexamide and chloramphenicol to inhibit bacterial growth

XVII. Nutrient Agar (NA)
A. Media used for the cultivation and transport of nonfastidious organisms

XVIII. Oxidation Fermentation Medium With Dextrose (OF)
A. Semisolid medium used to determine dextrose utilization in gram-negative bacteria

XIX. Urea Agar Slant (urea)
A. Used to determine urease production of bacteria
B. Positive result is indicated by the presence of a phenol red indicator

TYPES OF SPECIMENS

There are three types of areas of the body to consider when obtaining a specimen for microbiological culture.

Sterile Areas

I. Body areas or cavities that do not normally contain bacteria or fungi; any bacteria encountered in these specimens should be considered abnormal. The samples most commonly cultured include
A. Blood
B. Urine
C. Spinal fluid
D. Joint fluid
E. Solid organs
F. Milk
G. Lower respiratory tract

Nonsterile Areas

I. Body areas that, when healthy, contain resident bacteria and fungi (normal flora) that must be distinguished from disease-causing organisms; these areas include
A. Hair/fur
B. Skin
C. Sputum or saliva
D. Intestinal tract/feces
E. Ears
F. Upper respiratory tract, including nares and trachea

Abscessed Areas

I. Areas that the body has filled with exudative material in response to inflammation or irritation
A. Sterile abscesses have no bacterial etiology, and their culture will result in no growth
B. Primary infection abscesses usually contain only one type of pathogen (the cause of the original infection)
C. Secondary infection abscesses contain multiple opportunistic pathogens, bacterial or fungal, that invaded after the original infection

COLLECTION AND CULTURE OF SPECIMENS

Swab Specimen

I. Culturette or sterile cotton-tipped swab
A. Commonly used when culturing ears, nares, and abscesses
B. Liquid specimen may be squirted onto a swab, then submitted
C. Prepackaged sterile swabs may contain a small amount of liquid or gel used as a transport medium, which keeps the organisms viable while in transit (usually for up to 48 hours)
D. Use swab to inoculate one third of each plate: BAP, CNA, MAC
E. Place remaining swab into THIO broth. If swab is plastic or wood, break off cleanly against side of tube so that specimen end of swab is immersed in the medium (break off at a low enough height so that swab end does not protrude from tube). If swab is metal, use clean utility scissors to cut swab off at a good site and flame the cut end of the swab before allowing to rest in broth
F. Streak inoculated plates for isolation (Figure 5-1)
G. Gram stain can be made from the swab if a flamed, sterile slide is used. Smear sample onto the slide before the swab is placed in the broth. It is best to get a second swab for gram staining
H. Incubate overnight

Liquid Specimen

I. Aspirate in syringe, sterile tube, etc.
A. Typically, liquid specimens presented are abscess material, tracheal wash, bronchial wash, nasal discharge, joint fluid, or spinal fluid
B. Inoculate each of the plates (usually BAP, MAC, and CNA) with a small drop of specimen
C. Inoculate thioglycollate broth with a few drops of specimen
D. Use flamed, cooled loop to spread inoculant on one third of each plate; then streak each plate for isolation (see Figure 5-1)
E. Gram stain specimen from syringe/tube

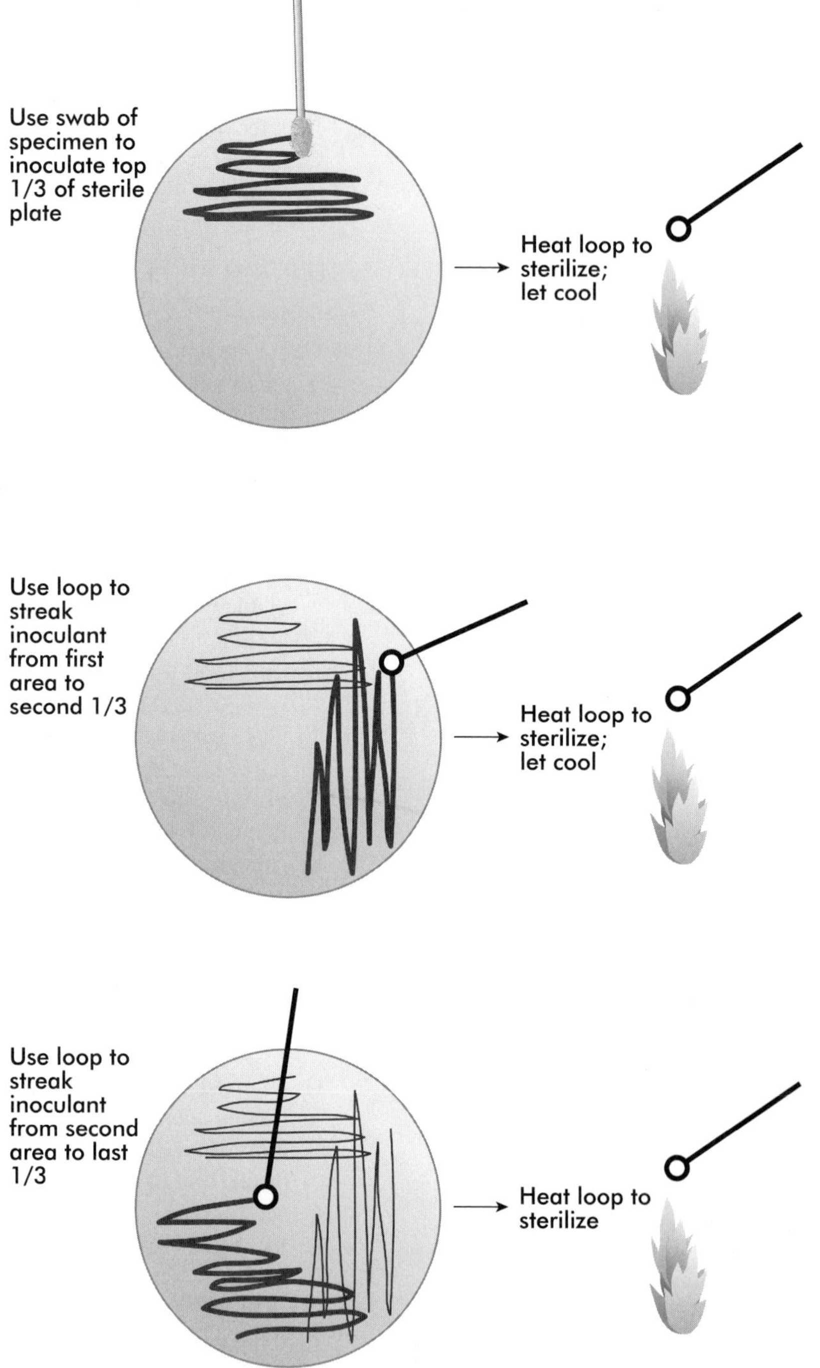
Use swab of specimen to inoculate top 1/3 of sterile plate
Heat loop to sterilize; let cool
Use loop to streak inoculant from first area to second 1/3
Heat loop to sterilize; let cool
Use loop to streak inoculant from second area to last 1/3
Heat loop to sterilize

Figure 5-1 Streaking for isolation. Goal of streaking for isolation is to obtain individual bacterial colonies that are far enough away from other colonies that they can be tested separately and identified.

Solid Specimen

I. Solid specimens include hard abscess material and tissue samples, including organs, skin, and scales

II. Usually the best way to culture these materials is to place a small amount in broth overnight, then subculture the broth onto the plated media

III. Use aseptic technique when collecting tissue samples, especially at necropsy

Urine Specimen

I. Best urine specimen for culture is obtained by cystocentesis; sterile catheterization may also be used. A specimen obtained by free catch may contain normal flora from the skin and genital area

II. Use a sterile, calibrated, nonreusable loop to inoculate 100 μL of urine on a BAP

III. Spread inoculant evenly over entire surface of plate. Any colonies that grow will be counted; the results multiplied by 10 will give bacteria per mL of urine
IV. Inoculate MAC and CNA plates as for liquid specimens
V. A urine sample is generally not placed in THIO because of the high incidence of false-positive readings from contamination (even cystocentesis)

Blood Specimen

I. Mammal
   A. Disinfect rubber tops of two TSB tubes and venipuncture site with a surgical preparation solution
   B. Collect blood directly into TSB tube from venipuncture (i.e., with Vacutainer). One tube is vented to allow aerobic growth; one is left sealed for anaerobic growth
   C. If patient/vein size does not allow direct venipuncture, place noncoagulated blood into broth via syringe (use clean needle if possible or remove needle from syringe before inoculating)
   D. If two tubes are inoculated, one is vented using aseptic technique with a Vacutainer needle (leave needle in place with cover on loosely)
   E. Tubes should be observed every day for hemolysis or cloudiness. Anaerobic activity may be indicated if lid pops off tube
   F. If signs of growth are observed, treat tubes as liquid specimens and subculture/gram stain
   G. Keep tubes at least 8 days, after which subculture to TSA plate and gram stain to confirm negative result
II. Avian, reptile, amphibian, and fish blood
   A. Most of these patients are small; if large enough, follow mammal protocol
   B. Place at least five drops of aseptically drawn blood into THIO broth. Avoid use of anticoagulants; may interfere with bacterial growth
   C. Observe tube daily. Treat as liquid specimen if signs of growth occur
   D. These specimens tend to look positive because of the presence of red blood cell nuclei; subculture is required to verify negative
   E. Confirm negatives at 8 days, as for mammals

Fecal Cultures

I. All fecal cultures are inoculated onto MAC and SS plates and into GN broth
II. GN broth, regardless of plate findings, is subcultured onto an SS plate at 24 or 48 hours
III. Be aware of species-specific pathogens when looking for possible pathogenic colonies: in most carnivores and hoofstock, *Salmonella* spp. are of main concern. In primates, one must also look for *Shigella* spp. Both are NLFs, but *Salmonella* spp. are H_2S producers and *Shigella* spp. are not
IV. Pathogenic H_2S-positive organism *Salmonella* can be distinguished from the common nonpathogenic H_2S-positive *Proteus* spp. by a simple urea test (*Proteus* spp. are urea positive)
V. Of concern in some primates and hoofstock is *Yersinia pseudotuberculosis*. This is an NLF that does not produce H_2S. This bacteria is urea positive, however, and could be overlooked if urea tests are performed to rule out pathogens. For this reason, any NLF colonies encountered in a primate or hoofstock fecal sample should be fully identified
VI. Gram stain all fecal specimens. *Campylobacter* spp., a curved gram-negative rod that can appear as "seagull" or "W" shapes, may be presumptively identified by its pathognomonic shape. Large quantities of large, spore-forming gram-positive rods may indicate a clostridial problem

Fungal Cultures

I. Examine specimen for fungal elements under the microscope, if possible
II. If the specimen is to be incubated for dermatophytes (hair and/or skin samples, most often) place into a small slant tube of DTM
III. All other fungal cultures are placed in Mycosel slants
   A. If the sample is liquid, as in tracheal or bronchial wash, a clean needle on the syringe is used to scratch a few lines in the fungal medium; then a couple of drops of the specimen are placed on the medium
   B. If the sample is on a swab, aseptically break the end of the swab off so it fits in the tube of medium; then gently embed the swab into the agar
   C. Pieces of hair or skin can be aseptically placed on top of the medium
IV. If unsure of the organism, place in both media (as in severe skin infections)
V. Cultures are placed at room temperature in a dark area and examined daily for fungal growth
   A. Dermatophyte fungi (which invade the hair and skin) will often grow within 3 or 4 days
   B. Saprophytic fungi (which are opportunistic environmental fungi) can take up to 3 weeks to grow
VI. Cultures should be held for 1 month to confirm negative results

BASIC DIAGNOSTIC TESTS

Coagulase Test

Place a sample of the colony to be tested into a small amount of liquid rabbit plasma with ethylenediaminetetraacetic acid (EDTA). Incubate overnight.

Coagulase-positive staphylococcus will cause the plasma to gel. Coagulase-negative staphylococcus will not affect the plasma's liquid state.

Gram Stain

Follow directions from the gram stain kit. Usual staining procedure is

I. Specimen is placed on a microscope slide
II. Colony from a plate is suspended in water, or a flamed, cooled loop is used to transfer a drop of thioglycollate broth
III. Allow to air dry
IV. Heat fix by passing quickly through a flame, specimen slide up, about four times
V. Flood slide with crystal violet stain; let sit 1 minute
VI. Rinse with tap water until water runs clear
VII. Flood slide with Gram's iodine; let sit 1 minute
VIII. Rinse with tap water until water runs clear
IX. Flood slide with decolorizer, rock back and forth about 10 seconds, and then rinse slide with tap water. Repeat if specimen is very dark but try not to overdecolorize
X. Flood slide with safranin counterstain, allow to sit for 30 to 50 seconds, and then rinse with tap water until water runs clear
XI. Dry on blotting (bibulous) paper or allow to air dry
XII. Observations under oil immersion (×100) objective: gram-positive bacteria stain purple or dark blue. Gram-negative bacteria stain pink. Overdecolorizing or using an old colony can cause false gram-negative reactions. Forgetting to decolorize or not decolorizing a heavy specimen sufficiently may yield a false-positive result

Catalase Test

I. Using a wooden applicator stick, smear a small amount of the colony to be tested on a clean glass slide
II. Place a drop of 3% hydrogen peroxide on the specimen
III. Observe for bubbling, which indicates a positive reaction

Oxidase Test

I. Using a wooden applicator stick, smear a small to moderate amount of colony to be tested on a piece of white filter paper
II. Place a drop of oxidase reagent on the paper
III. Smeared sample will turn dark blue if positive (some colonies appear blue when initially placed on the filter paper: watch closely for color change)
IV. Many colonies will turn dark after 5 or more minutes, so only record immediate color change

Bile Esculin

I. Inoculate a bile esculin agar slant with *Streptococcus* colony to be tested
II. Place in incubator
III. Examine within a few hours. If agar turns black, test is positive (enterococcal streptococci are positive)
IV. Incubate negative result overnight to confirm

Miniature Biochemical Test Kits (for Gram-Negative Identification)

I. Examples include Micro ID, Enterotube, Minitek, and API 20E
II. API 20E can be used as an example
    A. Each little cup of the API strip is actually a separate test (each test used to be performed separately but now the results can be assessed quickly and easily)
    B. The 0.85% saline suspension of bacteria used for setting up the API 20E is also used to inoculate the Mueller-Hinton plate for Kirby-Bauer sensitivity testing
    C. When the API 20E instruction sheet is followed correctly, the main causes for improper readouts are using mixed colonies of bacteria, using too few colonies, trying to identify a gram-positive colony, or using old, nonviable colonies
III. Other tests for identification of enteric bacteria exist; follow manufacturer's instructions

Kirby-Bauer Sensitivity

I. Bacteria to be tested is diluted in 5 mL BHI broth (or 5 mL 0.85% saline if an API strip is being set up) to match a 0.5 McFarland standard of cloudiness (which is available commercially)
II. Using a sterile cotton-tipped applicator, the sample is inoculated onto a Mueller-Hinton plate to cover the entire surface evenly (the opposite goal of streaking for isolation)
III. Antibiotic sensitivity disks are placed on the agar surface with the antibiotic disk dispenser. Disks must be tapped lightly onto the agar surface so they adhere to the media while the plate is being incubated (upside down)
IV. Inhibition zones are read with a millimeter ruler. Measure the complete clear zone across the antibiotic disk, where bacteria did not grow. Several readings can be taken if the zones are unclear or irregular

Acid-Fast Stain

I. Make a saline or water suspension of sample on slide (not too thick); allow to air dry
II. Heat-fix slide by passing through a flame, specimen side up, three or four times. Let slide cool to touch

III. Flood slide with carbol fuchsin stain; allow to sit for 5 minutes. Rinse with tap water until water runs clear

IV. Flood slide with malachite green counterstain; let sit for 50 to 60 seconds. Rinse under tap water and blot dry

V. Mycobacteria will stain as thin red or pink rods against a green or bluish background. A few yeasts will also stain pink; they are clearer and smaller

BACTERIAL IDENTIFICATION*

Examine bacteriological plates after overnight incubation. Observe the morphology of the colonies. Each colony of the same type of bacteria will look the same. Growth on the TSA and CNA plate indicates the bacteria are gram positive. Growth on the TSA and MAC plate indicates the bacteria are gram negative. Growth on the TSA plate only indicates a fastidious organism; gram stain a representative colony.

Gram-Positive Cocci (Figure 5-2)

Gram-positive cocci are composed mainly of three groups: staphylococci (staph), streptococci (strep), and micrococci. The micrococci are not often encountered in the veterinary laboratory.

I. *Staphylococcus* spp.
   A. Note if colony causes any hemolysis on the blood agar plate. Staphylococci are either hemolytic or nonhemolytic
   B. First test performed on any gram-positive colony is the catalase test (staphylococci are catalase positive)
   C. Coagulase test is performed on the colony (generally, the coagulase-positive staphylococci are more pathogenic)
   D. Mueller-Hinton sensitivity test is performed using BHI broth as a colony diluent
   E. Some samples (such as skin swabs) can be expected to have Staph growth. It may be wise to ask the requesting veterinarian if a sensitivity test should be performed
   F. Often staph colonies growing in a broth tube will resemble comets or shooting stars
   G. Staph, especially those that are coagulase positive, can cause skin or other infections

II. *Streptococcus* spp.
   A. Streptococci are catalase negative
   B. Note any hemolysis surrounding the colonies on the BAP; streptococci hemolysis is graded into
      1. α-Hemolysis (incomplete hemolysis): agar surrounding the colony is greenish
      2. β-Hemolysis (complete hemolysis): agar surrounding the colony is clear
      3. γ-Hemolysis (no hemolysis): agar surrounding the colony is unaffected
   C. Sensitivity is performed using BHI broth. (An MH plate with 5% sheep blood can be used to promote the growth of the streptococci)
   D. *Streptococcus* spp. that do not grow well on the MH plate, especially β-hemolytic *Streptococcus*, will be sensitive to most antibiotics
   E. Enterococci, or enterococcal streptococci, are found in the alimentary tract but are opportunistic pathogens (e.g., *Streptococcus faecalis*). To determine if a colony is an *Enterococcus*, a bile esculin test is performed; enterococci are bile esculin positive
   F. Many *Streptococcus* spp. will grow like stars suspended in the broth
   G. Streptococci can be responsible for many illnesses in animals, including pneumonia, mastitis, and septicemia

Gram-Negative Cocci

I. *Neisseria* spp.: often found as normal flora in the respiratory tract of many animals; as pathogens, they mainly cause concern in humans
   A. *N. gonorrhoeae* is the cause of human gonorrhea
   B. *N. meningitidis* causes human meningitis

Gram-Negative Rods (Figure 5-3)

I. Enterobacteriaceae, or enteric (gut) bacteria, are gram-negative rods that are isolated commonly in veterinary medicine

II. Gram-negative rods grow on the BAP and MAC plate (they will often overgrow gram-positive cocci on the BAP, which makes the CNA plate essential for recovering these)

III. Note the lactose reaction of the colony
   A. If the colony is a NLF, it will be clear. Perform an oxidase test
   B. LFs are dark pink or purple. All LFs are oxidase negative

IV. Colony is prepared for API 20E and sensitivity testing using sterile 0.85% saline

V. If searching for fecal pathogens, all NLFs must be identified and/or ruled out
   A. For example: *Proteus* spp. and *Salmonella* spp. are both NLF and H_2S positive. *Proteus*, however, is urea positive; a urea test can distinguish these bacteria within a few hours

*Note that these procedures are basic. They are described in greater detail in a clinical microbiology book, which is the final reference when identifying organisms.

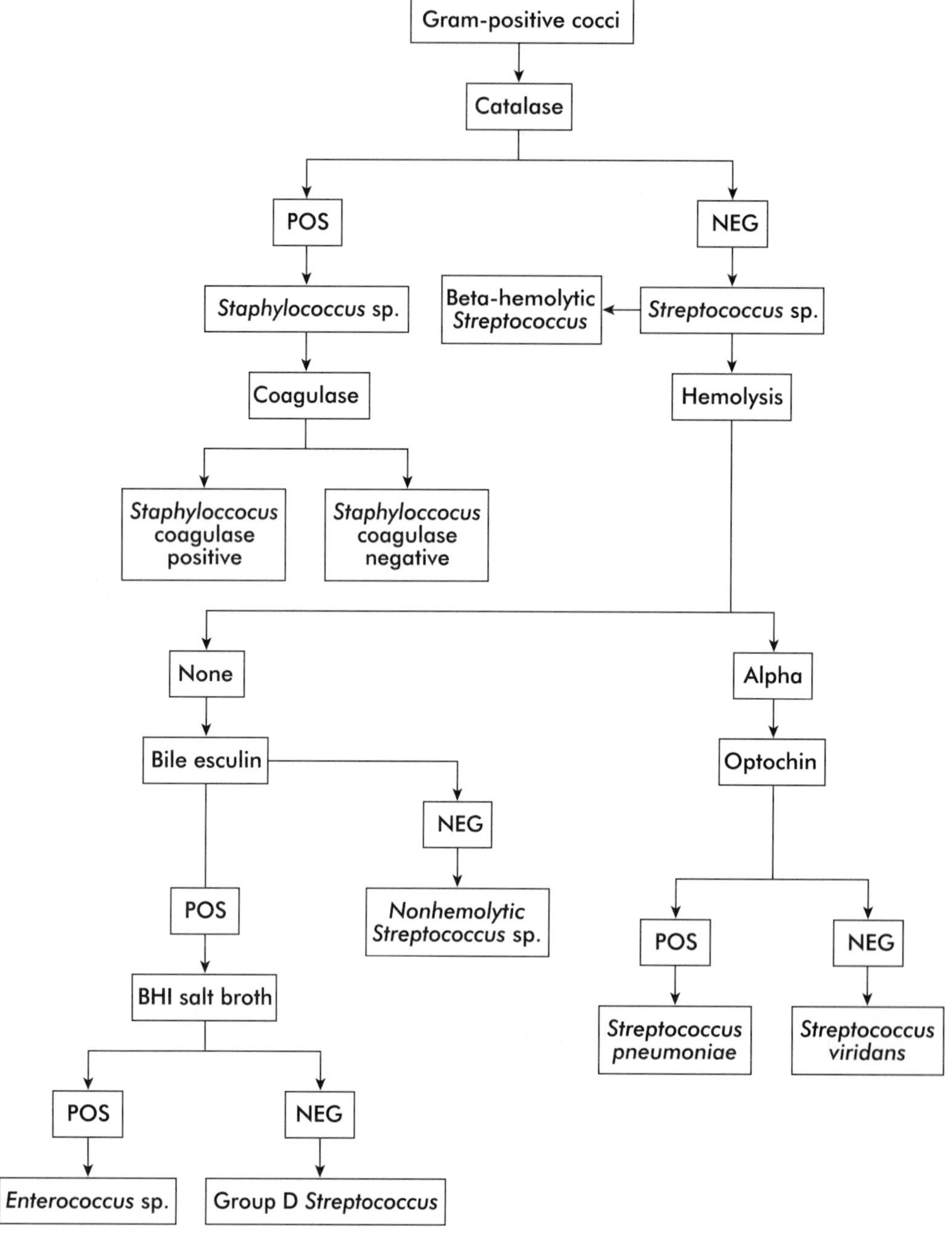

Figure 5-2 Gram-positive cocci.

B. *Shigella* and *Pseudomonas* look similar on an MAC plate. To rule out suspicious colonies, perform an oxidase test: *Shigella* will be oxidase negative

C. *Aeromonas* spp. are a light LF, appearing light creamy pink on an MAC plate. It is oxidase positive

VI. API 20E test is performed to identify gram-negative rods. Follow the directions from the package insert

VII. Enteral bacteria are found in many infections: they are opportunistic pathogens

VIII. Some of the nonenteral gram-negative rods such as *Pseudomonas* and *Aeromonas* spp. can be serious primary pathogens, especially in birds, reptiles, and amphibians

Gram-Negative Spirochetes

I. *Campylobacter* spp. are bacteria found in the digestive tracts of many mammals. In hoofed

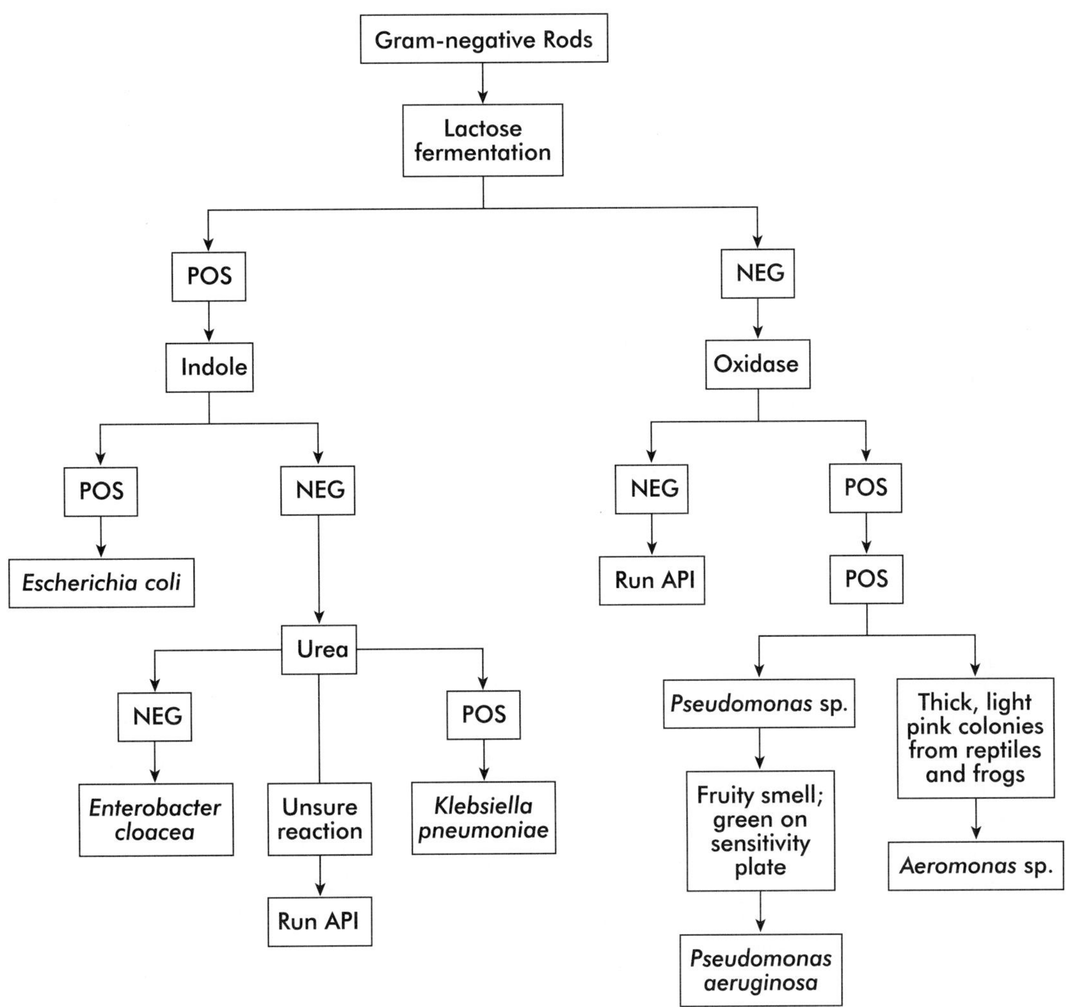

Figure 5-3 Gram-negative rods.

mammals they can be normal flora; in others (especially primates and carnivores) they can cause a chronic debilitating diarrhea

A. Shape of *Campylobacter* is often characteristic: two small, curved gram-negative rods join end-to-end to form a "seagull" or "W." These can be difficult to see on a gram stain and other forms may be present (spiraled), so a negative gram stain is not diagnostic

B. *Campylobacter* requires a microaerophilic environment to grow and often are overgrown by less fastidious organisms. Special media and growing conditions are required for culture

II. *Yersinia* spp. may be encountered in reptile/amphibian cultures and primate or ruminant fecal cultures. These bacteria are halophilic (requiring salt to grow). Most media has sufficient salt to enable the bacteria to grow and be identifiable by API

III. Other spirochetes examples include *Leptospira* spp., *Borrelia* spp., and *Helicobacter* spp.

Gram-Negative Coccobacilli

I. *Moraxella bovis* are large gram-negative cocci that sometimes resemble fat rods; they cause pinkeye in cattle

II. Gram-negative coccobacilli include *Bordetella* spp. and *Pasteurella* spp. These organisms are of concern to the veterinary microbiology laboratory because they can cause respiratory disease, especially in dogs *(Bordetella)* and in cats and rabbits *(Pasteurella)*

III. These organisms can be identified in the API system

IV. Care must be taken not to misidentify these as streptococci, as they may not grow on MAC. Any flat, shiny gray colony (especially if it has no lookalike on the CNA plate) should be gram stained

V. It can be difficult to tell coccobacilli from cocci, so it is best to work with young colonies. Older colonies of streptococci may lose their ability to hold a positive gram reaction

Gram-Positive Rods

I. Most small microbiology laboratories do not attempt to identify *anaerobic* gram-positive rods such as *Clostridium* spp.
II. Note their presence and whether they have spores on gram stain
III. They will grow anaerobically in THIO, toward the bottom, but not on regular plates. For this reason it is important to gram stain the broth
IV. Most common *aerobic* gram-positive rod encountered is *Bacillus* spp.
   A. These are large, parallel-sided rods that grow on the blood agar plate only
   B. Colonies often have a "grainy" *or* "mucoid" appearance and can be hemolytic and spore forming
   C. They grow at the top of the broth in the THIO tube
   D. Sensitivities can be performed but often are not necessary because *Bacillus* spp. are mostly found in culture as normal flora or environmental contaminants
   E. Prominent exception is *B. anthracis*, which causes sudden death in cattle and sheep, and skin and lung lesions in humans
   F. *B. piliformis* causes acute fatal enteritis in rodents and foals
V. *Corynebacterium* spp. are small gram-positive rods that are often curved and pleomorphic, giving them a "Chinese letters" look on gram stain
   A. In people and animals, they are often found as normal flora of the alimentary tract, especially the mouth and skin
   B. Pathogenic *Corynebacterium* include
      1. *C. equi* (foal pneumonia), *C. pseudotuberculosis* (caseous lymphadenitis in sheep and goats), and *C. renale* (urinary tract infections in cattle, pigs, and male sheep)
VI. *Listeria monocytogenes* and *Erysipelothrix rhusiopathiae* are also small rods
   A. *Listeria* spp. is a small, non–spore-forming rod that is catalase positive; *Erysipelothrix* spp. is a pleomorphic rod that is catalase negative
   B. *Listeria* spp. can infect the brainstem
   C. *Erysipelothrix* spp. is most commonly found in cases of septicemia and occasionally is a cause of endocarditis in dog
VII. *Mycobacterium* spp. are long, thin gram-positive rods that sometimes branch. These can be serious pathogens. They do not grow on typical bacteriological media
   A. *M. tuberculosis* causes pneumonia in humans and other primates
   B. *M. avium* causes a fatal, untreatable gastrointestinal and respiratory infection in birds
      1. These bacteria are difficult to culture: it takes months and specialized media
      2. Their presence in sputum or tissue can be demonstrated by their ability to retain an acid-fast stain, which is a test that can be performed in most veterinary laboratories

Mycoplasma

I. *Mycoplasma* spp. are small bacteria that lack a cell wall and therefore are not easily stained and observed in exudates
II. Pneumonia and arthritis are the most common diseases associated with *Mycoplasma* spp.
III. Identification of *Mycoplasma* spp. can be made only at a reference laboratory

FUNGAL IDENTIFICATION

Fungi are identified by their characteristic microscopic morphology.

I. Small piece of clear cellophane tape is pressed gently but firmly onto the fungal colony, sticky side down. The tape is placed, sticky side down, on a microscope slide to which a drop of saline or lactophenol cotton blue has been added. The slide is examined under the microscope for hyphal identification
II. Other specialized techniques and media can be used to identify fungi, but these are generally more time consuming and not commonly done in small laboratories
III. TSA plate will often grow yeast, if present in a sample. Therefore any colonies that are not easily recognized should be gram stained (or make a wet mount with saline) and examined microscopically
IV. In very heavy fungal infections (e.g., avian aspergillosis) the fungus will often grow on top of the THIO and/or the surface of the TSA plate. These colonies are usually readily identified as fungi by their dry, fuzzy appearance

Dermatophytes

I. Found in hair, skin, nails, and claws, they are the cause of ringworm in humans and animals
II. Main dermatophytes affecting animals are *Microsporum* spp. and *Trichophyton* spp.
III. Most dermatophytes cause a color change in dermatophyte test medium (from orange to red)

IV. These fungi are distinguished by their large macroconidia, visible microscopically. The shape of the macroconidia identifies the organism

Saprophytes

I. Saprophytic fungi are found in the environment and are opportunistic pathogens
II. The saprophytes include
   A. *Aspergillus* spp., which can cause pneumonia, especially in birds
      1. Some species can also cause disease by their presence in feed and hay
      2. They create a toxin known as aflotoxin, which can cause a severe immunosuppressive effect in animals ingesting affected feed
   B. *Mucor* spp. and *Rhizopus* spp. can cause lymph node, lung, and liver lesions in immunosuppressed animals

Yeast

A cream-colored colony growing only on the TSA plate could be a yeast.

I. *Candida* spp. can be found infecting mucous membranes, especially in the gastrointestinal tract (including the mouth), genital tract, respiratory tract, and ears
II. *Candida albicans* causes many diseases, especially when predisposing conditions exist such as
   A. Immunosuppression
   B. Primary bacterial infection
   C. Prolonged antibiotic use
   D. *Candida albicans* can be identified by means of the germ tube test
      1. An isolate of yeast is incubated in rabbit plasma with EDTA for 2 to 3 hours, and then examined microscopically
      2. *C. albicans* produces germ tubes, which grow from the side of the yeast like tiny hyphae
      3. True germ tubes do not "pinch in" at the point of attachment to the parent yeast cell
   E. Commercial agglutination tests also exist for identification of *C. albicans* and many other yeasts
III. *Cryptococcus neoformans* is an encapsulated yeast that can cause severe nasal infections in dogs and cats and meningitis in people (this is a very zoonotic organism)
   A. Cultures or nasal exudates can be examined under the microscope with a drop of India ink to highlight the thick capsule
IV. *Malassezia pachydermatis* is found in the external ear and is emerging as the cause of seborrheic dermatitis and hypersensitivity reactions
   A. It can be identified by its appearance on a gram stain of an oval, bottle-shaped budding yeast
V. Yeast can be normal flora in the ears, genitals, and oral cavity

Dimorphic Fungi

I. Dimorphic fungi exhibit yeastlike growth when in animal tissue and saprophytic fungus-type growth in the environment
II. These fungi are highly zoonotic and must be handled using protective measures
   A. They are identified by their characteristic microscopic appearance
   B. Infections can also be diagnosed by serology testing
III. Dimorphic fungi of special clinical concern
   A. *Histoplasma capsulatum:* causes respiratory tract infections in dogs, cats, and humans
   B. *Blastomyces dermatiditis:* causes blastomycosis, a respiratory and/or skin infection in dogs and humans
   C. *Coccidioides immitis:* causes respiratory disease in dogs and humans; can also affect bones and internal organs
   D. All of these organisms can be presumptively identified by cytological examination of the clinical specimen

Glossary

aerobic Requiring oxygen to live
agar Semisolid medium
anaerobic Requiring the absence of oxygen to live
aseptic technique Performed with as little opportunity for contamination as possible
broth Liquid medium
culture Deliberate growing of an organism under controlled conditions
differential medium Microbiological medium that contains compounds that identify certain characteristics of organisms grown on the medium
enteral bacteria Bacteria found in the gastrointestinal tract
halophilic Bacteria that require a high concentration of salt for optimal growth
microaerophilic Bacteria that require oxygen for growth but at a lower concentration than what is present in the atmosphere
nlf Non-lactose fermenters
normal flora Organisms found in a healthy animal
opportunistic pathogen Organism able to infect an area already compromised by injury or infection
optochin susceptibility test A test to distinguish between streptococcus pneumoniae from other alpha hemolytic streptococci
plate Flat, round container of agar

selective medium Microbiological medium that contains compounds that inhibit growth of certain types of organisms
slant Tube of agar that has been allowed to gel at an angle
tube Screw-top container that can contain broth or agar
zoonotic Capable of causing disease in animals and humans

Review Questions

1 An in-house microbiology laboratory must be
 a. Run without the veterinarian's input
 b. Completely autonomous
 c. Staffed by proficient personnel and have the most up-to-date equipment
 d. Cost effective, staffed by proficient personnel, and aware of clients' needs

2 The oculars (or eyepieces) of a microscope
 a. Have no magnification abilities
 b. Multiply the magnification of the objectives by 5, 10, or 15
 c. Add 10 to the magnification of the objectives
 d. Control the amount of light entering the microscope

3 Nutritive media
 a. Select for different types of bacteria
 b. Differentiate types of bacteria
 c. Grow most bacteria
 d. Are not used for most microbiological procedures

4 MacConkey agar is an example of
 a. A differential and selective medium
 b. A general nutritive and differential medium
 c. A general nutritive medium
 d. A selective medium

5 Sterile abscesses
 a. Are cleaned with a disinfectant before sampling
 b. Contain only one type of organism
 c. Contain many types of organisms
 d. Contain no bacterial or fungal organisms

6 Bacterial cultures are incubated
 a. At room temperature
 b. At the patient's body temperature
 c. At human body temperature
 d. In the refrigerator

7 The best specimen for urine culture is obtained
 a. Via aseptic catheterization
 b. Via free catch
 c. Via cystocentesis
 d. Off of the cage floor

8 Fungal cultures are incubated
 a. At room temperature
 b. At the patient's body temperature
 c. At human body temperature
 d. In the refrigerator

9 A streptococcal colony on a blood agar plate with a greenish zone around it is said to be
 a. Hemolytic
 b. α-Hemolytic
 c. β-Hemolytic
 d. Nonhemolytic

10 Dermatophyte fungi are found
 a. Infecting skin hair and nails
 b. To commonly cause pneumonia
 c. As normal flora on most animals
 d. As free-living fungi in the environment

BIBLIOGRAPHY

Baron E, Finegold S: *Bailey and Scott's diagnostic microbiology,* St Louis, 1989, Mosby.
Mahon CR, Manuselis G: *Textbook of diagnostic microbiology,* Philadelphia, 1997, WB Saunders.
McCurnin DM: *Clinical textbook for veterinary technicians,* ed 4, Philadelphia, 1998, WB Saunders.
Power D, ed: *Manual of BBL products and laboratory procedures,* Cockeysville, MD, 1988, Becton-Dickinson Company.
Pratt PW: *Laboratory procedures for veterinary technicians,* ed 3, Goleta, Calif, 1997, American Veterinary Publications.
Pratt PW: *Principles and practice of veterinary technology,* St Louis, 1998, Mosby.
Quinn PJ et al: *Clinical veterinary microbiology,* St Louis, 1994, Mosby.

CHAPTER 6

Clinical Chemistry

Joanne Hamel

OUTLINE

LEARNING OUTCOMES

After reading this chapter you should be able to:

1. Identify common laboratory tests used to evaluate kidney, pancreatic, and liver function, as well as electrolytes and minerals, in small and large animals.
2. Understand the significance of abnormal results of these tests.
3. Provide samples required and proper conditions under which the tests are performed.
4. Identify common tests that appear in various chemistry profiles.

It is essential that all blood samples destined for biochemical analysis be collected with care, using the correct anticoagulants or no anticoagulants. One must pay close attention to any special requirements when collecting blood samples. The results are only as good as the samples tested.

Evaluation of the chemical constituents of whole blood, plasma, and serum has become increasingly realistic in the practice setting. Instrumentation, equipment, and procedures have been greatly modified to allow relatively rapid and reliable diagnostics. Chemical components are routinely assayed by use of chemical reagent test strips or automated dry chemical analysis machines. Box 6-1 and Tables 6-1 to 6-3 at the end of the chapter provide the commonly requested tests, biochemistry reference values, a summary of function tests, and a conversion chart for SI and conventional units.

GENERAL INFORMATION

I. Components of whole blood
   A. Whole blood: composed of fluid and cellular components
      1. Plasma is the fluid portion
      2. Erythrocytes, leukocytes, and thrombocytes compose the cells
   B. Plasma: fluid portion of the blood in which cells are suspended; 90% water and 10% dissolved proteins, hormones, lipids, enzymes, salts, carbohydrates, vitamins, and waste materials
   C. Serum: fluid portion with fibrinogen protein removed; derived when whole blood is allowed to clot

II. Sample handling
    A. The following should be kept in mind when handling samples
        1. Samples should be collected from calm, fasted patients
        2. Avoid hemolysis by selecting needles of the correct size and dry syringes or new evacuated tubes
        3. To avoid chemical interaction with the specimen, serum is the sample of choice for all tests
            a. Blood samples taken for serum separation are allowed to clot, centrifuged, and separated
            b. Samples are allowed to clot at room temperature for 20 to 30 minutes
            c. Separate the clot by "rimming" with a wooden applicator stick around the inside of the tube
            d. Blood tubes are counterbalanced and centrifuged for 10 minutes at 2000 to 3000 rpm
                (1) Centrifuge as soon as possible and transfer the serum or plasma to chemically clean and properly labeled test tubes
            e. Several types of blood tubes and devices are designed to facilitate serum separation
            f. Serum is carefully pipetted or poured off into a suitable container and labeled
            g. Serum may be refrigerated or frozen; freezing may affect some test results
            h. Quality of serum
                (1) Lipemic serum: cloudy, excessive lipids, often due to diet, metabolic disease
                (2) Hemolytic serum: pink to reddish tint; caused by damage to red blood cells either physiological or iatrogenic
                (3) Icteric serum: yellow tinge; indicative of liver disease
        4. Samples for whole blood or plasma should be collected with an anticoagulant. If plasma is used, be sure that the anticoagulant chosen does not interfere with the tests requested
        5. Types of anticoagulants include
            a. Heparin: available in sodium, potassium, lithium, and ammonium salts
                (1) Good choice for plasma samples because there is little interference with chemical assays; use at 20 units/mL of blood
            b. Ethylenediaminetetraacetic acid (EDTA): anticoagulant of choice for hematological tests because it has little effect on morphology
                (1) Should not be used for chemical assays of plasma
            c. Sodium fluoride: a glucose preservative with some anticoagulant properties
        6. Samples should be analyzed immediately
            a. When this is not possible, samples should be refrigerated until tests can be performed (return to room temperature before testing)
        7. Collect sufficient sample for the tests requested
        8. Each laboratory should establish a set of normal values that will reflect test procedures and conditions used

KIDNEY FUNCTION

More than 70% of the glomeruli of both kidneys must be nonfunctional before serum chemistry changes occur. The nephron parts are so closely related that malfunction in one area will eventually affect another.

Creatinine

I. A byproduct of muscle metabolism that is produced at a constant rate and filtered out almost entirely by the glomeruli
    A. A constant small amount is produced daily
II. Increased serum creatinine levels are seen when there is a lack of functional glomeruli
III. Serum creatinine concentrations are influenced by
    A. Fluid and hydration levels
    B. Prerenal factors such as shock
    C. Postrenal factors such as bladder and urethral obstructions
IV. Used to evaluate glomerular function
V. Sample required
    A. Serum or plasma may be used
    B. Hemolysis does not influence the results
    C. Bilirubinemia will cause false increases

Urea (Urea Nitrogen)

I. Urea is an end product of protein metabolism and is excreted primarily by the kidneys
    A. Up to 40% is reabsorbed by the tubules for reexcretion
    B. Rate of reabsorption is inversely proportional to the amount of urine output
II. Evaluates glomerular filtration and function
III. Nonrenal causes of increased serum urea nitrogen include
    A. The amount of protein ingested and absorbed
    B. Fever

C. Corticosteroids
IV. Levels are increased in renal insufficiency
V. Etiology of increased levels include
A. Prerenal factors such as shock and dehydration
B. Postrenal factors such as obstruction in the ureters, bladder, or urethra
VI. May be decreased in anorexia, liver disease, tubular injury
VII. Sample required
A. Serum preferred
B. Plasma should not be collected with ammonium oxalate
1. False increases will be produced
C. Plasma should not be collected with fluoride
1. Decreases will be produced
D. Samples should be nonlipemic
E. It is recommended to fast the animal for 18 hours before testing
F. Serum or plasma should be tested as soon as possible because bacterial contamination will reduce the amount of urea in the sample

Water Deprivation/Urine Concentration Tests

I. The patient is gradually deprived of water over a 3- to 5-day interval until there is a stimulus for endogenous antidiuretic hormone (ADH) release
A. This usually occurs at about 5% weight loss
II. If sufficient ADH, specific gravity of normal urine concentration is 1.025
III. Failure to concentrate urine over the duration of the test is indicative of insufficient ADH or tubular dysfunction
IV. This test should never be performed on animals that are dehydrated or have increased serum urea

PANCREATIC FUNCTION

The pancreas has endocrine and exocrine functions. Pancreatic endocrine function involves the production of glucagon and insulin. Diabetes mellitus, or a deficiency of insulin resulting in hyperglycemia, is the most common endocrine disorder of the pancreas. Pancreatic exocrine function involves the production of lipase, amylase, and trypsin. Most pancreatic disturbances occur in the exocrine function of the pancreas. Dogs seem to have a greater incidence than cats.

Urine Glucose

I. Glycosuria (glucosuria) exists when blood glucose levels exceed the renal threshold for absorption of glucose in the proximal convoluted tubules
II. A diagnosis of diabetes mellitus is not made unless glycosuria accompanies hyperglycemia
III. Clinitest tablets (Ames) are not specific for glucose and will give a positive reaction with any reducing sugars
A. This is considered a screening test only
IV. Reagent sticks such as Clinistix, Chemstrip, and others are specific for measuring glucose
A. These sticks use glucose oxidase, peroxidase, and a color indicator
V. False-positive test outcomes in urine may result from
A. Ascorbic acid
B. Morphine
C. Salicylates
D. Penicillin
E. Tetracycline
F. Intravenous fluids containing glucose
G. General anesthetics, etc.
VI. Sample required
A. Freshly voided, morning sample

Serum/Plasma Glucose

I. Most test procedures use glucose oxidase, which is specific for measuring glucose in samples
II. Hyperglycemia may result from
A. Diabetes mellitus
B. Several nonpancreatic causes such as stress and hyperadrenocorticism (Cushing's disease)
III. Hypoglycemia may result from
A. Malabsorption
B. Severe liver disease
C. Prolonged contact of the serum or plasma with the cellular component of the blood
IV. Glucose tolerance tests may be used to determine how well an animal is able to utilize carbohydrates
V. Sample required
A. Serum is preferable
1. Sodium fluoride may be used if the plasma cannot be removed from the cells immediately
2. It is essential to collect and treat the sample properly to obtain meaningful results
B. Centrifuge sample immediately
1. Remove plasma or serum and transfer to another test tube
C. Blood cells will continue to utilize glucose at a rate of 7% to 10% per hour if allowed to remain in contact with the serum or plasma
D. A fasting sample is preferred 16 to 24 hours in dogs and cats
E. Ruminants should not be fasted

Serum Amylase

I. Amylase acts to break down starches and glycogen
II. Increased serum amylase levels are seen in

A. Acute, chronic, and obstructive pancreatitis
B. Hyperadrenocorticism
C. Liver disease
D. Upper gastrointestinal inflammation or obstruction
E. Renal failure

III. Animals have a greater serum amylase activity level than humans (10 times greater in the dog and cat) so it is recommended to dilute the serum with normal saline before testing if using tests designed for human samples
IV. Amyloclastic test: should be used for dogs because maltose does not influence the results
V. Amylase concentrations are not considered useful in cats
VI. Sample required
A. Nonlipemic serum or heparinized plasma
B. Hemolysis may elevate the values

Serum Lipase

I. Lipase breaks down the long-chain fatty acids of lipids into fatty acids and alcohols
II. Lipase is usually in low levels in serum but serum levels increase in cases of pancreatitis (chronic and acute)
III. Increased serum lipase is also seen in
A. Renal failure
B. Hyperadrenocorticism
C. Dexamethasone treatment
D. Bile tract disease
IV. Manual methods for measuring lipase are cumbersome, but with the newer colorimetric and new dry chemistry kits, it is easier to evaluate serum lipase levels
V. It is recommended to perform serum amylase and lipase tests on patients suspected of having acute pancreatitis
VI. Some cats with pancreatitis do not have elevated serum lipase levels
VII. Sample required
A. Nonhemolysed, nonlipemic serum or heparinized plasma

Trypsin-Like Immunoreactivity

I. Trypsin-like immunoreactivity on serum
A. Considered the test of choice
1. A highly specific and sensitive assay for exocrine pancreatic insufficiency in dogs
B. Trypsinogen, a trypsin-like substance, is synthesized in the pancreas and normally released in trace amounts into the circulation
1. By determining the amount of this hormone present using ligand assay techniques, it can be determined if the animal has exocrine pancreatic insufficiency (EPI)
C. Suspect animals are fasted for 12 hours; serum is collected and sent away for analysis
1. Normal TLI for the dog is 5.2 to 35 µg/L
2. Dogs with EPI have levels of less than 2.5 µg/L
D. EPI may result from chronic pancreatitis, juvenile atrophy, and pancreatic hypoplasia
1. Lack of functional tissue leads to maldigestion of food because inadequate amounts of lipase, trypsin, and amylase can be produced
E. This condition is a common cause of malabsorption in dogs but rarely occurs in cats

LIVER FUNCTION

No one test is totally satisfactory for determining the presence or absence of liver disease. A liver profile is usually ordered, and other special tests can be done as well. Seventy percent of the liver is nonfunctional before serum chemistry changes are noted.

Bilirubin

I. Bilirubin results from the metabolism of heme by the mononuclear phagocytic system (formerly called the reticuloendothelial system)
II. Hyperbilirubinemia refers to increased serum bilirubin levels
A. Hyperbilirubinemia can cause jaundice
III. Conjugated and unconjugated forms of bilirubin are found normally in serum or plasma
A. The unconjugated or initial form of bilirubin is lipid soluble, bound to serum proteins, and carried to the liver to be conjugated
B. The conjugated form is found mainly as glucuronic acid, which is water soluble and more readily excreted from the body via the biliary system to the intestines and kidney
1. Some is "regurgitated" back into the liver and circulatory system
2. The bile secretes the remainder conjugated to the intestines
a. The conjugated form is unbound to serum proteins so it can pass into the urine through the glomerulus
IV. Increases in the total amount of bilirubin are significant
V. Total bilirubin and conjugated (direct form) bilirubin are measured
A. The amount of unconjugated bilirubin is determined by subtraction
VI. Bilirubin measured in urine is always the conjugated form unless there is renal damage

VII. Increased unconjugated serum bilirubin levels indicate prehepatic jaundice, an inability of the liver cells to take up unconjugated bilirubin, or an inability to conjugate the bilirubin within the liver cells

VIII. Prehepatic jaundice is due to moderate to severe intravascular hemolysis and will be accompanied by a decreased hematocrit
  A. In cattle, most hyperbilirubinemia is caused by hemolysis
  B. Unfortunately, serum bilirubin levels rarely increase sufficiently to aid in diagnosis

IX. Increased serum conjugated bilirubin levels are seen with hepatic jaundice or cholestasis (posthepatic jaundice)

X. A more marked rise in conjugated bilirubin is noted with posthepatic jaundice

XI. Some dogs have a lower renal threshold for bilirubin
  A. Bilirubin in the urine is considered a sensitive indicator of liver disease in dogs
  B. Cat, pig, sheep, and horse do not normally have bilirubin in their urine
  C. Occasionally, normal cattle will exhibit biliuria

XII. Horses will have increased unconjugated serum bilirubin in prehepatic and hepatic conditions
  A. Increased unconjugated levels also will be seen in many nonhepatic diseases (cardiac insufficiency, constipation, colic)
  B. Unconjugated and conjugated serum bilirubin levels increase after fasting

XIII. In cattle, sheep, goat, and pig
  A. Even in severe liver diseases, only slight increases in total bilirubin will be noted
  B. Most increased total bilirubin levels are due to hemolytic disorders; thus serum bilirubin measurements are not useful indicators of liver disease

XIV. Most testing methods for serum contain diazo reagent, which reacts specifically with bilirubin
  A. Ictotest tablets contain diazo reagent and measure bilirubin in urine. This test
    1. Is highly specific
    2. Is sensitive to small amounts of bilirubin
    3. Rarely produces false-positive results
    4. May be semiquantitative with serial dilutions of the urine
  B. Reagent strips
    1. Examples: Ictostix, Multistix use diazo reagent
    2. Considered less sensitive to bilirubin in urine than Ictotest

XV. False-positive results are caused by some medications

XVI. Samples required
  A. Nonlipemic, nonhemolysed serum or plasma
  B. Remove serum or plasma from the clot or cells within 3 hours
  C. Store samples in the dark because up to 50% bilirubin will be lost in the first hour of collection if left in light
  D. Samples can be refrigerated or frozen
  E. Freshly collected urine must be tested immediately for bilirubin

Urine Urobilinogen

I. In small animals other than in cats and dogs the results are not as useful in pinpointing liver problems: testing is not routine

II. In humans and dogs, the amount of urine urobilinogen will increase in hepatocellular disease and decrease with obstructive problems

III. No urobilinogen or a decreased amount is a common finding in normal dogs

IV. Sample required
  A. Freshly voided urine sample
  B. Urine left sitting out converts to urobilin, which cannot be detected with tests used for urobilinogen

Total Serum/Plasma Proteins

I. Proteins in serum samples are easily subjected to denaturation from heat, exposure to strong acids or bases, enzymatic action, exposure to urea and other substances, and ultraviolet (UV) light

II. Total serum proteins (TSPs) and serum albumin are measured, and the serum globulins are determined by subtraction

III. Levels are affected by
  A. Altered rates of protein synthesis in the liver
  B. Altered breakdown or excretion of proteins
  C. Dehydration or over hydration
  D. Altered distribution of proteins in the body

IV. Serum protein indicates the hydration level in the animal
  A. Animal in shock or overhydrated animal will have decreased serum protein
  B. Dehydrated animal will have increased serum protein

V. TSP also can be used as a guide to the nutritional status of an animal

VI. Goldberg refractometer (American Optical Company, Greenwich, CT) is most commonly used to measure TSP in clinics
  A. Refractometer is considered a good screening method
  B. Results obtained are affected by electrolytes, lipids, hemolysis, urea, and glucose in the sample

C. It is essential to have a clear, unturbid sample

VII. Wet and dry chemistry methods for measuring protein, use the Biuret method for measuring serum proteins

VIII. Total dye binding is used in an automated serum analyzer to also measure total serum proteins

IX. Sample required
   A. Nonhemolysed, nonlipemic serum or plasma collected with EDTA or heparin
   B. Serum gives slightly lower values
   C. Avoid contact with detergents and UV light, which will denature the proteins

Albumin

I. Serum albumin and globulin levels change in response to several diseases

II. As a general rule, when changes occur, the albumin level decreases, whereas the globulin level increases to maintain a constant TSP level

III. Globulin fraction can be divided in subfractions

IV. TSP and albumin are measured, and the globulin fraction can be obtained by subtracting the smaller from the larger value

V. Albumin dye binding is used to measure serum albumin levels

VI. Increases in this fraction are rare; seen sometimes in shock

VII. Decreased albumin may occur in
   A. Chronic liver disease
   B. Starvation/malnutrition
   C. Malabsorption
   D. Enteritis, colitis, parasites
   E. Pregnancy and lactation
   F. Prolonged fever
   G. Uncontrolled diabetes
   H. Trauma
   I. Nephritis, nephrosis
   J. Ascites, protein losing enteropathy
   K. Blood loss

Globulins

I. Globulin fractions, along with albumin, can be separated out by electrophoresis
   A. The globulin fraction of serum proteins is quite complex and can be subdivided into α-globulins, β-globulins, and γ-globulins

II. Fibrinogen is one of the coagulation factors and is used in the clotting process
   A. Fibrinogen is part of the globulin fraction and is sometimes measured separately
      1. Plasma must be used
      2. This protein makes up about 4 g/L of the total plasma protein fraction

III. Electrophoresis shows relative increases and decreases in the different fractions
   A. These can be related to specific diseases

IV. Different species show different normal electrophoretic patterns

V. In general, increases in globulins may be seen with
   A. Inflammation/infections
   B. Antigenic stimulation
   C. Neoplasia or abnormal immunoglobulin production

VI. Globulin fraction usually increases when albumin decreases

Enzymes

Biological enzymes are classified as plasma/serum specific (normally present in plasma/serum) and non–plasma/serum specific.

I. Non–plasma specific enzymes
   A. Assayed during clinical diagnosis, because these enzymes increase in concentration in serum if
      1. Tissue cells are destroyed
      2. There is an increase in their production
      3. There is obstruction of their excretory route
      4. There is a decrease in circulation
   B. Test kits should contain all required substrates, coenzymes, and cofactors
   C. It is important to perform tests at the temperature indicated in the instructions
      1. This is usually 30° C
   D. It is important to handle samples carefully, paying careful consideration to any special requirements for anticoagulants and separation
   E. Historically there have been many units of measurement used for measuring the same enzymes (e.g., serum alkaline phosphatase) has been measured in Bodansky units, Bessy-Lowry-Brock units, King-Armstrong units, etc.)
      1. The international unit of measurement for enzyme assays replaces the old units used
         a. IU (the amount of enzyme that will catalyze the conversion of one micromole of substrate per minute)
      2. It is advisable for labs to establish their own normal values

II. ALT
   A. Also known as alanine aminotransferase or alanine transaminase
      1. Formerly called SGPT
   B. Found in large amounts in the hepatocytes of dog, cat, and primate
      1. Considered a useful and specific test for liver function in these species
   C. This enzyme is not present in large enough amounts in liver cells of horse, ruminant, or pig to be of diagnostic significance

D. Serum ALT increases if hepatocytes are damaged, but the damage may not necessarily be irreversible
   1. The increase is due to an isolated incident if the initial ALT is increased but declines on subsequent serial tests
   2. If ALT remains elevated or increases, the cause is chronic in nature
E. Some drugs can cause increased ALT in dog but not in cat
F. Sample required
   1. Nonhemolysed, nonlipemic serum or plasma collected with EDTA or sodium citrate
   2. Do not freeze

III. AST
A. Also known as aspartate aminotransferase or aspartate transaminase
   1. Formerly called SGOT
B. Present in all tissues of the body, especially in cardiac muscle, skeletal muscle, and the liver
   1. Not an organ-specific enzyme
C. AST assays should be run in conjunction with other enzyme assays, especially ALT, when evaluating liver function
D. For species in which ALT is not useful, AST is sometimes looked at as an alternative to ALT in diagnosing liver disease
   1. In this case other causes of increased AST should be ruled out before focusing on the liver
E. Horse has higher normal AST values than other species
   1. Test method used should be specific for this species
   2. Samples should be diluted before assaying
F. AST should be evaluated in conjunction with ALT for dog and cat
   1. Increased ALT with normal to mildly elevated AST may indicate reversible liver damage
   2. Marked elevations in ALT and AST indicate hepatocellular necrosis
   3. Increased AST with normal ALT may indicate that the source of AST is not liver
G. Samples required
   1. Nonhemolysed, nonlipemic serum or plasma
   2. Specimen should be centrifuged and removed from the cells immediately because AST will leak out of the red blood cells into the serum or plasma

IV. AP
A. Alkaline phosphatase
B. Present in almost all tissues of the body, especially in liver and bone
   1. Used as an indication of intrahepatic or posthepatic cholestasis
C. Increases in AP are due to increased production of the enzyme rather than reduced excretion of the enzyme through the bile system
   1. This enzyme is normally present in serum in small amounts
D. Increased AP is common in young animals due to the increased rate of bone growth
E. Increased AP in adult animals may be seen with bone injury or in obstructive liver disease
F. Glucocorticoids and some anticonvulsant drugs will give a marked increase in AP for up to 2 weeks after administration
G. Samples required
   1. Serum or heparinized plasma

V. LDH
A. Lactate dehydrogenase
B. Found in most tissues of the body, including liver, muscle, and red blood cells
C. Elevations in serum are considered nonspecific because they may be due to damage or necrosis of any tissues containing this enzyme
D. Samples required
   1. Serum or plasma collected with any anticoagulant other than EDTA or the oxalates

VI. GGT
A. γ-Glutamyltransferase
B. Found in liver, pancreas, and kidney
C. Elevations in serum usually caused by liver source
   1. GGT is elevated primarily in cholestasis but will be increased in all liver diseases
   2. In small animals, increased GGT will usually be accompanied by increased ALT
   3. GGT increase is a good indicator for small animal fatty liver disease
   4. Some medications also will cause an increase in GGT

VII. SD
A. Sorbitol dehydrogenase
B. Found primarily in liver cells; will be elevated in serum in cases of hepatocellular damage or necrosis
C. Sometimes used in large animals to replace ALT when diagnosing liver disease
D. Very unstable
   1. Much of the activity is lost within 8 hours of collection of the sample
   2. This is a limiting factor if samples are being processed by out-of-clinic laboratories

Bile Acids

I. Formed in the liver, secreted into the bile, and stored in the gallbladder between meals

II. Secreted into the intestinal tract where they aid in fat absorption and digestion
III. Most reabsorbed in the ileum, filtered from the blood by the liver, and recycled
   A. Mechanism is so efficient that normally serum values are very low
      1. Normal resting values: cat, 5 μmol/L; dog, 9 μmol/L
      2. Two-hour postprandial values: cat, 10 μmol/L; dog, 30 μmol/L
IV. Increased serum bile acid levels are noted in all forms of liver disease because the liver cannot clear the acids from the blood
V. Decreased serum bile acid levels are noted in delayed gastric emptying and ileal disease
VI. Sample required
   A. Serum

Serum Cholesterol

I. Mostly derived from liver synthesis
II. Increases usually associated with hypothyroidism
   A. Will also occur with lipemia
   B. Associated with diabetes mellitus, hyperadrenocorticism, nephrotic syndrome, some liver diseases, bile duct obstruction, and pregnancy
III. Not a liver-specific test
IV. Sample required
   A. Nonhemolysed serum or heparinized plasma; fasting is recommended

ELECTROLYTES AND MINERALS

General Information

I. Sodium, potassium, chloride, and bicarbonate are the four electrolytes in plasma
II. Minerals of importance are calcium, phosphate, and magnesium
   A. These two groups are often simply called electrolytes
   B. These are the anions (negatively charged ions) and cations (positively charged ions) found in the fluids of all animals
III. Electrolytes help to maintain water balance, osmotic pressure, and normal muscular and nervous functions; act as activators for enzyme reactions; and function in acid-base balance

Serum Sodium

I. Most abundant extracellular cation that plays a major role in the distribution of water and the maintenance of osmotic pressure of fluids in the body
   A. If sodium is retained, water is retained
II. Hypernatremia or increased serum sodium is rare unless the animal is deprived of water
III. Hyponatremia, or decreased serum sodium, is quite common and is seen in conditions such as renal failure, vomiting, or diarrhea; use of diuretics; excessive ADH; congestive heart failure; water toxicity; or excessive administration of fluids
IV. Sample required
   A. Nonhemolysed serum is preferred
   B. Plasma collected with lithium or ammonium heparin is also acceptable
   C. Remove from cells as soon as possible

Serum Potassium

I. Cation that is 90% intracellular
   A. Serum levels are so low that measurement of serum potassium does not give much information about the body's potassium levels
II. Hyperkalemia or increased serum potassium will be seen in adrenal cortical hypofunction, acidosis, or late-stage renal failure
III. Hypokalemia or decreased serum potassium will be seen in alkalosis, insulin therapy, or excess fluid loss due to diuretics, vomiting, and diarrhea
IV. Samples required
   A. Nonhemolysed serum or heparinized plasma (plasma preferred)
   B. Remove from the cells as soon as possible
      1. Especially important in cattle and horse, which have sufficient potassium in their red blood cells to alter serum chemistry results

Serum Chloride

I. It is the most abundant extracellular anion
   A. Chloride plays an important role in water and electrolyte balance and osmotic pressure
      1. Concentration is regulated by the kidneys
   B. There is a close relationship between sodium and chloride levels
      1. Hyperchloremia is increased serum chloride
         a. May be due to metabolic acidosis or renal tubular acidosis
      2. Hypochloremia is decreased serum chloride
         a. May be due to excessive vomiting, anorexia, malnutrition, or diabetes insipidus or in conjunction with hypokalemia
II. Samples required
   A. Nonhemolysed serum preferred
   B. Also heparinized plasma
   C. Remove serum from cells as soon as possible

Serum Calcium

I. About 99% of the body's calcium is in bone
II. Remaining calcium

A. Maintains neuromuscular excitability and tone
B. Acts as an enzyme activator
C. Is important in coagulation
D. Helps in transport of inorganic ions across cell membranes

III. Calcium and phosphorous levels are closely related and have an inverse relationship
A. Both are regulated by parathyroid hormone (PTH), calcitonin, and vitamin D

IV. Serum calcium levels vary with serum protein and serum albumin levels
A. These should be evaluated with serum calcium

V. Hypercalcemia or increased serum calcium seen in
A. Pseudohyperparathyroidism
B. Hyperparathyroidism
C. Excessive vitamin D intake
D. Bony metastases

VI. Hypocalcemia or decreased serum calcium may be seen in
A. Malabsorption
B. Eclampsia
C. Pancreatic necrosis
D. Hypoalbuminemia
E. Gastrointestinal stasis or blockage in ruminants
F. Postparturient lactation in cow, bitch, ewe, and mare
G. Hypoparathyroidism

VII. Sample required
A. Nonhemolysed serum or heparinized plasma

Serum Phosphorus

I. Most of the body's phosphorus (80%) is found in bone
A. Remaining 20% functions in the body in carbohydrate metabolism, energy storage, and release and transfer, and in the composition of important structures such as nucleic acids

II. Serum calcium and serum phosphorous are closely related and have an inverse relationship

III. PTH regulates serum phosphorus

IV. Hyperphosphatemia or increased serum inorganic phosphorous may be seen in renal failure, anuria, excessive vitamin D intake, ethyl glycol poisoning, and hypoparathyroidism

V. Hypophosphatemia or decreased serum inorganic phosphorous may occur in
A. Primary hyperparathyroidism
B. Malabsorption
C. Inadequate intake
D. Hyperinsulinism
E. Diabetes mellitus
F. Lymphosarcoma
G. Hyperadrenocorticism

VI. Sample required
A. Nonhemolysed serum or heparinized plasma
B. Remove serum or plasma from the cells as soon as possible

Serum Magnesium

I. Magnesium (cation) is found in all body tissues and is closely related to calcium and phosphorus

II. Imbalance in the calcium-magnesium ratio can lead to muscle tetany in cattle and sheep

III. Sometimes calcium and magnesium have a reciprocal relationship; other times they have a direct relationship

IV. Sample required
A. Nonhemolysed serum or plasma

MEASUREMENT OF ELECTROLYTES

I. Flame photometry: serum sodium and serum potassium

II. Ion-selective electrodes: all of the electrolytes

III. Coulometric methods: serum chloride

IV. Atomic absorption: serum calcium, serum magnesium

V. Colorimetric methods: serum calcium, serum phosphorus

Box 6-1 Summary of Function Tests

LIVER FUNCTION TESTS

AST (aspartate aminotransferase)
ALT (alanine aminotransferase)
AP (alkaline phosphatase)
Total serum bilirubin
Direct/conjugated bilirubin
Bile acids
Glucose
Cholesterol
Urine bilirubin
Urine urobilinogen
Total serum protein
Serum albumin
Electrophoresis: protein fractionation
Plasma fibrinogen
Hematology

KIDNEY FUNCTION TESTS

Serum creatinine
Blood urea nitrogen
Urine concentration/water deprivation tests
Endogenous creatinine clearance tests
Serum electrolytes and minerals: sodium, potassium, calcium, phosphorus, magnesium, chloride
Hematology

PANCREATIC FUNCTION TESTS

Endocrine Function

Serum glucose
Urinalysis; urine glucose
Glucose tolerance tests

Exocrine Function

Serum amylase
Serum lipase
Trypsin-like immunoreactivity assay

TESTS FOR MUSCLE DISEASE

Creatine kinase
AST
LDH

DIGESTIVE TRACT TESTS

Serum amylase
Serum lipase
Fecal trypsin
Examine feces for parasites, fat, starch, muscle fibers
Plasma turbidity test
Glucose tolerance test
Total serum protein
Hematology
Xylose absorption test
Serum folate
Serum B_{12}

ENDOCRINE FUNCTION TESTS

Parathyroid Gland

Parathormone (PTH)
Serum and urine calcium
Serum and urine phosphorus
Serum alkaline phosphatase

Thyroid Gland

Thyroxine: serum T_4
Triiodothyronine: serum T_3
Serum cholesterol
Serum protein

ADRENAL CORTEX FUNCTION TESTS

Serum glucose
Serum cholesterol
Alkaline phosphatase
Serum sodium
Serum potassium
Leukogram

ELECTROLYTES

Serum sodium
Serum potassium
Serum chloride

MINERALS

Serum calcium
Serum phosphorous
Serum magnesium

Table 6-1 Biochemistry reference intervals

	Unit	Canine	Feline	Bovine	Equine	Porcine
Albumin	g/L	29-43	30-44	34-43	30-37	27-39
Alkaline phosphatase	U/L	22-143	16-113	33-114	119-329	0-500
Alkaline transaminase	U/L	19-107	31-105	–	–	–
Amylase	U/L	299-947	482-1145	–	–	–
AST	U/L	–	–	56-176	259-595	–
Total bilirubin	µmol/L	0-4	0-3	0-5	21-57	0-4
Calcium	mmol/L	2.30-2.80	2.22-2.78	2.10-2.70	2.75-3.25	1.80-2.90
Chloride	mmol/L	104-119	114-123	91-103	95-104	99-105
Cholesterol	mmol/L	3.60-10.20	2.00-12.00	2.90-8.00	1.70-2.70	2.0-5.0
Creatinine	µmol/L	20-150	50-190	40-80	80-130	90-240
Glucose	mmol/L	3.3-7.3	4.4-7.7	2.1-3.8	3.7-6.7	3.6-5.3
Lipase	U/L	60-848	29-77	–	–	–
Magnesium	mmol/L	0.70-1.00	0.80-1.10	0.85-1.20	0.6-1.00	0.8-1.6
Phosphorus	mmol/L	0.90-1.85	0.80-2.29	1.46-2.83	0.73-1.71	1.6-3.4
Protein	g/L	55-74	66-84	70-94	58-75	61-81
Potassium	mmol/L	3.8-5.4	3.6-5.2	3.7-5.4	3.1-4.3	4.7-7.1
Sodium	mmol/L	140-154	147-157	134-149	136-144	140-150
Urea	mmol/L	3.5-9.0	6.0-12.0	3.0-8.3	4.2-8.9	3.0-8.5

Results vary from laboratory to laboratory and depend on the method used, as well as the animal's breed, sex, age, and environment.
Courtesy of the Animal Health Laboratory, Laboratory Services Division, University of Guelph, Guelph, Ontario, Canada.

Table 6-2 Biochemical reference values: conventional units

	Cattle	Sheep	Goat	Swine	Horse	Dog	Cat
Alanine aminotransferase (ALT; SGPT) (U/L)	–	–	–	–	–	17-69	34-55
Alkaline phosphatase (AP; SAP) (U/L)	41-94	0-140	42-775	–	83-283	5-73	14-25
Amylase (U/L)	–	–	–	–	9-34	700-1700	1000-1700
Aspartate aminotransferase (AST; SGOT) (U/L)	42-98	31-111	67-117	–	153-411	12-37	11-29
Bile acids (µg/mL)	–	–	–	–	0-5	0-5	0-5
Bilirubin							
Total (mg/dL)	0-1.9	0-0.4	0-0.1	0-0.2	0.2-6.0	0-0.4	0-0.5
Direct (mg/dL)	0-0.4	0-0.3	–	–	0-0.4	0-0.1	0-0.1
Calcium (mg/dL)	8.0-10.5	11.5-13.0	8.5-10.2	11.0-11.3	11.2-13.8	8.7-11.8	9.2-11.9
Chloride (mEq/L)	95-110	98-110	99-110	100-105	98-110	99-110	117-123
Cholesterol (mg/dL)	39-177	40-58	80-130	117-119	46-177	117-345	100-165
Creatine phosphokinase (CPK; CK) (U/L)	66-220	0-330	108-211	–	92-307	12-292	0-540
Creatinine (mg/dL)	1.0-2.7	1.2-1.9	–	1.0-2.7	1.2-1.9	0.7-1.6	1.2-2.1
Gamma glutamyltransferase (GGT) (U/L)	13-32	35-67	43-71	–	11-44	0-11	0-1
Glucose (mg/dL)	35-55	30-65	58-76	65-95	60-100	55-102	55-114
Iron (µg/dL)	57-162	166-222	–	91-199	73-140	94-122	68-215
Lipase (U/L)	–	–	–	–	40-78	52-305	–
Magnesium (mg/dL)	1.2-3.5	1.9-2.5	2.8-3.6	1.9-3.9	1.8-2.5	1.5-2.4	1.9-2.7
Phosphorus (mg/dL)	4.0-7.0	4.0-7.0	7.5-12.3	4.0-11.0	3.1-5.6	2.8-7.6	4.6-7.1
Potassium (mEq/L)	3.9-5.8	4.8-5.9	3.5-6.7	4.7-7.1	3.0-5.0	3.7-5.6	4.0-4.5
Sodium (mEq/L)	132-152	145-160	142-155	140-150	132-150	137-149	147-156
Sorbitol dehydrogenase (SDH) (U/L)	18-46	14-41	35-80	–	0-15	–	–
Triglycerides (mg/dL)	–	–	–	–	5-55	10-140	30-100
Urea nitrogen (mg/dL)	6-27	8-20	15-33	8-24	10-20	7-21	18-34
Acid-base							
Bicarbonate (mmol/L)	20-30	21-28	26-30	18-27	23-32	17-24	17-24
pH	7.35-7.50	7.32-7.50	–	–	7.32-7.55	7.31-7.42	7.24-7.40
Pco_2 (mm Hg)	34-45	–	–	–	38-46	–	–
Proteins							
Total protein (g/dL)	5.7-8.1	6.0-7.9	5.9-7.4	7.9-8.9	6.0-7.7	5.4-7.1	5.4-7.8
Albumin (g/dL)	2.1-3.6	2.4-3.0	2.7-3.9	1.8-3.3	2.9-3.8	2.6-3.3	2.1-3.3
α_1 Globulin (g/dL)	0.7-1.2	0.3-0.6	0.5-0.7	0.3-0.4	0.7-1.3	0.2-0.5	0.2-1.1
α_2 Globulin (g/dL)	–	0.3-0.6	–	1.3-1.5	0.7-1.3	0.3-1.1	0.4-0.9
β_1 Globulin (g/dL)	0.6-1.2	1.1-2.6	0.7-1.2	0.1-0.3	0.4-1.2	0.7-1.3	0.3-0.9
β_2 Globulin (g/dL)	–	–	0.3-0.6	1.3-1.7	–	0.6-1.4	0.6-1.0
γ_1 Globulin (g/dL)	1.6-3.2	0.9-3.3	0.9-3.0	2.2-2.5	0.9-1.5	0.5-1.3	0.3-2.5
γ_2 Globulin (g/dL)	–	–	–	–	–	0.4-0.9	1.4-1.9

All enzymes measured at 37° C. Reference values may be influenced by the method of measurement and by the animal's breed, sex, age, and environment. Hence these values are guidelines only.
Updated from first edition by B.W. Parry, University of Melbourne, Werribee, Victoria, Australia.
Reproduced from Blood DC, Studdert VP: *Saunder's comprehensive veterinary dictionary*, ed 2, Philadelphia, 1999, WB Saunders.

Table 6-3 Conversion factors for biochemistry data

Analyte	Conventional unit	Multiplication factor	SI unit	Multiplication factor	Conventional unit
Alanine aminotransferase	U/L	1	U/L	1	U/L
Albumin	g/dL	10	g/L	0.10	g/dL
Alkaline phosphatase	U/L	1	U/L	1	U/L
Amylase	U/L	1	U/L	1	U/L
Aspartate aminotransferase	U/L	1	U/L	1	U/L
Bicarbonate	mEq/L	1	mmol/L	1	mEq/L
Bile acids	μg/mL	2.547	μmol/L	0.3926	μg/mL
Bilirubin	mg/dL	17.10	μmol/L	0.058	mg/dL
Calcium	mg/dL	0.2495	mmol/L	4.008	mg/dL
Chloride	mEq/L	1	mmol/L	1	mEq/L
Cholesterol	mg/dL	0.02586	mmol/L	38.67	mg/dL
Creatine (phospho)kinase	U/L	1	U/L	1	U/L
Creatinine	mg/dL	88.4	μmol/L	0.011	mg/dL
Gamma glutamyltransferase	U/L	1	U/L	1	U/L
Glucose	mg/dL	0.0555	mmol/L	18.0	mg/dL
Iron	μg/dL	0.1791	μmol/L	5.583	μg/dL
Lipase	U/L	1	U/L	1	U/L
Magnesium	mg/dL	0.4114	mmol/L	2.431	mg/dL
Pco_2	mm Hg	0.1333	kPa	7.502	mm Hg
Phosphorus	mg/dL	0.3229	mmol/L	3.097	mg/dL
Potassium	mEq/L	1	mmol/L	1	mEq/L
Proteins	g/dL	10	g/L	0.10	g/dL
Sodium	mEq/L	1	mmol/L	1	mEq/L
Sorbitol dehydrogenase	U/L	1	U/L	1	U/L
Triglycerides	mg/dL	0.01129	mmol/L	88.6	mg/dL
Urea (nitrogen)	mg/dL	0.3570	mmol/L	2.80	mg/dL

From Blood DC, Studdert VP: *Saunder's comprehensive veterinary dictionary*, ed 2, Philadelphia, 1999, WB Saunders.

Glossary

amyloclastic test Method of measuring serum amylase by measuring the disappearance of a starch substrate

anion Negatively charged ions

anticoagulant Chemicals used to inhibit whole blood from clotting. The liquid portion of the sample harvested is plasma

azotemia Increased levels of urea in blood samples

bile A fluid produced by the liver and stored in the gallbladder that aids in digestion. This substance is primarily composed of bile acids or salts, bile pigments, and cholesterol

cation Positively charged ion

Cushing's syndrome Hyperactivity of adrenal cortices secondary to excessive pituitary excretion of adrenocorticotropin hormone

dry chemistry Method of chemical analysis. All the reagents needed for a particular test are incorporated into a multilayered film slide. These special slides are used in automated analyzers

electrolytes Ions capable of carrying an electric charge

electrophoresis Separation of ionic solutes, such as serum proteins, based on their rates of migration in an applied electric field

endogenous Something produced within an organism or caused by something within an organism

hemolysis Destruction of red blood cells, causing release of hemoglobin

hypercalcemia Excess calcium in the blood

hyperchloremia Excess chlorides in the blood

hyperglycemia Increased blood glucose levels

hyperkalemia Excess potassium in the blood

hypernatremia Excess sodium in the blood

hyperparathyroidism Excessive activity of the parathyroid glands

hyperphosphatemia Excessive phosphate in the blood

hypocalcemia Blood calcium levels below normal

hypochloremia Abnormally low levels of chloride in the blood

hypoglycemia Decreased blood glucose levels

hypokalemia Abnormally low potassium levels in the blood

hyponatremia Salt depletion or abnormally low levels of sodium in the blood

hypoparathyroidism Underactivity of the parathyroid glands

hypophosphatemia Blood phosphate levels below normal

icterus Jaundice; result of excess bilirubin in the blood

lipemia Excess lipids in the blood
malabsorption Impaired intestinal absorption of nutrients
malassimilation Gastrointestinal tract is unable to take up nutrients because of faulty digestion or impairment of the transport mechanisms across the intestinal mucosa
metastasis Growth of pathogenic organisms or abnormal cells distant from the primary site of development
osmotic pressure Hydrostatic pressure required to stop osmosis, which is the diffusion of molecules of a dilute solution passing through the walls of a semipermeable membrane into a more concentrated solution
plasma Liquid portion of blood in which proteins, cells, electrolytes, nutrients, and products of metabolism are suspended
prehepatic Before the liver
radioimmunoassay Technique that measures the rate of immune complex formation using radiolabeled isotopes
saccharogenic test Method for measuring serum amylase by measuring reducing sugars that are produced as a result of amylase action
serum Liquid portion of blood that has been allowed to clot; contains all the same constituents as plasma except fibrinogen, which is consumed in the clotting process
steatorrhea Large amounts of fat in the stool

Review Questions

1 Serum urea levels can be influenced by all except
   a. Amount of protein in an animal's diet
   b. Lipemia
   c. Hemolysis
   d. How well the glomeruli are filtering

2 Plasma samples collected for measurement of blood glucose levels
   a. Should ideally be collected right after an animal has eaten
   b. Should be collected using EDTA
   c. Should be centrifuged and the plasma removed from the cells as soon as possible
   d. Are preferred over serum samples because they are easier to collect

3 Which of the following is considered to be of little diagnostic value when evaluating cats for pancreatic insufficiency?
   a. Serum lipase levels
   b. Serum amylase levels
   c. Serum protease levels
   d. Bile acids

4 Total serum bilirubin levels are an important indicator of liver disease in some species but not in others. This is a useful test for which of the following species?
   a. Bovine
   b. Equine
   c. Canine
   d. Ovine

5 As a general rule, when the albumin and globulin fractions of blood proteins are measured
   a. Albumin fraction increases, globulin fraction decreases
   b. Globulin fraction increases, albumin fraction decreases
   c. Both the albumin and globulin fractions increase at the same time
   d. Ratios of each protein remain the same regardless of the disease state

6 Which of the following liver enzyme tests would likely not be part of a liver profile for a horse?
   a. AST
   b. ALT
   c. AP
   d. SD

7 Which of the following statements regarding samples used for liver profiles is not true?
   a. Any anticoagulant can be used when collecting for the profile
   b. Serum is the sample of choice for any blood chemistry tests
   c. Samples should be separated as soon as possible, because the levels of some of the chemicals will be altered if the serum or plasma sits on the cells
   d. Commercially prepared blood collection systems are preferred over reusable syringes

8 Which of the serum protein fractions rarely increases in a disease state?
   a. Albumin
   b. α-Globulins
   c. β-Globulins
   d. γ-Globulins

9 Bile acids
   a. Are usually found in high levels in the bloodstream
   b. Aid in the absorption and digestion of ingested fats
   c. Are removed from circulating blood by the duodenum
   d. Are stored in the liver

10 Which statement is false: when measuring urea levels in serum or plasma, these samples should be handled carefully because
   a. Ammonia in the room can produce false increases in results
   b. Ammonium oxalate anticoagulant will produce false increases in results
   c. Fluoride will inhibit the reaction used to measure urea
   d. Hemolysis will produce false decreases in the results

BIBLIOGRAPHY

Bishop ML, Duben-Engelkirk JL, Fody EP, editors: *Clinical chemistry: principles, procedures, correlations,* ed 4, Philadelphia, 2000, JB Lippincott.
Burtis CA, Ashwood ER, editors: *Tietz fundamentals of clinical chemistry,* ed 5, Philadelphia, 2001, WB Saunders.
Duncan JR, Prasse KW, Mahaffey EA: *Veterinary laboratory medicine: clinical pathology,* ed 3, Ames, 1994, Iowa State University Press.
Fenner WR: *Quick reference to veterinary medicine,* ed 2, Philadelphia, 1991, JB Lippincott.
Houston D: Lecture delivered at St. Lawrence College, 1991.

Kaneko JJ, Harvey JW, Bruss ML, editors: *Clinical biochemistry of domestic animals,* ed 5, New York, 1997, Academic Press.

Kaplan A, Szabo LL: *Clinical chemistry: interpretation and techniques,* ed 2, Philadelphia, 1983, Lea & Febiger.

McCurnin DM, Bassert JM, editors: *Clinical textbook for veterinary technicians,* ed 5, Philadelphia, 2002, WB Saunders.

Pratt PW, editor: *Laboratory procedures for veterinary technicians,* ed 3, St Louis, 1997, Mosby.

Simpson JW, Else RW: *Digestive disease in the dog and cat,* ed 2, London, 1996, Blackwell Scientific Publications.

Sirois M, McBride DF, editors: *Veterinary clinical laboratory procedures,* ed 1, St Louis, 1995, Mosby.

CHAPTER 7

Virology

Patricia L. Bell

OUTLINE

LEARNING OUTCOMES

After reading this chapter you should be able to:

1. Describe the composition of a virus.
2. Describe the process of virus replication.
3. Describe, in general, different types of viral infections.
4. Describe sampling techniques, including the collection of specimens and submission of samples.
5. Describe various diagnostic testing procedures commonly performed in the clinic.
6. Explain common techniques for the prevention of contracting a virus or reducing the effects of viral diseases.

This chapter begins by reviewing the basic features of viruses, including their composition, control, and replication. The chapter also contains a brief summary defining common methods of studying the collection, culturing, and submission of clinical specimens for diagnostic laboratory analysis and laboratory diagnostic techniques. A list of a few of the most common viral diseases for different species and their vaccine availability are provided at the end of the chapter.

COMPOSITION AND CONTROL

I. Viruses are not cellular
   A. Viruses consist of protein and nucleic acid; some have lipids and carbohydrates
II. Viruses do not possess a nucleus, cytoplasm, cell membrane, or cell wall
III. Viruses are obligate intracellular parasites
   A. Viruses depend on host cell metabolism for their reproduction
   B. Animal viruses are most commonly cultured in mice, embryonated chicken eggs, or tissue culture
IV. Virus sizes vary
   A. Largest is poxvirus (300 × 240 × 200 nm)
   B. Smallest is parvovirus (22 nm diameter)
   C. Prions are considered to be smaller life forms
V. Classification
   A. Viruses are classified on the basis of
      1. Their shape as seen on electron microscopy
      2. Composition of their nucleic acid core (genome)
      3. Whether the virus possesses an envelope
VI. Envelope
   A. Lipid membrane that surrounds the virus is termed the envelope
      1. Enveloped viruses are easily killed
         a. Hypochlorite (common household bleach) dissolves fats

b. Freezing and thawing process will render the virus inert due to the breakdown of the envelope by frozen water molecules

B. "Naked virus" does not possess an envelope
1. Naked viruses are more refractory
2. It is more difficult to disinfect an area where these viruses have been located
a. Steam sterilization is recommended to kill all viruses at the temperature of 121° C (250° F) at 15 pounds per square inch (psi) for 30 minutes
b. Many commercial viricidal compounds, designed to be used in a clinical setting, are available to destroy different types of viruses

VII. Genomes
A. Mammalian genomes are composed of double-stranded DNA (deoxyribonucleic acid), from which various RNAs (ribonucleic acids) are transcribed
B. Viral nucleic acid can be DNA or RNA; can also be double or single stranded
1. Viruses with a nucleic acid core composed of RNA also possess a reverse transcriptase enzyme to create DNA from their RNA when they infect a mammalian host cell
2. Oncogenic viruses are common in the group, which have an RNA nucleic core; they are potentially cancer-causing agents
C. Some double-stranded DNA viruses can incorporate their DNA sequences into host cell DNA and be replicated during mitosis
1. This does not cause cellular damage and therefore no clinical signs: these are termed latent infections
2. Virus may lie dormant for years until the host is stressed due to age, malnutrition, water deprivation, shipping, surgery, or trauma, when the virus reemerges to produce intact virions and disease

VIII. Replication—there are four basic stages of replication for most viruses: attachment, penetration-uncoating, replication, and assembly-release
A. Attachment
1. Virus must gain access to the host cell to which it can bind
2. This is done via the virus portal entry
3. Portal entry is usually the mucosal surface to the respiratory, urogenital, or gastrointestinal tract
4. Breaks in the integument are a rare method of entry except when insect vectors are involved
5. Cell membrane is bound in a complementary fashion by the viral binding proteins
6. Viral binding proteins determine the species affected and the type of pathology caused
B. Penetration-uncoating
1. Most viruses produce enzymes that degrade the host cell membrane sufficiently to permit the nucleic acid core to enter
2. As it does so, the core exits the capsid (the "outer shell of the virus"), which remains on the host cell exterior
3. Exiting of the capsid is the uncoating process and occurs simultaneously with penetration
C. Replication
1. Aim is for the virus to produce thousands of copies of itself to ensure survival, but it lacks the ability to do so on its own
2. So the virus's nucleic acid redirects the host cell DNA to ignore its own needs and to instead produce viral components such as capsid fragments and viral nucleic acid
3. This results in the breakdown of the host cell membrane, and this change initiates the immune response (see Chapter 8)
4. Because the virus is hidden in the host cell, the immune system is not able to respond to the virus specifically
5. Virus has already reproduced many copies of itself, which readily invade other cells and begin replication before the immune system is activated
D. Assembly-release
1. After all the various components of the virus structure have attained a critical concentration, assembly occurs spontaneously
2. Viral components come together to produce virions
a. Virions can be visualized on electron microscopy
b. They are cytoplasmic, nuclear, or both, depending on where they occur within the host cell
3. Virions almost immediately leave the cell
4. Most viruses exit the cell by causing it to rupture, termed the "lysogenic cycle"
5. Cell is destroyed; this causes the overall signs of disease
6. Most viruses that undergo replication are released from the host cell, spread to neighboring cells, and begin again the process of replication
7. Some viruses will be shed in secretions of the host body
8. Other viruses enter the systemic circulation and spread throughout the body; this

is called a "viremia"—such infections can cause overall bodily signs such as rashes

IX. Limitation of viruses
   A. Some viruses are restricted to certain body temperatures
      1. Nasal passages of mammalian respiratory tract average 2° C lower than that of the lower respiratory tract and therefore remain susceptible to upper respiratory tract infections
   B. Some viruses are limited by the surface proteins found on certain cell types (these form localized infections)
   C. Other viruses enter the systemic circulation and spread throughout the body; this is viremia

VIRAL INFECTIONS

I. Viral infections of any type can affect the host with regard to clinical signs in one of two ways
   A. Apparent infection: causes clinical disease
      1. This disease may be peracute to chronic
   B. Silent, nonapparent, or subclinical infection: does not result in overt signs
      1. This may result in a transient carrier state
      2. Such carriers are difficult to identify
         a. They therefore can sometimes infect a herd despite quarantine precautions

II. Examples
   A. Neurons in rabies victims or the T-lymphocytes in cats infected with the feline immunodeficiency virus (FIV)
      1. These are cells that have become inactive or malfunction due to a virus
   B. Equine infectious anemia virus causes an immunological reaction within the host in which the immune system does more harm than the virus
      1. Immune system attacks the red blood cells, resulting in the anemia

III. Viral infections predispose an affected animal to secondary diseases (usually bacterial in nature) that can be worse than the primary viral disease
   A. Oncogenesis occurs with some viruses
      1. Infected cells transform, resulting in neoplasm with potential for malignancy such as Marek's disease in chickens

NOMENCLATURE

I. Viral family names end in the suffix *-viridae*

II. Viral genus names end in suffix *-virus*

III. Names are not underlined or italicized

SAMPLING TECHNIQUES

I. Analysis of samples is not usually done within a veterinary practice but instead at a commercial, regional, or state diagnostic laboratory

II. Analysis of samples is not usually completed in time to treat the sick animal, but it is used to confirm a diagnosis and for epidemiological reasons

III. Laboratory test results are only as reliable as the quality of the samples submitted and the history provided

IV. Virus is most easily cultured from specimens just before the onset of signs and for a short time afterward

V. Animals that have been showing clinical signs for a few days generally are not sampled for viruses

COLLECTION OF SPECIMENS

I. Representative animal from a herd should be sent for full examination (i.e., necropsy)

II. Examine ill and contact animals and sample from both because the virus titer (concentration) is highest before signs

III. To identify a disease via an antibody titer
   A. Bleed at least six readily identifiable animals with early clinical signs
   B. Bleed the same animals 2 to 4 weeks later
   C. Change in titer means a positive diagnosis of a current disease and not immunity from previous recovery from the disease

IV. If unsure what samples to collect, take a wide range for the virologist to choose from, or call the laboratory and discuss sample collection with the personnel

V. Use one of the following transport media
   A. Sterile Hanks' balanced salt solution plus 10% bovine serum albumin
   B. Sterile skim milk
   C. Sterile charcoal transport medium, which is available commercially

VI. Note: A virus will survive 3 weeks without refrigeration and therefore will survive shipping

VII. Antibiotics may be added to control bacterial contamination

VIII. Keep specimens cool, 1° to 4° C (34° to 39° F), but do not freeze

IX. Postmortem tissues collected aseptically from several areas of the body can be used for histopathology
   A. Sections should be no larger than 3 to 5 mm (3/16 inch) thick
   B. Sections should be fixed in 10% formalin
   C. Less than 1 g of tissue in transport medium
   D. Do not freeze these samples

X. Collection from a live animal
   A. Heparinized plasma for immediate submission
   B. Serum may also be collected, which may be frozen

SUBMISSION OF SAMPLES

Most laboratories will provide submission forms. The following pertinent information is needed for diagnosis.

I. Sampling information
II. Animal species
III. Age and sex of the patient(s)
IV. Size of the herd, flock, and kennel involved where applicable
V. Number of animals affected
VI. Duration of the illness to date
VII. Clinical signs
VIII. Losses, if any
IX. Similar cases in the area
X. Vaccination history (if not available, note on form)
XI. Treatment given up to the time of sampling
XII. Disease suspected
XIII. Specimens submitted and labeled appropriately

IN-CLINIC LABORATORY TESTING OF SAMPLES

I. Viruses are identified initially on the basis of
    A. Clinical history
    B. Specimen sample submitted
    C. Immunoreactivity
    D. One or a combination of histopathology, advanced laboratory tests, and electron microscopy
II. In some instances the most commonly used techniques have been adapted to kit form so they may be used in a clinical setting or out in the field
    A. Fluorescent antibody (FA) test
        1. This test uses antibodies of known specificity that bind viral antigens
        2. Binding can then be visualized due to conjugation (labeled) with a fluorescent dye
        3. Such a procedure can be performed using frozen tissue sections, tissue imprints, tissue scrapings, and blood smears
        4. Selection depends on the viral life cycle within the host
        5. Often such results are available rapidly (in less than 1 hour)
            a. Accuracy depends on the application to appropriate specimens that are in good condition (fresh with little to no autolysis)
        6. This may not be an applicable test method if the required samples cannot be obtained from live animals
    B. Enzyme-linked immunosorbent assay (ELISA) test
        1. Popular test kit method in which a known specific antibody is adsorbed, usually in a small plastic well in a well plate or a specially designed membrane (kit dependent)
        2. These antibodies will have patient sample applied
        3. Common disease that is screened in this manner is feline leukemia virus (FeLV)
            a. Viral antigen, if present in the animal's serum, is tightly and specifically bound by the adsorbed antibodies
            b. Another antibody of the same specificity, which is labeled (most frequently with an enzyme), is applied to produce a sandwich formation
            c. Another alternative to the enzymatic label is a fluorescent label
            d. Very important wash step is then performed to remove any unbound labeled antibody (which would be the case if the animal does not possess the viral antigen in its serum and therefore is negative for FeLV)
            e. If the viral antigen is present, the labeled antibody will not be removed because the binding is very strong
            f. Substrate is then added; it must be one that reacts with the enzyme with which the second antibody is labeled
            g. Reaction produces a visible color change to permit the technician to recognize the unhealthy animal's state
            h. In some cases in which no vaccine is available, the viral antigen can be bound to the well or membrane to detect antibody in the patient's serum as an indicator of the disease; this technique is the one of choice in such cases and where the viral titer remains low in the body
    C. Latex agglutination (LA) test
        1. Another popular test kit; it uses the same principles as the ELISA test
        2. Antiviral antibodies are adsorbed to microscopic latex beads. If the applied sample contains the antigen (virus), it will be bound by these antibodies and produce agglutination
        3. Due to the granular appearance of the latex beads in solution, it is very important to run positive and negative controls simultaneously
        4. Such a method can be used to detect parvovirus from fecal samples of ill dogs or rotavirus in the feces of various species with rotaviral diarrhea

PREVENTION

There are three major factors involved in preventing occurrence or reducing the effects of viral diseases.

I. Health measures
   A. Good hygiene
   B. Prompt disposal of dead animals
   C. Proper nutrition
   D. Clean and adequate water supply
   E. Reasonable population density to reduce stress
   F. Screening and quarantine of new animals before their entry into the household or herd
II. Immunization if possible and maintenance of current vaccinations
III. Treatment of viral disease

COMMON VIRAL DISEASES AND VACCINE AVAILABILITY

Disease	Etiology	Vaccine available
	BOVINE	
Leukemia	Retrovirus	No
Spongioform encephalopathy	Prion	No
Viral diarrhea	Pestivirus	Yes, killed and modified live virus (MLV) (caution when using in pregnant cows and those incubating the disease)
Calf scours complex	Rotavirus and coronavirus	Yes, but best when given to the dam and passed through colostrum
Foot and mouth	Picornavirus	Yes, killed, resulting in short-term immunity; not always effective
Infectious rhinotracheitis	Herpesvirus	Yes, MLV and killed
Parainfluenza-3	Paramyxovirus	Yes, killed and attenuated-live
Respiratory syncytial virus	Paramyxovirus	No
Vesicular stomatitis	Vesiculovirus	No, not in North America
	PORCINE	
Encephalomyocarditis	Picornavirus	No
Hemagglutinating encephalomyelitis	Coronavirus	No
Hog cholera	Pestivirus	Yes, MLV
Porcine parvovirus infection	Parvovirus	Yes, killed and MLV
Pseudorabies	Herpesvirus	Yes, attenuated; effectiveness is low
Reproductive and respiratory syndrome	Arteriviridae	Yes
Rotavirus infection	Rotavirus	Yes, MLV and killed
Swine influenza	Orthomyxovirus	Yes, inactivated
Swine pox	Poxvirus	No
Transmissible gastroenteritis	Coronavirus	Yes, attenuated-live and killed planned infections are done in epidemic areas only
Vesicular exanthema of swine	Calicivirus	No
	OVINE AND CAPRINE	
Border disease	Pestivirus	No
Bluetongue	Orbivirus	Yes, MLV and killed (used in some countries—not in the United States, where import restrictions are used for control
Caprine arthritis-encephalitis	Lentivirus	No
Contagious ecthyma	Poxvirus	Yes
Progressive pneumonia of sheep	Lentivirus	No
Scrapie	Prion	No
	EQUINE	
Coital exanthema	Herpesvirus	No
Encephalomyelitis	Arbovirus	Yes, MLV
Influenza	Orthomyxovirus	Yes, killed
Infectious anemia	Nononcogenic retrovirus	No
Viral arteritis	Togavirus	Yes, MLV
Rhinopneumonitis	Varicellavirus	Yes, killed and MLV; caution—high abortion risk

COMMON VIRAL DISEASES AND VACCINE AVAILABILITY—cont'd

	CANINE	
Coronavirus infections	Coronoavirus	Yes, killed
Distemper	Morbillivirus	Yes, MLV; can use measles followed by distemper or a combination in very young pups
Herpesvirus infection	Herpesvirus	No
Infectious hepatitis	Adenovirus	Yes, MLV and killed
Infectious tracheobronchitis	Parainfluenza virus, adenovirus, morbillivirus, and simultaneous bacterial infections	Yes, polyvalent vaccines due to simultaneous infections
Parvoviral enteritis	Parvovirus	Yes, MLV; possibly not effective due to viral mutation
Rabies	Rhabdovirus	Yes, MLV and killed
	FELINE	
Calicivirus/rhinotracheitis	Calicivirus	Yes, polyvalent MLV
Infectious peritonitis	Coronavirus	Yes, MLV (not entirely effective)
Immunodeficiency virus	Lentivirus	No
Leukemia	Oncogenic retrovirus	Yes, effectiveness varies
Panleukopenia	Parvovirus	Yes, inactivated and MLV
	AVIAN	
Encephalomyelitis	Enterovirus	Yes, killed and MLV
Infectious laryngotracheitis	Herpesvirus	Yes, MLV
Influenza	Orthomyxovirus	No
Leukosis	Retrovirus	No
Coronal enteritis of turkeys	Coronavirus	No
Duck plague	Herpesvirus	No
Fowl pox	Poxvirus	Yes, attenuated-live
Infectious bronchitis	Coronavirus	Yes, killed and MLV polyvalent; full immunity may not occur
Marek's disease	Herpesvirus	Yes
Psittacine beak and feather	Circovirus	No
Newcastle disease	Paramyxovirus	Yes, MLV
Infectious bursal disease	Birnavirus	Yes, inactivated and MLV

See Chapter 8 for an in-depth explanation about types of vaccines.

Glossary

adsorbed To attract and retain other material on the surface

altered self Any change in the molecular configuration of one's cells and therefore attack by the immune system. This state may be a result of viral invasion of cells, cancer, radiation, or poisoning

autoclave Instrument with a chamber in which materials are rendered sterile via a treatment with the necessary steam heat and pressure for a specific period of time

autolysis Rupture and death of a cell

capsid Shell of protein that protects the nucleic acid of a virus

DNA Standard short form for deoxyribonucleic acid. The physical basis for the genetic code. It forms a double-stranded helix in animals. Under strict and specific physiological regulations, it codes for the production of RNA. In viruses it may be single or double stranded

genome Entire genetic complement of an organism. In animals it involves DNA and RNA, but in viruses it is one or the other

inactivated To render inert or nonfunctional by exposure to heat of sufficient temperature and duration

latent Quiescent state awaiting later reactivation, which may occur years later. In the case of latent viruses, they insert their DNA into the host cell DNA to be replicated together. Frequently stress is implicated in the viruses' resurgence and resultant disease state

lysin Agent that ruptures (bursts) and therefore kills host cells

lysogenic cycle Ability to cause lysis or produce lysins; ability to exit a host cell by rupturing that cell causing its death

nucleic acid core Molecule of DNA or RNA, either of which can be double or single stranded. The term is used synonymously with "viral genome"

obligate intracellular parasite A parasite that lives within a host cell. The host cell is its only means of survival

oncogenesis Production of tumors
parasite One organism that survives at the detriment of another
portal of entry Pathway by which a pathogenic agent gains entry to the body
prion Proteinaceous infectious particle, the smallest known microorganism. Still unseen on electron microscopy; laboratory tests indicate that although this microorganism does not possess any nucleic acid, it consists of protein and is capable of producing disease
psi Old, standard unit of pressure that is still widely in use; denotes pounds per square inch
refractory Resistant, capable of withstanding adverse conditions and surviving
RNA One form of nucleic acid, of which there are three forms: ribosomal, messenger, and transfer. It codes for the assembly of proteins. Some viruses, such as the retroviruses, possess only RNA in their genome but due to the possession of a reverse transcriptase enzyme they can "reverse code" for DNA
reverse transcriptase RNA Enzyme of RNA viruses that catalyzes the transcription of RNA to DNA, which is then incorporated into a genome of the host cell self-recognized by the immune system as one's own molecular configuration and therefore tolerated
subclinical Used to describe the early stages or a very mild form of a disease
titer Strength per volume of a volumetric test solution
T-lymphocytes Lymphocytes that do not produce antibody; rather they primarily act to destroy altered self in the body due to viral infection or neoplastic transformation
tolerance State of being tolerated by the immune system and therefore not attacked. In health this occurs to one's own body only; if it is conveyed to microorganisms, it will result in an immunodeficiency
viremia Stage of some infections where the virus enters the blood and spreads throughout the body
viricidal Term meaning virus killer; frequently used to describe disinfectant chemicals with this capacity
virion Intact, functional virus particle, capable of infecting a host cell

Review Questions

1 Which of the following statements is true about viruses?
 a. They are microscopic, cellular, parasitic organisms
 b. They are all readily destroyed by ordinary household soaps and other disinfectants
 c. They are obligate intracellular parasites
 d. All of the above

2 Which of the following is not a major factor in reducing the effects of or preventing viral disease?
 a. Treatment
 b. Immunization
 c. Replication cycle of the virus
 d. Health measures

3 Envelope viruses are rendered inert with
 a. Freezing and thawing
 b. Heat
 c. Soap and water
 d. None of the above

4 Which of the following is used to classify a virus?
 a. Their shape, as seen via electron microscopy
 b. Type of genome it possesses
 c. Presence or lack of an envelope
 d. All of the above

5 Autoclaving to sterilize a virally contaminated material requires the following same parameters, as for a bacterially contaminated material
 a. 121° C, 15 psi for 30 minutes
 b. 250° F, 150 psi for 15 minutes
 c. 121° C, 10 psi for 15 minutes
 d. 250° F, 100 psi for 30 minutes

6 Complete the following statement: "viruses are spread between contacts most effectively . . ."
 a. During the acute stage of the disease
 b. Before the onset of clinical signs and for a very short time afterward
 c. At the beginning of convalescence
 d. None of the above

7 When submitting samples to a diagnostic laboratory virology department, it is important to
 a. Include a thorough case history
 b. Use an approved shipping medium
 c. Take serum samples from readily identifiable animals, now and up to 4 weeks later
 d. All of the above

8 Viral diseases are treated by administering antibiotics
 a. True
 b. Only during the viremic stage
 c. Only as a supportive measure to control opportunistic infections
 d. Only if the disease is due to an enveloped virus

9 Viral diagnostic tests include
 a. Fluorescent antibody test
 b. Electron microscopic visualization
 c. Enzyme-linked immunosorbent assay
 d. All of the above

10 The following is an acceptable transport media for viruses
 a. Skim milk medium
 b. Sterile William's solution
 c. Sterile carbon transport medium
 d. Formaldehyde

BIBLIOGRAPHY

Black JG: *Microbiology principles and applications,* ed 3, New Jersey, 1996, Prentice-Hall.
Blood DC, Studdert VP: *Saunders comprehensive veterinary dictionary,* ed 2, Philadelphia, 1999, WB Saunders.
Gershwin LJ et al: *Immunology and immunopathology of domestic animals,* ed 2, St Louis, 1995, Mosby.

Quinn PJ et al: *Clinical veterinary microbiology,* Madrid, Spain, 1994, Mosby.

Roberts AW, Carter GR, Chengappa MM: *Essentials of veterinary microbiology,* ed 5, Philadelphia, 1995, Williams & Wilkins.

The Merck veterinary manual, ed 8, Whitehouse Station, NJ, 1998, Merck and Company.

Turgeon ML: *Immunology and serology in laboratory medicine,* St Louis, 1990, Mosby.

CHAPTER 8

Immunology

Patricia L. Bell

OUTLINE

LEARNING OUTCOMES

After reading this chapter you should be able to:

1. Briefly describe in general terms how the immune system defends the body from an infection.
2. Describe innate and adaptive immunity.
3. Compare and contrast primary versus secondary immune responses and how they relate to vaccine protocols.
4. List and describe antibody classes, their roles in the immune response, and how they are used in diagnoses.
5. Describe different types of acquired responses.
6. Describe hypersensitivities and cell-mediated and humoral immunodeficiencies.
7. Describe the types of vaccines and give advantages and disadvantages of each.
8. Explain the transfer of maternal immunity to the offspring, and explain the differences between the species.
9. Describe various components that can cause the immune system to not respond to a vaccine.
10. Recognize clinical signs of an immune response, including the response to a vaccine.
11. Recognize life-threatening reactions (anaphylaxis) to a vaccination.

This chapter deals with the general physiological mechanisms involved in an innate and adaptive immune response, as well as primary versus secondary immune responses. This is done so that the manipulations of the immune system by vaccines, which are discussed later, can be better understood. In the adaptive system the section on antibodies is expanded on so that the sections on maternal transfer of immunity to offspring, types of acquired immunity, and vaccines themselves are clear. Other sections included are immunopathological mechanisms and vaccine difficulties and precautions. Each section provides some background information and stresses clinical and diagnostic considerations.

INNATE OR NONSPECIFIC IMMUNITY

I. Definition: the immunity with which we are born
II. Includes physical and chemical barriers to an antigen such as
   A. Intact skin, stomach acids, commensal organisms, mucus production, cilia, lysozyme in tears, and body temperature
III. Also involves the humoral and cell mediated systems
   A. They include reactions involved in the inflammatory responses, particularly the functions of the phagocytes, which are the body's first line of defense for containing and halting the spread of the pathogen

B. Wound healing also occurs due to this process

IV. If the innate system is successful, the adaptive immune response will not be activated and antibody production will not occur

V. Especially important features of innate immunity

A. Occurs immediately after an antigen's entry (which is important because antibody production takes days)

B. Treats all antigens the same (no specificity involved)

C. Strength and speed of the response do not increase with subsequent encounters with the same antigen (no memory involved)

D. Common clinical signs of an innate system response are primarily due to the histamine release

1. Clinically seen as swelling or edema because plasma moves from the circulation into the tissues

2. Redness and excess heat from vasodilation and increased blood flow

3. Release of extra mucus occurs in some areas

ADAPTIVE OR SPECIFIC IMMUNITY

I. Definition: the response of the defenses of the body to a specific substance (antigen)

II. Individuals produce antibodies

III. Response is highly specific

IV. Adaptive immunity possesses a memory so the body's response becomes more rapid and stronger with each encounter with the same antigen

V. During the adaptive response, immunity is created

A. Cell-mediated immune response involves T-lymphocytes and the phagocytes (neutrophils, monocytes, and macrophages)

1. Macrophage engulfs the pathogen; digests it, rendering it dead; and presents a piece of it (epitope) on its surface

2. T-helper lymphocytes binds to the epitope presented on the macrophage surface

3. T-helper lymphocyte then presents the epitope to a B-lymphocyte

a. Macrophage and T-helper cell then produce specific cytokines (also called lymphokines)

b. Examples of lymphokines are

(1) Interleukin-1: produced from the macrophage that cause the T-helper cell to release more interleukins

(2) Interleukin-2: (causes more T cells to be produced)

(3) Also releases interleukin-4 and interleukin-6 (they cause the B-lymphocyte to clone and produce memory cells and antibodies)

B. Strength that the immune system attains and therefore the individual's level of immunity reached depends on

1. Genetics, general state of health, the dosage of antigen, the antigen's portal of entry and persistence (rate of clearance) in the body, and the number of times it has been encountered previously

VI. Antibody will bind and neutralize the antigen by providing a physical barrier between the antigen and the host cells

ANTIBODIES

I. Definition: noncellular components (they are glycoproteins) of the adaptive immune response that bind specifically to parts of the antigen called antigenic determinants or epitopes

II. By binding to the antigen, antibodies prevent the antigen from doing further harm (neutralizing) and they enhance other immune responses

III. Five classes of antibodies (also called immunoglobulins [Ig])

IgM

I. During the primary immune response to a particular antigen, stimulated (antigen-bound) B cells (also known as B-lymphocytes, plasma- or antibody-forming cells) secrete IgM antibody

A. Due to its large size, this antibody class is confined to the vascular system

B. It comprises about 10% of the antibody pool in most mammals

IgG

I. Most plasma cells produce IgG antibody molecules during secondary and subsequent immune responses (to the same antigen)

A. IgG can cross the placental barrier (transplacental immunity) in species with a lower number of placental membranes (dog, cat, rodent, and primate) to convey short-term immunity to the newborn

IgA

I. If a plasma cell resides in a lymph node that drains portals of entry such as the gastrointestinal tract, urogenital tract, or the conjunctiva of the eyes, it will produce IgA antibodies

A. Here it serves to bind the potential invader, blocking its ability to bind to the host tissue, and making it too large to pass through the mucosal membrane

B. This class of antibody is found in body secretions, including tears, mucus, and colostrum

1. After about 18 hours of life the neonate will begin to produce stomach acids and the antibodies of the colostrum will be digested, rendering them useless for immune purposes. So ingestion of the colostrum must occur very early in life or the neonate may not be protected

IgE

I. It is found in minute levels in the plasma of healthy animals
   A. IgE functions to boost local inflammatory reactions
   B. It also plays a role in protecting animals against helminths by attracting eosinophils to the site of infestation
   C. If an individual produces excess IgE, such a response may become damaging to self
      1. If the reaction is localized, it is termed an allergy
      2. When it acts systemically, it is a hypersensitivity reaction called anaphylaxis; it may induce anaphylactic shock, which can be fatal

IgD

I. It is found on lymphocyte membranes and in negligible amounts in body fluids
   A. Primary role is as an antigen receptor for B cells

PRIMARY VERSUS SECONDARY IMMUNE RESPONSES

I. There are two stages to the adaptive immune response
II. It is these stages that are manipulated by modern vaccine therapy
   A. Primary immune response occurs the very first time the adaptive response engages a particular substance (antigen) and only then; this could be due to disease or the first vaccination
      1. Response is slow and takes several days to become clinically detectable
      2. IgM antibody is produced
      3. Response is weak as the antibody titer remains relatively low
      4. Antibody does not last long in the body
      5. Clinical signs are longer lasting with a disease situation
   B. Secondary immune response occurs with the second or subsequent encounter with the same antigen; this could be due to disease or a booster vaccine
      1. Response is rapid, taking only 1 or 2 days to become clinically detectable
      2. IgG antibody is produced
      3. Response is strong as the antibody titer can be up to a 10^5 times higher than for the primary response
      4. Antibody persists in the system up to months or even years after the response has occurred
      5. Clinical signs are usually less severe and of shorter duration than those of the primary response with a disease situation
III. Physiology of these stages must be taken into account when using antibody titers to determine an animal's health status
   A. Blood samples are drawn to obtain data regarding a patient's antibody type and titer
      1. IgM antibody titer to a particular antigen infers either a recent initial vaccination for that disease (check the vaccination history) or a current disease state
      2. IgG antibody titer to a particular antigen infers either booster vaccines have been administered at some time previously (check the vaccination history), the animal has recovered from this disease at some time in the past (check the clinical history if available), or a current disease state. Retest in 2 to 4 weeks
      3. If the retesting of the titer shows the IgG antibody level to be close to the previous test level, then the animal has antibodies from a previous disease recovery (convalescent state) or a vaccine. If the titer is increasing the animal is currently ill (actively infected state)

TYPES OF ACQUIRED IMMUNITIES

I. Definitions
   A. Acquired immunities: occur after birth
   B. Natural immunity: without medical (human) intervention
   C. Artificial immunity: medically induced immunity
   D. Active immunity: the individual's own immune system produced the antibodies (and therefore long-term immunity occurs)
      1. This is known as a seroconversion
   E. Passive immunity: antibodies were "donated" and therefore the individual's immune system was not stimulated to produce the antibodies (nor any memory cells)
      1. This involves short-term immunity because these antibodies will be quickly catabolized and cleared from the body and no replacements will be synthesized
   F. Acquired natural active immunity

1. Usually induced by disease recovery

G. Acquired natural passive immunity
   1. Antibodies are passed to the fetus or neonate
      a. From the mother across the placental barrier (species dependent)
      b. Or via the ingestion of colostrum

H. Acquired artificial active immunity
   1. Via vaccination

I. Acquired artificial passive immunity
   1. Antibodies produced in one animal are infused into another animal
   2. Initial animal is administered a pathogen, vaccination series, or a bacterial toxin repeatedly until that animal is "hyperimmune" (possesses a very high antibody titer)
   3. During the hyperimmune state a portion or all of the animal serum is removed and the antibodies are harvested and can be used for the following
      a. To produce an antiserum, which can then be given to other animals to convey short-term immunity
         (1) Common example is in the treatment of people after exposure to the rabies virus
      b. To produce a toxoid (in the case of the use of a bacterial toxin on the initial animal), which can be administered to other animals
         (1) Common example is the antitetanus toxoid for potential *Clostridium tetani* exposure
         (2) It is also available for the treatment of other clostridial pathogens

TRANSFER OF MATERNAL IMMUNITY TO THE OFFSPRING INCLUDING THE ROLE OF VACCINES

I. Dam can pass on only the antibodies that she possesses
   A. Vaccines are important to neonatal health
      1. It is critical that the breeder female be fully vaccinated and that those vaccines are up-to-date. If not, her progeny may not have the needed immunity to survive until their own immune systems are finished developing
      2. Check the vaccine protocol carefully to determine when the mother should be vaccinated to provide maximum immunity to the young. Some cannot be administered during pregnancy; others must be given close to parturition
   B. Check the vaccine protocol with regard to immunizing young animals and follow them carefully
      1. If vaccines are given too soon, the maternal antibodies may block the neonate's immune system from responding, so no immunity occurs
      2. Neonate's immune system may not be ready to react to the vaccine, so no immunity occurs
      3. If given too late, the maternal antibodies may be gone and the disease can occur during the time the infant is left unprotected without any antibodies of its own

II. Route by which immunity (antibody) is transferred from mother to offspring is determined by the placental barrier, as well as the type of antibody involved
   A. It is the number of membranes, which comprise the placenta, that decides how much IgG antibody can cross from the maternal into the fetal circulation
      1. Three membranes allow 100% of the maternal IgG antibody to cross
      2. This type of placentation occurs in humans and other primates and protects them from systemic infections
      3. These neonates still require IgA antibody, which cannot cross the placental barrier but is obtained via the ingestion of colostrum. Such ingestion conveys immunity to the gastrointestinal tract to help prevent neonatal diarrhea
      4. Dog and cat possess four membranes in their placentas, and therefore most of their maternal immunity is conveyed through the ingestion of colostrum
      5. Ruminant has five, whereas pig, horse, and donkey have six membranes in their placentas. These numbers block all antibodies from crossing. As a result, colostrum is the only source of immune transfer in these species. Such ingestion is crucial in these species

IMMUNOPATHOLOGICAL MECHANISMS

I. Disorders result from inappropriate or inadequate immune responses and are labeled as hypersensitivities, autoimmune reactions, or immunodeficiences

II. Immunoproliferative disorders can also occur where the proliferation of the leukocytes becomes aberrant, excessive, and functional
   A. Example: lymphosarcoma, for which the theory of an oncogenic viral etiological agent has been proposed

1. This type of pathology is usually studied as a hematological disorder even though it severely compromises the immune system's ability to function

III. Four types of hypersensitivity reactions (some of which occur in isolation but more often more than one type occurs simultaneously)
   A. Type 1 involves the animal producing an excess of IgE antibody
      1. If this is a genetically based condition, it is known as an atopy
      2. It can produce very problematic, even fatal, conditions
         a. Too much IgE antibody means too many mast cells degranulate and in turn too much histamine is released
         b. This results in allergies of various forms dependent on the allergen's (an antigen that induces an allergic response) portal of entry, such as
            (1) Inhalation, ingestion, or topically
            (2) It may result in an allergy or anaphylactic shock and death
      3. Unfortunately allergies are relatively common in animals and can occur to almost any compound from feedstuffs and pharmaceuticals to environmental items, and POTENTIALLY EVEN VACCINES!
         a. Common examples: canine atopic dermatitis and contact dermatitis (classic flea bite hypersensitivity and sweet itch fit here) but the latter does not involve atopy
   B. Type 2 occurs when an animal produces antibodies against its own cells that are then lysed by complement
      1. Results in an autoimmune disorder
      2. Examples: autoimmune hemolytic anemia, equine infectious anemia, immune-mediated thrombocytopenia, pemphigus, and systemic lupus erythematosus
   C. Type 3 occurs when antibodies bind to an antigen and form large complexes that become deposited in body tissues; often joints and vessel walls or kidneys are involved
      1. It produces inflammation and tissue necrosis at these sites
      2. A common example: rheumatoid arthritis
   D. Type 4 is the result of the actions of the cell-mediated immunity (CMI)
      1. They infiltrate the area in which the allergen occurs. Then redness, hard lump formation, and necrosis occur
      2. These create a granuloma
      3. Example: flea collar sensitivities

IV. Immunodeficiences
   A. Definition: lack of a particular immune system component and/or a malfunction
   B. Types
      1. Congenital, cell-mediated immunodeficiency
         a. Example: cyclic neutropenia in gray collies and their crosses
         b. They experience a cyclic decrease of all cellular elements (most notably the neutrophils), during which time they have a very low resistance to infection
      2. Congenital, humoral immunodeficiencies include the inability to produce certain classes of antibody
         a. IgG deficiency in cattle, IgM deficiency in horse, Doberman pinscher, and basset hound, and IgA deficiency in other dogs
      3. Combined immunodeficiency can be seen in some Arabian horses and basset hounds that do not possess a thymus, no lymphoid organs, and a very low number of lymphocytes
         a. Such animals survive their first few months primarily because of the antibodies received from their mothers
         b. Usually they succumb to adenoviral pneumonia (horse) or the distemper vaccine (dog)
      4. Deficiencies due to cell-mediated immunity alone are rare
      5. Acquired deficiencies (occurring after birth)
         a. These are common especially in the cat due to feline leukemia and feline AIDS viruses
         b. They occur in animals that do not receive colostrum or that nurse from mothers with poor immunity and therefore produce low-quality colostrum
         c. Also in old age as the immune system weakens and deficiencies begin to develop
   C. Other general causes of inappropriate immune reactions
      1. Breakdown of tolerance to usually "ignored" material such as dust (i.e., chronic alveolar emphysema in horses or autoimmune disease occurs)

TYPES OF VACCINES

I. Vaccines are important in the preventative health care program as they reduce the chances of a particular disease occurring
II. Ideal vaccine would be safe and effective and have no undesirable side effects

III. There are many types of vaccines
   A. Killed or inactivated vaccines
      1. Organisms (bacteria or virus) used to produce these vaccines are killed, often by chemical treatment
      2. These are safe, stable (store well) vaccines
      3. They require repeated dosages to maintain protective immunity, and this increases their cost
      4. Immunity conveyed may be weak due to the effects of killing the organism
      5. Adjuvants (compounds to boost the immune response) are often added, which can cause severe reactions at the site of administration
   B. Attenuated-live/modified-live vaccines (MLVs)
      1. These use live but attenuated or otherwise avirulent organisms
      2. They convey strong, long-lasting immunity
      3. They can cause abortions, mild immunosuppression or residual virulence can cause mild disease (rare)
   C. Recombinant vaccines
      1. These are produced through DNA technology
      2. They possess a high degree of efficacy and safety
      3. Not many are available, and they are expensive
      4. Types include subunit, gene deleted and vectored
   D. Monoclonal/polyvalent vaccines
      1. Monoclonal vaccines produce immunity directed against a specific pathogen only
      2. Polyclonal vaccines produce immunity directed against more than one pathogen simultaneously
         a. These are also termed "-way" vaccines, such as three-way or four-way depending on the number of diseases it protects against
         b. They contain a mix of antigens
   E. Other similar therapies include
      1. Use of bacterial toxins; such vaccines are termed toxoids
         a. Animal still produces its own antibodies; therefore the immunity is long-lived
      2. Use of antitoxins that contain antibodies directed against the toxins produced by the pathogen
      3. Use of antisera that contains antibodies directed against the pathogen itself
         a. In the above two situations, the animal is "given" antibodies from another already immune animal and therefore this type of immunity is short-lived

Vaccine Difficulties

I. Vaccines are not guaranteed to work, because an individual may react to carried over proteins from the culture environment of the virus or to chemicals used to kill it, or even the adjuvant itself
   A. Adjuvant may not perform adequately, the epitopes may be altered during processing, or they may not be very immunogenic in the first place
II. Usually vaccines are sold as a lyophilized powder to which a particular amount of sterile distilled water is added
   A. Amount of water must be correct because the concentration is important in inducing a good response
   B. Do not mix vaccines in the same syringe unless the protocol states it is safe to do so as the resultant combination could be inactivated
   C. It must be handled gently after reconstitution so that no mechanical damage occurs, and it must be delivered to the appropriate area in the body for which it was designed to work
      1. Some are to be injected subcutaneously; others are for intramuscular injection
      2. If administered incorrectly there may not be sufficient inflammation or the vaccine may be cleared so rapidly that it does not stimulate the immune system
      3. Nonstimulation can occur with accidental intravenous administration but it could also result in anaphylaxis
      4. Use of excessive quantities of alcohol at the injection site has also been implicated
III. Vaccine must be stored properly during shipping because temperature extremes can cause a loss of antigenicity
IV. After all proper precautions are taken, there is still no guarantee the vaccinated animal will respond appropriately
   A. Young animal that is immunologically compromised may succumb to illness to a live vaccine or may not develop immunity to killed or other vaccines
   B. Even if an animal does not become ill from the administration of a vaccine, there is no way of knowing what the animal's immune status is unless an antibody titer is done
   C. Vaccines may not be effective when administered to certain populations of animals, such as animals that are
      1. Immunosuppressed
      2. Heavily infested with parasites

3. Very stressed
4. Malnourished
5. Incubating disease
6. Showing signs of an abscess at the site of inoculation

V. Viruses are capable of a process called "antigenic drift"
   A. Example: canine parvovirus
   B. Such a virus mutates its genome and its epitopes so that preexisting antibodies from previous vaccines are now unable to bind and therefore are useless
   C. As a result, a previously ill and recovered animal or a previously vaccinated animal is no longer immune

Vaccine Precautions

I. Following the recommended vaccination schedule increases an animal's chances of developing a protective immunity

II. If a vaccine is given too early in life, the maternal antibodies in the circulation may prevent the young animal's immune system from properly responding to the vaccine, lessening its efficacy
   A. Neonate's immune system may not be sufficiently developed to respond

III. Boosters must be administered at correct times to maintain the necessarily high level of immunity to prevent disease

ADVERSE VACCINE REACTIONS

I. These are rare; when they do occur, they are usually mild and/or localized
   A. Common clinical signs include
      1. Slight fever, lethargy, soreness at the injection site, and possibly anorexia
      2. These clinical signs usually subside in a day
      3. Client must be warned of the possibility of such an occurrence but educated so as not to be alarmed
   B. Common causes include
      1. Cell culture (that the viruses are grown in) proteins carried over into the vaccine
      2. Adjuvants added
   C. Severe reactions involving anaphylaxis are rare; common clinical signs include
      1. Vomiting
      2. Salivation
      3. Incoordination
      4. Dyspnea
      5. Epinephrine may be used to treat these potentially life-threatening cases
   D. Vaccines have been implicated in cases of fibrosarcoma in cat and immune-mediated hemolytic anemia in dog
      1. These situations are currently under investigation
      2. Occurrence is rare
      3. Benefits of vaccines still greatly outweigh the risks involved
      4. Protocols may be altered to less frequent administrations to help prevent these problems from occurring

Glossary

adjuvant Substance added to vaccines to enhance their antigenicity

allergen Material that invokes an allergic response, usually localized in an individual

antigen Material capable of eliciting an antibody response in an animal

antigenic drift Process of mutation whereby an antigen changes its epitopes, thereby rendering previous immunity (and vaccines) useless or clinically reduced. A common occurrence in influenza viruses; occurred recently in the canine parvovirus

antiserum Serum containing antibodies directed against the various epitopes of an antigen that elicited their production

atopy A hereditary condition involving immunoglobulin E hypersensitivity

autoimmune reaction Occurs when tolerance to self breaks down and the immune system attacks self; it is usually an unhealthy state

avirulent Without disease-causing properties; this may be induced by multiple subculturing of some pathogens

cell-mediated immunity Branch of the immune system where cells, rather than antibody, play the predominant role. It occurs in both the innate and adaptive branches of the immune system

colostrum "First milk" secreted by a mother. In many species it is high in proteins, including antibodies, and therefore is a form of passive natural immunity

commensal Living on or within another organism and deriving benefit while befitting or not harming the host

congenital Born with; possibly but not necessarily hereditary

epitope Structural component of an antigen against which immune responses are made and to which an antibody binds; also called antigenic determinant

etiological agent Cause of the disease

fibrosarcoma Tumor from collagen-producing fibroblasts

gene-deleted Specific genes are removed from the pathogen so it is now harmless and can produce a safe vaccine that elicits strong immunity

genome Genetic inventory

granuloma Dysfunctional tissue filled with eosinophils, fibroblasts which produces a scar, and large macrophages

hypersensitivity Normal reaction of the immune system, which for one reason or another becomes exaggerated and does damage to self

immunodeficiency Lack of all or part of the immune system's function with varying degrees of compromise to the animal's health; may be fatal

immunoproliferative disorder Characterized by the rapid production of lymphoid cells producing immunoglobulins

lyophilized Freeze-drying

memory One of the unique components of the immune system; it permits the recognition of an antigen that has been encountered before; due to the production of a greater number of B-cells (memory cells), the response is therefore faster and stronger. It goes hand-in-hand with specificity

necrosis Breakdown and death of cells, usually a result of inflammation

pemphigus A group of immune mediated diseases of skin and mucous membranes

phagocyte White blood cell of the innate immune response that recognizes material as foreign to the body and engulfs it for digestion to render it harmless to the body

self One's own cells and molecules that the immune system, in health, does not attack but tolerates

seroconversion Changeover from a nonexistent or low antibody titer to one that is elevated; it usually implies an immune level

specificity Increased speed and strength of the immune system when encountering the same antigen for a second or subsequent time

sub-unit Genes from a pathogen are placed in another microbe so as to clone pathogen products. These gene products are then extracted, isolated, and purified for use in vaccine production

sweet itch Dermatitis of horses caused by hypersensitivity to the bites of *Culicoides* spp. characterized by intense itching along the middle of the back

tolerance Lack of responsiveness by the immune system. Tolerance is healthy when it occurs to self but is immunosuppressive when it occurs to antigens; can be induced by drugs such as steroids

toxoid A toxin treated to destroy its toxicity without destroying antigenicity

vectored Specific pathogenic material is inserted into a non-pathogenic organism as a carrier for vaccine production

Review Questions

1 Innate immunity
  a. Is recognized by the clinical signs of fever and chills
  b. Is solely created by the actions of the neutrophils
  c. Occurs after the adaptive immune response
  d. Type of immunity with which one is born and does not develop after birth

2 Which are clinical signs of anaphylaxis?
  a. Vomiting
  b. Dyspnea
  c. Incoordination
  d. All of the above

3 Booster vaccines are given to
  a. Elicit a primary immune response
  b. Cause the production of IgM antibodies
  c. Stimulate the innate immune system
  d. Elicit a secondary immune response and a higher antibody titer

4 Which of the following is false with regard to vaccine therapy?
  a. Vaccines may not be effective when given to a patient that is currently not showing clinical signs but is incubating a disease
  b. Vaccines may be responsible for certain types of anemia in dogs
  c. Vaccines are an example of acquired natural active immunity
  d. Recombinant vaccines are very effective and safe

5 When administering a vaccine, to ensure the maximum immunity possible in the patient, it is important that you
  a. Follow the timing given by the manufacturer in the written protocol
  b. Use the correct route of administration
  c. Store the vaccines correctly and reconstitute them according to the manufacturer's instructions
  d. All of the above

6 Which of the following species receive no maternal antibody during gestation?
  a. Cat
  b. Cow
  c. Dog
  d. Primate

7 It is important that all neonates receive colostrum within what time period?
  a. The first 18 hours of life
  b. The first 24 hours of life
  c. The first 2 days of life
  d. The first week of life

8 An example of acquired natural active immunity is
  a. Ingestion of colostrum
  b. Recovery from disease
  c. Vaccination
  d. Maternal antibodies crossing the placental barrier in cats

9 The following statement describes an allergy
  a. It involves the excess production of IgE antibody and release of histamine
  b. It is rare in all species of animals but when it occurs it is always hereditary in nature
  c. It is a localized reaction to an allergen in animals that produce too much IgA antibody to that compound
  d. It is a type 2 hypersensitivity reaction

10 The only antibody that can enter tissue spaces and cross the placental barrier in some species is
  a. IgG
  b. IgA
  c. IgD
  d. IgM

BIBLIOGRAPHY

Alberts B et al: *Molecular biology of the cell,* ed 3, New York, 1994, Garland Publishing.

Facts on File Conference Highlights Agricultural Biotechnology International Conference, June 11-14, 1996, Saskatoon, Canada.

Gershwin L et al: *Immunology and immunopathology of domestic animals,* ed 2, St Louis, 1995, Mosby.

Janeway CA, Travers P: *Immunobiology, the immune system in health and disease,* London, 1994, Garland Publishing.

Roitt I, Brostoff J, Male D: *Immunology,* ed 4, London, 1996, Mosby.

Steinberg M, Cosloy S: *The Facts on File dictionary of biotechnology and genetic engineering,* New York, 1994, Facts on File Inc.

Tizard I: *Veterinary immunology, an introduction,* ed 6, Philadelphia, 2000, WB Saunders.

PART II

Clinical Applications

CHAPTER 9

Restraint and Handling

Teresa Sonsthagen

OUTLINE

Dog Restraint
- Danger Potential
- Behavioral Characteristics
- Considerations for Restraint
- Restraint Equipment

Cat Restraint
- Danger Potential
- Behavioral Characteristics
- Considerations for Restraint
- Restraint Equipment

Horse Restraint
- Danger Potential
- Behavioral Characteristics
- Approaching a Horse
- Capturing a Horse
- Leading a Horse
- Tying
- Restraint for General Examinations
- Restraint for Dental Procedures
- Distraction Techniques
- Tail Tie
- Picking Up Feet
- Foals
- Casting

Cattle Restraint
- Danger Potential
- Behavioral Characteristics
- Restraint

Sheep Restraint
- Danger Potential
- Behavioral Characteristics
- Anatomy and Physiology
- Restraint

Goat Restraint
- Danger Potential
- Behavioral Characteristics
- Anatomy
- Restraint

Pig Restraint
- Danger Potential
- Behavioral Characteristics
- Anatomy and Physiology
- Restraint

Knots

LEARNING OUTCOMES

After reading this chapter you should be able to:

1. Know the danger potential of each species so that your safety is kept in mind when restraining successfully.
2. Predict the common behavioral characteristics so that the most successful method of restraint will be used.
3. Keep in mind the considerations of restraint so that the animal is handled safely and will recover as soon as possible after the restraint procedure.
4. Be comfortable with the restraint equipment available for the species and use the proper tool for the procedure.

This chapter will reacquaint you with some of the basic restraint techniques taught in most veterinary technology programs. Without good basic knowledge of behavior, safety measures, and proper restraint techniques, the patient could injure the veterinary technician, veterinarian and the owner, or injury could result to the patient. Restraint should be safe and firm, yet gentle. Restraint should be safe for the animal, safe for the person performing the restraint, and safe for the person performing the procedure.

This chapter will cover the restraint of cats, dogs, horses, cattle, sheep, goats, and pigs and is designed to refresh your memory on how the basic restraint techniques are performed, how most animals behave, and some safety measures that should be used to ensure no one is injured. Restraint of rabbits and rodents will be covered in Chapter 17.

DOG RESTRAINT

Danger Potential

I. Canine teeth are a main means of defense
II. Toenail scratches are painful but not usually serious

Behavioral Characteristics

I. Determined by breed, training, previous experiences, and human association
  A. The normal dog is a well-cared-for, sociable animal
    1. The pet or working dog is recognized by a happy attitude—tail wagging, comes to greet you
    2. It has been taught definite social behaviors—sit, stay, down, and off
    3. Clients with new puppies should be advised on how to teach social behavior
    4. About 90% of clients will fall into this category
    5. Dogs are usually docile but can be pushed into biting with painful procedures or harsh treatment
  B. Nervous, frightened dogs
    1. Recognized by anxious expression, rapid head movement, sclera evident, grimacing, trembling lips, avoidance of eye contact, and shivering. They may cower or they may be boisterous
    2. Convince them to come to you on their own time, never push them into a corner
    3. Some nervous dogs nip out of excitement
    4. Expect these dogs to bite
      a. Approach them slowly, let them come to you
      b. After they allow you to touch them, quickly but gently, restrain their heads and snuggle them close
  C. Vicious or aggressive dogs
    1. Recognized by head held low, hackles raised, tail straight out
    2. Dogs will bite, especially if challenged
    3. These dogs will try to make eye contact with you. This is a challenge
      a. If they look away it usually means they have backed off
      b. The best action on your part is to slowly back away and avoid eye contact
      c. Challenge definition: looking the dog in the eye, body faced forward
      d. To avoid challenging keep body sideways to the dog, look out the corner of your eye, and do not crouch
    4. Both small and large dogs are capable of inflicting serious damage
      a. Small dogs can be more aggressive than large but keep in mind that a large dog can cause more damage
    5. Dogs do not always exhibit obvious characteristics of aggressiveness; some will attack without much warning

Considerations for Restraint

Look at the type of animal, behavior, and past treatment received from humans to determine what type of restraint will be needed. Keep in mind the following seven points while restraining.

I. Rough handling will usually provoke retaliation; if the animal is pushed too far you will cause it to defend itself
  A. Minimal restraint is often the best way to start, moving up to more restrictive forms as necessary
II. If injured and in pain, a dog can be confused and disoriented, which makes determining its behavior unpredictable
  A. Always muzzle these dogs; the only exception is a dog with head injuries
    1. Apply the muzzle tightly or not at all
    2. The muzzle should not be left on longer than 20 minutes without a break
  B. When manipulating a dog, avoid putting pressure on the injured area; pressure can cause more damage or more pain, which in turn can cause the animal to go into shock or retaliate
III. Aggression and hostility
  A. Do not take chances with aggressive and hostile dogs; use the restraint tools necessary to keep yourself safe. These tools include
    1. Capture poles or rabies stick
    2. Gloves
    3. Blanket if the dog is small
    4. Cage or run doors as a shield
IV. Fear and/or nervousness
  A. Attempt to reason and soothe the dog but exercise caution
    1. Use muzzles or rope leashes to remove them from cages or runs
    2. Sometimes you have to sedate these animals before they are brought into the clinic
V. Old/young
  A. Special care is required when dealing with the very old and the very young
    1. Geriatric animals have to be handled with care and consideration
      a. If hospitalized, they will miss human contact; visits by the owners should be encouraged
      b. They are sensitive to stress

c. They are most likely arthritic, so manipulation and pressure placed on joints can be very painful
d. Comfort measures, such as a soothing voice, blankets or pads, and treats, are a must
2. Puppies are difficult to hold onto because they are full of boundless energy and curiosity
a. You must always maintain contact with them
b. A fall from the examination table can cause fractures or dislocations
c. When carrying them, keep a secure hold

VI. Pregnant animals should be treated the same as a geriatric patient
A. Pregnant animals are prone to injury from increased weight, which puts pressure on hips, spine, and shoulders
B. Pressure to the abdomen can be traumatic and should be avoided
C. Stress and physiological changes may cause the bitch to abort

VII. Pets that are dominant are usually difficult to handle if their owners are present, because the pets have not learned to be submissive to people
A. Owners may be asked to leave the room
1. Most dogs calm down because they do not know what to expect from strangers
2. If the owner refuses to leave, explain that the dog will have to be muzzled to protect the staff and the owner and that a muzzle will also have a calming effect on the dog
B. When the owner is not present and the dog is still misbehaving
1. Speak to the dog in a commanding voice
2. It may be necessary to rap it under the chin or use a choker collar
3. Be firm, consistent, and very persistent in getting the dog to behave
4. If the dog wins the first battle, you will lose the war

Restraint Equipment

I. Choker collars are used only as a discipline tool
A. The correct use is to sharply snap the collar closed and then release; this correction should be done immediately after bad behavior
B. If not placed on the neck correctly, pressure will not be released
1. Hold the collar so that it makes a "D" and slip it over the dog's neck
2. Check for proper release. When pulling up on the collar and letting it loose, the loop around the neck should loosen up immediately
C. Do not pull and tug continuously on the choker collar because the dog will get used to the stimulus and not react
D. Never use a choker collar as an everyday collar. Many animals have been caught on fences and have hung themselves because the loops can get caught in chain link and other nooks and crannies

II. Gentle Leaders/Promise/Halti Collars
A. These collars are used for training and for behavior modifications
B. They work on the premise of a bitch making corrections to a puppy with pressure behind the ears and over the muzzle
C. These collars must be fitted properly to each individual to work properly

III. Two types of leashes
A. Leather leashes should be at least 6 ft (2 meters) long and are ideal for training with choker collars, because they do not give and seldom break or tear
B. Nylon, flat or round, rope leashes are usually 4 to 5 feet (1.5 to 2 meters) in length, with a choker collar like loop that will loosen when the standing part is released. They are used in several ways
1. A nervous or vicious dog can be removed from a cage by using the rope leash
a. A large noose is flipped over the dog's head; the dog can be pulled to the edge of the cage, keep the leash taut, grab a back leg, and quickly lower the dog to the floor
b. Never just drag the dog out of the cage and let it drop to the floor; this can cause injury to the neck, back, and legs
2. For vicious dogs, rope leashes can be used to cross-tie them
a. Two leashes are placed around the dog's neck and held taut in opposite directions. This allows you to approach the rear for an injection or to place a muzzle
C. Chain or hard rope leashes should be avoided as they will cause injuries to the hands

IV. Capture pole or rabies pole is a long pole with a rope or covered wire protruding from the end to form an adjustable noose. The noose is slipped over the head of an aggressive animal
A. Slide the noose in and out several times before using to make sure it is working correctly and can be quickly released in an emergency

B. Once the animal is captured, the head can be controlled well enough to apply a muzzle or give an injection in the rear leg

V. Muzzles: two types of muzzles
   A. The commercially prepared muzzle should be fitted to the dog at the store
      1. If not a proper fit, the dog may bite with its incisors
   B. The gauze muzzle is a temporary muzzle constructed of roll gauze
      1. Tear off enough gauze to go around the nose of the dog twice and up behind the ears
      2. Make the first loop by tying a large open, loose overhand knot centered in the gauze; quickly slip this loop over the dog's nose
      3. Crisscross the gauze under the muzzle
      4. Bring the ends up behind the ears and tie with a bow
      5. If the dog is a brachycephalic breed, like a boxer, tie the ends behind the ears with an overhand knot. Bring one end of the gauze between the eyes, then under the loop around the nose, and tie to the other end in a bow, which will end up on top of the head. This prevents the loops from slipping off
         a. This same method is used to muzzle cats

VI. A harness works extremely well for small dogs
   A. They cannot slip out of them
   B. If necessary you can lift them out of harm's way

VII. Voice commands. Fortunately, of all the animals we have to deal with, the dog will respond readily to the human voice
   A. A soft crooning voice comforts and calms and should be used throughout a restraint procedure
   B. The tone of voice should not be high pitched
      1. A high-pitched voice tone simulates the yelps and barks of littermates, which can make the dog think it is dominant over you
   C. A sharp, low, commanding voice tone often gets the dog's attention; this is similar to the low barks or growls of a dominant bitch or dog
      1. Avoid a yelling tone, which can frighten or cause aggression
   D. Always be consistent with your vocal tones so you do not confuse the dog
      1. If you are a littermate 1 minute (high pitched voice) and then yelling at the dog the next, this can cause it to become very confused and it may act out

CAT RESTRAINT

Danger Potential

Of all domestic animals, the cat is one of the most difficult to handle because of its agility and formidable weaponry.

I. Teeth are capable of inflicting serious wounds that often become infected

II. Claws are razor sharp; all four feet can be used simultaneously and are the main means of defense

Behavioral Characteristics

I. Normal behavior
   A. Cats are aloof independent creatures; they are not pack animals and do not have the pack instinct like a dog
   B. They are, however, social animals and will live peacefully with an established pecking order in a group of cats
   C. They are highly intelligent and curious creatures, often getting in serious situations because of it!
   D. Cats are extremely territorial and mark their territory by spraying urine and rubbing scent glands (found by the commissure of the lips and at the base of the tail) on furniture, the boundaries of their yard, and their owner
      1. New places are thoroughly investigated; cats will explore everything and mark it as their territory
      2. When confined to a small space like a cage or small room, a cat's first instinct is to escape
         a. If escape is impossible the cat will defend the area as its own territory. This often explains why a placid cat turns aggressive when that territory is "invaded"
   E. Most cats are placid and friendly in general, especially if well treated

II. Depressed behavior
   A. A depressed cat may stop eating and drinking
   B. The cat may be depressed as a result of boarding or removal from a familiar environment
      1. Depression results from lack of freedom and interaction with people
   C. It may sit in the litter box or huddle in the corner under newspapers or a towel
   D. If depression continues, the cat can become weak and could turn hostile if pushed
   E. These cats can/should be handled gently and often

III. If hostile, pound for pound, cats are among the most fearsome animals alive

A. Hostile cats are difficult to handle—they do not respond or submit to restraint, and if they escape they are very difficult to capture
B. They will fight until they are too weak to fight anymore. You should handle these cats with restraint tools such as gloves, towels, nets, or capture poles
C. You can recognize them by observing their body language
   1. Ears pinned back or flat
   2. Vocalizing from hissing, low growls to screams
   3. Fur on tail and hackles raised
   4. Pawing at you

Considerations for Restraint

Cats in general are not difficult to handle if you understand their actions. Observe each cat to determine the best method to use.

I. Make sure all doors and windows are locked. Cats can squeeze through very small openings and are extremely difficult to catch when they are on the floor and running
II. With a calm cat begin with the least amount of restraint and become firmer as the situation demands. Make your adjustments in small increments—too firm too fast will often anger the cat
III. Do not begin restraint until all participants are ready to begin as cats tolerate manipulation for only a very short period of time
IV. Stay calm but firm and be consistent with your voice and the restraint techniques chosen
V. Few cats attack without warning so angry cats should be covered with a large towel or blanket and scooped up. Wearing protective gloves is a must when doing this as the blanket will not prevent bites or scratches
VI. If one is aware of the instinctive territorial trait, many problems can be avoided
   A. Cornered cats will attempt to escape and if unable to do so will fight
   B. Allow the cat to leave its territory by walking out of the cage under its own power or quickly reach in with rope leash, capture pole, or gloved hands and remove it
VII. Distraction techniques work very well on the cat; this involves inflicting mild pain to a certain area so the cat does not pay attention to what is going on elsewhere. Do not start the techniques too early because it can backfire and make them angry fast
   A. "Caveman" pets, vigorous pats on the head or body
   B. Tapping or blowing on the nose
   C. Vigorous rubbing on top of the head

Restraint Equipment

I. A rope leash as the one described in canine restraint is used in the same manner
   A. You occasionally capture one or both front legs, along with the neck. If you are gentle it still works well
II. A towel, pillowcase, or small blanket can be used to surround a hostile cat
   A. One method is to center the towel over the cat and then sweep the flaps of the towel under the cat, wrapping its legs in the folds of the towel similar to the way a taco is wrapped
   B. A second method is to place the towel on the table, depositing the cat in the first third of the towel, wrapping the other two thirds tightly around the cat, and tucking in the end closest to the tail, much like a burrito is wrapped
III. Gloves are made of thick leather that should cover your arms up to the elbow
   A. Disadvantages of gloves
      1. The loss of tactile sense, which may result in applying too much pressure
      2. They will not protect you from bites but do reduce the number of scratches you receive
   B. Use of gloves
      1. Place your hand partially in one gauntlet
      2. Offer that hand to the cat while it is trying to bite or scratch
      3. Reach in with your other hand, fully encased in a gauntlet, and grab the animal by the scruff of the neck. This same technique can be used on small to medium-sized dogs
IV. Feline restraint bag (cat bag) is usually made of canvas or thick nylon. This bag completely encloses the body of the cat. The head is held in place and there are access zippers or Velcro strips to allow the legs to be brought out. Never leave the cat unattended as it can roll off the table
   A. Advantages to using a cat bag
      1. It usually has a calming effect; after a cat realizes it cannot escape, it will calm down
      2. The feet are taken out of action for use against you
   B. Disadvantages
      1. The cat can still bite
      2. You must be careful not to get the fur and skin caught in the zipper
      3. Large and/or angry cats are difficult to place into the bag
      4. The jugular vein is not easily accessible

5. To prevent spread of disease and ectoparasites, the bag should be disinfected after each use

V. If you are alone and need to perform a simple and painless procedure, floral tape or Vet wrap works well to bind the legs together
  A. First tape front legs together and then tape rear legs together
    1. A towel over the head may also prove beneficial
  B. When removing tape, do so with the back legs first and then the front legs
  C. Never leave cat with legs bound like this alone on top of a table because it could roll off and severely injure itself
  D. The use of adhesive tape could pull and remove hair

VI. Muzzles such as leather/nylon or gauze muzzles work well and protect the handler from bites
  A. Most commercial muzzles also cover a cat's eyes
  B. Reusable muzzles should be disinfected to prevent spread of respiratory diseases

VII. An Elizabethan collar can also be effective to protect the handler from bites

HORSE RESTRAINT

Danger Potential

I. Rear feet
  A. The kicking range of the hind feet is 6 to 8 feet (2 to 2.5 meters) straight out, with the furthest extension of the foot the most dangerous for handlers
  B. The aim is usually very accurate
  C. To pass safely behind a horse you can either
    1. Stay at least 10 to 12 feet (3.5 to 4 meters) behind or to the side
    2. Stay in direct physical contact with the horse by placing a hand on the rump

II. Front feet
  A. If a horse rears it can knock a person to the ground
  B. It can strike a handler's head and arms with or without rearing

III. Teeth
  A. Front incisors can cause major injuries as they can "lock" their jaws, which will cause further damage as the bitten area is pulled from the horse's mouth
  B. Discipline is a must if a horse bites
    1. This may include a sharp jerk on the halter or a firm pop on the nose

Behavioral Characteristics

I. The horse is nervous and suspicious by nature. It is quick to detect threats and react to them in a manner that may be dangerous to humans
  A. As part of its flight instinct, if suddenly frightened or hurt, reactions may include rearing, biting, kicking, or running away, all without obvious warning
  B. Keep alert and never treat a horse complacently
  C. Always move slowly and deliberately. Quick motions and loud noises will almost always frighten a horse into evasive action

II. Horses often show some warning signals that should be heeded to prevent possible injuries. The most expressive parts of a horse are the ears; however, the tail, eyes, and mouth are also useful indicators of behavior
  A. Ears
    1. If the horse is alert, the ears are pricked forward
      a. The horse sees what is coming and usually will not become startled
    2. If the horse is nervous or uncertain, the ears are constantly moving back and forth
      a. Offer comforting words and be ready for a flight response
    3. If the horse is angry or fearful, the ears are pinned back
      a. Expect these horses to strike, kick, or rear up
    4. If the horse is concentrating, the ears are pinned back (out to the sides)
      a. It is usually busy performing what it is meant to do
  B. Tail
    1. Nervousness is indicated by wringing or circling. Comfort measures are also appropriate: gentle pats and quieting talk
    2. When the horse is in pain or sleeping, the tail is straight down. If in pain, a harsh stimulus may cause a "fight-or-flight" response. If sleeping and startled, expect the same
    3. Fear is shown by the tail being clamped tight between the gluteals. Comfort measures are a must with this horse. Be ready for the fight-or-flight response

Approaching a Horse

I. Approach from the front and slightly to the left side
  A. Horses are accustomed to being handled from this near (left) side
  B. The right side is referred to as the far side

II. Move slowly without sudden movements or loud noise

    A. If the horse moves away, stop. If you do not stop, the horse will think it is being chased and will flee

III. Talk to the horse and perhaps offer it some grain so it will approach you; a quick hand can get a rope around its neck while its head is in the bucket!

IV. Some horses will need to be put in a smaller pen to catch them
    A. Luring them into the pen with grain is a much better method than chasing them

V. When approaching a horse from the rear
    A. Begin talking to it before you get close. A startled horse may kick or jump forward and injure itself or you

Capturing a Horse

I. Check the halter and lead rope for splits or fraying
    A. A horse can easily break a defective lead rope and/or halter

II. Slip the lead rope around the horse's neck and tie a single overhand knot to keep the rope from slipping off. Proceed to put the halter on the horse

III. Hold the neck strap of the halter in the left hand, reach under the horse's neck, and hold the head still so the right hand can bring the halter over the horse's neck

IV. Slide the nose band of the halter onto the nose and buckle the neck strap behind the ears
    A. Keep your movements slow and deliberate

V. Check to make sure the halter is settled correctly on the horse's face

VI. Attach the lead rope to the center ring of the halter under the chin. Untie the end of the lead rope from around the neck. The left hand should hold the loose end of the rope in neat loops with the entire rope held in front of you
    A. Never wrap the loose end of the lead rope around your hand
    B. Never have the rope loose behind you

Leading a Horse

I. Gather the lead rope in your left hand. Do not wrap it around your hand in case the horse bolts; it could snag, causing a severe injury

II. Always walk on the left side of the horse with your right hand on the lead rope approximately 5 to 6 inches (12 to 15 cm) from the halter ring

III. Stay close to the shoulder
    A. Do not get too far in front of the horse because it can rear up and strike with a front foot or it can accidentally step on the back of your heels as it walks. It can also bite you on the shoulder or back
    B. When stopping, stand facing the same direction as the horse

Tying

I. A horse should always be tied to a sturdy, vertical object with a well-fitting halter and suitable lead rope

II. The knot used to tie the lead rope should be a quick release knot such as the halter tie
    A. The horse can be released quickly if it gets into trouble

III. Allow about 2 to 3 feet (0.75 to 1 meter) of lead rope so the horse can adjust the angle of its neck and shift its position as it desires
    A. The horse may tangle its front feet in the rope if a longer rope is left
    B. A shorter rope may frustrate the horse enough to cause it to attempt to free itself

IV. Check the area around your tied horse for possible hazards that could cause serious injuries

V. Never pass under the neck of a tied horse to get to the other side. This is a very dangerous practice that could result in serious injuries if the horse is startled

Restraint for General Examinations

I. Stand on same side of horse as the person who is working on the animal
    A. By standing on the same side, the horse has the option of moving away from both of you to escape
        1. If there are people on both sides, the animal will pick the smallest of the barriers and try to move over that. Unfortunately, that may be a person bending or kneeling

II. Never stand directly in front of the horse
    A. It can rear up and come down on top of you
    B. It can strike out with its front feet
    C. It can run you over in an effort to escape

III. Hold head level with the withers; if the head is held higher, the horse has an advantage and can easily escape

IV. Cross tying
    A. Used to prevent a horse from rearing and from moving its forequarters from side to side
    B. The horse can still strike with its front feet and move its rear quarters
        1. Snap a lead rope onto the cheek piece ring on each side of the halter. Tie each lead rope to the side of the stanchion, to stocks, or to beams
        2. Tie the ropes high enough to prevent the horse from rearing and entangling its feet in the ropes
        3. Use a quick release knot such as the halter tie or use a quick release buckle

4. Cross tying allows you access to the horse's entire body but does not prevent it from swinging its rear end

V. Stocks
   A. A narrow stall with removable or semi open sides and a gate at both ends
      1. Lead the horse through the back gate and close the front after it is in the stocks
      2. Do not go into the stocks with the horse; pass the rope around the bars as needed to keep the horse moving
      3. Stocks are used usually for rectal and uterine examination or procedures on the head

VI. Blindfolds
   A. Can be used to control an obstinate or a fearful horse
   B. The horse will usually calm down and depend on you to guide it wherever you want it to go
   C. Work slowly and talk constantly to reassure the horse

Restraint for Dental Procedures

I. Place your left hand on the bridge of the horse's nose with your thumb under the nose band of the halter and the right hand placed on the nape of the neck; push head down

II. To hold the tongue, reach in at the commissure of the lips, grasp the tongue, and slowly pull it out to the side through the diastema of the lower jaw

Distraction Techniques

I. Twitches are used on obstinate horses that will not allow procedures to be performed
   A. Through the release of endorphins, which mask the pain, twitches distract the horse's attention from other procedures by applying a mild pain to the upper muzzle
   B. Of the three types (chain, humane, and rope), the chain is most common
      1. Place the loop of chain over your left hand, catching one side of the loop between your little finger and ring finger
      2. Grasp as much of the horse's upper lip with your left hand as possible, press the bottom edges together to protect the delicate inner surface, and quickly slide the handle up so the chain loop rests high up around the lip
      3. Tighten the chain by twisting the handle until the twitch is fitted snugly on the lip so lip curls upward
      4. Tighten and loosen the chain on the muzzle to keep the twitch effective. If steady pressure is applied the muzzle would lose circulation, thereby reducing sensitivity of the muzzle and rendering the twitch ineffective
      5. Many horses will attempt to get away or resist the twitch when it is first applied; stay with them by moving with their motions. If they shake you off the first time it will be more difficult to place the twitch again
      6. After the twitch is removed, massage the muzzle to restore circulation
   C. A humane twitch is a hinged pair of long handles that squeeze over the sides of the lip and then can be secured at the bottom
      1. Once applied it need not be held
      2. The pressure is mild and may be ignored by horses

II. Lead shank is a long leather strap with about 2 feet (0.75 meters) of flat chain attached to it with a snap on the end
   A. It is used as a distraction device, or if more restraint than just a halter is needed. It is used as a training device and on stallions for added control
   B. There are several ways to use a chain shank
      1. With the halter in place, pass the chain end through the ring on the cheek piece
         a. Pull it across the bridge of the nose to the ring on the other side of the head (Figure 9-1)
         b. Pull it under the jaw. This method is not ideal because this may cause the horse to throw its head up
         c. Place it under the top lip over the upper gum. This is very effective in directing the horse's attention away from other procedures, but it is painful and may inflict injury

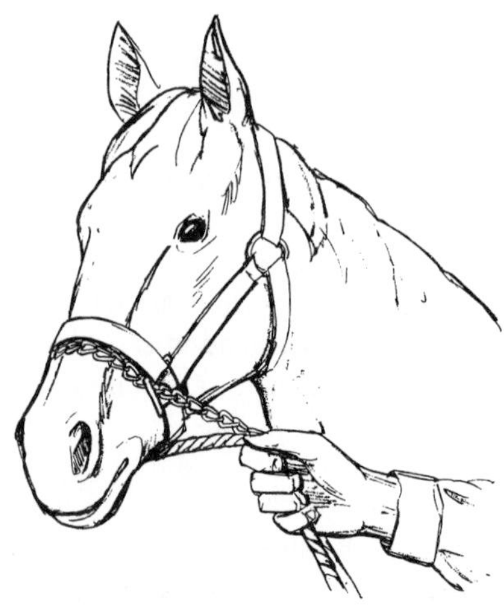

Figure 9-1 Chain shank across the bridge of the nose. (From Sonsthagen TF: *Restraint of domestic animals,* St Louis, 1991, Mosby.)

d. Put the chain in the mouth like the bit of a bridle and clip it to the ring on the other side

C. Be careful not to jerk excessively on the chain shank because injury may result

III. Eyelid press involves gently placing fingers on the upper eyelid and pressing down; it is a very gentle distraction technique that can be used for injections or to keep the horse still

IV. Shoulder roll is done by grasping a large fold of skin with both hands just over the shoulder and wiggling or moving it from side to side or up and down; it works very well for intravenous injections

V. "Caveman pets," or somewhat heavy swats, are excellent ways to distract a horse

VI. Pick up or tie up the opposite foot from the one being radiographed or bandaged

VII. Grasp the base of the ear with the heel of your hand touching the head. Squeeze or rotate the ear in a small circle

A. It is best to use this only as a last resort

1. If done incorrectly it could cause the horse to become sensitive and make it afraid of having its ears touched

2. This can cause the owner of a show animal a lot of frustration when the hair in the ears needs to be trimmed

B. Do not apply so much pressure to the ear that damage occurs to the cartilage, which can result in the ear flopping over

VIII. A cradle is a device that is placed around a horse's neck to prevent it from chewing or licking at wounds; it prevents the horse from bending or turning the neck

Tail Tie

I. Always tie the tail to the animal's own body

II. Secure a cord or rope to the hair on the tail using a "sheet bend" or "tail tie" knot

III. Pull the tail to the side of the buttocks and pass the rope to the opposite front leg

IV. Use a quick release knot to secure the other part of the rope to the neck or front leg

V. Purpose is to move the tail out of the way for rectal/uterine or obstetric procedures (see Figure 9-12)

Picking Up Feet

I. Front feet (Figure 9-2)

A. Stand lateral to the shoulder and parallel to the horse, facing the caudal end

B. Place your closest hand on the horse's shoulder; gently but firmly run it down to the fetlock

C. Grasp the fetlock by placing your palm on the underside of the fetlock and wrapping your fingers around the joint

D. Squeeze and lift the foot; at the same time lean into the horse to make it shift its weight to the other three legs

E. After raising the foot up, bring it slightly out to the side. Position your body close to the horse's body so that your knees are slightly bent. Place the foot between your legs so it rests on top of your knees, allowing both hands to be free. Flex fetlock and hoof toward yourself

II. Rear feet (Figure 9-3)

A. Approach in the same manner as the front feet

B. After you have lifted the foot, extend the leg out to the rear and place it on top of your bent knee closest to the horse

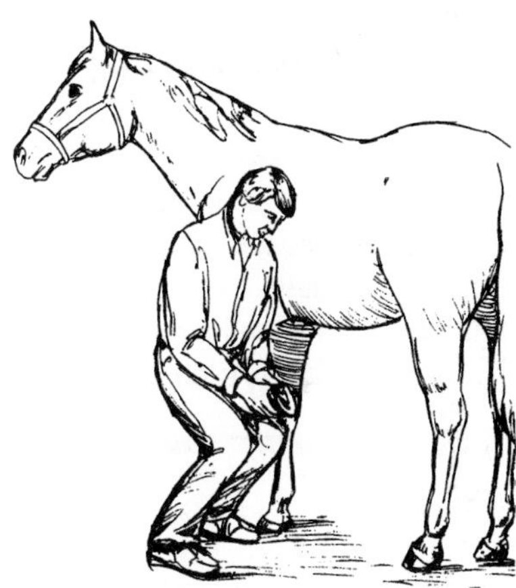

Figure 9-2 Picking up a front foot. (From Sonsthagen TF: *Restraint of domestic animals,* St Louis, 1991, Mosby.)

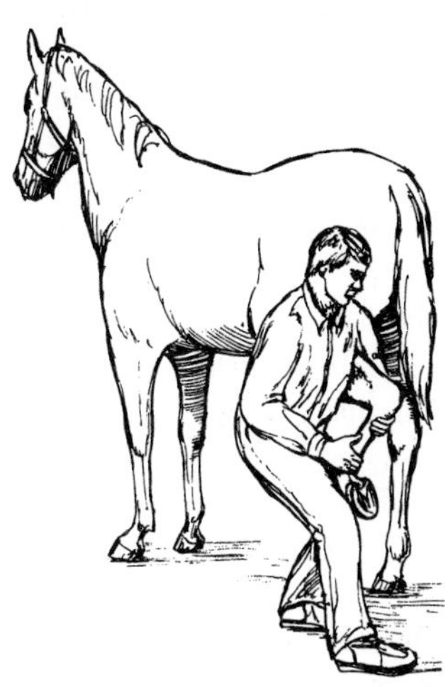

Figure 9-3 Picking up a back foot. (From Sonsthagen TF: *Restraint of domestic animals,* St Louis, 1991, Mosby.)

Foals

I. Capture and restraint
  A. Keep the foal in sight of the mare. Place the mother in a large box stall (the mare often needs to be restrained as well) so that she can see her foal but is not be able to get at you
  B. Grasp the foal around the front of the chest with one arm, and around the rump with the other arm, or grasp the tail. Quickly move the foal clear of the dam
  C. Use your arms to form a "mini corral" and keep the foal encircled with your arms
  D. Do not lift the foal off its feet; this makes it very nervous and it will struggle
  E. Always talk to and comfort a foal when handling it

Casting

I. Laying a horse in lateral recumbency
  A. Anesthesia drugs are used almost exclusively
  B. Key to a smooth drop is to maintain control of the horse's head. Lift it up and to the side when it starts to go down
  C. Once the horse is down, pad the side of the head facing the ground and place a knee on the neck to keep the horse recumbent
  D. Ropes are usually used to secure three of the four legs to prevent kicking
    1. Clove hitch or variations are often used

CATTLE RESTRAINT

Danger Potential

I. Head
  A. Horned animals can fatally gore a handler by quick thrusts forward and sideways
  B. Be constantly aware of the swinging arc and the extent of reach from side to side and forward
  C. Butting is done by polled and horned animals
    1. This can be a rushing motion, pinning you against a fence, wall, or ground
    2. It can be a swing of the head, knocking you down and holding you down
II. Body
  A. Cattle can pin restrainers against a wall or fence or between other cows (dairy cows in stanchions)
III. Feet
  A. Front feet are seldom used as weapons
    1. Cattle do paw the ground to show aggression
    2. The split toe can cause serious damage to human toes and feet if they step on you
  B. Hind feet are very dangerous and very accurate
    1. Cattle usually kick by bringing the foot forward, arching out to the side and then backward (cow kicking)
    2. They can kick straight back, like a horse, but seldom do
    3. Usually kick is one legged, not a two-legged kick like horses
  C. The safest place to stand is at the shoulder, but remember that bovine can kick past its shoulder
IV. Tail
  A. The tail is useful to cattle for swatting flies and for attending to other twitches
  B. The tail is an annoyance and can cause injury to the restrainer's or examiner's eyes during procedures
    1. To prevent injury, remove awns or burrs from the tail by dipping it in mineral oil. Melt frozen ice and feces by dipping the tail in a warm bucket of water and then tying it up to the cow's body
  C. The tail is very fragile
    1. Never tie the tail to anything but the animal's body
    2. Use the same procedure as with horses; you just do not have as much hair with which to work
V. Cattle seldom bite because they lack upper incisors
  A. If they do bite, it is more of a pinch than a bite and is usually an accident

Behavioral Characteristics

Cattle differ markedly in their reactions to manipulations and the presence of humans as a result of the breed, handling, and gender.

I. Dairy cows are accustomed to being handled and are the most docile of the bovine breeds
  A. Restraint is usually done in stanchions or by tying to a fence. Talk to and treat dairy cows gently
  B. They may become nervous and vigorously resist handling if not treated gently
II. More so than any other animal, dairy bulls require special restraint techniques because they are extremely unpredictable
  A. If handled correctly, the unpredictability can be minimized
  B. Nose rings, in addition to halters, are often used in bulls for more control while leading
    1. Do not tie the bull fast to stationary objects by the nose ring; the halter and lead rope is used
III. Beef cows are easily frightened because of little association with people
  A. Restraint involves chutes (with head gates) and alleyways

IV. Beef bulls are handled the same as females; be careful around beef bulls when the females are in heat

Restraint

I. Approach
  A. Avoid quick movements so as not to startle the animals; use slow deliberate actions
  B. Talk to them so they are aware of your presence
    1. A low command to move is much preferred over sharp yelling
  C. Do not approach from the front because it is a natural instinct for cattle to charge. Cattle can not charge if they are in a squeeze chute and head gate, or tied in a stanchion
    1. Remember they can still stretch their necks and butt you if you are too close
II. Herding
  A. Flight zone (this is true in cattle, sheep, goats and horses). Most prey animals have a large field of vision with blind spots directly behind them and a few degrees to the right and left of the rump
  B. To make these animals move forward, stand inside their field of vision, which is just behind the point of the shoulder
  C. If you stand in their blind zone and suddenly talk loudly or slap them with a whip or strap, they may bolt or kick
III. Head
  A. If using chutes, always check the operation of the chute before use
    1. Familiarize yourself with the operation
    2. Repair if necessary
  B. Rope halters are the basic tool of restraint
    1. The part that tightens is placed around the nose, with the loop down. The lead rope should be on the left side of the cow's head
    2. The head then can be tied to a post, fence, or part of the chute
    3. The position of the head is generally up and to the side
    4. Tie the end of the rope with a snubbing hitch or halter tie
    5. Procedures, like blousing, stomach tubing, dehorning, or eye examinations
  C. Cattle have a sensitive nasal septum that can be used to produce a mild pain that acts as a distraction technique. Pressure can be applied manually or with instruments
    1. Thumb and index finger can be used for very short periods of time (your fingers will tire quickly)
    2. Nose leads (tongs) are commercially manufactured
      a. Make sure that the balls on the tongs are smooth and not too close together
      b. Close tong handles together to adequately hold onto the nose without pinching too much
      c. Have a holder grasp the tongs or secure it to the halter
  D. Examination of eye requires the head to be rotated so that the afflicted eye is parallel with the ceiling
    1. This is usually accomplished with a halter or nose tong
  E. Passing a stomach tube requires application of a halter and a mouth speculum (such as a Frick's speculum) to hold the jaws apart while passing the stomach tube into the esophagus
    1. If the speculum is not used, the cow may clamp down on the tube
IV. Hobbles
  A. Used to prevent kicking—just above the hocks or close to the ankles
  B. Place on the back legs
    1. Place on the leg opposite you first, then the one closest to you
    2. Keep the legs "square" so the cow can maintain its balance
    3. Hobbles can be padded straps held with a chain or an angled piece of metal that slips on the back side of the legs just above the hocks
V. Feet and legs
  A. Examination of hind legs or trimming hooves can be performed
    1. Cast the cow in lateral recumbency by using the burley or double half hitch method and administration of a sedative
    2. A hydraulic lift table can be used to place the animal in lateral recumbency—again with the administration of a sedative
      a. Lead the animal in front of the table, strap on, and then lower the table to a lateral recumbency
    3. The legs can be raised by the use of ropes and pulleys, either in a chute or stanchion
VI. Tail
  A. "Jacking" the tail up acts as a distraction technique (Figure 9-4)
    1. Is done by lifting the tail straight up and forward from the base
      a. Should be ventral and over the midline so handler can keep balance

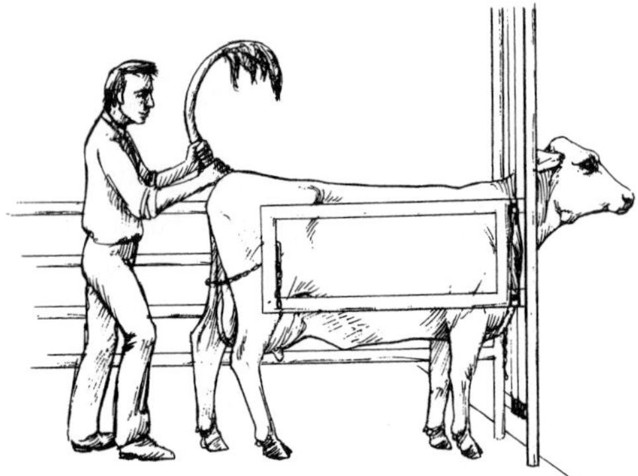

Figure 9-4 Tail jacking a cow in a squeeze chute. (From Sonsthagen TF: *Restraint of domestic animals,* St Louis, 1991, Mosby.)

b. Hold the tail about one third of the way down from the base
2. Pressure on the spinal column removes sensation to the rear
3. Make sure that the animal is secured from moving forward or from side to side
4. Used for intravenous venipuncture or rectal examination

B. The jacking should not be performed for more than a few minutes due to possible fracture of coccygeal vertebrae

VII. Casting: laying an animal in lateral recumbency
   A. Important for the animal to have a sturdy harness
   B. Avoid incorporating the udder of the cow or testicles of a bull into the flank rope
   C. All knots should be positioned dorsally
   D. Two methods could be used
      1. Burley or half hitch method
         a. A bowline knot around the neck and a set of half hitches distal to the front legs and rear legs, proximal to the flank
         b. Not appropriate for mature cattle, but if used, watch the udder and testicles
         c. One person can easily pull down acow
      2. Crisscross method
         a. Divide the rope in half and place the middle part of the rope over the neck; then pass it between the front legs near the sternum
         b. Cross the ropes over the back and between the rear legs
         c. Two people are needed
         d. This is appropriate for mature cattle

VIII. Flank restraint
   A. A lariat can be tightened around the flank area just cranial to the tuber coxae to prevent kicking. Avoid excess pressure; otherwise the animal may fall
   B. A metal clamp often known as an "anti-kicker" can be placed over the dorsum and along the sides in the same location

IX. Calf restraint
   A. Newborns are guided from place to place by placing one hand under the neck and grasping the tail head or placing the other hand around the hindquarters
   B. Calves up to 200 lb (91 kg) can be put into lateral recumbency by "flanking or legging" the calf down. After it is down, apply a three-legged tie: place one knee on its neck and the other knee in front of the closest hind leg to hold it down
   C. Never turn your back to the calf's mother: she is extremely protective of her young and could potentially kill a careless handler

SHEEP RESTRAINT

Danger Potential

I. Head is used as a battering ram with most injuries consisting of serious bruises

Behavioral Characteristics

I. Sheep have allelomimetic (strong flocking instincts), causing them to move as a group, which makes them easy to handle

II. Move slowly when working with sheep; their first line of defense is speed and flocking to flee, which makes them startle easily

Anatomy and Physiology

I. Sheep are not the jumpers that goats are, although they can jump up to 1.2 m (4 ft)
   A. Exceptions are range sheep and cheviots (harder to handle)

II. Sheep can have problems when worked in hot weather; normal body temperature can be as high as 104° F (40° C)
   A. Running, struggling, and crowding, plus their heavy wool, can very quickly result in hyperthermia

III. Never grab the wool when restraining sheep because it pulls out easily; damage to the fleece, the skin, and subcutaneous layers can result

Restraint

I. Trained sheepdogs are your best tool; they save a lot of steps when herding the sheep to specific spots

II. Herding
   A. Flight zone similar to cattle: move as a group
   B. Get one sheep to move in the direction you want, and the rest will follow

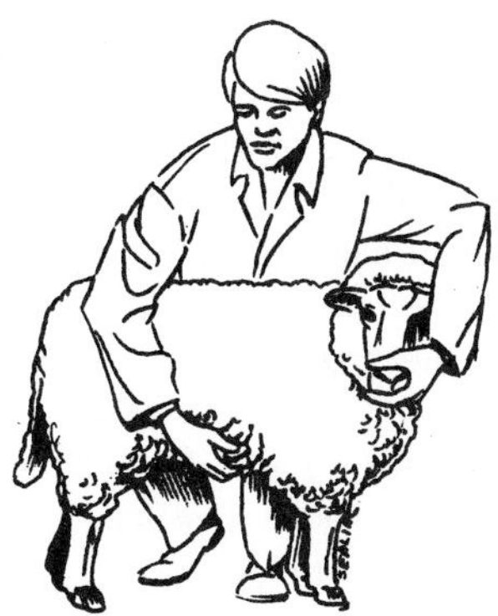

Figure 9-5 Hand positions for setting a sheep on its rump. (From Sonsthagen TF: *Restraint of domestic animals,* St Louis, 1991, Mosby.)

III. Crowding the flock into a small pen or area, with portable gates, is usually the best way to work a group or to capture a single sheep
   A. Mark sheep with a wax crayon as it is medicated so that double dosing does not occur
IV. To capture a single sheep
   A. Approach slowly, quietly, and deliberately
   B. Reach down and limit the forward movement with a hand under the chin
   C. Quickly reach for the dock or flank fold with the other hand to stop backward motion
   D. Move wherever you wish by applying pressure on the chin or dock
   E. Turning can be done by grasping the muzzle and turning the head toward the shoulder
V. A shepherd's crook is a handy tool for catching a sheep
   A. It is used to "snare" a hind leg proximal to the stifle (hock)
VI. "Setting-up" (also referred to as "rumping" or "docking") a sheep allows you to examine the underside of the sheep, shear, vaccinate, or trim the hooves of the sheep (Figures 9-5 and 9-6)
   A. Move the sheep so it is standing sideways in front of your legs
   B. Plant your left leg by the sheep's shoulder
   C. Grasp the chin with one hand and the flank with the other
   D. Lift up on the flank, turn, and push the sheep's head into its shoulder; pivot on your left leg and move your right leg back. This throws the sheep off balance and onto its dock
   E. Lean the sheep back between your legs and release your hands
   F. Make sure the hocks are off the ground
   G. If done properly, the sheep will not be able to get to its feet. Your hands are free to perform whatever procedure you choose

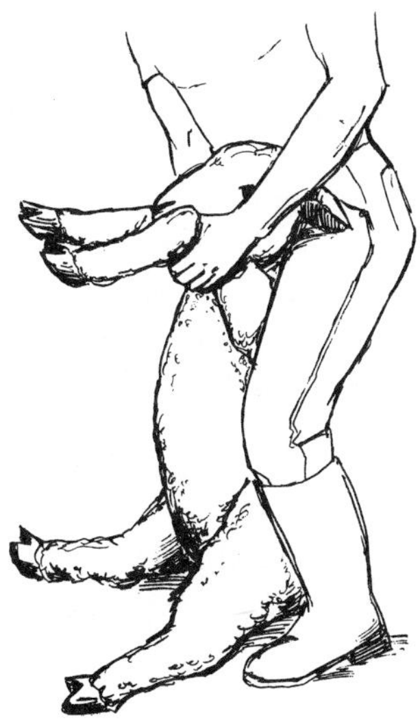

Figure 9-6 Setting a sheep on its rump. (From Sonsthagen TF: *Restraint of domestic animals,* St Louis, 1991, Mosby.)

VII. Halters can be used but the sheep's short nose makes it difficult to prevent the nose piece from sliding down and occluding the nares
VIII. Lambs are held by supporting them beneath their chest with your forearm between their front legs
   A. For castrations and tail docks, the lamb can be held by grasping a front and back leg in one hand and the opposite front and back leg in the other hand, resting the lamb's back against your chest. The head will hang down between the legs

GOAT RESTRAINT

Danger Potential

I. Goats use their heads as battering rams
   A. If annoyed they will rear up on their hind legs and slam into you with their heads
II. Most goats are disbudded or dehorned at a young age
   A. Horned goats do not like to have their horns held and will swing their heads back and forth viciously if held
   B. The horns add power to the butt and can cause injury

Behavioral Characteristics

I. Goats are very vocal
   A. The kids sound like human babies when handled, and the entire herd will come to investigate any fuss
   B. The herd may try to protect the kid or other members of the herd in danger
II. They respond to gentle treatment and become quite tame if handled a lot
   A. Rough handling may make them nasty

III. Intact males have scent glands at the base of the horns that secrete a very disagreeable long-lasting odor that attracts females during breeding season
   A. When in rut, intact males will mark their territory by urinating on their beards, legs, neck, and body and then rubbing those parts on objects around the farmyard. This odor lasts throughout the breeding season
IV. Goats are good escape artists and will work loose knots and chains
   A. Make sure all gates are properly locked

Anatomy

I. Their delicate bones are easily fractured and dislocated if grasped incorrectly
II. Goats are very hardy animals that can take a lot of stress
III. They are very good jumpers but will rarely be able to jump over 6 ft (2 m)
   A. If they try to jump over you, you may be hit at chest or shoulder height

Restraint

I. Capture
   A. To capture a single goat, it is best to place the entire herd in a small pen
      1. Because goats do not have the strong flocking instinct of sheep, it is best to lure them in with grain
      2. After the goats are in the small pen, move slowly and deliberately toward your intended patient
      3. Grasp around the neck or catch by the collar, with the other hand on the goat's dock to move it
         a. If unable to grasp as above, try capturing by the front leg. This usually makes them stand still
         b. Once caught, grasp the head behind the ears and under the chin and back the goat into a corner
      4. If you are using chain collars, make sure they are the flat chains to prevent the goat from getting caught on fences
      5. It is best to use plastic link "breakaway" collars
II. Head
   A. To restrain the head with no "neck" wear, you can place both hands on either side of the cheeks and wrap your fingers around the lower jaw
   B. The handler can push the goat sideways onto a wall or fence, securing the head by holding the jaws firmly at an upward angle. It works even better if in a corner to prevent the goat from backing up
   C. The beard can be grasped with one hand, with the other hand placed on top of the head
III. Goats cannot be set on their haunches because they are much more agile than sheep and will struggle
   A. They can be flanked similar to a calf or be placed against a fence and have their legs lifted similar to a horse
   B. Dairy goats can be placed in a milking stanchion for restraint or secured to a fence using a quick release knot
IV. Dehorning and castration
   A. To disbud kids, hold them like a lamb, then sit down, folding the kid's legs under its body and cradling its head in both hands so the thumbs hold down the ears
   B. To castrate, hold the kid the same as described for lambs
V. Pick feet up as you would pick up a horse's hoof

PIG RESTRAINT

Danger Potential

I. Teeth
   A. Newborn piglets have sharp needle-like deciduous teeth (canines and third incisors, called "needle teeth") that can damage the sow's udder and handlers
   B. Clipping of the teeth, along with other management techniques, is done soon after birth
      1. Wounds made by the canines (called tusks) are almost always septic
   C. Adults have very strong jaws and can tear flesh easily. A male with tusks is quite dangerous
II. Adult pigs can push and knock down a handler with their head and body

Behavioral Characteristics

I. Herding instincts are virtually nonexistent, but the entire herd will converge to the rescue of a screaming mate. Sows reacting to perceived danger to their piglets are extremely dangerous
II. Pigs are stubborn and contrary, but you can use this behavior to your advantage during restraint procedures
III. They are unpredictable and can become aggressive without warning
IV. They enjoy being talked to and petted or scratched gently. Simple procedures can sometimes be done while gently rubbing the ventral

abdomen and while they are lying down, but be careful

V. They are extremely vocal

Anatomy and Physiology

I. Pigs have streamlined bodies that were designed to run through underbrush, making it very easy for them to slide under objects such as fences or between your legs

II. Strong neck muscles developed to root enable the pig to lift with considerable force such items as fencing panels or even a handler

III. Thin legs can easily be fractured or dislocated if held in the wrong manner

IV. Because of a thick layer of subcutaneous fat, pigs overheat easily

Restraint

I. Small enclosures are the easiest way to handle large numbers of pigs for injections
   A. Each pig is marked with a wax crayon as the injection is administered

II. Squeeze pens and farrowing crates are ideal but they can be extremely dangerous. Never get into a small pen with a pig (especially a sow and litter) without checking for an escape route with an easy access

III. Moving
   A. A cane, light plastic pipe, leather or canvas strap, or flat stick can be used to move or direct the pig
      1. A gentle slap on the rear will make a pig move forward; a tap on the side of the head will turn it in the opposite direction
      2. Sound, more than pain, is what makes a pig move. Never use any of the objects to inflict pain because it can anger the pig and the pig may attack you
   B. A bucket placed over the pig's head will cause the pig to back up
      1. By grabbing the tail you can direct it
   C. Hog panels or hurdles/shields/barriers are made of solid sheets of plywood, plastic, or aluminum and are used to move and direct pigs
      1. The hurdles should be solid and wall-like to prevent the pigs from running through or raising the panel
      2. To move pigs using a hurdle, place it between you and the pig and start walking
      3. To turn the pig, set the barrier down on the opposite side of the pig's head
      4. If a pig charges, set the barrier between you and the pig and tilt the top of it toward you
      5. A tap on the snout with a cane or strap may stop a charging pig

IV. Hog snare
   A. This is the restraint tool of choice when working with pigs
   B. Use of the snare is easy
      1. Place the loop in front of the pig's snout
      2. Allow the pig to mouth the loop and then quickly slip the noose over the top jaw all the way back to the commissure of the lips
      3. Pull back on the handle, applying pressure to the nose; the pig's response will be to pull back in the opposite direction and squeal. The pig is immobilized by its own stubbornness
   C. The snare can be used for restraint when vaccinating, drawing blood samples, or examining pigs
   D. Length of time used should be 15 to 20 minutes maximum because it can have a tourniquet effect on the upper jaw
   E. Release of the snare should be quick; if the snare gets caught on a tusk, the pig will jerk the snare out of your hands and start swinging its head until the snare comes loose

V. Lifting
   A. Newborns (to 15 lb [7 kg]) are lifted by a back leg and then held with a hand under the chest and abdomen
      1. They will squeal when picked up, so you should move them quickly to your hand or out of the hearing range of the sow
   B. Larger pigs (less than 60 lb [27 kg]) can be grasped by a hind leg to capture them. Once caught, the other hind leg is held; the pig is held upside down with your legs supporting the back. They can then be examined or transported
   C. Use the same method for pigs up to 125 lb (57 kg), but two people are necessary, with each holding one leg

VI. Recumbency
   A. You can cast a pig a number of ways with the use of ropes; one method is described here (Figure 9-7)
      1. Capture pig with hog snare
      2. Place a rope on a front and back leg on the same side of the pig
      3. Pass the ropes under the abdomen to the opposite side of the pig, moving to that side of the pig
      4. Pull the ropes toward you, pulling the legs out from under the pig; the person controlling the hog snare will have to move with the pig so the snare does not injure the upper jaw
      5. Use the ropes to tie together three of the pig's legs
      6. If the procedure is prolonged, every attempt should be made to make the pig

comfortable to prevent nerve and muscle damage

B. V-troughs are made of wood and are V shaped
   1. Depending on the size of the trough, a 50- to 70-lb (23- to 32-kg) pig can be placed in the trough on its back, where it will remain until you are finished
   2. This may be used for castrations or umbilical hernias
   3. The feet are often left untied or just held out of the way because the pig can not roll out of the trough; however, you can tie with a loop around the foot and a half hitch to the legs

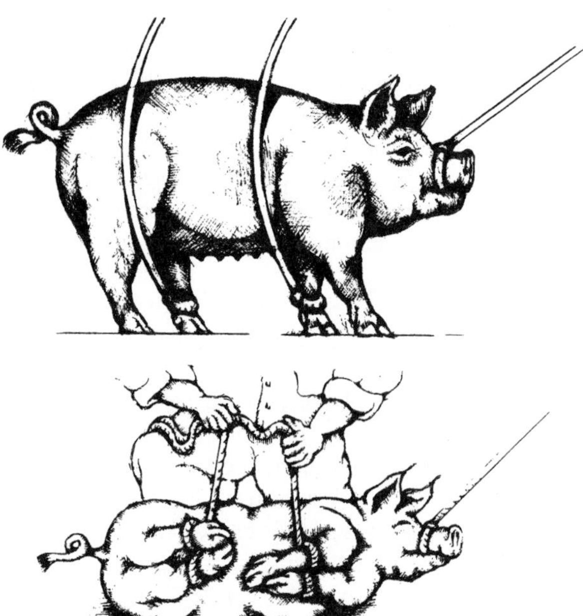

Figure 9-7 Placing a pig in lateral recumbency. (From Sonsthagen TF: *Restraint of domestic animals,* St Louis, 1991, Mosby.)

KNOTS

I. Square knot is a nonslip, noose-forming knot (Figure 9-8)
   A. It is important to test the loop to make sure the knot is tied correctly. If it slides open or closed, the knot should be redone
   B. There are variations, such as reefer's knot, surgeon's knot, and tom fool knot (Figures 9-9 to 9-11)

II. Sheet bend knot can be used to tie together two pieces of rope, one of which can be of different diameter (Figure 9-12)
   A. It can be used to tie an animal's tail out of the way
   B. Use the hair on the tip of the tail as one of the "ropes"

III. Bowline is the universal knot of restraint (Figure 9-13)
   A. It is a secure knot, yet can be easily untied even with excessive tightening
   B. Can be used around necks or legs as temporary rope halters, casting ropes, and breeding hobbles

IV. Quick release or halter tie is a knot that can be completely undone by quickly pulling on the end (Figure 9-14)
   A. This knot is the only one to be used to tie animals to inanimate objects. Any other knot takes too much time to untie and can tighten up so much that the rope has to be cut

V. Hitches: half hitches are usually stacked one on top of another to hold a rope in place either on a fence post or around a cleat (Figure 9-15)
   A. Cleats usually associated with sailing and boating are often found on surgery tables

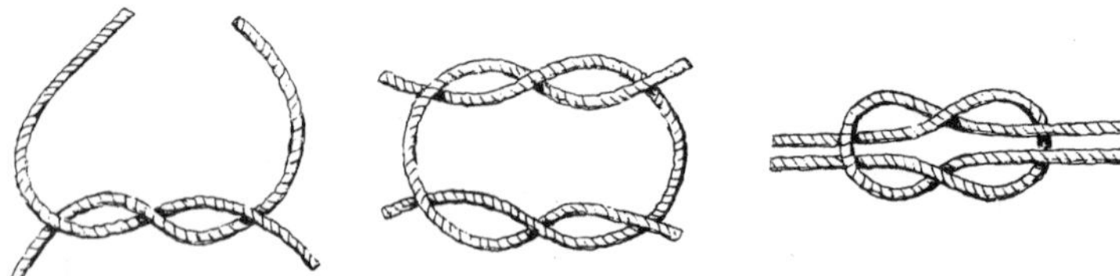

Figure 9-8 Square knot. The rope used to make the first throw should also be used to make the second. (From Sonsthagen TF: *Restraint of domestic animals,* St Louis, 1991, Mosby.)

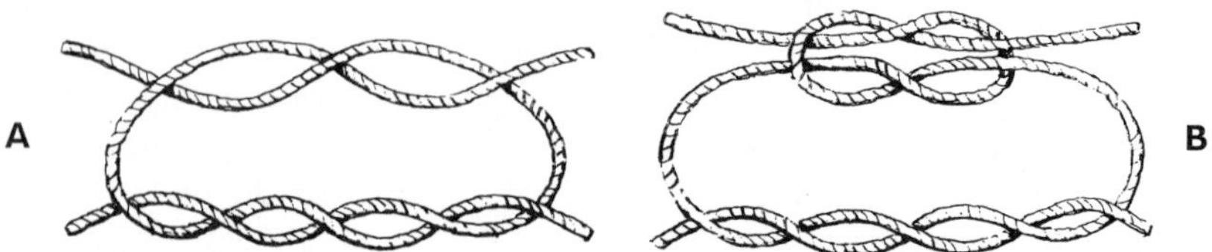

Figure 9-9 **A,** Surgeon's knot. **B,** A square knot is placed on top of the surgeon's knot to make it more stable. (From Sonsthagen TF: *Restraint of domestic animals,* St Louis, 1991, Mosby.)

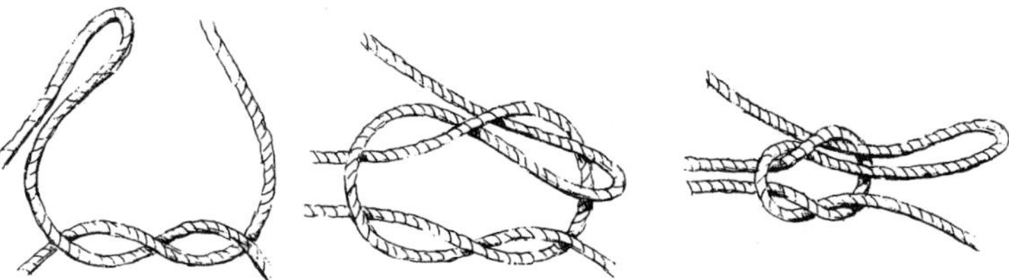

Figure 9-10 Reefer's knot or single bow knot is a quick release knot. (From Sonsthagen TF: *Restraint of domestic animals,* St Louis, 1991, Mosby.)

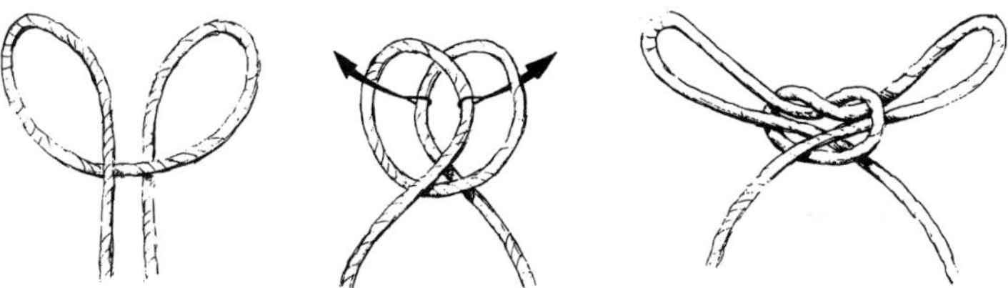

Figure 9-11 Tom fool or double bow knot is useful for hobbles on small animals. (From Sonsthagen TF: *Restraint of domestic animals,* St Louis, 1991, Mosby.)

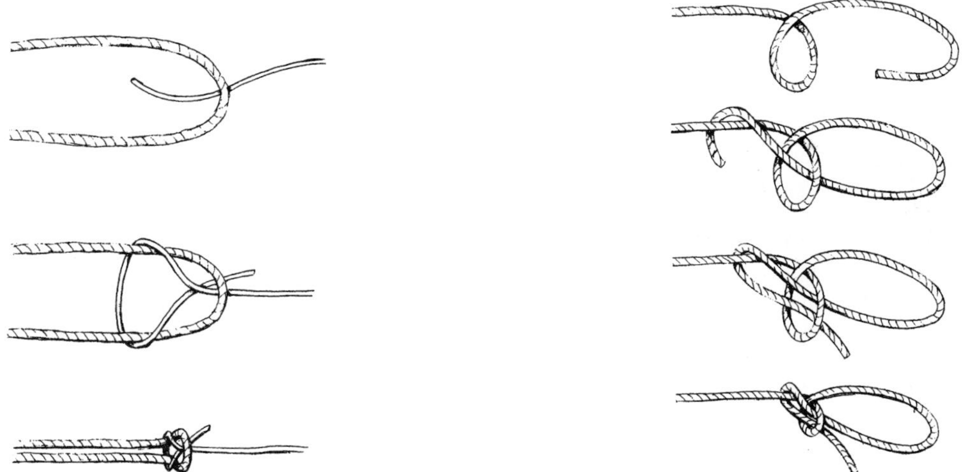

Figure 9-12 The sheet bend is a useful knot for tying together two ropes of different sizes. (From Sonsthagen TF: *Restraint of domestic animals,* St Louis, 1991, Mosby.)

Figure 9-13 Bowline knot provides a nonslip knot. (From Sonsthagen TF: *Restraint of domestic animals,* St Louis, 1991, Mosby.)

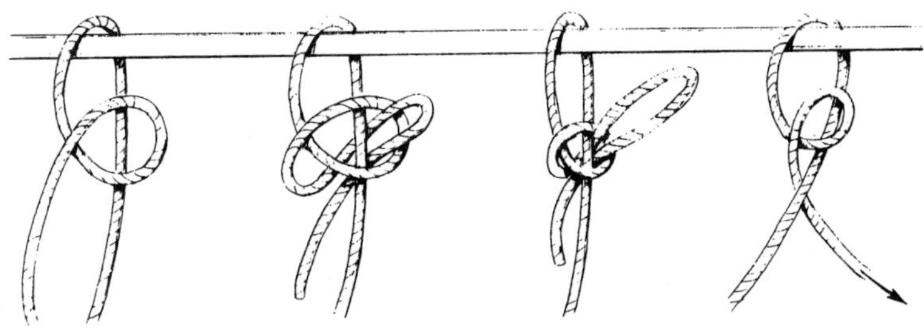

Figure 9-14 Halter tie or quick-release knot is used to tie an animal to an immovable object.

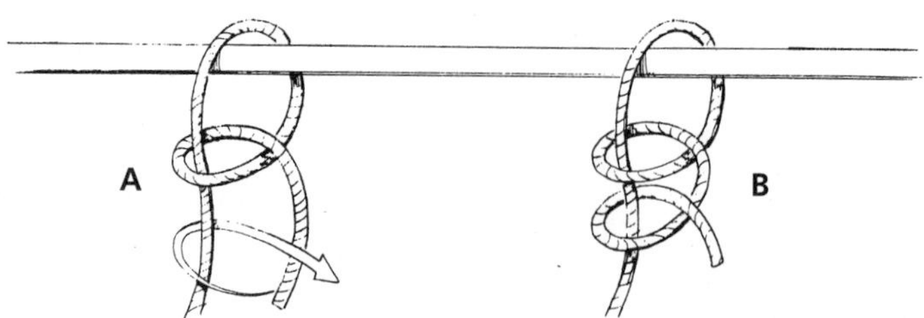

Figure 9-15 **A,** Half hitch. **B,** Two half hitches around a rope. (From Sonsthagen TF: *Restraint of domestic animals,* St Louis, 1991, Mosby.)

Glossary

allelomimetic Mimicking behavior usually associated with sheep, whereby what one sheep does, the rest will follow; can be used to advantage for restraint

anti-kicker Device shaped like a giant C clamp, which is squeezed over the flank of cattle to prevent them from kicking

balling gun Metal or plastic device used to pill large animals such as sheep and cattle

bight Sharp bend in the rope

breakaway collar Collar that will release if excessive force is applied

casting Laying an animal down on its side for restraint purposes

"caveman pets" Heavy swats usually around the shoulder region of an animal to provide minor distractions

cradle Device placed around a horse's neck to inhibit bending of the neck or turning of the head to prevent the horse from licking or chewing at its wounds

cross tying Method of securing a horse to two sides of a stanchion or stocks by use of two lead ropes, one attached to each side of the halter. This is used to prevent rearing or movement of the front quarters from side to side

diastema Space between two adjacent teeth in the same dental arch; in this case, the large space between the lower incisors and the molars on the lower jaw of a cow

disbudding Process of removing horn tissue of young goats or cattle with caustic paste or the use of a hot iron

dry An animal that is not lactating; usually in reference to the last 60 days of gestation of dairy cattle

end Part of the rope that is the short end or the end that can be freely moved around

farrowing In swine, the act of giving birth

far side Opposite or right side of the horse

flanking Method of restraint usually used in calves. Pressure is applied over the flank region just proximal to the rear legs. Used to cast an animal to the ground into lateral recumbency

half hitch or loop Complete circle formed in the rope when tying a knot or hitch

headgate Mechanical device at the end of a chute that secures an animal's head on both sides of the neck between the jaws and shoulder

hitches Temporary fastening of a rope to a hook, post, or other object, with the rope arranged so that the standing part forces the end against the object with sufficient pressure to prevent slipping

hobble Device placed on caudal aspects of the hocks of large animals to restrain hind legs

hog snare Device made out of rope, cable, or wire and placed around the pig's upper snout so that the head can be secured

jacking Term used in reference to grasping a bovine tail at the base and elevating it dorsally to distract the animal from painful procedures elsewhere on the body

knot Intertwining of one or two ropes in which the pressure of the standing part of the rope prevents the end from slipping

lactation Period of time during which an animal is producing milk

lead shank Lead rope with a snap of some sort attached to the halter of an animal such as a horse

near side Left side of the horse, from which it is accustomed to being handled

needle teeth Term applied to the eight deciduous teeth (canines and third incisors) that pigs are born with and that are removed within 1 to 2 days of birth

overhand knot Base knot for a number of different knots, made by making a half hitch and then bringing the end through the resulting loop

poll Area directly behind the ears on a large animal

polled Term used to refer to cattle that are not born with the ability to grow horns

rut Annually recurrent state of sexual excitement in males

setting up Applied to sheep. Also referred to as docking or rumping; sheep are set up into a sitting position on their hind legs so that they lean against the restrainer's legs

squeeze chute Enclosed device into which large animals are individually restrained; these chutes often have various attachments to effectively restrain the head and provide access to other body parts

stanchion Area in a barn usually used to tie dairy cattle or goats

standing part Part of the rope that is the longer end of the rope or the end attached to the animal

stocks A closed-in area used to place a large animal for rectal and head examinations

throw When one rope or a section of rope is wrapped around another to make part of a knot

twitch Used in horses; a handle with a loop of rope or chain on one end that is tightened over the upper lip or muzzle for restraint

Review Questions

1 Which of these behaviors is not a normal behavior for cats?
   a. Hiding under the papers in a cage
   b. Investigating a new room
   c. Being fairly aloof and independent
   d. Rubbing on the leg of a chair

2 Which of these is not a sign of warning from a cat?
   a. Hissing
   b. Ears lowered
   c. Swiping at you with a paw
   d. Looking the other way

3 As a restraint tool, a towel is used to
   a. Wrap up an angry cat
   b. Let the cat curl up and go to sleep
   c. Let the cat hide under
   d. Protect you from bites and scratches

4 Always muzzle an injured, conscious dog except if it has
   a. Huge gaping wounds on the neck
   b. A spinal injury
   c. A leg injury
   d. A head injury

5 Horses show many emotions through body language. Which ear movement can mean concentration or anger?
   a. Pricked forward
   b. Constantly moving back and forth
   c. Held erect
   d. Pinned back

6 Serious injury is most likely to occur from a kick if you are within this range while standing behind a horse
   a. 1 to 2 ft
   b. 3 to 5 ft
   c. 6 to 8 ft
   d. 10 to 12 ft

7 In a horse, a chain twitch is best applied to the
   a. Upper muzzle
   b. Lower muzzle
   c. Ear
   d. Tongue

8 A nose lead or tong in cattle is applied to the
   a. Left nostril
   b. Right nostril
   c. Upper muzzle
   d. Nasal septum

9 "Jacking" the tail is
   a. Twisting it to the side
   b. Bending it straight up
   c. Holding it straight out
   d. Kinking the end of it

10 To move a newborn calf from one spot to another
   a. Place a halter on its head and neck and lead it
   b. Place your arms around the neck and rump, and guide it
   c. Place a lariat around its shoulder and drag it
   d. Use a whip against its lumbar region and herd it

BIBLIOGRAPHY

Aanes WA: Restraint of cattle: head restraint. *Mod Vet Pract* 5:498, 1987.

American Veterinary Medical Association: *Medication and force feeding a cat at home,* Schaumburg, IL, Client Information Series, 1985.

Blanchard S: Here's how to read your horse's body language, *Pet Health News* 5:25, 1989 (Mission Viejo, CA, Fancy Publication Inc).

Catcott EJ (ed): *Animal health technology,* Santa Barbara, CA, 1977, American Veterinary Publications.

Crow SE, Sally WO: *Restraint of dogs and cats: manual of clinical procedures in the dog and cat,* Philadelphia, 1997, JB Lippincott.

Edwards LM: Behavior and diseases of the dairy goat, *Vet Tech* 4:294, 1983.

Evans JM: Developing canine social skills, *Dogs USA Annual* 3:64, 1988.

Faler K, Faler K: Restraint of sheep, *Mod Vet Pract* 6:562, 1987.

Fowler ME: *Restraint and handling of wild and domestic animals,* Ames, 1995, Iowa State University Press.

Gilbert SG: *Pictorial anatomy of the cat,* New York, 1984, Crescent Books.

Kazmierczak K: *Bandage management in small animals,* Continuing education article No. 2, 3:309, 1982.

Kocab JM: Restraint of pigs, *New Methods J Anim Health Technol* 2:12, 1983.

Leahy JR, Barrow P: *Restraint of animals,* Ithaca, 1953, Cornell University Campus Store, Inc.

McBride DF: *Learning veterinary terminology,* St Louis, 1996, Mosby.

Moran HC et al: Basic cat handling techniques, *Lab Animal* 3:29, 1988.

Neil DH, Kese ML: Restraint and handling of animals. In McCurnin DM, Bassert JM (eds): *Clinical textbook for veterinary technicians,* ed 5, Philadelphia, 2002, WB Saunders.

Nelson B: Restraining horses, *Western Horseman* 10:89, 1980.

Sayer A: *The complete book of the cat,* New York, 1984, Crescent Books.

Sonsthagen T: *Restraint of domestic animals,* St Louis, 1991, Mosby, pp 65-84.

Strickland C: How to tie your horse safely and securely, *Horse Illustrated* 5:39, 1988.

Vail C: Tips on equine dentistry. *Nordon News* Summer:15, 1980.

Vaughan JT, Allen R Jr: Restraint of horses, part I: head restraint, *Mod Vet Pract* 6:373, 1987.

CHAPTER 10

Sanitation, Sterilization, and Disinfection

Margi Sirois

OUTLINE

LEARNING OUTCOMES

After reading this chapter you should be able to:

1. List the classes of pathogenic organisms in order of their resistance to destruction.
2. Differentiate between sanitation, disinfection, and sterilization.
3. List the different ways that microbial control methods destroy or inhibit pathogenic organisms.
4. List the five categories of physical methods of microbial control.
5. Name and describe the physical methods of microbial control.
6. Identify the level of microbial control achieved with each of the physical methods.
7. State an example of the application of each of the physical methods of microbial control.
8. List the properties of the "ideal chemical agent" for microbial control.
9. Name and describe the classes of microbial control chemicals.
10. Identify the level of microbial control achieved by the chemical classes.
11. State an example of each of the chemical classes of microbial control.
12. List three advantages and two disadvantages of the autoclave in animal care facilities.
13. Explain the function of the autoclave.
14. Compare the gravity displacement autoclave and the prevacuum autoclave.
15. Describe the preparation of each of the following for processing in the autoclave: linen packs, pouch packs, hard goods, liquids, and contaminated objects.
16. List the guidelines for loading the autoclave chamber.
17. Compare the three different autoclave cycles.
18. List and define the five methods of quality control for sterilization.
19. List and define the two methods of quality control for disinfection.

The objective in sanitation, sterilization, and disinfection is to control microorganisms, or pathogens, in the environment, thus protecting patients and staff from contamination and disease, and thereby promoting optimum healing and wellness. Improper application of methods of sanitation, sterilization, and disinfection can lead to microbial resistance and increase the risk of nosocomial infection.

LEVELS OF MICROBIAL RESISTANCE

I. Pathogens are microorganisms that cause disease
II. Different classes of pathogens vary in their resistance to destruction by chemical methods (Figure 10-1)

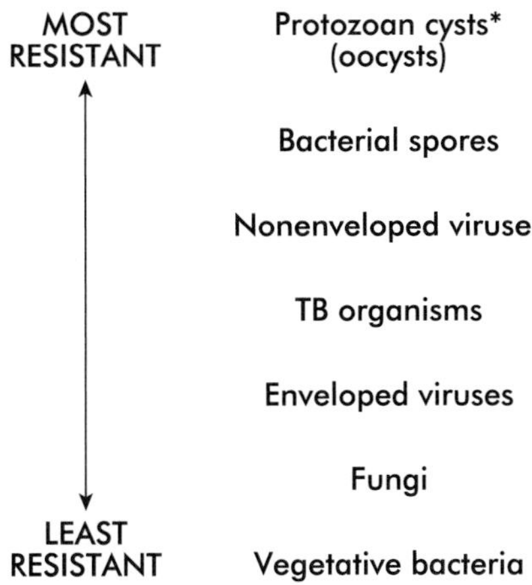

*No chemical disinfectant carries a claim for killing oocysts; the best method for eliminating them is to use heat and agitation (or the autoclave).

Figure 10-1 Ranking of microorganisms according to resistance to destruction by chemical methods. (Courtesy S. McLaughlin)

III. Microbial control is achieved by using methods of sanitation, disinfection, and sterilization to a degree that is practical, efficient, and cost effective
  A. Sterility is used only when necessary
  B. In many situations sanitation and disinfection create acceptable levels of microbial control

DEGREES OF MICROBIAL CONTROL

I. Sterilization is the elimination of all life from an object, or complete microbial control
II. Asepsis is a condition in which no living organisms are present; free of infection or infectious material
III. Disinfection, sanitization, and cleaning remove most microorganisms
  A. Most disinfectants are microbicidal; that is, they kill microbes. Some disinfectants are bacteriostatic; they inhibit the growth of microbes
  B. Disinfectants can be classified according to their spectrum of activity as
    1. Bacteriocidal (kills bacteria)
    2. Bacteriostatic (inhibits growth of bacteria)
    3. Sporicidal (kills bacterial spores)
    4. Virucidal (kills viruses)
    5. Fungicidal (kills fungi)

HOW MICROBIAL CONTROL METHODS WORK

Mode of Action

Different physical and chemical methods destroy or inhibit microorganisms in several ways.

I. Damage cell walls or membranes
II. Interfere with cell enzyme activity or metabolism
III. Destroy microbial cell contents through oxidation, hydrolysis, reduction, coagulation, protein denaturation, or the formation of salts

Efficacy of Microbial Control

The effectiveness of all microbial control methods depends on the following factors.

I. Time: most methods have minimum effective exposure times
II. Temperature: most methods are more effective as temperature increases
III. Concentration and preparation: chemical methods require appropriate concentrations of agent; disinfectants may be adversely affected by mixing with other chemicals
IV. Organisms: type, number, and stage of growth of target organisms
V. Surface: physical and chemical properties of the surface to be treated may interfere with the method's activity; some surfaces are damaged by certain methods
VI. Organic debris or other soils: if present, will dilute, render ineffective, or interfere with many control methods
VII. Method of application: items may be sprayed, swabbed, or immersed in disinfectants; cotton and some synthetic materials used to apply or store chemicals may reduce their activity

METHODS OF MICROBIAL CONTROL

Physical Methods

I. Dry heat (mode of action: oxidation)
  A. Incineration (efficacy: complete sterilization)
    1. Material or object is exposed to a hot fire
    2. Object must become red hot as in "loops" for microbiology
    3. Used to dispose of tissue or carcasses; must be burned to ashes
  B. Hot air oven (efficacy: complete sterilization)
    1. Sterility requires 1 hour of exposure at 170° C (340° F)
    2. Useful for powders and nonaqueous liquids such as paraffin or Vaseline
    3. Used in some animal care facilities
    4. Useful for domestic applications (e.g., the kitchen oven)
  C. Drying (efficacy: incomplete sterilization)
    1. Most organisms require humidity to survive and grow
II. Moist heat (mode of action: denatures microbial protein)
  A. Hot water (efficacy: incomplete sterilization)

1. Used to clean and sanitize surfaces
2. Addition of detergents increases efficacy by emulsifying oils and suspending soil so they are rinsed away

B. Boiling (efficacy: may be complete sterilization)
1. Requires 3 hours of boiling to achieve sterility
2. Boiling for 10 minutes will destroy vegetative bacteria and viruses but not spores
3. Addition of 2% calcium carbonate or sodium carbonate will inhibit rust and increase efficacy
4. Useful for "field work"

C. Steam (efficacy: incomplete sterilization)
1. Similar to boiling because the temperature is the same
2. Exposure to steam for 90 minutes kills vegetative bacteria but not spores

D. Steam under pressure (efficacy: complete sterilization)
1. Autoclave: most efficient and inexpensive method of sterilization for routine use in animal facilities

III. Radiation (mode of action: damages cell enzyme systems and DNA)

A. Ultraviolet (UV) (efficacy: may be complete sterilization)
1. Low-energy UV radiation is a sterilant when items are placed at close range; UV radiation has no penetrating ability
2. Used to sterilize rooms
3. Very irritating to eyes

B. Gamma radiation (efficacy: complete sterilization)
1. Ionizing radiation produced from cobalt 60 source
2. Good penetrating ability in solids and liquids
3. Used extensively in commercial preparation of pharmaceuticals, biological products, and disposable plastics

IV. Filtration (mode of action: physically traps organisms that are too large to pass through the filter)

A. Fluid filtration (efficacy: can be complete sterilization)
1. Fluid, by means of positive or negative pressure, is forced through a fiber filter or more commonly a screen filter
2. Used to sterilize culture media, buffers, and pharmaceuticals
3. Pore size of 0.45 μm removes most bacteria, but microplasmas and viruses require 0.01- to 0.1-μm pore size
4. May be used in conjunction with a prefilter to remove larger particles

B. Air filtration (efficacy: can be complete sterilization)
1. Used extensively in animal care facilities in surgical masks, laboratory animal cage tops, and air duct filters
2. Fibrous filters made of various paper products are effective for removing particles from air
3. Efficacy is influenced by air velocity, relative humidity, and electrostatic charge
4. HEPA: high efficiency particle absorption; filters are 99.97% to 99.997% effective in removing particles over 0.3 μm
5. Surgical masks are designed to protect the patient from the wearer and not the wearer from the patient; special masks are available for protecting personnel from pathogens in animals
   a. Masks must fit snugly on the face, stay dry, and be changed at least every 4 hours to be effective

V. Ultrasonic vibration (mode of action: coagulates proteins and disrupts cell walls)

A. Cavitation (efficacy: incomplete sterility)
1. High-frequency sound waves passed through a solution create thousands of cavitation "bubbles"
2. Bubbles contain a vacuum; as they implode or collapse, debris is physically pulled from objects
3. Effective as an instrument cleaner

Chemical Methods

Many chemicals are available to sterilize, disinfect, or sanitize, but none is the "ideal" agent. Chemicals penetrate organism cell walls and react with cell components in various ways to destroy or inhibit growth. Many chemicals are disinfectants with varying levels of activity (Table 10-1); a few are sterilants. Figure 10-2 ranks chemicals in order of their ability to destroy specific classes of microorganisms.

I. Ideal chemical agent

A. Effective against a broad spectrum of pathogenic organisms
B. Does not damage or stain surfaces
C. Stable after application
D. Effective in a short time
E. Nonirritating and nontoxic to surfaces and tissues
F. Inexpensive and easy to store and use
G. Not affected by organic debris or other soil
H. Effective at any temperature
I. Nontoxic, nonpyrogenic, nonantigenic

Table 10-1 Levels of disinfection

Some manufacturers refer to low-medium- and high-level disinfectants. Higher level products are effective against a greater variety of organisms. They must kill hydrophilic and lipophilic viruses. They must also kill spores. Medium-level disinfectants must be tuberculocidal. Low-level products kill vegetative bacteria.

	Bacteria			Viruses		
Level	Vegetative	Acid-fast	Spores	Lipophilic	Hydrophilic	Example
High	+	+	+	+	+	Aldehydes, VPHP, chlorine-dioxide
Medium	+	+	0	+	+/–	Alcohols, phenols, 7th-gen quats
Low	+	0	0	+/–	0	Quats

Courtesy McLaughlin S.

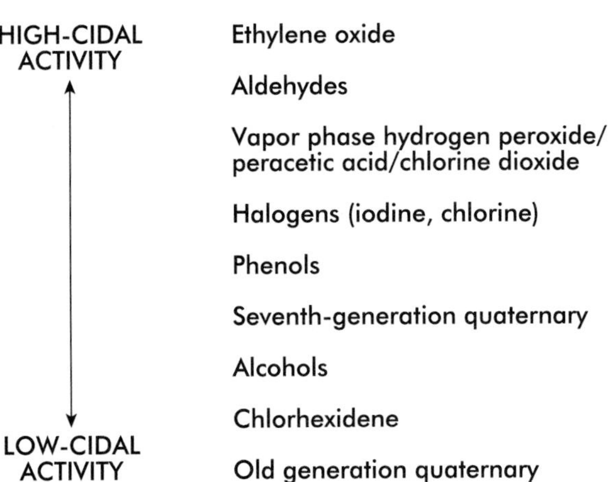

Figure 10-2 Ranking of chemicals according to *–cidal* activity. (Courtesy S. McLaughlin.)

J. Residual and cumulative action

II. Chemicals

A. Soaps
1. Anionic cleaning agent made from natural oils
2. Ineffective in hard water
3. Does not mix well with quaternary ammonium compounds and diminishes the effectiveness of halogens
4. Minimal disinfectant capability and is not antimicrobial

B. Detergents
1. Synthetic soaps
2. Anionic, cationic, or nonionic; anionic combined with cationic will neutralize both
3. Anionic and nonionic soaps are good cleansers; cationic soaps are better disinfectants
4. Most are basic; a few are acidic
5. Emulsify grease and suspend particles in solution
6. May contain wetting agents

C. Quaternary ammonium compounds (quats) (e.g., Centrimide, benzalkonium chloride, Zephiran, Quatsyl-D, Germiphene)
1. Effective against gram-positive and -negative organisms and enveloped viruses
2. Low toxicity and generally nonirritating
3. Prolonged contact irritates epithelial tissues
4. Reduced efficacy in presence of organic debris, soap, detergents, and hard water
5. Ineffective sporicide and fungicide
6. Organically substituted ammonium compounds
7. Inactivated by organic material, soap, hard water, cellulose fibers
8. Bacteria not destroyed may clump together; those inside are protected
9. More effective in basic pH
10. Cationic detergent
11. Deodorizes
12. Dissolve lipids in cell walls and cell membranes

D. Phenols (e.g., phenol, carbolic acid, coal tar phenols, cresol)
1. Active against
   a. Gram-positive bacteria
   b. Enveloped viruses
2. Developed from phenol or carbolic acid
3. Synthetic phenols are prepared in soap solutions that are nontoxic and nonirritating
4. Prolonged contact may lead to skin lesions
5. Toxic to cats because cats lack inherent enzymes to detoxify
6. May be toxic to rabbits and rodents
7. Activity decreased by quats
8. Not inactivated by organic matter, soap, or hard water

E. Aldehydes (e.g., gluteraldehyde, formaldehyde)
1. Active against
   a. Gram-positive bacteria
   b. Gram-negative bacteria

c. Most acid-fast bacteria
d. Bacterial spores
e. Most viruses
f. Fungi
2. Considered to be a sterilant but may require 12 hours of contact
3. Gluteraldehyde (Cidex)
 a. Noncorrosive
 b. Supplied as an acid, activated by adding sodium bicarbonate
 c. Good for plastics, rubber, lenses in "cold sterilization"
 d. Not inactivated by organic material or hard water
 e. Irritating to respiratory tract and skin
4. Formaldehyde (Formicide)
 a. Aqueous solution 37% to 40% (w/v) formaldehyde
 b. May be diluted with water or alcohol
 c. Irritating to tissue and respiratory tract; toxic
 d. A vapor phase surface disinfectant that slowly yields formaldehyde
5. Biguanide (e.g., chlorhexidine gluconate [Hibitane, Precyde])
 a. Active against
  (1) Gram-positive bacteria
  (2) Most gram-negative bacteria
  (3) Some lipophilic viruses
  (4) Fungi
 b. Efficient disinfectant, used mostly as an antiseptic
 c. Some reduction of activity in presence of organic material and hard water
 d. Has immediate, cumulative, and residual activity
 e. Precipitates to an inactive form mixed with saline solution
 f. Used as a surgical scrub and hand wash
 g. Low toxicity

F. Halogens (e.g., chlorine, iodine, fluorine, and bromine)
1. Active against
 a. Gram-positive bacteria
 b. Gram-negative bacteria
 c. Acid-fast bacteria
 d. All viruses
 e. Fungi
2. Iodine most common; used in solution with water or alcohol
 a. Iodophors: iodine plus carrier molecule that acts to release iodine over time
 b. Surgical scrub (Betadine): iodophor plus detergent
 c. Tinctures and solutions: iodines and iodophors without detergents
 d. Nonstaining and nonirritating
 e. Inactivated by organic material
 f. Aqueous forms are staining, irritating, and corrosive to metals, especially if not diluted properly
3. Chlorine and chlorine-releasing compounds (e.g., chlorine gas, chlorine dioxide)
 a. Commonly available as sodium hypochlorite (household bleach)
 b. Least expensive and most effective chemical disinfectant
 c. Available chlorine equals oxidizing ability
 d. Damages fabrics, corrosive to metals
 e. Inactivated by organic debris
 f. May require several minutes of contact to be effective
 g. Skin and mucous membrane irritant if not diluted properly or rinsed well

G. Alcohols (e.g., ethyl alcohol, isopropyl alcohol, methyl alcohol)
1. Active against
 a. Gram-positive and gram-negative bacteria
 b. Enveloped viruses
2. Most effective when diluted to 60% to 70% (isopropyl), 70% to 80% (ethyl)
3. Used as a solvent for other disinfectants and antiseptics
4. Most commonly used skin antiseptics
5. Low cost and low toxicity
6. Irritating to tissues and painful on open wounds
 a. Repeated use dries skin
 b. Forms coagulum in presence of tissue fluid
  (1) Coagulum consists of layer of tissue fluid whose proteins have been denatured by alcohol
  (2) Facilitates survival of bacteria under coagulum
7. Fogs lenses, hardens plastics, dissolves some cements
8. Inactivated by organic debris
9. Ineffective after evaporation
10. Defatting agent

H. Peroxygen compounds (e.g., peracetic acid)
1. Active against
 a. Gram-positive and gram-negative bacteria
 b. Acid-fast bacteria
 c. Fungi

d. Classified as a sterilant; may not kill pinworm eggs
e. No virucidal activity
2. Oxidizing agent
a. Reacts with cellular debris to release oxygen; kills anaerobes
3. Applied as a 2% solution for 30 minutes at 80% humidity
4. Explosive and can damage iron, steel, and rubber
5. Irritating to healthy tissues

I. Ethylene oxide (EO)
1. Active against
a. Gram-positive and gram-negative bacteria
b. Lipophilic and hydrophilic viruses
c. Fungi
d. Bacterial spores
e. Classified as a sterilant
2. Effective sterilant for heat-labile objects
3. EO is a colorless, nearly odorless gas
a. Diffuses and penetrates rapidly
4. Flammable and explosive
5. Toxic, carcinogenic, and irritating to tissue
6. Used in a chamber with a vacuum
7. May be mixed with CO_2, ether, or freon
8. Used at temperatures of 21° to 60° C (70° to 140° F) (works more quickly at higher temperatures); exposure times of 1 to 18 hours
9. Requires minimum relative humidity of 30% (40% is optimum)
10. Items must be clean and dry and may be wrapped in muslin, polyethylene, polypropylene, or polyvinyl
11. Sterilized items must be ventilated in a designated area for 24 to 48 hours to remove residual EO

AUTOCLAVE

Advantages

I. Consistently achieves complete sterility
II. Inexpensive and easy to operate
III. Safe for most surgical instruments and equipment, drapes and gowns, suture materials, sponges, and some plastics and rubbers
IV. Safe for patients and personnel
V. Established protocols and quality control indicators are easy to access

Disadvantages

I. Staff may overestimate the ability of the autoclave; sterility depends on saturated steam of the appropriate temperature having contact with all objects within the autoclave for a sufficient length of time
II. Requires a thorough understanding of techniques to ensure that the above occurs

Function

I. Heat is the killing agent in the autoclave
II. Steam is the vector that supplies the heat and promotes penetration of the heat
III. Pressure is the means to create adequately heated steam
IV. Complete sterilization of most items is achieved after 9 to 15 minutes of exposure to 121° C (250° F)
V. The temperature of steam at sea level is 100° C (212° F); an increase in pressure results in an increase in the temperature of the steam
VI. The minimum effective pressure of the autoclave is 15 pounds per square inch (p.s.i.), which provides steam at 121° C (250° F)
VII. Many autoclaves attain pressures of 35 p.s.i., which creates a steam temperature of 135° C (275° F)
VIII. Exposure times must allow penetration and exposure of all surfaces to 121° C (250° F) steam
IX. Exposure time is decreased by increasing pressure, which increases steam temperature (Table 10-2)

Types

I. Gravity displacement autoclave
A. Water is heated in a chamber; the continued application of heat by an electric element creates pressure within the chamber; this pressure raises the boiling point of the water and thus the ultimate temperature of the steam
B. Known as gravity displacement autoclave because the steam gradually displaces the air contained within the chamber; the air is forced out through a vent
C. Timing of the cycle begins when the temperature in the chamber reaches at least 121° C (250° F)

Table 10-2 Steam sterilization temperature/pressure chart

	Temperature		
Pressure (psi)	°C	°F	Time (min)
0	100	212	360
15	121	250	9-15
20	125	257	6.5
25	130	266	2.5
35	133	272	1

Modified from Minshall D: *CALAS training manual*, 1995.

D. After sufficient exposure time, the steam is exhausted through a vent into a reservoir
E. Air that has been sterilized within the jacket and then filtered is admitted into the chamber to replace the exhausting steam
F. If the chamber is improperly loaded or there is insufficient steam, there will be air pockets remaining in the chamber that will interfere with steam penetration and result in nonsterile areas
G. Load must be dried within the autoclave

II. Prevacuum autoclave
A. Usually a much larger and more costly machine; equipped with a boiler to generate steam and a vacuum system
B. Air is forced out of the loaded chamber by means of the vacuum pump
C. Steam at 121° C (250° F) or more is introduced into the chamber; the steam immediately fills the chamber to eliminate the vacuum
D. Exposure time starts immediately
E. At completion of exposure cycle, the steam is vacuumed from the chamber and replaced by hot, sterile, filtered air, which dries the contents
F. Air pockets are eliminated and processing times are reduced due to use of vacuum
G. Often equipped with readout and/or printout of chamber temperatures and pressures

Operation

I. Preparation of load
A. Linen packs
1. All instruments in packs are scrupulously cleaned and rinsed in deionized water
2. Instruments are disassembled and ratchets are usually left closed and unlocked
3. Appropriate linens are in good repair and freshly laundered
4. Disposable linens (drapes, wrappers, etc.) are not reused
5. A chemical sterilization indicator is included in every pack
a. Chemical sterilization indicators provide verification that the inside of the pack was exposed to appropriate sterilization temperatures for the correct amount of time
6. The pack is wrapped using at least two layers of material
a. The shelf-life of the sterilized pack varies with the type of outer wrap (Table 10-3)
7. Pack is sealed with autoclave tape and labeled with date, contents, and operator

Table 10-3 Recommended storage times for sterilized packs*

Wrapper	Shelf-life
Double-wrapped, two-layer muslin	4 wk
Double-wrapped, two-layer muslin, heat-sealed in dust covers after sterilization	6 mo
Double-wrapped, two-layer muslin, tape-sealed in dust covers after sterilization	2 mo
Double-wrapped nonwoven barrier materials (paper)	6 mo
Paper/plastic-peel pouches, heat-sealed	1 yr
Plastic-peel pouches, heat-sealed	1 yr

*Note that sterilized items from hospitals adopting event-related sterility assurance have an indefinite shelf-life.
Modified from Pratt PW: *Principles and practice of veterinary technology*, St Louis, 1998, Mosby.

a. Autoclave tape provides verification that the *outside* of the pack was exposed to appropriate sterilization temperatures
8. Pack should not exceed 30 × 30 × 50 cm (12 × 12 × 20 inches) in size
9. Pack should not exceed 5.5 kg (12 lb) in weight
10. Pack should not exceed 115.3 kg/m^3 in density

B. Pouch packs
1. Used for single instruments, sponges, etc.
2. Above guidelines apply (see Linen packs)
3. Pouches are heat sealed or ends are rolled and securely taped with autoclave tape
4. Labeled as above

C. Hard goods
1. Stainless steel or other hard instruments, trays, bowls, laboratory cages, and other equipment may be autoclaved without wrapping
2. Must be physically clean and rinsed in deionized water
3. Syringes and barrels are separated before autoclaving

D. Liquids
1. Contained in Pyrex flask three times larger than contents require
2. Cover with loosely applied lid or parafin wrapping film, or place a needle through stopper to allow air exchange (the sterility of liquids processed in the autoclave is in question; removing liquids from the chamber is hazardous to personnel)

E. Contaminated objects
1. Used before disposal to decontaminate syringes, culture plates, etc., that contain biohazardous waste

2. Place objects in appropriate container for disposal; special autoclavable biohazard bags are available

II. Loading the chamber
   A. Must allow free circulation of steam; use perforated or wire mesh shelves
   B. Linen packs have 2.5 to 7.5 cm (1 to 3 inch) space between; place multiple packs on edge instead of stacking
   C. Paper/plastic pouches are placed in specially designed baskets that support them on edge with paper side of each package facing the plastic side of the adjacent package
   D. Solid bowls or basins are placed upside down or on edge
   E. Mixed loads (hard goods and wrapped goods) have wrapped goods on upper shelf

III. Autoclave cycles
   A. Wrapped goods
      1. Has "dry" cycle that allows wrapped packs to dry
      2. Used for most surgical packs
   B. Hard goods
      1. Has no dry cycle; used for trays, bowls, cages, etc. that will not be maintained in a sterile condition
      2. Also used for "flash autoclave" to quickly sterilize instruments that are needed immediately
   C. Liquids
      1. Exhausts steam more slowly than other cycles
      2. Used for liquids that would be forced from containers during a faster exhaust

QUALITY CONTROL FOR STERILIZATION AND DISINFECTION

The effectiveness of any method of microbial control must be monitored regularly. Verification of the effectiveness of microbial control should be performed at least monthly.

Sterilization

I. Recording thermometer
   A. Displays temperature of autoclave chamber; operator observes for correct temperature during cycle
   B. Some autoclaves are equipped with printed tape of chamber temperatures and pressures

II. Thermocouple
   A. Used in steam, dry heat, and chemical sterilization chambers
   B. Temperature sensors are placed in the part of a test pack that is most inaccessible to steam penetration

III. Chemical indicator
   A. Definition: paper strips impregnated with sensitive chemicals that change color when conditions of sterility are met
   B. Used with autoclaves and ethylene oxide systems
   C. Placed deep inside packs before autoclaving

IV. Biological testing
   A. Bacterial spores are exposed to autoclave or ethylene oxide and then cultured
   B. Recommended method for verification of proper autoclave operation in veterinary clinics

V. Bowie Dick Test
   A. Tests prevacuumed autoclaves for complete removal of air and uniform steam penetration
   B. Uses a pack made to specific dimensions with a cross of autoclave tape in the center

VI. Surface sampling
   A. Surface to be tested is swabbed with a sterile applicator and transferred to a suitable media plate for growth
   B. Surface or item may be rinsed with sterile solution, which is examined for contaminants
   C. "Contact plate" of media is touched to surface and incubated
   D. Recommended method for ensuring proper disinfection of surgical suites in veterinary clinics

VII. Serology
   A. The presence of viruses in the environment is monitored by serological testing of animals to determine the presence of antibodies
   B. Animals maintained for this purpose are referred to as sentinel animals
      1. Rabbits are commonly used as sentinel animals due to their readily accessible veins for blood collection

ACKNOWLEDGEMENT

The editors and author recognize and appreciate the original work of Pat Carter on which this chapter is based.

Glossary

anion An ion carrying a negative charge

antiseptic Antimicrobial chemical that is applied to the skin or mucous membranes

aspesis Condition in which no living organisms are present; free of infection or infectious material

bacteriostat Agent that stops or inhibits the growth of bacteria but does not necessarily kill the bacteria

cationic Positively charged ion

cavitation Cleaning method that uses sound waves passed through a solution to remove debris from materials

-cide, -cida Suffix denoting death or destruction; used after bacteria, virus, spore, etc. to denote "death to"

cleaning Physical removal of organic and inorganic soils and many microbial contaminants
coagulum Gel-like substance composed of tissue fluid and organic debris formed in the presence of alcohol on an open wound
disinfectant An agent, usually chemical, that is applied to inanimate objects to destroy or inhibit the growth of microorganisms
efficacy Effectiveness of an agent
fungicide Agent capable of destroying fungi
HEPA High-efficiency particle absorption filter; removes particles over 0.3 μm in size
hydrolysis Addition of water
hydrophilic Affinity for water
lipophilic Affinity for fat
microbicidal Destroying microbes
microorganism Microbe, especially pathogenic bacterium
oxidizing agent Chemical that releases oxygen when in contact with organic material; usually kills anaerobic organisms
pathogen Any disease-producing microorganism
sanitize Process of removing infectious material and reducing numbers of pathogens in an environment to promote health; the application of a detergent combined with a disinfectant
sentinel Animal that is used for surveillance of an environment
sporicide Agent capable of killing bacterial spores
sterilant Agent that destroys microorganisms
sterilize To eliminate all forms of life, including viruses and spores
viricidal Killing or destroying a virus

Review Questions

1 The following microorganisms are listed from most to least resistant:
a. Fungi, spores, protozoan cysts, vegetative bacteria
b. Spores, protozoan cysts, lipophilic viruses, vegetative bacteria
c. Protozoan cysts, TB organisms, fungi, vegetative bacteria
d. Spores, protozoan cysts, lipophilic viruses, hydrophilic viruses

2 Disinfection controls (kills) _________ of the microorganisms on an object.
a. 90%
b. 99%
c. 98%
d. 95%

3 An agent that stops or prevents the growth of microorganisms but does not necessarily kill them contains the suffix:
a. *–cidal*
b. Pathogen
c. *–stat*
d. *–biotic*

4 A chemical antimicrobial that is applied to the skin or mucous membranes is a/an:
a. Antiseptic
b. Disinfectant
c. Antibiotic
d. Germicide

5 The efficacy of boiling as a method of microbial control is increased by adding _________ to the water.
a. Sodium chloride
b. Calcium chloride
c. Sodium bicarbonate
d. Sodium carbonate

6 Hibitane is an example of which class of disinfectant?
a. Phenols
b. Quaternary ammonium compounds
c. Biguanides
d. Halogens

7 The following chemicals are classified as sterilants:
a. Ethylene oxide, peroxygen compounds, alcohols
b. Ethylene oxide, aldehydes, quaternary ammonium compounds
c. Aldehydes, peroxygen compounds, halogens
d. Aldehydes, peroxygen compounds, ethylene oxide

8 The killing agent in the autoclave is:
a. Steam
b. Heat
c. Pressure
d. Time

9 The minimum effective pressure in an autoclave is _____________.
a. 5 p.s.i.
b. 20 p.s.i.
c. 25 p.s.i.
d. 15 p.s.i.

10 At 135° C (275° F), microorganisms are destroyed in __________ minute(s).
a. 3
b. 2
c. 1
d. 5

BIBLIOGRAPHY

Kagan KG: Care and sterilization of surgical equipment, *Vet Tech* 13, 1992.
McCurnin DM, Bassert JM, editors: *Clinical textbook for veterinary technicians,* ed 5, Philadelphia, 2002, WB Saunders.
Pratt P, editor: *Principles and practices of veterinary technology,* St Louis, 1998, Mosby.
Tracy DL: *Small animal surgical nursing,* ed 3, St Louis, 2000, Mosby.

CHAPTER 11

Radiography

Marg Brown

OUTLINE

LEARNING OUTCOMES

After reading this chapter you should be able to:

1. Understand some of the basic principles involved with x-rays and their production.
2. Describe the anatomy of the x-ray tube.
3. Briefly explain the components of the x-ray machine.
4. Understand the principles of accessory x-ray equipment and image receptors used in veterinary practice so that diagnostic radiographs are consistently produced.
5. Properly process radiographs based on your understanding of darkroom principles.
6. Explain what is meant by radiographic quality, including density, contrast, and detail, and the factors influencing these.
7. Identify common technical errors and artifacts and know how to prevent or correct them.
8. Understand the concepts involved with setting up a technique chart.
9. Describe the effects that could occur if proper radiation safety is not practiced.
10. State the units of radiation and the maximum permissible dose allowed.
11. List practical methods that can be used to reduce radiation exposure.
12. List and define proper directional terminology used in radiography.
13. List basic guidelines for veterinary radiographic positioning and restraint.
14. Explain what is meant by contrast media, giving examples.

Radiography is an important diagnostic tool available to veterinary practice. To arrive at a proper diagnosis, high-quality images must be produced. This chapter discusses basic but essential information needed to produce diagnostic radiographs. Radiation physics, positioning and restraint, technique charts, and specialized procedures are discussed briefly and can be further investigated by consulting the excellent texts listed in the Bibliography.

X-RAY PRODUCTION

I. Definition of radiation: propagation of energy through space and matter

II. Three types of radiation
  A. Particulate radiation
    1. "Particles" of the atom
      a. Examples: neutrons, protons, electrons, alpha particles, beta particles
      b. Some particles may have a positive, a negative, or a neutral charge
    2. Cannot reach the speed of light
    3. Process that occurs in the x-ray machine is an example
  B. Electromagnetic radiation
    1. Definition: transport of energy through space without matter
    2. Examples: radio waves, television waves, microwaves, x-rays, gamma rays
    3. Has wavelength: defined as the distance from one crest of a wave to the next
    4. Has frequency: the number of crests passing a particular point per unit of time. It is measured in Hertz (Hz)
    5. Energy associated with electromagnetic radiation is the ability to do work and is measured in electron Volts (eV)
    6. Electromagnetic radiation is measured in frequency, energy, and wavelength
      a. Wavelength and frequency are inversely related
        (1) The shorter the wavelength, the greater the energy
      b. The greater the energy, the greater the ability to penetrate
    7. When matter and electromagnetic radiation interact, wave and particle behavior can be described
    8. X-rays have similar physical properties as other forms of electromagnetic radiation
  C. Ionizing radiation
    1. Definition: particulate and electromagnetic radiation with sufficient energy to cause ionization
    2. Radiation must have greater energy than the electron binding energy
    3. Ionization causes damage to tissues
III. Definition of x-rays
  A. X-rays are a form of radiation that result when the energy of the electrons is converted to electromagnetic radiation
  B. X-ray beam is composed of bundles of energy or quanta referred to as photons that travel in a wave
  C. Photons have no mass or electrical charge
IV. Production of x-rays
  A. X-rays are produced when the fast moving electrons or particulate radiation collide with matter
  B. This is best achieved in an x-ray tube. The tube consists of a negative electrode known as the cathode and a positive electrode called the anode
  C. A cloud of electrons (negative particulate radiation) forms at the cathode and accelerates across the tube where the electrons interact with the target material at the positive anode
  D. This interaction forces the high-speed electrons to lose their energy, resulting in the production of 1% x-radiation and 99% heat
  E. The electrons that travel across the tube have different energies, measured in kilovoltage peak or potential (kVp)
  F. A setting on the x-ray machine determines the kVp of the electrons and thus the x-ray penetrating power
  G. Thus to produce x-rays, one needs a source of electrons, a method of accelerating electrons, a directed path, a target, and an envelope to provide a vacuum, all of which are provided in the x-ray tube
V. Discovery of x-rays
  A. Wilhelm Conrad Roentgen on November 8, 1895
  B. Used a cathode ray tube (Crookes), which was an evacuated glass tube with two electrodes through which an electrical current was passed
  C. X-rays were used almost immediately for medical and surgical diagnoses
  D. Changes in skin color, similar to sunburn, due to radiation exposure were reported as early as April 1896

X-RAY TUBE

I. Cathode (electrically negative portion of the x-ray tube; Figure 11-1)
  A. Provides the source of electrons and a directed path
  B. The filament is a coiled wire that emits electrons when heated up
    1. When heated, electrons are held less tightly by the nucleus of the atom. After the binding energy of the electrons is exceeded, an electron cloud available for travel is formed
      a. The flow of current to the filament is controlled by the step-down transformer, which is regulated by the milliamperage (mA) control
    2. The filament is constructed of tungsten, which has a high melting point and atomic number
    3. Most machines contain a small and a large filament
  C. The focusing cup is a cavity in which the filaments sit

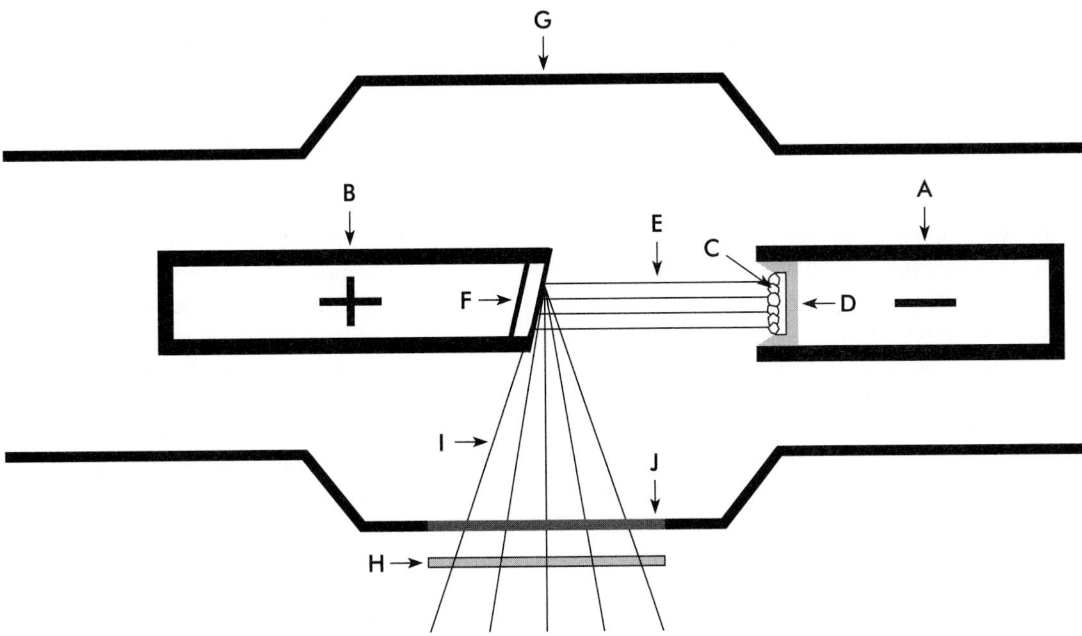

Figure 11-1 Anatomy of an x-ray tube. *A,* Cathode. *B,* Anode. *C,* Tungsten filament. *D,* Focusing cup. *E,* Accelerating electrons. *F,* Tungsten target. *G,* Glass envelope. *H,* Aluminum filter. *I,* Generated x-rays. *J,* Beryllium window. (From Pratt PW: *Principles and practice of veterinary technology,* St Louis, 1998, Mosby.)

1. It is maintained at the same negative potential as the heated filament
2. Because like charges repel, the electron beam is directed to a small area on the anode

D. Acceleration of the electrons is controlled by the kVp

II. Anode (electrically positive portion of the x-ray tube)
   A. Provides the target for the interaction of the electrons
   B. Composed of the target and a copper stem
   C. Tungsten is used also for the target material to dissipate the high temperatures while the copper stem conducts the heat away from the target
   D. The actual area on the target that the electrons hit is the focal spot
      1. Size of the spot affects the x-ray image
      2. Size is determined by the filament size chosen
         a. The smaller the focal spot the sharper the image but there is less heat dissipation
      3. Because of the target angle, more x-rays leave the cathode side of the x-ray tube than from the anode side, resulting in an uneven distribution of x-rays on the image (this is known as the "heel effect")
         a. Most noticeable when using largest film size, short source image distance (SID) and low-kVp techniques
         b. May be advantageous to place the thickest part of the animal toward the cathode side
   E. Two types of anodes: stationary anode and rotating anode
      1. Stationary anodes are found in dental and small portable units used in large animals
         a. These units have a small capacity for x-ray production and are unable to withstand a lot of heat
         b. Consists of a beveled target angled toward the window embedded on a cylinder of copper
      2. Rotating anode
         a. An approximate 3-inch disk-shaped anode rotates on an axis through the center of the tube
         b. Filament from the cathode directs electron stream against the beveled edge of this tungsten disk mounted on a molybdenum spindle
         c. Position of the focal spot remains fixed while this circular ring rotates rapidly (3350 times per minute), using a larger target area for the electrons to dissipate their heat

d. Can use higher tube currents, shorter exposure time, and smaller filament

III. Tube envelope
   A. Traditionally made of Pyrex glass that has been evacuated to form the vacuum necessary for x-ray production
   B. Window is the thin segment of the glass that allows maximum emission of x-rays and minimum absorption by the glass (also called aperture)

IV. Tube or machine housing
   A. Metallic structure that covers and protects the x-ray tube or, in the case of portable units, the entire machine
   B. Lined internally with lead and contains insulating oil

V. Causes of x-ray tube failure
   A. More than 95% is due to operator error
   B. Most damage is related to heat accumulation in the tube, which may lead to filament evaporation, broken filaments, cracked anodes, anode melting or pitting, and burned-out or frozen bearings

VI. Tube rating chart
   A. Provided by all manufacturers of x-ray tubes
   B. Composite graph that shows the maximum combination of kVp, mA, and exposure time that can be used safely in a single exposure to avoid injury to the x-ray tube from excessive heat production

X-RAY MACHINE

I. Electrical circuits for x-ray tube control
   A. High-voltage circuit
      1. Purpose is to provide high electrical potential needed to accelerate the electrons from the cathode to the anode
      2. High potential (kVp peak or potential) generated by a step-up transformer
         a. Incoming wall voltage (110 or 220 V) must be changed to kilovolts (1000× greater)
         b. Most machines have a range of 40 to 120 kVp
      3. kVp selection switch controlled by autotransformer
      4. Line voltage compensator also associated with circuit
   B. Low-voltage (filament) circuit
      1. Purpose is to provide electricity (amperage) needed to heat the filament
      2. Tungsten filament needs minimal energy so a step-down transformer is needed to reduce incoming voltage
      3. Connected to the mA control
   C. Timer switch
      1. Purpose is to control the length of exposure time during which high voltage is applied across the tube
      2. Best to have exposure times of less than one thirtieth of a second (0.03 second) to minimize potential of patient movement
   D. Rectification circuit
      1. Purpose is to change the alternating current coming into the tube into direct current to ensure that there are no negative deflections of the wave when no electrons are generated
      2. Various possibilities exist, depending on the type of x-ray machine

II. Technique selection or control panel
   A. Quality (energy, penetrating ability) of x-rays produced, controlled by kVp potential, whereas mA and time (sec) control the quantity (intensity)
   B. Product of mA and time is milliampere-seconds (mA × sec = mAs)
   C. Depending on the machine, operator can control
      1. kVp, mA, and sec
      2. kVp and mAs
      3. kVp only

III. Tube stand
   A. Apparatus that supports x-ray tube

IV. Accessory x-ray equipment
   A. Filtration
      1. Total filtration is result of inherent (filtering by glass envelope) and added (aluminum disk placed over window) filtration
      2. Purpose is to selectively remove less-energetic, less-penetrating (nondiagnostic) x-rays from primary beam
      3. Filtered primary x-ray beam decreases the amount of undesirable patient exposure by increasing the mean beam energy but decreasing the overall beam intensity. This necessitates increasing the exposure time or mA
   B. Collimation
      1. Beam-restricting device that limits the primary beam
      2. Purpose is to prevent unnecessary patient exposure and to decrease production of scatter (secondary) radiation
         a. This results in greater patient safety, increased operator safety, and an improved quality radiograph
      3. Beam-restricting devices include lead aperture diaphragm, lead cone, lead cylinder, and adjustable lead aperture shutter
      4. Most regulatory agencies require some evidence of collimation on the films
   C. Grids (Figure 11-2)

A

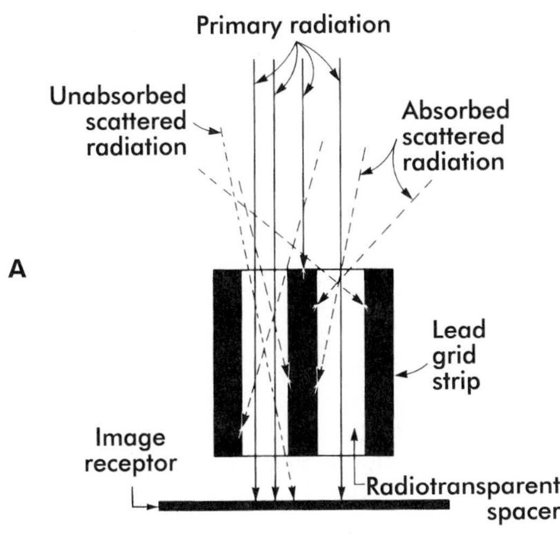

B

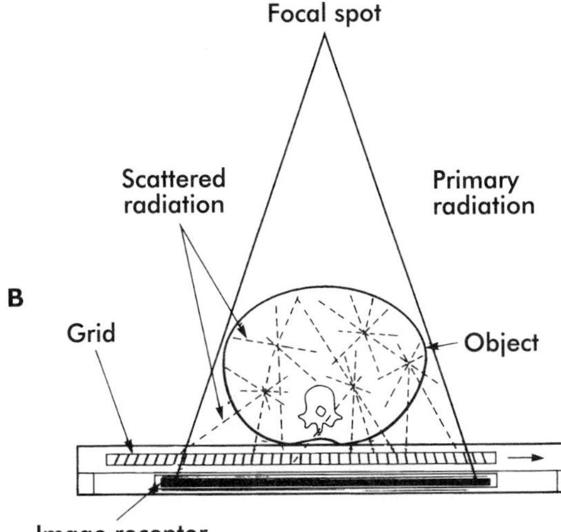

Figure 11-2 Cross section of a grid. **A,** Diagram of a small section of a grid showing how a large proportion of the scattered radiation is absorbed and image-forming primary radiation passes through to the image detector. **B,** Diagram of focused Potter-Bucky diaphragm being moved toward the right. (From Eastman Kodak Company: *The fundamentals of radiography,* ed 12, Rochester, NY, 1980, Eastman Kodak Company, Radiographic Markets Division.)

1. Series of thin linear strips of alternating radiodense (lead) and radiolucent (plastic or aluminum) materials encased in an aluminum protective cover
2. Placed between patient and film
3. Generally used when area radiographed is greater than 9, 10, or 11 cm, depending on the reference source. The author uses 10 cm
4. Purpose is to prevent scatter radiation from reaching the film. This improves quality of the radiograph
5. Part of the primary beam is also absorbed so exposure needs to be increased (usually mA or sec)
6. Characteristics
   a. Grid ratio: relationship of the height of the lead strips to the distance between them (e.g., if the lead strips are eight times as high as the space between them, the ratio is 8:1)
      (1) The greater the ratio, the better the absorption of scatter radiation, but the disadvantages of a higher ratio are greater exposure needed, more perfect centering required, and narrower focusing range permitted
   b. Grid pattern: determined by orientation of lead strips
      (1) Linear grid: lead strips in one direction (most common)
      (2) Crossed grid (crosshatch): two linear grids sandwiched together so that the strips are at right angles to each other
   c. Types of grids
      (1) Parallel grid: strips perpendicular to face of grid and parallel to each other
      (2) Focused grid: strips placed parallel to the primary x-ray beam. Angle begins at 90 degrees to the surface at the center of the grid and progresses to greater angles toward both edges of the film
         (a) Most common
   d. Lines per centimeter or inch (grid frequency)
      (1) As the number of lead strips per centimeter or inch increases, they become narrower, which means the lines will be less objectionable on the radiograph
      (2) The increased frequency also means less absorption of scatter, increased exposure factors, and increased cost
   e. Mode of movement
      (1) Stationary grid: the grid does not move, which means that the grid lines are identifiable on the radiograph
      (2) Moving grid (Potter-Bucky diaphragm): through a mechanical device the grid lines are blurred, resulting in a clearer radiograph

IMAGE RECEPTORS

I. Definition
   A. Mechanisms involved with transferring the invisible ionizing radiation into a visible image
II. Cassette

A. Rigid film holder designed to keep the intensifying screen and the film in close contact
B. The front, which is made of plastic, light metal, or carbon fiber, must face the x-ray tube
C. The back is made of heavy steel to sustain the weight of the patient if necessary
D. Do not drop the cassette, and keep it clean

III. Intensifying screens
A. Layers of tiny luminescent phosphor crystals bound together on a plastic base and covered with a protective coating
B. X-ray film is sandwiched between the two intensifying screens that are positioned on the inner surfaces of the cassette
C. When the phosphor crystals in the screen are struck by x-radiation, they fluoresce and emit light
1. This visible light exposes the light sensitive emulsion of the x-ray film
2. More than 95% of exposure to film is due to this light emitted from the intensifying screens (indirect imaging)
D. The primary purpose is to reduce the amount of exposure required to produce a diagnostic image
E. Screen construction
1. Base material for support
2. Reflective layer to redirect light toward the film to increase efficiency of film
3. Phosphor layer composed of calcium tungstate or rare earth crystals to convert the energy of the remnant x-ray beam into visible light
a. These phosphorescent crystals
(1) Have a high atomic number
(2) Have a high level of x-ray absorption
(3) Must have high x-ray–to–light conversion with suitable energy and color
(4) Should stop emitting light when the x-ray exposure ceases
4. Protective coating applied to phosphor to prevent abrasion and allow transmission of light
F. Care of intensifying screens
1. Important to clean regularly (monthly) with a cleaner that is recommended (best) or 70% alcohol
2. Make sure surface is dry before loading films
3. Any debris on screen surface will cause artifacts
4. Avoid "digs and scratches" on the screen surface when loading and unloading film

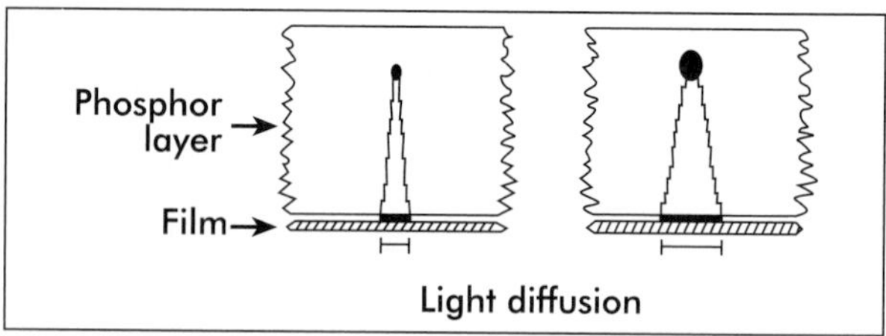

Figure 11-3 Increasing the size of the phosphor crystals increases the speed of the screen. However, the image appears more grainy.

G. Phosphor types
1. Calcium tungstate phosphor
a. Emits blue light
b. Has good x-ray absorption ability but lacks in light conversion efficiency
c. Traditionally used in phosphor layer
2. Rare earth phosphors
a. Primarily emit in the green light spectrum
b. Greater x-ray–to–light conversion, resulting in decreased exposure required
c. Because of greater absorption and conversion, rare earth screens can produce a better degree of radiographic detail than calcium tungstate with less radiation exposure
H. Screen speed (Figure 11-3)
1. Relative term referring to the measure of exposure necessary to produce a diagnostic film
2. Screen speed ratings
a. Slow (high definition, ultra-fine, fine grain): designed for optimal detail with minimal concern for exposure time
b. Medium (regular, mid speed, normal, par speed): good resolution with relatively low exposures
c. Fast (high speed) used when reduced exposure time or increased patient penetration required
3. Fast screens
a. Require less radiation exposure than slower speed screens to produce the same degree of blackness on the film
b. Generally have larger crystals to increase the x-ray absorption and light conversion
c. Usually have a thicker phosphor layer
d. The larger crystals and thicker layer mean more blurriness (high grain) and less detail
4. Quantum mottle resulting in a spotty or mottled radiograph is a disadvantage of increased film speed

IV. X-ray film
  A. Purpose is to provide a permanent diagnostic record
  B. Film composition
    1. Transparent polyester base
    2. Adhesive that attaches emulsion to base
    3. Emulsion that consists of gelatin and silver halide crystals (appear as tiny grains under the microscope [billions per mL])
    4. Protective coating to protect emulsion from scratching
  C. Latent image
    1. Definition: an invisible image on the x-ray film after it has been exposed by ionizing radiation or visible light before the film has been processed
    2. On a screen-type film, the grain of silver halide absorbs the emitted light photon and begins to split apart
    3. The partially split crystals will convert to metallic silver and turn black after the film is developed
    4. The greater the number of converted silver halide crystals, the blacker the film
    5. Unexposed crystals will be cleared away by the fixer
  D. Film types
    1. Screen film
      a. Silver crystals are more sensitive to wavelengths of light emitted from the intensifying screens than from direct ionizing radiation
      b. Less exposure needed to produce a diagnostic radiograph
      c. Must be sensitive to the light emitted by the intensifying screens
      d. Depend on size of the crystal
      e. Generally the smaller the crystal, the wider the latitude or exposure factors that can be used without significantly changing the film density (Table 11-1)
        (1) Also the greater the resolution
      f. Medium film represents a compromise between fine grain and speed; it is mostly used in veterinary radiography
    2. Nonscreen film
      a. Designed to be more sensitive to direct ionizing radiation
      b. Greater exposure factors required because there is no intensification of the x-ray beam
      c. Packaged in a light-tight heavy envelope
        (1) Dental film speed that is available is usually designated as D or E
        (2) E film speeds are faster

Table 11-1 Comparison of film speed

Characteristic	Fast film (ultraspeed)	Slow film (high detail)
Crystal size	Larger crystals	Smaller crystals
Exposure required	Lower needed	More needed
Film latitude	Less latitude	Greater latitude
Image	More grainy image	Less grainy image
Definition	Less resolution	Greater resolution

  E. Film care
    1. Store film boxes on end so film is in a vertical position
    2. Store in a cool (10° to 15° C or 50° to 59° F) room with low relative humidity (40% to 60%)
    3. Use before expiration date to prevent radiographic fogging
    4. Film can be placed in a plastic bag and stored in a refrigerator or freezer to prolong usefulness

V. Film-screen systems
  A. Combined speed determines exposure requirements
  B. Must determine most desirable system for your clinic based on image detail and speed requirement
  C. Numeric value is assigned to each film and screen combination
  D. Numerical value differs for each company so that proper comparisons can be made only for that particular company
  E. As a rule 300-400 speed is medium speed and considered most versatile
  F. Speed of the system is inversely related to the mAs setting: as you increase the speed (higher number), you decrease the mAs
  G. Values are similar to ISO (ASA) of photographic film

VI. Legal records and identification
  A. Must be properly identified (in film emulsion) to be legal
  B. Identification should include
    1. Patient identification
    2. Owner identification
    3. Date of examination
    4. Name of hospital
  C. Numeric system using a patient case number or file number facilitates record keeping
  D. Methods of labeling a radiograph include
    1. Lead markers
    2. Lead-impregnated tape
    3. Photoimprinting label system
    4. Miscellaneous markers
      a. Right (Rt) or Left (Le) is essential

b. Labeling of front (F) or hind (H) limbs and medial (M) or lateral (L) in equine radiography
c. Time sequence labels for special procedures
d. Position markers
e. Technician identification markers

VII. Film filing
A. Must be properly labeled and filed for future referral or follow-up examinations
B. Because these are legal records, provincial and state associations require a minimum file and retrieval period before they are allowed to be discarded
1. Varies with the state or province

DARKROOM AND PROCESSING TECHNIQUES

Radiography begins and ends in the darkroom, where films are loaded into cassettes and returned for processing into finished radiographs. Most mistakes made in animal radiography are related to the processing of radiographs.

Darkroom Considerations

I. Cleanliness is absolutely essential
II. Good ventilation and temperature control
III. Lightproof so that film fogging does not result
IV. Darkroom safelight
A. Filter must match sensitivity of film used
1. Amber for blue sensitive film
2. Dark red (e.g., Kodak GBX) can be used for blue and green sensitive film
B. Correct wattage (usually 7 to 15 W)
C. At least 4 feet from working area
D. Work as quickly as possible
V. Fogging due to light leakage or improper safelight illumination can be evaluated as follows
A. Place a nonradiographed film on the counter
B. Cover three fourths of it with a piece of cardboard for 1 minute
C. Move the cardboard covering one half of the film for 1 additional minute
D. Shift the cardboard so that only one fourth of the film is covered for 1 additional minute
E. Remove the cardboard and expose the entire film for 1 additional minute (4 minutes in total)
F. Process normally
G. Darkened areas are indicative of fogging
VI. Organize into a wet and dry area to minimize processing artifacts
VII. State, provincial, or federal regulations require proper use of gloves, protective eye wear, eye wash bottle (Workplace Hazardous Materials Information System [Canadian] [WHMIS]/ Occupational Safety and Health Act [United States] [OSHA])

Manual Film Processing Pointers

I. Basic steps include developing, rinsing or stop bath, fixing, washing, and drying
II. Chemical solutions are usually required by manufacturer to be diluted; follow steps carefully
III. Keep all solutions at required temperature
A. Optimum temperature is 20° C or 68° F
B. Less activity occurs at lower temperatures; greater activity occurs at higher temperatures
IV. Make sure chemicals are well mixed before using
V. Carefully follow manufacturer's suggestion for time-temperature development
VI. Agitate film intermittently in solutions to prevent air bubbles
VII. Avoid letting liquid drain back into chemical solutions when removing from the tanks
VIII. Keep lids on the solution tanks whenever possible to prevent oxidation
IX. Developer: primarily functions to reduce or convert the exposed silver halide crystals of the film to black metallic silver
A. pH is alkaline in a range of 9.8 to 11.4
B. Solution needs replacing when it turns brown to green or when the processed radiographs do not have the expected density or contrast
C. Maintain level of solution with fresh replenisher
1. Daily replacement is suggested
X. Purpose of the rinse bath is to stop the developing process and to prevent contamination of the fixer
A. Rinse in circulating water for about 30 seconds
XI. Fixer: primary functions are to remove and clear away the unexposed, undeveloped silver halide crystals and to harden the film to make it a permanent record
A. Fixer consists of clearing or fixing agent, preservative, hardener, acidifier, buffer, and a solvent
B. pH is acidic
C. Film can be briefly viewed after it is cleared (about 1 minute but it is safer to wait at least 2 minutes)
1. Must be returned and fixed in total for about double the development time
2. This ensures proper hardening
D. Change fixer when time required for the film to change from cloudy to clear exceeds 2 to 3 minutes
E. Replenish when solution is low as evidenced by film artifact (Box 11-1)

Box 11-1 Artifacts and Other Technical Areas

BLACK MARKS
- Film scratches usually after exposure but before processing
- Crescent marks: rough handling, fingernail
- Folding of film
- Light leak: defective cassettes, storage in bin
- Static electricity: linear dots or tree pattern from too low humidity or improper handling
- Developer drops before processing
- Fingerprints due to developer on hands during loading or unloading
- Film stuck together while in fixer

Heavy lines due to
- Grid cutoff: grid out of focal range, upside down, not perpendicular to beam and not aligned to center beam
- Damaged grid
- Roller lines of automatic processor
- Film jammed in automatic processor

YELLOW RADIOGRAPH
- Exhausted fixer solution
- Fixing time too short
- Inadequate rinsing: residual fixer oxidizes to yellow powder and also destroys image
- Film sticking together during fixer process

SLOW DRYING
- Waterlogged films due to: prolonged washing, water too warm or improper hardening by the fixer
- Air too humid or cool
- Automatic processor
- Thermostat malfunction
- Too low dryer temperatures
- Improper hardening
- Inadequate air venting

WHITE MARKS OR CLEAR AREAS
- Film emulsion scratched off usually before exposure or during processing
- Debris in cassette
- Defective screens (pitted, scratched)
- Smudges of fixer on fingers before developing
- Grit due to remnant fixer not washed
- Increased atomic number of object (e.g., positioning device, lead contrast media on cassette)
- Air bubble on film during developing procedure
- Developing solution low
- Film touching side of tanks during manual developing
- Reticulation due to improper stirring of solutions
- Blank film: unexposed or fixed before developed
- Evidence of collimation
- Positive contrast media spilt on table or cassette

BRITTLENESS OF FINISHED RADIOGRAPH
- Excessive drying temperature, time
- Excessive hardening in fixer

ORIGINAL FILM COLOR
- Processing solutions low
- Two films stuck together during processing

XII. Wash bath: purpose is to remove processing chemicals from the film, thereby preventing film discoloration and fading over time
   A. Wash in clean, circulating water about 15 to 20 minutes

XIII. Drying
   A. Place hanger in drier or hang on rack
   B. Avoid dusty areas

XIV. Maintenance and replenishing
   A. For optimum chemical efficiency, it is suggested to daily remove 8 oz (250 mL) of developer and fixer, and replenish same amount
   B. Solutions should be changed at least every 3 months or when 15 gallons (60 L) of working replenisher has been used

Automatic Film Processing

I. Mechanized film processing is a more accurate term

II. Films carried from solution to solution and through the dryer by a roller assembly

III. Processing times vary from 90 seconds to 8 minutes depending on temperature
   A. 77° to 96° F (20° to 35° C) with temperature inversely related to length of processing times

IV. Chemicals are more concentrated with similar properties and procedures to the manual processing, but there are a few exceptions
   A. A hardener is included in the developer
   B. No rinsing occurs between developing and fixing

V. Keep processor clean at all times, especially rollers, roller racks, and crossover rollers

VI. Change chemicals as required

VII. As cost of units decrease, automatic processing will become more popular in veterinary clinics

RADIOGRAPHIC QUALITY

Definition

I. That "feature of a diagnostic radiograph that describes to what degree the shadows identified on the film clearly depict the anatomical features under investigation"[1]

II. A film of good diagnostic quality should have optimal density, correct scale of contrast, and excellent detail with minimal magnification and distortion
   A. See Table 11-2 for technical errors related to density

Radiographic Density

I. Definition: the degree of darkness or blackness on the film

II. Determined by the number of photons that have affected the film: the greater the number, the darker the film

III. Influenced by several factors, including
   A. Total number of x-rays that reach the film (mAs) (Figure 11-4)
      1. mAs is a quantity factor that controls the number of x-rays produced (beam intensity)
      2. If more x-rays are produced, the film will be darker
   B. Penetrating power of the x-rays (kVp)
      1. kVp is a quality factor that affects the energy of the x-rays
      2. At higher kVp settings, more x-rays with more energy are produced, there is a better penetration through the tissue, and as a result the film density increases
   C. Developing time and temperature
   D. Forms of beam attenuation such as filters or grids
   E. Tissue density and patient thickness (Figure 11-5)
      1. Tissue and film density are inversely proportional
      2. Presented in order of increasing film density (white to black) and decreasing tissue density (most dense to least): metal, bone, water (organs), fat, gas

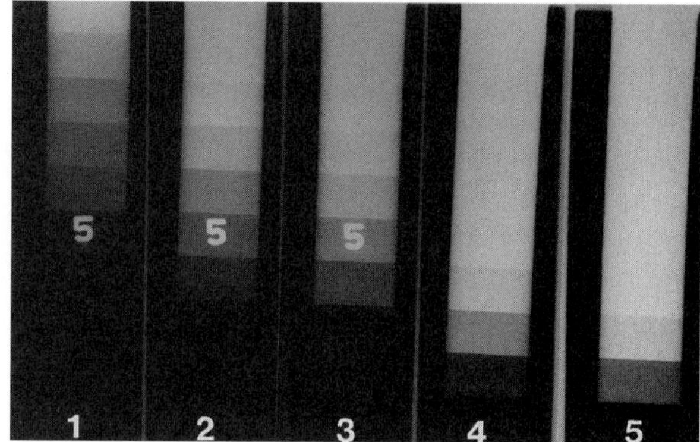

Figure 11-4 Image 1 displays more radiographic density than image 5. This means image 1 was exposed with a higher mA value. (From Han CM, Hurd CD: *Practical diagnostic imaging for the veterinary technician,* ed 2, St Louis, 2000, Mosby.)

Table 11-2 Technical errors that will or may cause change in film density if the factors are not compensated for

	Decreased film density (film too light)	Increased film density (film too dark)
Machine factors	Underexposure: too low kVp, mAs	Overexposure: too high kVp, mAs
	Drop in incoming line voltage	Surge in incoming line voltage
	Equipment malfunction	Equipment malfunction
Physical factors	Undermeasurement of anatomical part	Overmeasurement of anatomical part
	Increased subject density	Decreased subject density
	Source image distance (SID) too great	SID too short
	Grid used	No grid
	Positive contrast media used	Negative contrast media used
	Slow speed screen/film used	Fast speed screen/film
	No exposure	Double exposure
	Cassette not positioned in Bucky tray properly	
	Bucky tray not positioned directly under primary beam	
Processing factors	Underdevelopment	Overdevelopment
Wet tank	Developer time too short	Developer time too long
	Developer temperature too cold	Developer temperature too high
	Exhausted developer	Inaccurate thermometer
	Contaminated developer	Solutions too concentrated
	Diluted developer	Bromide missing from developer
	Developer improperly mixed	Defective thermometer
	Defective thermometer	Overreplenishment
Automatic processors	Underreplenishment	Developer temperature too high
	Developer temperature too low	Light leak from cover or in darkroom
	Exhausted developer	Rollers malfunctioning
	Developer improperly mixed	

F. Other physical factors are film and screen speed, use of contrast agents, and SID (formerly called focal film distance)

IV. Can be measured with a densitometer

Contrast

I. Definition: refers to the visible difference between two adjacent radiographic densities

II. See Table 11-3 for technical errors related to contrast

III. Can be divided into radiographic contrast and subject contrast

A. Radiographic contrast

1. Refers to the various shades of black, gray, and white on a radiographic film and the differences between them
2. High contrast film means a very black and white film with few grays
   a. Referred to as having a short latitude or scale of contrast
      (1) Fewer, but bigger steps
   b. Preferred for spine and extremity films
3. Long latitude or scale films have a larger number of shades of gray but little differences or contrast between them
   a. More but smaller steps
   b. Preferred for soft tissue
4. Kilovoltage has the greatest influence on radiographic contrast
   a. X-ray beam is polychromatic, which means that it contains a spectrum of energies (average energy is one half to one third the peak energy)
   b. At lower kVp there are more lower energy photons and a greater difference in energy levels
   c. As kVp increases, the difference between the energy levels lessen, allowing for greater penetration of the x-ray beam through the tissue
   d. The absorption of the x-ray beam by the various tissues at higher kVp is more uniform, resulting in lower radiographic contrast
5. Scatter radiation (non–image-forming radiation that is scattered in all directions resulting from objects in the path of the beam) adds a grayness to the film
   a. Inappropriate areas of the film are being exposed, thus decreasing contrast
6. Processing factors and other physical factors (beam attenuation, fogging, etc.) affect radiographic contrast

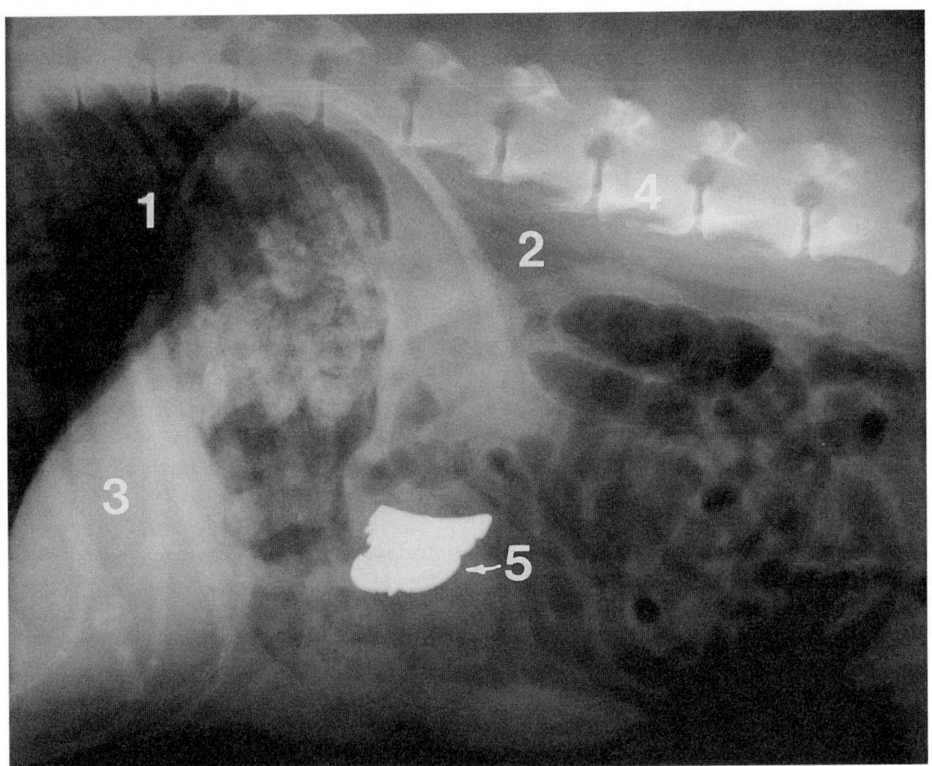

Figure 11-5 Subject densities: *1,* Air. *2,* Fat. *3,* Water. *4,* Bone. *5,* Metal. Air is least dense, allowing x-rays to penetrate and expose the film. Metal is the most dense, absorbing most of the x-rays and allowing only a few to penetrate, exposing the film. (From Han CM, Hurd CD: *Practical diagnostic imaging for the veterinary technician,* ed 2, St Louis, 2000, Mosby.)

Table 11-3 Technical factors affecting radiographic contrast

	Low contrast (film gray)
Machine factors	Overpenetration from too high kVp
Physical factors	Slower speed screens, film or those manufactured with lower levels Fog due to • Light leak such as safelight wattage or filter, while in cassette, or during loading or unloading • Scatter radiation if not using a grid for thick parts • Direct or scatter radiation: if left lying near machine during other exposures or if film bin exposed • Film stored in too hot or too humid place • Outdated film No grid used with high kVp exposure Beam not collimated Underfiltration Double exposure Negative contrast used Low subject contrast Excessive pressure on emulsions of unprocessed films
Processing factors Wet tank	Chemical fog • Prolonged development • Developer temperature too high • Solutions contaminated or exhausted • Fixed for too short of time or turning on light too soon • Luminous clocks and watch faces
Automatic processors	• Prolonged development • Developer temperature too high • Exhausted or contaminated solutions

Table 11-4 Common errors relating to lack of radiographic detail or definition (penumbra)

Machine factors	• Too large a focal spot used • Focal spot damaged
Physical factors	Motion unsharpness • Motion of patient, cassette, machine • Too slow time used
Geometric unsharpness	• Poor contact of intensifying screen and film • Increased object-film distance (OFD) • Decreased subject-image distance (SID) • Patient too thick • Rounded area of interest • Poor screen-film contact • Double exposure
Geometric distortion and magnification	• Patient/part not parallel to the film • Patient/part not perpendicular to the beam • Primary beam not centered over the area of interest • Area of interest not close to the film
Radiographic noise	• Film graininess (film speed too fast) • Structure mottle (intensifying screen speed too fast) • Quantum mottle (too few photons producing an image)

7. mAs does not affect contrast if sufficient quantity is used because an increase or decrease in mAs affects the number of x-rays evenly
   a. SID does not affect contrast either for the same reason

B. Subject contrast is defined as the difference in density and mass between two adjacent anatomic structures
   1. Subject contrast depends on the thickness and density of the anatomic part
   2. Subject contrast affects radiographic contrast
      a. High subject density means high tissue density
      b. The greater the subject density (e.g., bone), the greater the difference between the blacks and whites on the radiograph
      c. High subject contrast then increases radiographic contrast

Radiographic Detail or Definition (Table 11-4 and Figures 11-6 to 11-8)

I. Refers to definition of the edge of an anatomic structure

II. Image sharpness, clarity, distinctness, and perceptibility are synonymous

III. Lack of detail or penumbra may be due to many factors

TECHNICAL ERRORS AND ARTIFACTS

Several errors in handling x-ray film, manipulating exposure factors, or setting up a procedure could result. See Box 11-1 for artifacts and other errors.

DEVELOPING A TECHNIQUE CHART

A technique chart is a table with predetermined x-ray machine settings that enables one to select the correct machine settings based on the thickness of the tissue and the anatomical portion to be radiographed.

I. Each machine requires its own technique chart

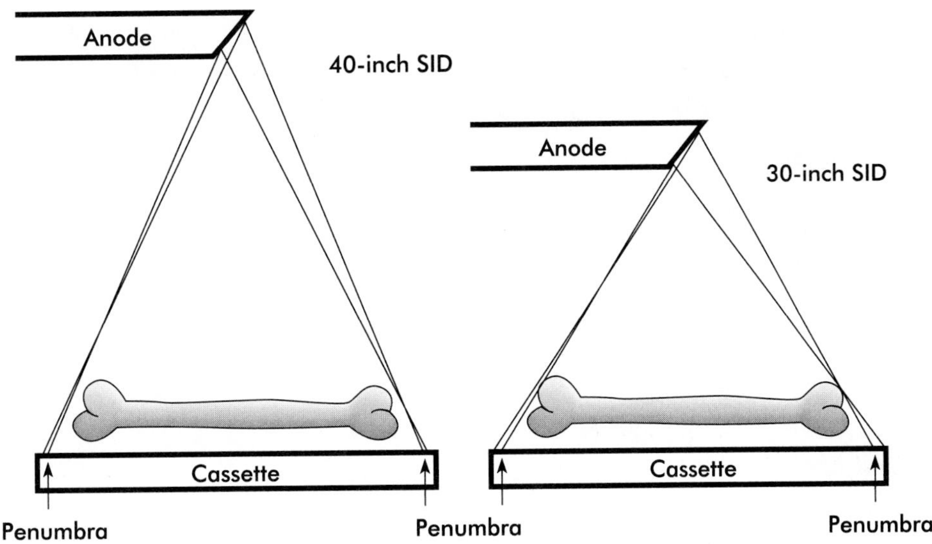

Figure 11-6 Increasing the source image distance (SID) decreases the amount of penumbra, increasing the radiographic detail. (From Pratt PW: *Principles and practice of veterinary technology,* St Louis, 1998, Mosby.)

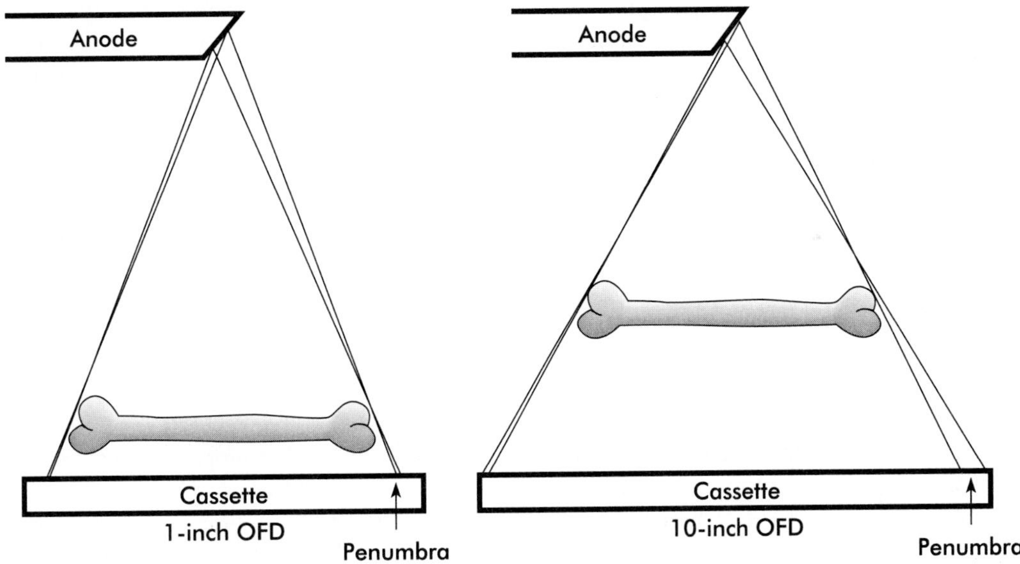

Figure 11-7 Increasing the object-film distance (OFD) increases the amount of penumbra, decreasing the radiographic detail. (From Pratt PW: *Principles and practice of veterinary technology,* St Louis, 1998, Mosby.)

II. Several charts may be needed (screen/nonscreen, grid/no grid, species specific, anatomy specific, various film/screen combinations)

III. Can use variable kVp chart, variable mAs chart, or a combination of both

IV. Whatever method is used, certain concepts should be kept in mind

   A. Standardize as many factors as possible (speed of screens, age of screens, speed of film, SID, beam filtration, temperature, age and time of processing, type of grid)

   B. Keep in mind that mAs is directly proportional to film density but it does not appreciably alter film contrast if the density is correct

   C. Kilovoltage is directly proportional to film density and inversely proportional to film contrast; low kVp means a high scale of contrast

   D. SID squared is inversely proportional to film distance

      1. Change in SID means a change in film density
      2. SID does not alter film contrast if film density is correct

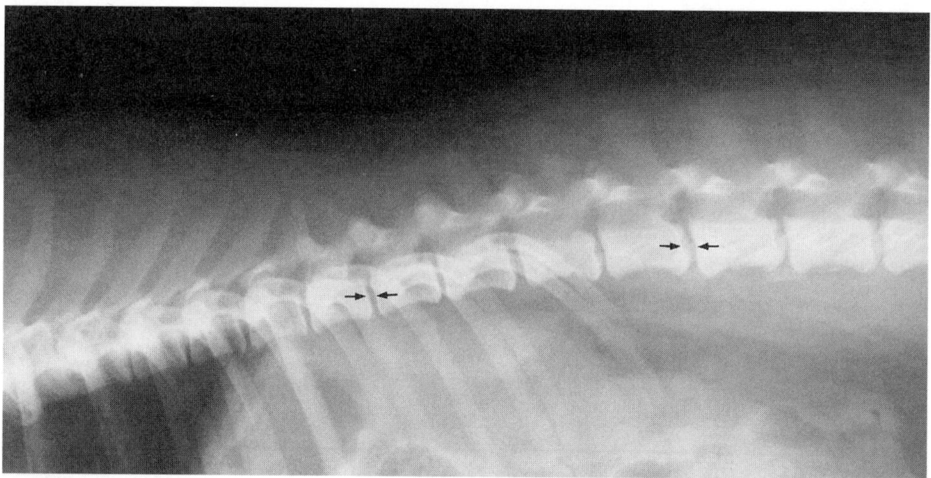

Figure 11-8 The intervertebral spaces appear narrow toward the edges of the radiograph *(arrows)* compared with the spaces in the center of the radiograph. (From Han CM, Hurd CD: *Practical diagnostic imaging for the veterinary technician,* ed 2, St Louis, 2000, Mosby.)

3. Also referred to as focal-film distance (FFD)

E. Change in thickness requires a change in kVp setting. For each additional thickness in patient centimeter, add
   1. 2 kVp if less than 80 kVp
   2. 3 kVp if 80 to 100 kVp
   3. 4 kVp if more than 100 kVp
F. A general relationship exists between mAs and kVp
   1. If film density is too dark, to correct the error
      a. Halve mAs setting or subtract 10 kVp (in range of 70 to 90)[1]
      b. Decrease mAs 30% to 50% or kVp 10% to 15%[2]
   2. If film density is too light, to correct error
      a. Double mAs setting or add 10 kVp (in range of 70 to 90 kVp)[1]
      b. Increase mAs 30% to 50% or kVp 10% to 15%[2]
G. Exposure factors must also be increased for conditions such as
   1. Pleural fluid/cardiomegaly
   2. Ascites
   3. Obesity
   4. Plaster cast
   5. Special positive radiographic procedures
H. To determine if kVp or mAs should be changed
   1. If film is too dark but contrast has not significantly been altered (i.e., soft tissue is dark but bones are relatively white), mAs should be decreased
   2. If film is too dark and bones are gray, then the problem is overpenetration or too much kVp
   3. If film is too light and anatomical parts, especially in cranial abdomen, are not clearly visible, an increase in penetration or kVp will improve density and contrast
   4. If film is too light and anatomical parts, especially in cranial abdomen, are clearly visible, an increase in mAs will improve density

RADIATION SAFETY

The major objective of a veterinary practice that uses ionizing radiation should be to obtain the maximum amount of information with the minimal exposure to all concerned. "Radiation should be respected, not feared."[2]

Responsibilities

I. It is the practice owner's responsibility to
   A. Ensure that proper radiation safety measures are observed
   B. Meet state or provincial requirements: dosimetry devices, proper protection devices, registration, room design, etc.
      1. Usually regulated by the department of health
   C. Instruct personnel in proper radiation safety and use

Hazards of Ionizing Radiation

I. All tissues are sensitive to ionizing radiation
   A. Ionizing radiation refers to the excitation of orbital electrons in an atom so that the atoms are separated into charged particles
      1. Molecules may break or alter
      2. Charged molecules may function improperly or not at all
   B. Interaction between x-rays and tissues occurs at the atomic level, but it is theorized that visible injury results from molecular derangements of macromolecules and water

Table 11-5 Maximum permissible dose: Whole body dose for occupationally exposed over 18 years of age*

Time period	MPD	Dose
Weekly	0.001 Sv	(0.1 rem)
Quarterly	0.03 Sv	(3 rem)
Calendar year	0.05 Sv	(5 rem)
Accumulated over lifetime	0.05 (age − 18) Sv	(5[age − 18]rem)

*ICRP 1986. Some states and provinces have adopted the 1991 schedule which gives 0.02 Sv (2 rem) as MPD.
Age for calculation in years.

C. Injury to cells, tissues, and organs occurs at the time of exposure but may require hours, days, or generations to show damage

II. Types of cellular damage in the body
   A. Genetic damage occurs to DNA (genes) of reproductive cells
      1. Manifestation not detectable until future generations
   B. Somatic cell damage occurs in all other cells and becomes evident at some point in the individual's life, although it may never become obvious due to tissue repair
   C. Nucleus of proliferating somatic and genetic cells is considered to be the area of the cell most sensitive to the ionizing effects
   D. Greater sensitivity occurs with
      1. Younger tissues and organs
      2. Higher metabolic activity
      3. Greater proliferation rate of cells and growth rate of tissues
   E. Organ tissues considered critical because of their sensitivity are dermis, thyroid, eye, lymphatics, blood-forming tissues, bone, and germinal epithelium or gonads

Radiation Measurement

I. Absorbed dose is the unit of ionizing radiation that measures the energy transferred by this radiation to a body part
   A. SI unit is Grey (Gy) = 100 rads
II. Dose equivalent makes allowances for the fact that ionizing radiation affects all tissues differently
   A. SI unit is Sievert (Sv)
   B. Previous unit was rem (1 Sv = 100 rem)

Maximum Permissible Dose

I. See Table 11-5 for specific maximum permissible dose (MPD)
II. Definition: maximum dose of radiation that a person may receive in a given period
III. Set by the National Committee on Radiation Protection and Measurement (NCRP) under the recommendations of ICRP (International Commission on Radiological Protection)
IV. NCRP and most provincial and state regulations allow occupationally exposed persons to restrain and position animals when absolutely necessary, but other states or provinces prohibit any manual restraint
V. Various dosimeters or personal exposure monitoring devices are available, but these and MPD are meaningless unless
   A. Each individual involved in taking radiographs properly wears the dosimeter every time he or she takes radiographs
   B. Dosimeters are routinely sent to a federally approved laboratory for evaluation
VI. For more information contact the radiation protection service of the department of health of your state or province

Safety Practices

I. Exposure and damage to tissue can occur from
   A. Primary beam: never allow any part of the body to be in the primary beam even if properly protected
      1. Primary beam will penetrate lead aprons and gloves
   B. Secondary or scatter radiation that is produced when the primary beam interacts with objects in its path
      1. Amount and direction of scatter depend on kVp level, volume of tissue irradiated, field size, and composition of tissue
   C. X-ray machine leakage
II. Important safety practices
   A. Never permit anyone younger than 18 years or pregnant women in the room during exposure
   B. Remove unnecessary personnel and rotate personnel during procedures
   C. Use nonmanual restraint such as chemical restraint, sandbags, sponges, tape, and restraining devices whenever possible. A little patience and creativity will go a long way
   D. Always wear protective gloves, thyroid protector, and aprons
      1. Minimum 0.5-mm lead equivalent
      2. Routinely inspect and radiograph for any damage
   E. Never permit any part of the body, even if it is shielded, to be in the primary beam
      1. Even if shielded, you could still receive 25% of the primary beam
   F. Consider use of protective goggles (0.25-mm lead equivalent) and larger shielding devices
   G. Collimate so there is at least an unexposed border on each film, proving that the primary beam is limited and scatter radiation reduced

H. Wear dosimeter outside of apron near the collar
I. Never hand hold an x-ray machine
J. Do not direct the x-ray beam at any individual or occupied adjacent room
K. Use 2.5-mm aluminum filter to remove the lower energy portion of the x-ray beam
L. Have the machine calibrated and checked regularly
M. Use fastest film-screen systems compatible with obtaining diagnostic radiographs
N. Plan each procedure carefully to avoid retakes
O. Keep an exposure log identifying the patient, study, and exposures
P. Follow state and provincial radiation safety codes

III. Remember the big three methods of radiation safety
  A. Time: avoid retakes, do it correctly the first time
  B. Distance: keep as far as possible from patient and x-ray beam
  C. Shielding: always wear protective apparel

IV. NCRP developed a program known as ALARA
  A. This stands for "as low as reasonably achievable"
  B. Always aim to keep this policy in mind when restraining animals and taking radiographs

POSITIONING TECHNIQUES

Proper positioning is essential to obtain diagnostic radiographic examinations. Refer to texts that thoroughly explain specific procedures for various species.

Basic Principles

I. Common terms and abbreviations used (based on American Committee of Veterinary Radiologists and Anatomists) (Figure 11-9)
  A. Left (Le), right (Rt)
  B. Medial (M), lateral (L)
    1. In reference to limbs
  C. Cranial (Cr)
    1. Toward head
    2. Also for limbs proximal to carpus/tarsus
  D. Cd (caudal), toward tail
    1. Also for limbs proximal to carpus/tarsus
  E. Dorsal (D)
    1. Toward back
    2. Also cranial portion of limb distal to carpus/tarsus
  F. Ventral (V)
    1. Toward abdomen
  G. Palmar (Pa)
    1. Caudal portion of pectoral limb from carpus distally
  H. Plantar (P1)
    1. Caudal portion of pelvic limb from tarsus distally
  I. Oblique (O)
    1. Less than 90° to axis
    2. Could be in a medial or lateral direction
  J. Rostral (R)
    1. Used for head: toward the nares

II. Beam direction
  A. Lateral: side closest to the film is marked (i.e., side it is lying on)
    1. For example: Rt L = lying on right side
  B. Abbreviated term indicates direction of beam: first letter is where the x-rays enter the body, second letter is where x-rays leave the body (part that lies against the film)
    1. For example: VD (ventrodorsal): the x-rays enter the ventral aspect of the animal while the film is against the dorsal aspect

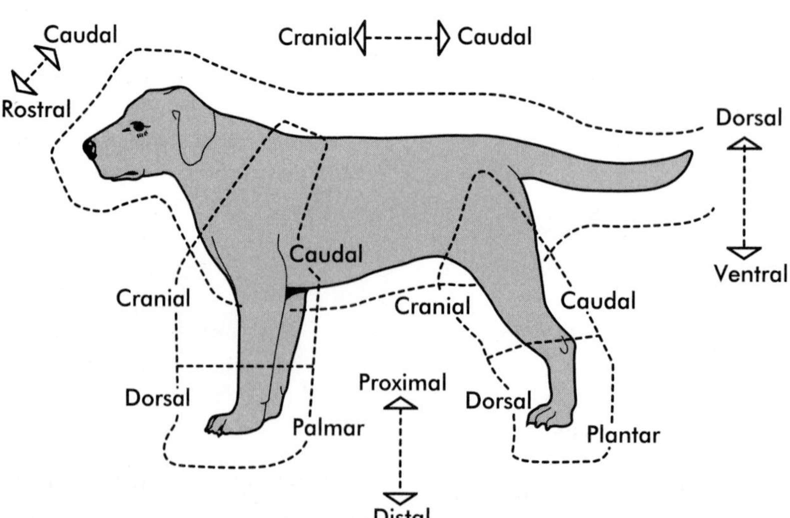

Figure 11-9 Veterinary anatomic terminology. (From Han CM, Hurd CD: *Practical diagnostic imaging for the veterinary technician,* ed 2, St Louis, 2000, Mosby.)

2. The animal would be lying in dorsal recumbency or on its back
C. Oblique views are usually in reference to limbs
1. The first two letters indicate where the beam enters the body, the next two letters indicate where it exits (the body part that is specifically against the film)
2. First letter in each pair describes cranial or caudal; second letter of each pair describes the side of the limb
3. For example: dorsomedial-palmarolateral oblique (DMPaLO) of the carpus
a. Carpus is rotated (O) so that the x-ray beam is aimed at the cranial part of the limb (D) toward the medial side (M). This faces the x-ray tube
b. This means that the beam exits from the caudal portion of the limb (Pa) so that the opposite side (L) faces or is against the film

Basic Criteria and Principles of Positioning and Restraint

I. Keep comfort and welfare of patient in mind
A. Be prepared before patient positioning
B. Use steady, slow, gentle movements
C. Use minimum restraint through chemical and/or mechanical assistance
II. Minimize exposure to radiation of assistants by using nonmanual restraint whenever possible
A. When using positioning aids, minimize placing radiopaque devices over the area of interest
B. Position devices so that the animal has the illusion it is being held
1. Strategic locations are usually head, shoulders, pelvis, and limbs
2. Be creative and patient
3. Stay with the animal until the rotor is depressed and move away quickly
a. Time is sufficient for most positions, especially laterals
III. Measure the area of interest in centimeters with calipers
IV. Have two views at right angles
A. Exceptions are thoracic views, contrast studies, and equine radiography, which often require more views
B. Injury may also only allow one view
V. Have the area of interest as close to the film as possible
VI. Center the beam to area of interest and include specific anatomy for each anatomic area
VII. Keep the area of interest parallel to the film and perpendicular to the x-ray beam
A. Bisecting angle technique is used in dental radiography (see Chapter 26)
VIII. Collimate using the smallest field size possible to accommodate essential anatomy
IX. When taking radiographs of extremities, include the proximal and distal joints of the long bone being radiographed
A. If radiographing a joint, include at least one third of the long bones distal and proximal to that joint
X. Make sure patient is adequately prepared
XI. Plan your procedure carefully to avoid retakes

CONTRAST RADIOGRAPHY

Basic Concepts

I. Used to enhance the visualization of individual organs and structures that are not adequately visible on the survey radiographs
II. Contrast means density difference

Media

I. Two classes of contrast media
A. Positive contrast (radiopaque) such as barium and iodine
1. Absorb more x-rays than bone so appear even whiter on a radiograph
2. May be classified as
a. Insoluble: barium, which is used mainly for gastrointestinal studies. Never give barium parenterally
b. Soluble: all other positive contrast media; contains iodine that can be used for renal, articular, vascular, myelographic, and gastrointestinal studies
c. Soluble iodinated contrast agents are hyperosmotic and, although rare, may cause toxic reactions
B. Negative contrast (radiolucent) such as air and carbon dioxide
1. No x-rays are absorbed so the medium appears black on the radiograph
C. Double contrast studies incorporate positive and negative contrast media

Patient Preparation

I. Depending on the procedure, the patient may have to
A. Have food withheld 12 to 24 hours
B. Be given an enema or a cathartic 4 to 12 hours before the procedure
II. Have a survey radiograph completed before the procedure

Positioning and Specific Studies

Please refer to the excellent references available for actual positioning as well as further information on special studies.

Glossary

absorbed dose Amount of energy that tissue receives when it is bombarded by ionizing radiation, measured as Grey (Gy) or rads

actual focal spot Area of the focal spot when viewed from 90 degrees to the target

amperage Term used to describe the flow of electrons through a current

anode Positive electrode in the x-ray tube that contains the target

artifact That which decreases the diagnostic quality of a radiograph

binding energy Energy that must be surpassed before an electron can be removed from its orbit

calipers Measuring device to determine patient thickness

cathode Negative electrode in the x-ray tube that supplies the electrons

caudocranial (CdCr) Directional term indicating that the x-ray beam enters from toward the tail and exits toward the head. Opposite is CrCd. Usually in reference to limbs, proximal to the carpal and tarsal joints

detail Part of film quality indicating clear resolution and definition of the shadows on the radiographic image

distal Farther away from the point of origin; opposite is proximal

dorsopalmar (DPa) Directional term that refers to limbs distal to and including the carpus. The beam enters from the front of the limb and exits at the back of the limb; opposite is PaD

dorsoplantar (DPl) Directional term that refers to limbs distal to and including the tarsus (see above)

dorsoventral (DV) Directional term that indicates that the x-ray beam enters from the back of the animal and exits out its abdomen. The animal would be lying in ventral recumbency (on its abdomen); opposite is VD

dosimeter Device used to measure the radiation exposure that personnel receive

effective focal spot Area of the focal spot as seen through the x-ray tube window and directed on the film

electromagnetic radiation Propagation of ionizing energy through space in the form of photons

electron Negatively charged particle of the atom that circles around the nucleus

electron beam Beam of electrons that is accelerated from the cathode to the anode by a high electrical potential in the x-ray tube

filament Coiled wire of the cathode that emits the electron beam

film contrast Characteristic of the film that influences radiographic contrast. Often film contrast and latitude are inversely related

film graininess Loss of detail caused by the size of the individual silver halide crystals; usually more pronounced in faster speed film; also referred to as radiographic mottle

film latitude Exposure range that will produce acceptable density on the film

focal range Distance from the grid to the x-ray tube that will minimize grid cutoff

fogging Overall grayness that does not contribute to the diagnostic quality of the film; may be caused from chemicals as well as undesirable radiation

geometric unsharpness Loss of detail due to geometric distortion also referred to as penumbra

grid cutoff When a grid is not used correctly and the primary beam is absorbed more than normal

grid ratio Ratio of the height of the lead strips as compared to the space between them ($r = h/d$)

heel effect Due to the angle of the target, a greater intensity of x-rays is emitted from the cathode side, rather than from the anode side

ionization Process of transferring sufficient energy to an atom so that the outer electron is removed; the atom is positively charged

kilovoltage peak (kVp) Maximum energy of the x-ray beam that determines the quality or penetrating power of the beam

latent image Invisible image produced on the x-ray film after exposure and before processing

maximum permissible dose (MPD) Maximum amount of radiation that an individual is allowed over a given time period

milliampere-seconds (mAs) Amount of current flowing through the tube times the exposure time in seconds; 1 milliampere = 1/1000 ampere

object film distance Space between the film and the part being radiographed

penumbra Loss of detail due to geometric unsharpness

photon Bundle of radiation energy, also known as quanta

polychromatic beam X-ray beam that has a broad spectrum of energies; depends on the kVp: the lower the kVp, the more polychromatic the beam

quality Term referring to the average energy of the x-ray beam or its penetrating ability (kVp)

quantity Term that refers to the total number of x-ray photons (controlled by mA)

quantum mottle Loss of radiographic detail that occurs in faster screens because of the uneven distribution of the phosphor crystals within the screen

radiodense or radiopaque Object or tissue that absorbs radiation so that the image on the film is lighter

radiographic contrast Variation in degree of darkness between two adjacent areas on the film

radiographic density Degree of darkness found on the radiograph

radiographic quality How well the shadows on the radiograph are clearly identified

radiography Making of radiographs

radiology Use of radiant energy in the diagnosis and treatment of disease

radiolucent Tissue or device that allows most of the x-ray beams to pass through unaffected

rectification Process of changing alternating current to current flowing in one direction only (direct current)

remnant beam Primary radiation emitted from the x-ray tube

scatter radiation or secondary radiation Caused by interaction of the primary beam with tissue or matter in its path

source image distance (SID) Formerly called focal-film distance, it is the distance from the focal spot or source of the x-rays to the image receptor or film

speed Exposure required to produce a diagnostic film density

structure mottle Loss of radiographic detail that occurs because of phosphor variations found in intensifying screens; more noticeable with fast-speed screens

subject contrast Contrast resulting from the difference in density, mass, and atomic number of adjacent tissue structures

thermionic emission Heating of the filament so that the energy produced forces the electrons to be released from their atomic orbits

thermoluminescent dosimeter Form of personnel monitor device that indicates dosage to radiation exposure

x-ray SA short-wavelength, high-energy form of electromagnetic radiation

Review Questions

1 What is the usual maximum permissible dose (MPD) or radiation that the whole body is allowed in 1 year?
 a. 5 SV (5.00 mRem)
 b. 0.05 (N-18) SV [5(N-18) rem]
 c. 0.05 SV (5 rem)
 d. 0.03 SV (3 rem)

2 Which factor does not appreciably affect contrast?
 a. kVp
 b. mAs
 c. Film speed
 d. Processing

3 For a diagnostic radiograph, what will a "high plus" speed film need in comparison to a par speed film?
 a. Use of a grid
 b. Longer processing time
 c. More mAs or kVp
 d. Less mAs or kVp

4 The main purpose of the developer is to
 a. Remove unexposed, undeveloped silver halide crystals
 b. Reduce exposed silver halide crystals to black metallic silver
 c. Change the calcium tungstate crystals to black calcium
 d. Create a latent image

5 Density is decreased on a film by
 a. Increasing the kVp
 b. Decreasing the tissue density
 c. Decreasing the mAs
 d. Increasing the processing chemical temperatures

6 A higher grid ratio means that
 a. The lead plate is thicker
 b. Less scatter radiation is absorbed
 c. More scatter radiation is absorbed
 d. Less primary radiation is absorbed

7 X-rays
 a. Are a type of electromagnetic radiation
 b. Have less energy than radio waves
 c. Have longer wavelengths than radio waves
 d. Are measured in meters

8 There will be more scattered radiation noticed on the film with
 a. Use of a grid
 b. Increased kVp
 c. Decreased kVp
 d. Decreased patient thickness

9 A radiograph using 70 kVp and 10 mAs is too dark. Which technique would be most reasonable for the repeat?
 a. 80 kVp and 5 mAs
 b. 85 kVp and 10 mAs
 c. 60 kVp and 20 mAs
 d. 70 kVp and 5 mAs

10 If an animal had its right side against the film, this view is known as a
 a. Right lateral
 b. Side view
 c. Ventrodorsal
 d. Left lateral

REFERENCES

1. Morgan JP: *Techniques of veterinary radiography,* ed 5, Ames, 1993, Iowa State University Press.
2. Lavin L: *Radiography in veterinary technology,* ed 2, Philadelphia, 1999, WB Saunders.

BIBLIOGRAPHY

Curry TS, Dowdy JE, Murray RC: *Christensen's physics of diagnostic radiology,* ed 4, Philadelphia, 1990, Lea & Febiger.

Darby ML, editor: *Mosby's comprehensive review of dental hygiene,* ed 3, St Louis, 2002, Mosby.

Eastman Kodak Company: *The fundamentals of radiography,* ed 12, Rochester, NY, 1980, Eastman Kodak Company, Radiographic Markets Division.

Han C, Hurd C: *Practical diagnostic imaging for the veterinary technician,* St Louis, 2000, Mosby.

Kleine LJ, Warren *RG: Small animal radiography,* St Louis, 1982, Mosby.

McCurnin D: *Clinical textbook for veterinary technicians,* ed 5, Philadelphia, 2002, WB Saunders.

NCRP: *Radiation protection in veterinary medicine,* #36, Bethesda, MD, 1970, NCRP.

NCRP: *Structural shielding design and evaluation or medical use of x-rays and gamma rays of energies up to 10 meV,* #49, Bethesda, MD, 1976, NCRP.

Owens JM: *Radiographic interpretation for the small animal clinician,* St Louis, 1998, Ralston Purina Company.

Rendano VT et al: Radiation safety-transparent leaded-plastic panels: a product evaluation, *J Am Anim Hosp Assoc* 23:141, 1987.

Rendano VT, Ryan G: Technician assistance in radiology, Part II. Basic consideration and radiation safety, *Comp Contin Educ* 9:547, 1988.

Ryan GD: *Radiographic positioning of small animals,* Philadelphia, 1981, Lea & Febiger.

Smallwood JE et al: A standardized nomenclature for radiographic projections used in veterinary medicine, *Vet Radiol J* 26:2, 1985.

CHAPTER 12

Ultrasonography

Pierry McLean

OUTLINE

LEARNING OUTCOMES

After reading this chapter you should be able to:

1. Have a better understanding of the basic physics of ultrasound.
2. Be familiar with the basic functioning of the ultrasound machine.
3. Understand the concepts of image physics.
4. Have an understanding of the concepts of the final image and artifacts.
5. Differentiate between the sonographic appearance of anatomical features and artifacts.
6. Properly prepare a patient for routine ultrasonography.
7. Explain the equipment controls responsible for the images.

Ultrasound is a diagnostic modality used to image various organs in the living body. By noninvasive means, the veterinary technologist may use ultrasound to determine and compare the location, size, and echogenicity of certain structures. Imaging can be done easily to most animals without tranquilization, so even the most critically ill patient can tolerate the examination. It is important to understand the basic fundamentals of physics concerning ultrasound. Without this knowledge, it would be difficult to understand the applications and limitations of ultrasound. In this chapter, the ultrasound machine, organ characteristics, artifacts, and patient preparation are discussed.

BASIC PHYSICS OF ULTRASOUND

Definition: waves of sound that are of a frequency beyond the range of human hearing.

Image Production

I. Waves travel through media, transferring energy from one location to another

II. Sound waves are reflected back to the transducer, analyzed by a computer, and displayed on a screen

Sound Waves (Figure 12-1)

I. Wavelength (λ)
   A. Definition: the distance that a wave must travel in one cycle
   B. Ultrasound has a shorter wavelength than that of audible sound
   C. Wavelength is determined by the characteristics of the transducer

II. Frequency (f)
   A. Definition: the number of cycles per unit of time (seconds)
   B. As frequency increases, the wavelength decreases
   C. Ultrasound waves are in the 2- to 10-MHz range compared with human hearing, which is around 20,000 Hz

III. Velocity (v)
   A. Definition: the speed at which sound travels through an object = frequency × wavelength
   B. When the sound wave returns, the computer records the time
   C. The computer will use the time taken for the echo to return to calculate the depth at which the sound was reflected

IV. Amplitude: intensity or loudness of a wave

V. Period (T): time needed to produce one cycle

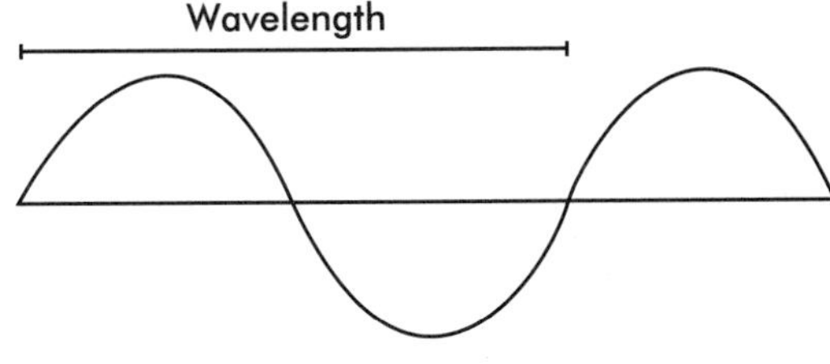

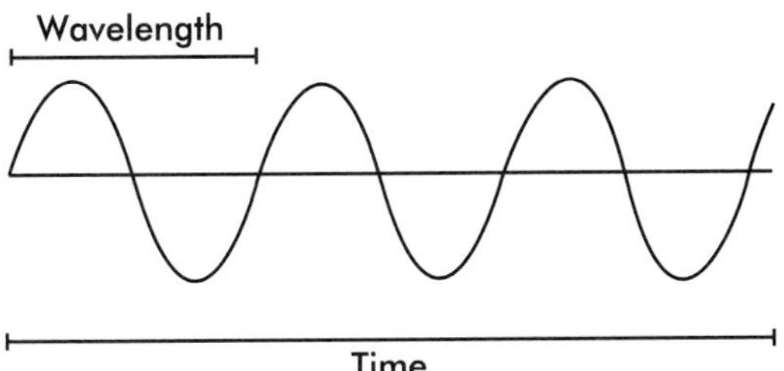

Figure 12-1 Frequency and wavelength are inversely related. As the wavelength increases, the frequency decreases. (From Han CM, Hurd CD: *Practical diagnostic imaging for the veterinary technician,* St Louis, 2000, Mosby.)

Attenuation

I. Definition: the loss of intensity of the ultrasound beam as it travels through tissue due to
   A. Absorption: production of heat as sound passes through soft tissue, causing loss of energy
   B. Scattering: sound is reflected in different directions from dissimilar tissue interfaces
   C. Reflection: the return of a part of the ultrasound beam toward the transducer

Acoustic Impedance

I. Definition: the ability of tissue to resist or allow the transmission of sound

II. Impedance depends on the density of certain tissue

III. Air and bone have high acoustic impedance, hindering the passage of the ultrasound wave, whereas tissue, with low acoustic impedance, is favorable

ULTRASOUND MACHINE

Transducers

I. Definition: the part of the ultrasound machine used to scan a patient
   A. Devices that convert one form of energy to another
   B. They send out a series of sound pulses and collect the returning echoes

II. Pulsed-wave transducers
   A. A short burst of sound is emitted from this transducer. It waits until the echo comes back before sending another one
   B. Most common
   C. One transducer alternately transmits and receives

III. Continuous-wave
   A. Contains two transducers: one transducer constantly sends sound waves while the other one "listens"

Transducer Crystals

I. Definition: the active element required to promote the conversion of electrical energy to ultrasound
   A. Natural crystals: quartz, tourmaline, rochelle salt
   B. Synthetics: most common; lead zirconate titonate, barium titanate, and lithium sulfate
   C. The crystal produces sound by vibrations through the piezoelectric effect
   D. After pulses are sent, the crystals are dampened to stop vibrations
   E. Struck by the echoes returning, they start to vibrate again
   F. Crystals convert echoes into electrical energy

Piezoelectric Effect

I. Definition: the conversion of electrical energy to pressure energy (ultrasound or acoustic)
II. Piezoelectric means pressure electricity

Bandwidth

I. Definition: the entire range of frequency
II. A transducer can produce more than one frequency above or below its center frequency

Types of Transducers

I. Mechanical sector
   A. Consists of one or more crystals mechanically steered to produce a "pie-shaped" image
II. Linear array
   A. Consists of a small row of crystals sequentially pulsed
   B. Produces parallel lines and allows the image to be rectangular
   C. Ideal for transrectals and equine tendons
III. Phased array sector scanner
   A. Contains about 20 crystals, which are electronically steered through a sector
   B. Commonly used in echocardiography
   C. Usually small and expensive
IV. Broad bandwidth transducer
   A. New type of transducer
      1. An advantage is that it is lighter weight with lower acoustic impedance
         a. More efficient transmission of sound waves through tissue
   B. The transducer element consists of piezoelectric ceramic and epoxy type of material
   C. These transducers have wide frequency bandwidths, therefore can operate at different frequencies or emit pulses of short duration

Equipment Controls

The ultrasound machine has many controls for adjusting the image. Improper use may decrease quality of the image and possibly produce lesions that in fact do not exist.

Brightness and Contrast

I. Display monitor controls should be adjusted so that black, white, and all different shades of gray can be seen

Gain and Power

I. Affects brightness of the image
II. The higher the overall gain or power, the brighter the image
III. Increasing the power increases the intensity of the sound leaving the transducer and the waves returning to it, because gain amplifies the returning echoes

Time-Gain Compensation

I. Time-gain compensation (TGC) adds increasing amounts of electronic gain to the more distant echoes
II. It enables the returning echoes from different depths to have the same brightness on the monitor
III. TGC consists of near-field, far-field, gain, and delay controls

IMAGE PHYSICS

Resolution

I. Definition: the ability to separately identify small structures on the ultrasound image
   A. The frequency of the transducer dictates the resolution of the image
   B. The higher the frequency (i.e., 7.5 MHz), the shorter the wavelength and thus the better the resolution
II. Lateral resolution
   A. The ability of the ultrasound beam to separate two structures lying perpendicular to the beam; depends on the beam diameter (width)
   B. The distance between two interfaces must be greater than the beam width for each interface to be identified separately
III. Axial resolution
   A. Depends on the wavelength of the sound frequency used
   B. Ability of the ultrasound beam to separate two structures lying along the path of the beam
   C. By using the narrowest beam width possible, one can achieve the best resolution

Sound Beam Zones

The dimensions and design of the transducer determine sound beam zones.

I. Near field
   A. The portion of the sound beam where the beam width narrows as the distance increases until it reaches the narrowest portion
   B. The area of the beam closest to the crystal
II. Focal point
   A. Where the beam reaches its narrowest point
III. Far field
   A. The area of the beam in which the boundaries diverge

Focusing

I. Definition: the method of moving the focal point closer to the image, to narrow the width and improve resolution

II. Transducers are focused by shaping the crystal, addition of a lens, or combining both concepts

THE DISPLAY

Display Format

I. Definition: how the returning echo, or the image, appears on the screen
  A. Can be rectangular or sector
II. A-mode (amplitude mode) (Figure 12-2)
  A. One-dimensional graphic display
  B. Returning echoes are viewed as a series of peaks on a graph
  C. The greater the intensity, the higher the peak
III. B-mode (brightness mode) (see Figure 12-2)
  A. Depicts dots on a screen as a two-dimensional image
  B. Brightness of the dot depends on the intensity of the returning echo
  C. The position of the dot on the baseline depends on the depth of the reflecting structure
IV. M-mode (motion mode) (Figure 12-3)
  A. A two-dimensional display of a reflector over time
  B. The position of a reflector is displayed on the vertical axis, and time is displayed on the horizontal axis
  C. Stationary objects result in straight lines while moving ones will be wavy
  D. Mainly used in cardiology to assess cardiac valves, walls, and chamber size

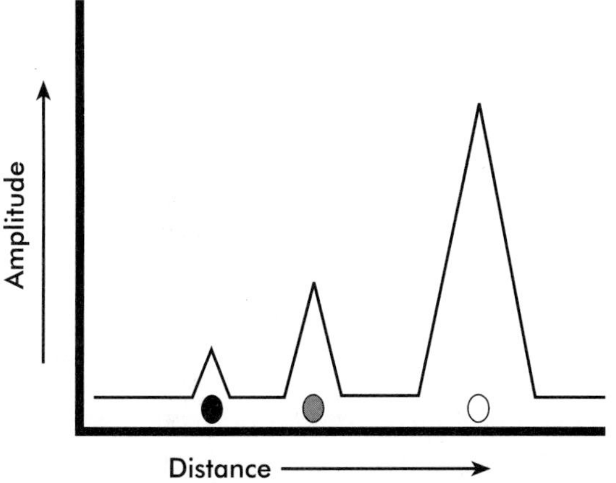

Figure 12-2 Where A-mode uses peaks on a graph to depict the strength of the returning echoes, B-mode uses bright pixels, or dots, on a monitor. The brighter the pixel, the stronger the returning echo. (From Han CM, Hurd CD: *Practical diagnostic imaging for the veterinary technician,* St Louis, 2000, Mosby.)

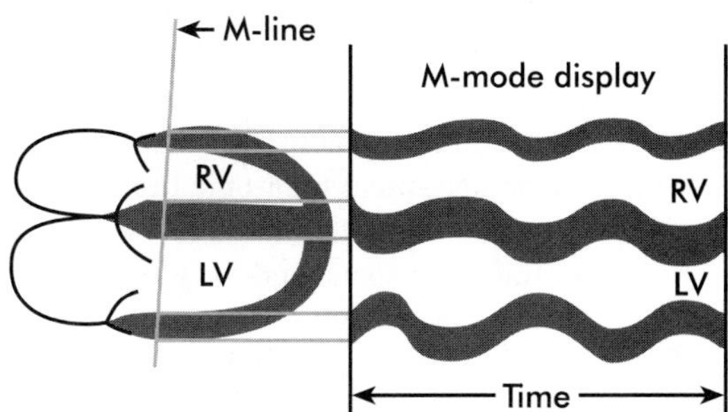

Figure 12-3 M-mode displays the motion of a thin slice of an organ over time. *RV,* Right ventricle; *LV,* left ventricle. (From Han CM, Hurd CD: *Practical diagnostic imaging for the veterinary technician,* St Louis, 2000, Mosby.)

FINAL IMAGE

Image Characteristics (Figure 12-4)

The format used for ultrasound display is a black background on which echo information appears in white. Size, shape, and margins of the organs should be known so that any deviation from the normal can be documented.

I. Echogenic (echoic)
  A. Tissue that produces sufficient echoes to return to the transducer to be displayed
  B. Appears white on the screen
  C. The greater the difference between two adjacent organs, the greater the echo reflection between them
II. Sonolucent
  A. Majority of the sound is penetrating deeper into the tissue, with only a few echoes being reflected back
III. Anechoic
  A. Describes tissue that transmits all the sound to deeper tissue
  B. Appears black on the screen and is usually fluid filled
IV. Hyperechoic

Hyperechoic

Hypoechoic

Isoechoic

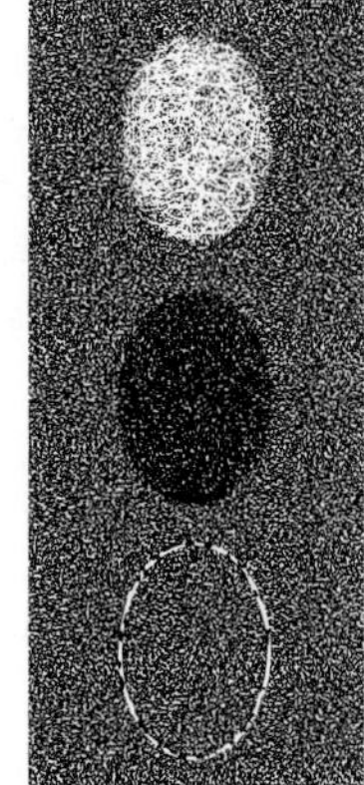

Figure 12-4 An area within an organ or the whole organ that is brighter or whiter than surrounding tissue is described as hyperechoic. Areas that are darker than surrounding tissue are described as hypoechoic. Areas that are the same as surrounding tissue are described as isoechoic. (From Han CM, Hurd CD: *Practical diagnostic imaging for the veterinary technician,* St Louis, 2000, Mosby.)

A. Appears brighter than surrounding tissue and thus more echogenic
B. Tissue that reflects more sound back to the transducer than the area around it

V. Hypoechoic
A. Area appears darker than surrounding tissue
B. Reflects less sound back than the area of tissue around it

VI. Isoechoic
A. Tissue equal in appearance to that of surrounding tissue

Organ Appearance

I. Contour
A. Is the organ outline smooth, rough, or irregular?

II. Texture
A. Is the organ parenchyma homogeneous?

III. Shape
A. Does the organ have its proper shape?

IV. Size
A. Specific organs should be measured to determine whether they are within normal parameters

Scanning Planes

The animal should be scanned laterally or in dorsal recumbency and the organs should be scanned in two planes.

I. Sagittal (longitudinal) or long axis
A. Transducer marker should be constantly held to the cranial or caudal end of the animal

II. Transverse (short axis)
A. Transducer marker should be 90 degrees to the longitudinal plane

ARTIFACTS

Definition: refers to something seen on an ultrasound image that anatomically does not exist.

I. Artifacts occur during imaging
II. Some are a direct benefit; others are not
III. It is important to distinguish between artifacts and real structures

Propagation Artifacts

I. Reverberations
A. Appear as many linear echoes
B. Occur when sound is reflected constantly between a strong reflector (i.e., bone or air and the transducer surface)

II. Refraction
A. Occurs when the sound beam changes direction as it passes from one medium to another
B. Allows the organ to appear in different positions

III. Mirror image
A. Appears when an organ lies next to a reflector on the image; the organ appears to be present on both sides of the reflector
B. Often occurs in the region of the diaphragm and liver

Attenuation Artifacts

I. Acoustic shadowing
A. Occurs when sound is totally reflected or absorbed by an object
B. Prevents sound from traveling to a greater depth
C. Calculi, bowel gas, etc. can cause this posterior shadowing

II. Enhancement
A. Echoes beside a fluid-filled structure will not be as strong as the ones behind it
B. Enhancement occurs because sound transmitted through fluid is less attenuated than the tissue beside it
C. This artifact can determine if the lesion is a hypoechoic mass or a cyst

Other Artifacts

I. Ring down
A. Similar to reverberation
B. Produces many parallel echoes
C. Associated with gas bubbles

II. Comet tail
A. Similar to reverberation
B. Caused by a strong reflector
C. Consists of thin lines with close echoes

DOPPLER IMAGING

I. Valuable in diagnosing moving structures such as blood flow

II. Where there is motion between a sound source and listener, the frequency heard by the listener usually differs from the source

III. The received frequency is either higher or lower than that transmitted by the source
A. Dependent on whether the listener and source are moving toward or away from each other
B. Information about the velocity of the structure is provided
1. Based on a Doppler shift in frequency of a continuous-wave ultrasonic beam reflected from a moving structure
a. Either by sound audible to the ear or by analysis with an instrument
C. Variety of uses in veterinary ultrasound
1. Can determine if a lesion is a mass or a vessel
2. Helps in the detections of portal systemic shunts

3. Provides data on cardiac output and structural abnormalities

THREE-DIMENSIONAL ULTRASOUND

I. State-of-the-art technique
II. Displays the total area rather than sections; therefore reduced image capture time
III. Improved diagnostic ability with enhanced visualization
IV. Surfaces can be reconstructed with computer capabilities
V. Useful for surgical applications, horse tendons, and prostate glands in small animals

EXAMINATION

Preparing the Patient

I. Shaving
   A. Essential, because the ultrasound beam would otherwise pass and reflect through air-filled hair coat before penetrating the skin
   B. For abdominal ultrasound, the abdomen should be shaved, from the xiphoid process to the pubis and then laterally, from the rib cage to the flanks, using a No. 40 clipper blade
   C. For cardiac ultrasound, the cardiac region is shaved using a No. 40 blade
   D. Alcohol can be used to wipe away residual dirt and hair
II. Positioning
   A. Small animals should be placed in dorsal recumbency in a padded V-shaped trough for abdominal ultrasounds
   B. Small animal cardiac patients are placed in sternal or lateral recumbency with the shaved cardiac region situated over a hole in the table so that the transducer may be passed through it
   C. Ultrasound is usually performed with large animals in a standing position
III. Acoustic coupling gel should be used so that no air is present between the transducer and the skin surface
IV. Physical and/or chemical restraint should be used as needed
V. Each ultrasound examination should be done in the same systematic order so as not to miss anything
VI. Small dogs and cats can be scanned using a 7.5-MHz transducer
   A. It provides better detail and greater attenuation
   B. Less depth penetration
VII. Larger dogs can be scanned with a 5-MHz transducer
VIII. The lower frequency increases the depth of penetration but results in less detail and attenuation

SONOGRAPHIC APPEARANCE OF ORGANS

Heart

I. Can use either M-mode or two-dimensional B-mode
II. Important to obtain both long- and short-axis directional views
   A. Doppler is useful to assess turbulence and velocity of red blood cells
III. Usually examined between fourth and fifth ribs
IV. Best in right lateral recumbency with an opening to allow the transducer to come from underneath
V. Walls and valves are most hyperechoic

Spleen

I. Most hyperechoic
II. Uniform, granular appearance
III. Surrounded by a bright capsule
IV. Seen best on left side of the patient
V. Lies close to the surface

Liver

I. Less echogenic than the spleen
II. Contains many vessels and bile channels
III. Overtexture is coarse
IV. Contains gallbladder

Gallbladder

I. Anechoic with a bright wall
II. Sometimes contains sludge
III. Can be large in an animal that has fasted

Kidneys

I. Ovoid shape
II. Surrounded by a bright capsule
III. Cortex is hypoechoic
IV. Medulla is anechoic
V. Bright central area is pelvic fat
VI. A saggital view should be measured to assess size

Bladder

I. Anechoic with a hyperechoic wall
II. Debris often seen

Prostate

I. Can be visualized by following the urethra into the pelvic inlet
II. Surrounds urethra and is bilobed with a bright appearance

Uterus

I. If enlarged, can be seen adjacent to the bladder
II. Wall is hypoechoic

III. Optimal time for pregnancy detection is 30 days of gestation in small animals and 11 days of gestation in horses
   A. Identify gestational sacs with viable embryos
   B. Because of superimposition of bowel gas, hard to determine number of foeti

Stomach and Bowel

I. Difficult to image due to gas
II. Walls seen as white or dark gray
III. Rugal folds can be visualized in the stomach

Pancreas

I. Adjacent to duodenum and between stomach and spleen

Adrenal Gland

I. Hypoechoic
II. Uniform gray color
III. Found medial and cranial to, or beside, the cranial pole of the kidneys
IV. Caudal pole of the adrenal is next to the renal artery as it joins the aorta

LESIONS

Disease can appear as an alteration in echo texture in an organ.

Appearance of Lesions

I. Focal changes
   A. Readily identified
   B. Can be in one specific area of the organ
II. Diffuse
   A. Can be subtle changes
   B. Can affect the whole organ; thus texture needs to be assessed by comparisons with other organs

Classification of Lesions

I. Cystic
   A. Well-defined borders
   B. No internal echoes
   C. Shows posterior enhancement
II. Solid
   A. Contains many echoes, which can be spread throughout
   B. No posterior enhancement
III. Mixed
   A. Contains cystic and solid lesions
   B. Borders may be irregular

Other Imaging Techniques

I. Computed tomography
   A. One of most expensive diagnostic tests in veterinary medicine
   B. Primarily for central and peripheral nervous system diseases
   C. Patient is placed on long moveable table
      1. Table then moves the patient through the circular gantry that contains the x-ray tube and detectors
      2. Can be moved 360 degrees around the patient
   D. Single cross-sectional slice of data is obtained with every movement of the scanner
      1. Photons emerging from the patient are absorbed by the scanner
      2. Converted to electronic signals that vary in intensity depending on attenuation
      3. Computer reconstructs information into a picture display
   E. General anesthesia is required
II. Nuclear scintigraphy
   A. Small amount of radioactive material or radionuclide is given intravenously, transcolonically, or by aerosol insufflation
   B. A gamma scintillation camera is used to detect the gamma emissions from the radionuclide
      1. A black-and-white image of the selected organ is printed on x-ray film
   C. Detects functional or physiological, pharmacological, and kinetic data
      1. Not the same visual images found in other modalities
   D. Clinical applications include thyroid, bone, and liver studies
   E. Often used for horses
   F. Animals are sedated
   G. Proper radiation protection is required
      1. Excretion of the radiopharmaceutical occurs through the urine and feces
      2. Usually an animal can be discharged 24 to 72 hours later
      3. Depends on the specific state or provincial safety and protection laws
III. Magnetic resonance imaging
   A. Similar to computed tomography in that the image is a thin slice of cross-sectional anatomy
   B. Differs in that no ionizing radiation is used
      1. Patient is placed in a magnetic field
      2. Signals are transmitted and received by the surrounding coils
      3. Detailed information on soft tissues is constructed by the computer
   C. Greater image resolution, differentiation of anatomy, and sensitivity to distinguish between tissue composition than CT
   D. Primarily used for head and spine evaluation

Glossary

A-mode Demonstrates returning ultrasound beam as peaks on a graph; the more intensified the beam, the higher the peak

acoustic impedance Ability of tissue to hinder the transmission of sound

amplitude Intensity or loudness of an ultrasound wave

anechoic Waves are transmitted to deeper tissue; none are reflected back

attenuation Loss of intensity of the ultrasound beam as it travels through tissue, caused by absorption or scatter

axial resolution Ability of the ultrasound beam to identify separate structures

B-mode Uses bright dots or pixels on the screen to identify the intensity of ultrasound echoes; the position of the dot depicts the depth of the reflecting structure

computer tomography (CT) Mode of alternate imaging in which the patient moves through a circular gantry. Photons emerging from the patient are absorbed by the scanner and are converted to electronic signals that vary in intensity depending on attenuation

cystic lesion Has a well-defined border with no internal echoes and shows posterior enhancement

diffuse Subtle changes that can affect an entire organ

Doppler shift Change in perceived frequency of a sound wave due to relative motion between the source and listener or transducer and reflector

echoic Tissue that produces enough echoes when it is returned to the transducer and displayed

focal changes Readily identified lesions found in a specific area of an organ

frequency Number of cycles per unit of time

gamma rays Electromagnetic radiations that are of nuclear origin

gantry Term applied to a unit that houses the computer tomography x-ray tube and detectors

hyperechoic Tissue that reflects more sound back to the transducer than the surrounding tissues; appears bright

hypoechoic Tissue that reflects less sound back to the transducer than the surrounding tissue; appears dark

isoechoic Tissue that has the same ultrasonic appearance as that of the surrounding tissue

lateral resolution Ability of the ultrasound beam to identify separate structures that lie in a plane perpendicular to the sound beam

linear scanner Scanner that produces a rectangular image

magnetic resonance imaging (MRI) Type of alternate imaging in which the patient is placed in a magnetic field and radiofrequency signals are transmitted, received, and constructed into detailed cross-sectional images

m-mode Mode of ultrasound that displays a two-dimensional image over a timed baseline

mixed lesion Borders are irregular and contain cystic and solid areas

nuclear scintigraphy Type of noninvasive imaging procedure that uses radioactive material to obtain an image

piezoelectric effect Conversion of electrical energy to ultrasound

radionuclide Radioactive material

sagittal Transducer marker is held to the cranial or caudal end of the animal; provides a scan of the long axis of an organ

sector scanner Scanner that produces a "pie-shaped" image with a narrow near field and a wide far field

solid Contains many echoes spread throughout

transducer Part of the machine that actually scans the patient, emits pulses of sound, and receives the returning echoes

transverse Transducer marker held 90 degrees to the longitudinal plane; provides short-axis view of organs

ultrasound Method of sending high-frequency sound waves into tissues and receiving the returning echoes as an image; a noninvasive diagnostic procedure

velocity Speed at which sound travels through an object

wavelength Length that a wave must travel in one cycle

Review Questions

1 A hyperechoic lesion appears
   a. Brighter than surrounding tissue
   b. Darker than surrounding tissue
   c. Dark with posterior enhancement
   d. Same as surrounding tissue

2 Piezoelectric refers to
   a. Acoustic impedance
   b. Pressure electricity
   c. Bandwidth
   d. Time-gain compensation

3 Bandwidth is best defined as
   a. Attenuation
   b. Half the range of frequency
   c. The entire range of frequency
   d. Image resolution

4 A Doppler shift is best explained as a change in _____ as a result of motion
   a. Loudness of a perceived sound
   b. Perceived frequency
   c. Loudness of the sound source
   d. Acoustic impedance

5 The type of transducer that images by transmitting beams in parallel lines is
   a. A broad bandwidth
   b. A phased array
   c. A annular array
   d. A linear array

6 These extra image artifacts are common next to reflective surfaces
   a. Mirror
   b. Refraction
   c. Acoustic shadowing
   d. Acoustic enhancement

7 Sound waves have difficulty traveling through
   a. Tissue
   b. Blood
   c. Fluid
   d. Bone

8 Three-dimensional ultrasound provides
   a. Less visualization
   b. Enhanced visualization

c. B-mode
d. M-mode

9 The normal adrenal glands on ultrasound are best described as
a. Hyperechoic
b. Cystic
c. Hypoechoic
d. Ceramic

10 The number of cycles per second is the
a. Wavelength
b. Wave period
c. Doppler shift
d. Frequency

BIBLIOGRAPHY

Han C, Hurd C: *Practical diagnostic imaging for the veterinary technician,* ed 2, St Louis, 2000, Mosby.

Kremkau FW: *Diagnostic ultrasound: principles and instruments,* ed 6, Philadelphia, 2002, WB Saunders.

McCurnin DM, Bassert JM, editors: *Clinical textbook for veterinary technicians,* ed 5, Philadelphia, 2002, WB Saunders.

Odwin C, Dubunsky T, Fleischer A: *Appleton and Lange's review for the ultrasonography exam,* ed 2, Norwalk, CT, 1993, Appleton and Lange.

Zagzebski JA: *Essentials of ultrasound physics,* St Louis, 1996, Mosby.

PART III

Patient Management and Nutrition

CHAPTER 13

Genetics, Theriogenology, and Neonatal Care

Karen Anderson *Monica M. Tighe*

OUTLINE

LEARNING OUTCOMES

After reading this chapter you should be able to:

1. Understand the basic definitions associated with inheritance.
2. Define monohybrid and dihybrid cross and complete a Punnett square for each type.
3. Describe the difference between outbreeding, back cross, inbreeding, and line breeding.
4. Describe the characteristics of X-linked genes.
5. Describe chromosomal abnormalities.
6. Define lethal gene and its consequences.
7. Have an understanding of the basics of transgenesis.
8. Define the basics of bovine, canine, caprine, equine, feline, ovine, and porcine reproductive characteristics.
9. Define the neonatal bovine, canine, caprine, equine, feline, ovine, and porcine nursing requirements.

This chapter contains the basics of genetics and animal breeding. Students often find genetics difficult. The difficulty could be due to the new terminology that novices must learn to understand the subject. The best suggestion when studying genetics is to approach the genetics parts of this chapter one step at a time and to understand the definitions before continuing on to the next section.

This chapter also briefly describes the reproductive cycles of small and large animals. It includes information such as puberty onset, estrous cycles, breeding soundness examination, semen collection techniques and characteristics, gestation/stages of parturition, pregnancy diagnosis, causes of dystocia, and neonatal care.

Karen Anderson wrote the theriogenology and neonatal portions of this chapter and Monica Tighe wrote the genetics section.

Genetics

GENES AND VARIATIONS

The monohybrid cross or the crossing of a single gene is obviously the simplest cross. Note that in most cases multiple genes are usually the case in inheritance.

Monohybrid Cross

I. Definitions
   A. Homozygous: having identical alleles, e.g., BB
   B. Heterozygous: having different alleles, e.g., Bb
II. Example: the Punnett square for the cross between cattle
   A. Two black individuals are crossed
   B. Their genotype is Bb (heterozygous)
      1. "B" represents the dominant allele of black
      2. "b" represents the recessive allele of red

Punnett square for the cross Bb × Bb

	B	b
B	BB	Bb
b	Bb	bb

   C. According to the Punnett square, the F_1 generation, or first familial generation, will be made up of 25% genotype BB, 50% genotype Bb, and 25% genotype bb
      1. Ratio is 1:2:1
   D. However, 75% of the F_1 generation will have the phenotype or physical trait of black color because the B allele is dominant over the recessive allele b
      1. There are 2 Bb (heterozygous) individuals produced who will be black and 1 BB (homozygous) individual produced who will also be black
      2. Only 25% of the F_1 generation will be red, or bb
      3. This 3:1 ratio (3 black to 1 red) is used to trace the heterozygous and homozygous genes of the parents
III. The following matings are possible
   A. Homozygous black to homozygous black will produce only black offspring
   B. Homozygous black to heterozygous black will produce all black: 50% of the offspring will be homozygous and 50% will be heterozygous
   C. Homozygous black to homozygous red will produce all heterozygous black
   D. Heterozygous black to heterozygous black will produce 25% homozygous black, 50% heterozygous black, and 25% red
   E. Heterozygous black to homozygous red will produce 50% heterozygous black and 50% red
   F. Red to red will produce only red homozygous because all genes are recessive

Dihybrid Cross

The crossing of two independent alleles.

I. Example: bantam chickens
   A. R (rose comb), r (single comb), B (black), b (white)
   B. Cross of a rose comb, black and a single comb, white produces only rose comb, black chickens (F_1 generation)
      1. RRBB × rrbb will produce only RrBb (F_1 generation)
      2. If two of the F_1 generation are crossed, they will produce the ratio of approximately 9 rose comb, black; 3 rose comb, white; 3 single, black; 1 single, white

		RrBb			
		RB	Rb	rB	rb
RrBb	RB	RRBB	RRBb	RrBB	RrBb
	Rb	RRBb	RRBb	RrBb	Rrbb
	rB	RrBB	RrBb	rrBB	rrBb
	rb	RrBb	Rrbb	rrBb	rrbb

C. F_2 generation or the second familial generation is produced from the breeding of the F_1 generation, or RrBb × RrBb

D. This ratio is the standard ratio in any F_2 generation when two independent pair of alleles are involved

II. Variable expressivity: the term used for traits that show continuous variation
   A. Example: orange tabby cats that display the phenotype of light ginger to deep red in color
   B. Example: some dogs are 80% spotted and 20% white; other dogs of the same breed are 20% spotted and 80% white

III. Polygenic traits: traits that are due to the interaction of several gene pairs
   A. Polygene inheritances produce phenotypes that vary quantitatively over a wide range
      1. Example: IQ, height, or eye color
      2. These traits are due to a polygenic effect or many genes acting collectively to produce variations

IV. Incomplete dominance or intermediate inheritance: a cross where both genes are expressed equally
   A. Heterozygote has a phenotype in between those of the homozygous dominant and homozygous recessive individuals
      1. Example: roan cattle
         a. Roan cattle are produced by breeding a red shorthorn and a white shorthorn
         b. When these two colors are crossed, they produce a red and white-haired individual
      2. Other examples include merle color in collies, foxes, Great Danes, and sheepdogs that have a characteristic black/gray color
         a. Color consists of irregular blotches of dark pigment against a lighter background of the same pigment

V. Codominance: a cross where each allele makes a comparable contribution to the phenotype
   A. Example: human blood type AB. This blood grouping contains the antigens A and B equally

VI. Epistasis: a masking of one allele over the genes on another locus
   A. Epistasis is different than dominance; epistasis masks independently inherited genes
   B. Example: black cats still carry tabby stripes
      1. Stripes are visible at certain ages of development in specific lights
      2. Striping is masked by the black color allele
   C. Example: an agouti mouse (AACC) crossed with an albino mouse (aacc)
      1. A (agouti), a (nonagouti), C (full color), c (albino)
      2. Note: (_) designates the dominant or recessive form of the gene
      3. Resulting F_1 generation is AaCc, or an agouti mouse with full color
      4. If the F_1 generation is crossed, the F_2 generation consists of 16 animals in the following color combinations: 9 A_C_, agouti; 3 A_cc, albino; 3 aaC_, nonagouti; 1 aacc, albino
   D. In this case, c, or the albino gene, masks any and all other pigment genes

X-LINKED INHERITANCE (ALSO CALLED SEX-LINKED INHERITANCE)

Definitions

I. Sex chromosomes
   A. Females have the designation XX, meaning two X chromosomes
   B. Males have the designation XY, meaning one X chromosome and one Y chromosome
   C. When a male inherits an X-linked recessive allele, it is always expressed because there is no corresponding allele (even though it is a "single dose")
   D. Females must have X-linked recessive alleles to express the trait
   E. X-linked traits are usually passed from mothers to sons; fathers do not pass an X chromosome to their sons, thus only a Y chromosome is passed from father to son
   F. X-linked: the gene in question is located only on the X chromosome
   G. Autosomal: refers to chromosomes not involved with sex determination

Identification of Autosomal or X-linked Genes

I. X-linked dominant familial characteristics
   A. Normal female will have two X-linked chromosomes; males have only one X-linked gene
   B. Because the X chromosome of the male is always transmitted to his daughters, affected males will pass the trait to daughters but not to sons
   C. Carrier females are heterozygous for a recessive X-linked gene and therefore will pass it on to 50% of their sons and 50% of their daughters (who will be normal but carriers)
   D. Example: color blindness in humans

II. X-linked recessive
   A. Disease appears in males whose mothers are unaffected but are heterozygous carriers of the mutant recessive allele
   B. Each son of a carrier female has a 1:1 chance of being affected
   C. Affected male never transmits the gene to his sons; however, he will transmit to all of his daughters, who will be carriers
   D. Unaffected males never transmit the gene
III. Autosomal dominant
   A. Dominant alleles will transmit disease from one affected individual to their offspring; there will be no skipping of generations unless penetrance is reduced
   B. There will be an approximately equal number of each sex affected with the disease
   C. Fifty percent of the progeny of each affected individual will be affected (due to Aa × aa matings)
   D. Dominant allele can be transmitted by the mother or father
IV. Autosomal recessive
   A. Parents and remote relatives of an affected individual will not be affected (often skips generations)
   B. In matings producing an affected offspring, approximately 25% of the progeny will be affected
   C. There should be an equal number of females and males with the defect or trait
   D. If both parents are affected, offspring will most likely be affected

Example: X-linked Heredity in Cats

I. Tortoiseshell pattern in cats is an example of X-linked genetics
II. There are very few male tortoiseshell cats; nearly all tortoiseshell cats are female
III. G symbolizes the ginger or orange coat color, which is carried on the X chromosome
IV. Male cats have only one X chromosome, so their genotype can be only G (yellow) or g (nonyellow)
V. Female cats have two X chromosomes, so females can be three genotypes
   A. GG (yellow), Gg (tortoiseshell), gg (nonyellow)
VI. Tortoiseshell is heterozygous and has a unique coat color
VII. Color variation is due to the influence of both the G and g genes in different parts of the animal at the same time
VIII. Important point to remember is that a male can transmit only one gene (G or g) in 50% of the gamete; the other 50% carries a Y chromosome that does not possess a G locus

		Gametes from tortoiseshell female Gg	
		X_G	X_g
Gametes from yellow male GY	X_G	X_GX_G Yellow female	X_GX_g Tortoiseshell female
	Y	X_GY Yellow male	X_gY Black male

BREEDING GENETICS

I. Definitions
   A. Pedigree chart: a chart that shows the ancestry of a particular family
      1. Specific symbols are used to designate different individual characteristics
         a. Open symbols indicate the individual does not possess the trait
         b. Solid symbols indicate the presence of a trait under study or an individual having the trait
         c. Half of a solid symbol indicates the individual is a carrier of the trait
         d. Male: symbolized by a square
         e. Female: symbolized by a circle
         f. Unknown sex: symbolized by a diamond
         g. A number in the symbol indicates the number of individuals
         h. Two symbols joined by a line indicate marriage or mating
      2. Byconstructing a pedigree, recessive allele carriers may be identified and eventually culled from the stock, depending on the trait in question
II. Test cross: this cross is used to determine the genotype of a particular phenotype
   A. Usually the unknown phenotype is crossed with a homozygous recessive individual
      1. Example: black Doberman pinscher phenotype of either BB or Bb
      2. Genotype B represents black color, and the genotype b represents brown color
      3. Cross will be B_ × bb (a homozygous recessive individual)
      4. If the dog is Bb, the cross will produce 50% bb (brown Dobermans) and 50% Bb (black Dobermans)
      5. If the dog is BB, all of the offspring will be black or Bb

	B	b
b	Bb	bb
b	Bb	bb

III. Heterosis, or hybrid vigor
   A. An F_1 generation is produced by crossing two different inbred strains
   B. Heterosis usually results in increases in size and weight gain; reproductive ability and resistance to disease are also increased
   C. Two individuals from the F_1 generation cannot be bred because this breeding will produce variables in the phenotype
IV. Outbreeding, or random breeding
   A. This type of breeding is considered to keep the gene pool as large as possible; mating to other strains maintains an increasing amount of heterozygous genes
   B. This type of breeding keeps all fitness traits such as resistance to disease at high levels
   C. In general, this type of breeding is between two animals who are unrelated
V. Back cross: the pairing of an F_1 generation hybrid with an organism whose genotype is identical to the parental strain
VI. Inbreeding: breeding together of closely related individuals to produce ever-increasing similarities in the offspring
   A. This breeding will produce as many homozygote individuals as possible
   B. Advantages: the breeding will be "true" and it is possible to fix mutant alleles into a line or strain of animals
   C. Disadvantage: recessive alleles may be revealed, such as lethal genes
VII. Line breeding: breeding of related individuals to guarantee similar traits in the offspring
   A. Types
      1. Brother × half-sister
      2. Parent × offspring
VIII. Inbreeding depression: relates to traits of fitness such as early growth, resistance to disease, or fertility, which are all multifunctional traits
   A. If an individual becomes homozygous, inbreeding depression occurs
   B. To reduce inbreeding depression
      1. Inbreed slowly and be stringent in selection of mating
      2. Do not breed poor phenotypes
   C. If inbreeding depression occurs
      1. Introduce a new sire or male with as many desirable traits as possible
      2. Outcross within your population to minimize inbreeding
      3. Always select healthy animals with good reproductive ability
IX. Harem mating: a mating where one male is mated to five females
   A. Generally used in some lab animal colonies

CHROMOSOMAL ABNORMALITIES

Definitions

I. Translocation: the breakage of two chromosomes, resulting in repair in an abnormal arrangement
II. Deletion: a part or all of a chromosome is missing
III. Duplication: an allele is duplicated, for example, human trisomy 21 or Down's syndrome—there are three chromosomes rather than two at location 21 in the karyotype
IV. Anomalies: deviations from normal
   A. There are many examples of anomalies in small animal breeding
   B. Examples: malocclusions, hip dysplasia, collie eye, Perthe's disease, hemophilia, diabetes mellitus, microphthalmia, deafness, entropion, and dwarfism

Lethal Genes

I. Definition: a gene that will cause the death of the embryo or serious impairment or death sometime after birth (sometimes called a delayed lethal)
II. Semilethal gene causes the individual to have abnormal traits
III. Lethal gene is expressed as a homozygous recessive, usually in the F_2 generation
   A. Genotype will be in the ratio of 1:2 instead of 1:2:1 (one individual will die)
IV. Dominant lethal gene is usually expressed only once and cannot be proved to be inherited genetically

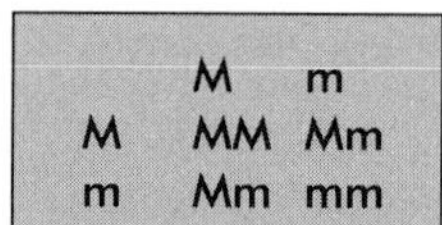

	M	m
M	MM	Mm
m	Mm	mm

   A. However, there are some dominant disorders in which the individual is only impaired and is still able to reproduce
      1. Example: achondroplasia (dwarfism)
         a. Most lethal genes are recessive
         b. An incomplete dominance lethal gene: homozygous dominant individuals will die but heterozygous individuals will show clinical signs, such as the Manx cat and many human lethal genes
   B. Example: Manx cat
      1. MM (lethal), Mn (tailless or Manx), mm (normal tail)
      2. Resulting ratio of the cross Mm × Mm is 25% of the kittens will die (MM), 50% will be the genotype Manx (Mm), and 25% will have genotype normal tail (mm)

TRANSGENESIS

I. Definitions
  A. Transgenesis is the transfer of genes from one individual into the genome of another, who passes it onto future generations
  B. Transgenic organism is an organism derived from a cell that has a genome that has been altered by the addition of exogenous DNA
    1. DNA may be from another species that has a desirable trait or may be modified from the same species
II. Purpose
  A. Useful for basic research because the alterations to the animals' genotypes facilitate specific experimentation
  B. Functions absent in a recipient as a result of a bad gene can be corrected by adding it to a vector, which inserts itself into the chromosomes of the recipient, thereby creating a transgenic animal that has been cured through genetics
  C. Transgenic plants, fungi, and animals are being used for research due to the added scope that this approach gives to the development of profitable genotypes

Theriogenology and Neonatal Care

FELINE

Puberty

I. Queen
  A. Average age, 5 to 9 months
  B. Long-haired cats reach puberty later than short-haired breeds
II. Tom
  A. Sexual maturity about 9 months

Breeding Soundness Examination

I. Examination of the male
  A. Scrotum and testes
    1. Testes should be symmetrical bilaterally in size and shape, firm and smooth
    2. Orchitis can be caused by traumatic injuries or can occur secondary to various viruses or bacteria
    3. Cryptorchidism is not common but may be inherited
    4. Testicular tumors are not common
  B. Penis and prepuce
    1. Major concerns are trauma and feline lower urinary tract disease (FLUTD)
      a. FLUTD can cause penile trauma due to the obstructive process, licking, and the relieving of the blockage
    2. Mating without penetration may be due to the accumulation of hair around the glans penis
      a. This can be removed by sliding the hair ring over the glans after retracting the sheath
  C. Semen evaluation
    1. The semen can be collected and evaluated

Semen Collection Techniques and Semen Characteristics

I. Semen Collection
  A. Artificial vagina (AV)
    1. An estimated 20% of tom cats can be trained to use an AV
  B. Electroejaculation
    1. Not commonly used
    2. Teflon rectal probe has been used to collect from tom cats that are under total anesthesia
  C. Natural breeding
    1. After natural breeding has occurred, a moistened cotton swab can be placed into the vaginal vault, rolled onto a slide, and examined for sperm
II. Semen characteristics
  A. Volume: 0.01 to 0.7 mL
  B. Concentration: 50 to 60 million/mL
  C. Motility: 80% progressively motile

Estrous Cycle

I. First estrous cycle is usually around 9 months
II. Polyestrus
III. Estrus periods may last 3 to 6 days, although they may last up to 10 days if mating does not occur
IV. Ovulation is not spontaneous; it is "induced" or "reflex"
  A. Ovulation occurs only when a cat is mated or the cervix is stimulated by an instrument such as a glass rod
V. Ovulation can be induced by treatments of hormones such as human chorionic gonadotropin (hCG), luteinizing hormone (LH), or gonadotropin-releasing hormone (GnRH)

Signs of Estrus

I. Vocalization
II. Crouching and rolling on the floor, called "lordosis"
III. Tail deflection

Pregnancy Diagnosis

I. Abdominal palpation: 3 to 4 weeks postbreeding
II. Ultrasound
  A. 11 to 16 days: gestational sacs
  B. 16 to 32 days: fetal heartbeats
III. Radiographs: 45 days' gestation

Gestation/Stages of Parturition

I. Gestation: approximately 63 days
II. Zonary placentation

III. Mammary gland develops during the last week
IV. Last few days of gestation, milk can usually be expressed from the nipples
V. Stages of parturition
  A. Stage 1
    1. Restlessness
    2. Vocalization
    3. Nesting behavior can be obvious for up to 48 hours before queening
  B. Stage 2
    1. Few obvious contractions and loud vocalizing by the queen may signal the birth of the first kitten
      a. This may take up to 60 minutes
    2. Between kittens, the queen will remove and eat any placental tissue, sever the umbilical cord, clean the kittens and her vulvular area
    3. Some queens may nurse newborns while continuing with parturition
    4. It is uncommon, but parturition may take up to several days
      a. This is not considered abnormal but must be differentiated from dystocia
  C. Stage 3
    1. Placenta is usually expelled after the delivery of each kitten
      a. It is possible for two placentas to be passed after the birth of two kittens

Causes of Dystocia

I. Rare
II. Fetal dystocia
  A. May be due to abnormal positioning
  B. Fetal oversize
  C. Fetal deformities
III. Maternal dystocia
  A. May be due to a congenitally small pelvis
  B. Queen may have previously fractured her pelvis
  C. Uterine torsion of the uterus, a single horn, or a portion of a horn
  D. Inguinal hernia
  E. Uterine inertia

Neonatal Care

I. Temperature, 38° to 39° C (100° to 102° F); pulse, 140 to 170/min; respiration, 30 to 50/min
II. Tomcats should be kept away from kittens
III. Hand-fed kittens should be fed 15% to 20% of their body weight divided into three daily feedings
IV. Unable to thermoregulate for the first 6 days
V. Kittens consume between 5 and 7 mL of milk per feeding by the second week of life and have doubled their birth weight
VI. Eyes open at 8 to 10 days of age
VII. After each feeding the queen cleans and grooms each kitten. She also stimulates them (by licking) to urinate and defecate; she then consumes the urine and feces
VIII. By 3 weeks of age, the activity level of the litter has increased, and they are now urinating and defecating some distance from their nest
IX. Solid food is supplemented in the diet by the fourth week
X. Kittens are weaned between 5 and 8 weeks of age

CANINE

Puberty

I. Bitch
  A. Average 8 months
  B. Puberty varies by breed and size from 6 to 18 months of age
  C. Smaller breeds reach puberty earlier than larger breeds
  D. Bitch should not be bred during her first estrus; she may be sexually mature but not yet anatomically mature
II. Stud
  A. Approximately 9 months

Breeding Soundness Examination

I. History
  A. Complete medical history of all organ systems must be obtained before breeding because infections and neoplasias of other organ systems (e.g., urinary tract) may cause secondary problems
  B. Alteration of secretory patterns of hormones such as testosterone, follicle-stimulating hormone (FSH), LH, and GnRH may affect the ability of the male to breed
  C. Administration of drugs (e.g., corticosteroids, cimetidine), stress, trauma, or a history of systemic illness can all affect the overall function of the reproductive tract
II. Examination of the reproductive tract
  A. Scrotum
    1. Normal scrotum should be lightly covered with hair, smooth and soft to the touch, have freely moving skin over the testes, be pain free, and be of consistent thickness
    2. Look for signs of inflammation, trauma, or swelling
  B. Testes
    1. Testes should be palpated for size, shape, and consistency with the left testicle sitting caudal to the right

2. Presence of an irregular surface, nodules, or scrotal adhesions may suggest chronic inflammation, infection, or neoplasia
3. Soft, spongy testes may suggest testicular degeneration, and hard testes may indicate neoplasia or acute orchitis

C. Epididymis and spermatic cord
1. Should be palpated for areas of thickening, enlargement, epididymitis, adenomyosis of the epididymis, or an inguinal hernia

D. Penis and prepuce
1. Discharge of blood, pus, or urine from the prepuce may be a cause for concern
2. Penis should be freely moveable within the prepuce and can be easily revealed by retracting the prepuce caudal over the bulbus glandis
3. Penis should be examined for the presence of infection, trauma, foreign bodies, and masses
a. The mucosa of the penis should be pink, white, and smooth
4. Os penis should be palpated for congenital deformities and fractures

E. Prostate gland
1. Only accessory gland in the dog
2. Palpate for abnormal size, asymmetry between lobes, and abnormal consistency

F. Semen evaluation
1. The semen can be collected and evaluated

Semen Collection Techniques and Semen Characteristics

I. Semen collection
A. Teaser bitch
1. It is easiest to collect semen from a male by allowing him to mount a teaser bitch
2. Once the male has mounted the female, the penis can be deviated into a collection device or an AV
B. Masturbation
1. Semen can be collected using this technique if there is no teaser bitch
C. Electroejaculation
1. Not commonly used
2. Male must be anesthetized

II. Semen characteristics
A. Volume: total volume about 20 mL but may vary from as little as 2 mL to 60 mL
B. Concentration: 200 to 3000 × 10^6/ejaculate
C. Motility: 60% to 90% motile sperm

Estrous Cycle

I. Nonseasonal

II. Phases of estrous cycle
A. Proestrus: usually lasts 5 to 9 days
1. Hemorrhagic vulvar discharge
2. Vulva is swollen
B. Estrus: usually lasts about 9 days
1. Receptive to the male
2. Usually ovulates 24 to 48 hours after the LH surge
3. Clear serous discharge
C. Metestrus: average 90 days
1. Occurs in unmated bitches
D. Anestrus: sexual inactivity between cycles

III. Signs of estrus
A. Clear serous discharge
B. Receptive to male

Pregnancy Diagnosis

I. Abdominal palpation: 3 to 4 weeks postbreeding
II. Ultrasound: 24 to 28 days postbreeding
III. Transabdominal ultrasound: 24 to 28 days postbreeding

Gestation/Stages of Parturition

I. Average gestation: 63 days
II. Zonary placentation
III. Drop in body temperature to less than 37° C (98.6° F) when parturition is imminent
IV. At 12 to 24 hours before whelping, milk can normally be expressed
V. Produce colostrum for up to 3 days postparturition
VI. Stages of parturition
A. Stage 1
1. Starts at the onset of uterine contractions and finishes when the cervix is completely dilated
2. Nervous anorexia
3. May vomit occasionally
4. Decrease in body temperature (other animals have elevated body temperatures)
B. Stage 2
1. Starts with full dilation of cervix and ends with the expulsion of the fetus
2. Bitches may deliver pups over a period anywhere from a few hours to 24 to 36 hours
3. When each pup is passed, the chorioallantoic membrane ruptures or the bitch removes the membrane by chewing or licking it away
4. Bitch must also remove the amniotic membrane, which the pup is more likely to still have at birth
C. Stage 3
1. Begins with the expulsion of the pup and is completed by the passing of the placenta
2. Placenta is usually passed 5 to 15 minutes after the birth of the pup
D. Dark green discharge the first 12 to 24 hours after parturition

Causes of Dystocia

I. Uterus
  A. This may include uterine weakness if lack of uterine force to propel the fetus through the birth canal
    1. Primary uterine inertia
    2. Secondary uterine inertia
    3. Miscellaneous causes
      a. A nervous or frightened bitch may actually interfere with her own whelping
II. Pelvis
  A. Birth canal may be too small
    1. May be a congenital problem where the pelvis is too small
    2. May be acquired, such as a pelvic fracture
III. Fetus
  A. Fetal oversize
    1. Most likely cause is a single fetus
  B. Abnormal fetal presentation
    1. Causes can be a head-first presentation with the legs back, presentation of a single leg, and flexion of the head back along the body
  C. Vaginal vault
    1. A puppy wedged in the vaginal vault, due to fetal oversize or a small pelvis, may be the problem
    2. Vault may be too small due to a vaginal stricture

Neonatal Care

I. Temperature, 38° to 39° C (100° to 102° F); pulse, 120 to 150/min; respiration, 25 to 50/min
II. Should be suckling by 3 hours postwhelping to receive optimum amounts of colostrum
III. Pups can be hand-fed three times a day
IV. Newborns can take 10 to 20 mL/feeding, depending on the breed
V. Unable to thermoregulate for the first 6 days
VI. Eyes open between 5 and 14 days of age, and the external ear canals open 1 to 2 days later
VII. Puppies should gain 2 to 4 g/day/kg of expected adult weight
VIII. After each feeding, the bitch stimulates the puppies to urinate and defecate and cleans each puppy
IX. By 18 days of age, the puppies are moving around and exploring their environment
X. Should be encouraged to consume solid food by 3 to 4 weeks of age
XI. Weaning is at 6 to 8 weeks of age

EQUINE

Puberty

I. Mare
  A. Approximately 12 months
  B. Low energy intake may delay puberty
II. Stallion
  A. Seldom used for breeding before 2 years of age
  B. Approximately 12 to 18 months
  C. Libido decreases during winter months

Breeding Soundness Examination

I. Conducted mainly to evaluate infertility
  A. Require a complete health history and any drug therapy the stallion has been receiving during the previous 2 months
II. General examination
  A. Observe stallion in a small corral or pasture to detect any musculoskeletal or other physical problems that may exist
    1. Chronic degenerative joint problems
    2. Chronic laminitis
    3. Back disorders
  B. Penis
    1. Avoid the use of promazine tranquilizer due to risk of penile paralysis
    2. Examine distal portion of penis for trauma or neoplasia (squamous cell carcinoma)
    3. Scarring or injuries may occur farther up the penis but are not common
  C. Scrotum, testicles, and epididymis
    1. Easily performed postbreeding
    2. Scrotum is rarely affected by disease
    3. Note any abnormalities in size, consistency, and symmetry in the testicles and epididymis
      a. It is common to discover one testicle may be slightly smaller
  D. Accessory sex glands (vesicular and bulbourethral glands, prostate)
    1. There have been few reported pathological changes involving these glands
    2. Can be palpated rectally but may be difficult to locate
  E. Swabs can be taken of the penis and prepuce if there is a chance of bacterial infection
  F. Stallion's libido, manners, ease of ejaculation, and ability to service the mare should also be taken into consideration
  G. Semen evaluation
    1. Semen can be collected and evaluated

Semen Collection Techniques and Semen Characteristics

I. Semen collection
  A. Artificial vagina (AV) and phantom mare
    1. Preferred technique
    2. Most commonly used
  B. Condoms, vaginal collection, and dismount sample
    1. Dismount sample can be collected from the urethra and used, but contamination is

common from the vagina and penis and may reduce mobility
a. The advantage of these techniques is that samples may be collected routinely, preserved, and monitored during breeding season
II. Semen characteristics
A. Volume: gel free, volumes vary from 20 to 250 mL/ejaculate
B. Concentration: 30 to 600 million/mL; average 120 million/mL
C. Motility: at least 60% progressively motile sperm is desirable

Estrous Cycle

I. Generally seasonally polyestrus
II. Estrus activity can be induced by increasing the exposure to light (natural or artificial)
III. Estrous cycle is usually 21 to 22 days, with estrus being 5 to 6 days
IV. Estrus cycle is divided into two phases
A. Follicular phase: 5 to 6 days
B. Luteal phase: about 16 days
V. Most ovulate 1 to 2 days before the end of estrus
VI. Approximately 9 days postfoaling, mares will have a fertile heat, also called "foal heat"

Signs of Estrus

I. Squatting, vulvar winking, raising tail, and urination
II. Usually show signs only in presence of a stallion

Pregnancy Diagnosis

I. Rectal palpation
II. Transrectal ultrasound: as early as 14 days postbreeding
III. Progesterone assay: 18 to 21 days postbreeding
IV. Estrone sulfate: after 80 days postbreeding

Gestation/Stages of Parturition

I. Gestation: approximately 336 days (11 months)
II. Diffuse and microcotyledonary placentation
III. Corpus luteum maintains pregnancy 90 to 100 days, then the placenta produces progesterone
IV. Waxing of teats and possible discharge of milk
V. Stages of parturition
A. Stage 1
1. Pacing in stall
2. Abdominal discomfort
3. Sweating
4. Pawing
5. During this stage, the final positioning and posturing of the foal occur
6. End of stage 1 is indicated by the rupture of the chorioallantoic membrane and the escape of the allantoic fluid
B. Stage 2
1. Signs are more obvious
2. May sit up and lay down many times and is generally sweating
3. When laying down, the legs may be extended and the head may be stretched outward from the rest of the body
4. May urinate/defecate due to the pressure from the contracting uterus, and may roll to try to lessen the pain and/or position the fetus
5. Stage 2 takes about 20 minutes from when the chorioallantoic membranes rupture to the delivery of the fetus
C. Stage 3
1. Begins with the foaling and ends with the expulsion of the placenta. This should occur within 3 hours
2. Mare should be allowed to lie quietly for the first hour after parturition

Causes of Dystocia

I. Not common in mares, less than 1% of equine parturition
II. Fetal causes are the most common form
A. Primary cause is postural abnormalities due to the long fetal extremities
B. Positional and presentation abnormalities may also occur but to a lesser degree
III. Round shape of the mare's pelvis, compared with that of a cow, decreases dystocia due to large fetuses
IV. Uncommon causes of fetal dystocia are fetal anasarca, ascites, fetal tumor, hydrocephalic fetus, fetal monster, and mummified fetus
V. Maternal causes of dystocia may be uterine torsion, small pelvis, uterine inertia, immaturity, constriction of the vagina or cervix, and other causes unrelated to the fetus

Neonatal Care

I. Foal should be standing and suckling within 3 hours
II. If not suckling by 4 to 5 hours, 250 to 500 mL of colostrums should be administered
III. Physical examination of the foal
IV. Navel should be dipped with 0.5% chlorhexidine diacetate and repeated in 4 to 6 hours
V. Blood sample should be taken at 18 to 24 hours of age to measure IgG, to make sure there is sufficient immunoglobulin absorption, and treated appropriately by intravenous plasma transfusion
VI. Temperature, 37.5° to 38.5° C (99.5° to 101° F); pulse, 80 to 120/min; respiration, 14 to 15/min
VII. If there are some signs of sepsis, blood cultures should be aseptically collected, and appropriate antibiotic treatment should be started

VIII. Foals will nurse from the mare every 30 to 40 minutes
 A. Failure to do so may indicate disease in the foal
 B. Healthy foals should gain 1.0 to 2.5 kg/day or 2.2 to 5 lb/day

IX. Foals are susceptible to a variety of problems
 A. Constipation due to meconium impaction, abnormal intestinal distention as a result of enterocolitis
 B. Ruptured urinary bladder causing uroperitoneum
 C. Profound anemia due to neonatal isoerythrolysis
 D. As a result of being premature, they may develop pulmonary insufficiency
 E. They are also susceptible to gastric ulcers when placed under stressful conditions

BOVINE

Puberty

I. Heifer
 A. Approximately 9 to 10 months
 B. Age of puberty is directly related to body weight
 C. Breed heifer at 15 months of age or 1000 lb (450 kg) of body weight
 D. A female is not called a "cow" until she gives birth to her first calf, at approximately 2 years of age

II. Bull
 A. Scrotal circumference is correlated with fertility

Breeding Soundness Examination

I. Breeding capacity test
 A. Measure breeding capacity under natural field conditions using ink chin-ball markers and/or constant observation

II. Locomotor abnormalities
 A. Any physical abnormalities that prevents or limits breeding
  1. On the feet, look for corns, hoof cracks, evidence of founder, overgrown hooves, and arthritis
  2. Look at structural faults such as sickle hocks, post-legged conditions, narrow chests, and weak pasterns
   a. These faults will make mounting and locomotion more difficult, therefore decreasing breeding capacity
  3. Injuries such as back injuries, sprains, spavins, bruises, and dislocated hips may also affect locomotion and breeding capacity

III. Reproductive abnormalities
 A. Penis and prepuce
  1. Reproductive organs such as the penis and prepuce may be examined by electroejaculation, which will cause the penis to extend, thus allowing a complete external examination
  2. Possible penile defects may include hair rings, attached frenulum, lacerations, growths, enlarged glans, scar tissue, deviations, coiled penis, and urethral fistulas
 B. Scrotum and testicles
  1. Scrotal circumference should be taken as it is related to paired testes weight, and this in turn is related to daily sperm production and semen quality traits
  2. Examine the scrotum for testicular defects with minimal restraint
  3. Look for testicular firmness, uniform size and shape, lumps, cysts, scar tissue, and excessive heat
  4. Epididymis tails can be palpated and should feel full but not swollen and hard
 C. Libido
  1. Bulls with a high libido are aggressive breeders and are physically fit for high breeding capacity
   a. These bulls are considered the dominant breeders
  2. Sometimes bulls with a particularly high libido may continue to attempt to breed even after their ability to produce viable sperm is exhausted
  3. Bulls with low libido will breed less frequently, are less socially aggressive, and therefore are less likely to become the dominant breeder

IV. Semen evaluation
 A. Semen can be collected and evaluated

V. Bull to cow/heifer ratio
 A. Length of breeding season, climate, access to feed, and terrain may all affect the conception rates
 B. Bulls are expected to breed 25 to 30 cows/heifers over a 60- to 90-day breeding period

Semen Collection Techniques and Semen Characteristics

I. Semen collection
 A. Electroejaculation
 B. Massage
  1. Quiet, sexually rested bulls are best candidates
  2. This technique may be used if there is some type of injury of the back, feet, or legs

C. Artificial vagina (AV)
1. Performed almost exclusively at artificial insemination (AI) centers
2. Bulls must be halter broke and nose ring trained
3. May require a female in estrus to be successful

II. Semen characteristics
A. Volume: 2 to 15 mL
B. Concentration: 300 to 2500 million spermatozoa/mL
C. Motility: rapid vigorous wave motion

Estrous Cycle

I. 21-Day estrous cycle
II. Estrus: 18 to 24 hours
III. Ovulates 10 to 11 hours after the end of estrus, unlike other farm animals, which ovulate during estrus
IV. Breeding should occur approximately 12 hours after the first signs of estrus or standing heat
V. Metestral bleeding occurs about 24 hours after ovulation

Signs of Estrus

I. Stands still while being mounted by other cows
II. Bawling
III. Clear mucus discharge from the vulva (bull stringing)

Pregnancy Diagnosis

I. Rectal palpation: 30 to 40 days postbreeding
II. Progesterone assay: 19 to 24 days postbreeding
III. Rectal ultrasound: after 25 days postbreeding
IV. Abdominal ballottement: after 5 months postbreeding

Gestation/Stages of Parturition

I. Gestation: 278 days (9 months)
II. Cotyledonary placentation: a combination of maternal caruncles and fetal cotyledons
III. Four to 5 days before calving, a clear mucous discharge from the vulva can be seen
IV. Vulva enlarges the last week of gestation, and sacrosciatic ligaments relax and cause the gluteal muscles to sink
V. Stages of parturition
A. Stage 1
1. Will last anywhere from 6 to 24 hours in heifers
2. Various signs such as anorexia, restlessness, shifting of weight, and an arched back with a tail that is extended
3. If able, most dams will separate themselves from the herd
4. There may be some minor abdominal straining during the latter portion of stage 1, thus making the change from stage 1 to stage 2 unclear
5. The end of this stage is marked by the rupture of the chorioallantois and the expulsion of the allantoic fluid

B. Stage 2
1. Average length of this stage is 2 to 4 hours in pluriparous cows and longer in heifers due to the greater effort required to dilate the birth canal tissues
2. Oxytocin stimulates myometrial contraction, which forces the calf into the cervical canal and stretches the tissues
3. Appearance of an intact amnion as a fluid-filled sac will usually rupture while the dam is recumbent
a. This will bring on more forceful and frequent abdominal contractions
4. When the contractions become more forceful, the dam will roll to lateral recumbency to deliver the calf
a. Pluriparous dams may deliver their calves while standing, but most deliver while lateral
5. Much force is required to deliver the calf's head through the vulva
a. The remainder of the calving should require very little effort

C. Stage 3
1. Detachment and expulsion of the placenta
2. Can occur anywhere from a few minutes to 12 hours
3. Dam may stand and start grooming the calf during this stage

Causes of Dystocia

I. Maternal dystocia is caused by the dam's ability to impede or prevent the delivery
A. Decreased expulsive force and abnormalities of the birth canal
B. Primary uterine inertia
C. Secondary uterine inertia
D. Birth canal abnormalities
1. Causes may be inadequate size or deformities of the pelvis
2. Incomplete dilation of the cervix
3. Vaginal cystocele, neoplasms of the vulva and vagina
4. Uterine torsion

II. Fetal causes
A. Abnormal fetal position, posture, and presentation

1. Position refers to the dorsum of the fetus versus the quadrants of the maternal pelvis
2. Posture is the relationship of the fetal extremities to the body of the fetus
3. Presentation refers to the relationship of the fetal spinal column to that of the dam and the portion of the fetus that is approaching the birth canal

B. Fetal monsters
  1. May be caused by schistosomus reflexus and perosomas elumbus

C. Fetal oversize
  1. Most common cause
  2. Most common in heifers where fetus is normal size but the maternal pelvis is undersize

Neonatal Care

I. Temperature, 37.5° to 39.5° C (99.5° to 103° F); pulse, 100 to 150/min; respiration, 30 to 60/min
II. Clear mucus from the upper airway
III. Sneezing can be stimulated by tickling the nostrils with straw
IV. Calf should be suckling 2 to 5 hours after birth
V. Colostrum may be administered if calf has not suckled (5% to 8% of its body weight)
VI. Dip umbilical stump in tincture of iodine to prevent navel ill or omphalitis
VII. Dystocia is the most significant factor affecting perinatal calf survival
  A. Direct losses are from parturient asphyxiation and injury
  B. Indirect loss is that of calves weakened by dystocia
  C. Calves that are hypoxic or injured are not as able to consume adequate colostrum
  D. Trauma may result from excessive use of obstetrical force
    1. Musculoskeletal injuries are common, such as fractures of the metacarpus, metatarsus, femur, ribs, and spine and luxations of the spine and coxofemoral joints
    2. Neurological damage such as spinal injuries and trauma to femoral and radial nerves
    3. Soft tissue trauma such as glossal edema and umbilical evisceration may be encountered

CAPRINE

Puberty

I. Doe
  A. Average age 6 to 7 months (pygmy goats could reach puberty as early as 3 months)
II. Buck
  A. Fertile at 6 to 7 months

Breeding Soundness Examination

I. Physical examination
  A. Buck should be in good body condition with a little more flesh than normal due to a possible weight loss during the breeding season
  B. Look for structural faults as diseases of the hind limbs will decrease the ability of the buck to service the does
  C. Check for footrot and foot abscesses
II. Reproductive tract examination
  A. Testes
    1. Testes should be examined for size, symmetry, and consistency
    2. Consistency of the testes during breeding should be firm to the touch, oval, and of equal size
      a. This criterion may change during the nonbreeding season or may be an indicator of poor health
  B. Epididymis
    1. Note any changes in the size, form, and consistency. Gross alterations are rare
  C. Penis
    1. Penis can be extended for examination either manually or by electroejaculation
    2. Look for any abnormalities
III. Libido
  A. Libido is difficult to measure during a routine breeding soundness examination
  B. A carefully collected history must be taken to assess libido
IV. Semen evaluation
  A. Semen can be collected and evaluated

Semen Collection Techniques and Semen Characteristics

I. Semen collection
  A. Artificial vagina (AV)
    1. No exogenous stimulus is required when using an AV
    2. The buck must be trained to use the AV by using a mount animal
  B. Bailey ejaculator or electroejaculation
    1. Due to the response by the buck, the Bailey ejaculator is not used
      a. Use of these machines results in increased vocalization and excessive muscle contractions of the hind limbs
    2. There is a greater volume of semen collected but a lower concentration of sperm using these methods

3. A combination of rectal massage with the electroejaculator and the use of direct stimulation is usually successful

II. Semen characteristics
   A. Volume: low, approximately 1 mL/ejaculate
   B. Concentration: very high
   C. Motility: swirling masses of spermatozoa are seen
      1. This swirling mass is called the wave motion

Estrous Cycle

I. Estrous cycle is approximately 21 days and is divided into two phases
   A. Follicular phase: 3 to 4 days
   B. Luteal phase: 17 days
II. Estrus (heat) is 30 to 40 hours, and ovulation occurs near the end of estrus
III. Optimal breeding time is 12 to 24 hours after the onset of estrus
IV. Seasonally polyestrous
   A. Estrous cycle is limited to the fall and winter under natural conditions
   B. Manipulations of light cycles offers year-round breeding capability of does and bucks

Signs of Estrus

I. Restlessness
II. Vocalization
III. Rapid tail wagging
IV. A "buck jar"
   A. A jar containing a rag that has been rubbed on the scent glands of the buck's horns; may be used to enhance the signs of estrus

Pregnancy Diagnosis

I. Progesterone assay: 21 days postbreeding
   A. Serum should be used instead of milk (milk gives false-negative results)
II. Estrone sulfate: 50 or more days postbreeding
III. External transabdominal ultrasound: 40 or more days postbreeding

Gestation/Stages of Parturition

I. Gestation: 149 days
II. Maintenance of pregnancy depends on luteal progesterone rather than placental progesterone
III. Cotyledonary placentation
IV. Stages of parturition
   A. Stage 1
      1. May last from 2 to 12 hours depending on the age of the dam
      2. Signs exhibited may be those of abdominal discomfort, standing and lying down, pawing at bedding, and frequent bouts of urination and defecation
      3. Appearance of the cervical seal, thick, yellow-brown mucus that indicates the cervix has relaxed
      4. Fetus, placenta, and fetal fluids are pushed forward to dilate cervix and contact the vagina
   B. Stage 2
      1. Starts with the abdominal press that indicates active labor
      2. This will last 1 to 3 hours
      3. Are routinely in lateral recumbency, but older does may stand to deliver
      4. Chorioallantois ruptures in the vagina
         a. The amnion is pushed through the vulva and ruptures, and the kid is delivered
      5. Doe may rest between kids or may continue to deliver
   C. Stage 3
      1. Delivery of the placenta or placentas and involution of the uterus occur
      2. Placenta should be passed within 1 hour of kidding
      3. After 12 hours, the placenta is considered retained
      4. Involution of the uterus may take up to 12 days
      5. There may be lochia present for up to 3 weeks

Causes of Dystocia

I. Only 3% to 5% of births require help
II. Causes
   A. Deviation of position, posture, and presentation
   B. Fetomaternal disproportion
      1. Fetal origin disproportion is when the fetus is too large to pass easily through the pelvis or vaginal canal
         a. Most often encountered with single-fetus pregnancies
      2. Maternal origin is most common in first fresheners that have not grown adequately before parturition
         a. Pelvis is not large enough for the fetus to pass through easily
         b. Other causes may be injury, ankylosis of the tail, and abscesses or tumors around the vagina
   C. Cervical dilation failure
      1. Also known as ringwomb
      2. Common cause of dystocia
      3. Predisposing causes may include hypocalcemia, hormonal or mineral imbalance, twinning, and season or breed

4. Previously dilated cervix can further complicate dystocia

D. Uterine torsion
   1. Occasional cause
   2. Typical in single-fetus pregnancies

E. Uterine inertia
   1. Primary uterine inertia
   2. Secondary uterine inertia

Neonatal Care

I. Temperature, 38.5° to 40.5° C (101° to 105° F); pulse, 80 to 120/min; respiration, 12 to 20/min

II. Umbilicus should be dipped several times in 7% tincture of iodine

III. Observe kids for normal respiration, evidence of respiratory acidosis, and other signs of fetal distress such as meconium staining

IV. Assess adequate colostrum intake
   A. Observe kids nursing from does
   B. Palpate abdomen of kid
   C. Hand feed colostrum if necessary
   D. If using cow colostrum, make sure it is free from *Mycobacterium paratuberculosis*

V. After treatment with colostrum, kids can be fed pasteurized milk or heat-treated colostrum if available

VI. Doe and kids must have an available, draft-free shelter to protect them from temperature extremes
   A. Shelter decreases the risk of hypothermia, heat stress, or pneumonia

VII. Concerns for kids
   A. For the first few days, a neonatal kid should be checked for hypothermia, hypoglycemia, and colibacillosis
   B. Cryptosporidiosis and floppy kid syndrome can be seen in kids between 3 and 10 days of age
   C. At 2 to 4 weeks of age, clinical signs of white muscle disease, copper deficiency, *Pasteurella haemolytica* pneumonia, mycoplasmosis, and coccidiosis can occur
   D. Dam-reared kids can be weaned after the age of 3 months

OVINE

Puberty

I. Ewe
   A. Average age: 6 to 7 months
   B. Minimum of 60% of their adult body weight
   C. Nutrition is important in puberty
   D. Mutton breeds tend to reach puberty earlier than wool breeds
   E. Age of puberty in ewes can be influenced by selecting a ram with a large scrotal circumference

II. Ram
   A. Fertile as early as 7.5 to 9 months but should not be considered to have adult capacity until they are at least 2 years old

Breeding Soundness Examination

I. Physical examination
   A. Structural soundness
      1. Refers to the ability of the ram to remain sound during the breeding season
      2. Examine the feet, legs, and teeth for soundness
   B. Physical soundness
      1. Refers to the overall health of the ram
      2. Examine the ram for diseases or conditions that may be transmitted to the ewe or may prevent optimal performance of the ram, such as foot rot, lip and leg ulcerations, and pizzle rot
      3. Body condition score of the ram should be a value of between 2.5 to 3.5

II. Reproductive tract examination
   A. Testes and epididymis
      1. Palpate the testicles for tone and symmetry
         a. Note any swelling, atrophy, and lack of tone or symmetry
      2. Palpate the epididymis for enlargement due to inflammation and fibrosis
         a. *Brucella ovis* is a major infective agent in epididymitis
      3. A scrotal tape should be used to measure the testes and scrotum
         a. This is an estimate of potential sperm production and fertility
         b. It is recommended by the Western Regional Coordinating Committee on Ram Epididymitis
            (1) Ram lambs over 60 kg (132 lb) should have a scrotal circumference of greater than 30 cm (12 in)
            (2) Yearling rams (12 to 18 months) should have a circumference of greater than 33 cm (13 in)
            (3) Breeding stock rams over 113 kg should have a circumference of greater than 36 cm (14 in)
   B. Prepuce and Penis
      1. Prepuce should be examined for open or ulcerated lesions at the orifice
      2. Penis should be extended and examined for injury or disease

III. Semen evaluation
   A. Semen can be collected and evaluated

IV. Ram to ewe/ewe lamb ratio

A. A healthy ram, under most range conditions, can breed 100 females in a 17-day breeding cycle

Semen Collection Techniques and Semen Characteristics

I. Semen collection
 A. Electroejaculation
 1. It is important to collect the semen in as clean a manner as possible
 a. Cells and cellular debris can interfere with proper evaluation
 2. Collection is done by alternating massage with the rectal probe and electrical stimulation
 3. Poor technique, inadequate electroejaculator stimulation, or too much voltage can affect the quality of semen collected
II. Semen characteristics
 A. Volume: low, approximately 1 mL/ejaculate
 B. Concentration: very high
 C. Motility: swirling masses of spermatozoa are seen and are called the wave motion

Estrous Cycle

I. Estrous cycle is approximately 17 days long and is divided into two phases
 A. Follicular phase: 3 to 4 days
 B. Luteal phase: 13 days
II. Estrus (heat) is 10 to 30 hours, and ovulation occurs near the end of estrus
III. Optimal breeding time is 12 to 18 hours after the first signs of estrus
IV. Ewes tend to cycle only during periods of short daylight; breeding season is usually from September to December
 A. Most breeds of sheep are seasonally polyestrus; they undergo a series of estrous cycles only during the fall
V. Shortly before or at the onset of breeding season, a ram is introduced to the ewes and the ewes will begin cycling 5 to 6 days later
 A. This is known as the "Whitten effect"

Signs of Estrus

I. Ewes will seek out the ram and remain immobile while being investigated
II. Tail wagging
III. Without a ram present, it is almost impossible to tell if a ewe is cycling

Pregnancy Diagnosis

I. Use a teaser ram (castrated male) to detect ewes returning to estrus
II. Progesterone assay: 17 to 18 days postbreeding
III. Rectal ultrasound: 30 or more days postbreeding
IV. External transabdominal ultrasound: 40 or more days postbreeding
V. Estrone sulphate: 50 or more days postbreeding

Gestation/Stages of Parturition

I. Gestation: 145 to 155 days (5 months)
II. Nutrition should be increased by 50% in the last trimester
III. First third of pregnancy depends on the corpus luteum for progesterone; after 50 days progesterone is mainly produced by the placenta
IV. Cotyledonary placentation
V. Mammary development the last 2 weeks of gestation
VI. Colostrum can be expressed 2 to 3 days before lambing
VII. Body temperature drops 0.5° C (1° to 2° F) during the last 48 hours
VIII. Stages of parturition
 A. Labor lasts approximately 1 to 4 hours
 B. Stage 1
 1. Signs of restlessness, decreased appetite, and a swollen vulva
 2. Characterized by increasing myometrial activity and the start of contractions
 3. As the cervix is dilating, myometrial activity is increasing intrauterine pressure and forcing the fetal membranes up to the cervix, causing them to rupture
 C. Stage 2
 1. As the fetus enters the cervical canal and vagina, there is a release of oxytocin, thereby increasing the myometrial contractions
 a. Aided by maternal abdominal contractions, the fetus is expelled and the risk of anoxia is minimized
 D. Stage 3
 1. Fetal membranes should be expelled within 2 hours

Causes of Dystocia

I. Fetal causes
 A. Head-only presentation
 1. Head may become swollen and edematous due to an extended time in lambing
 B. Fetopelvic disproportion
 1. Large lambs occur more often in ewes that are bred as lambs than in older ewes
 C. Malposition of the head
 1. Lateral deviation of the head and neck is more common in multiple births than in single births
 2. Plastic lamb puller can be used to correct and deliver the lamb

D. Elbow lock
E. Malposition of the forelegs
   1. Important, in multiple births, to determine that the correct fetal appendages are positioned and delivered
   2. Can palpate head and neck to determine fetal appendages
F. Breech
   1. Possible to rupture lamb's liver and fracture the ribs when delivering in this position
G. Transverse presentation
   1. Lamb's vertebral column is presented at the maternal opening
   2. Hypoxia and lamb death are common with caudal and transverse presentations
H. Ringwomb
   1. Incomplete dilation of the cervix occurs often with no known cause
   2. More common in ewe lambs

Neonatal Care

I. Temperature, 37.5° to 39.5° C (99.5° to 103° F); pulse, 100 to 150/min; respiration, 30 to 60/min
II. Lambs should be given a complete physical examination
III. Common defects
   A. Cleft palate
   B. Umbilical herniation
   C. Entropion
IV. Umbilicus should be dipped in 7% tincture of iodine
V. If lambs have not suckled within 3 hours after being born, they should be given 30 mL of colostrum
VI. Should stand and nurse within 20 minutes of delivery
   A. Maternal factors affecting the lambs attempt to nurse may be a long wool coat, pendulous udder, and enlarged teats
   B. Weak lambs or lambs born after the first of the litter may be ignored by the ewe, therefore increasing the risk of hypothermia and hypoglycemia
VII. Confine ewes and lambs to a claiming pen for the first 24 hours to optimize mothering
VIII. Health management of neonatal lambs
   A. Colostrum
      1. Require 50 mL/kg of body weight of colostrum within the first 2 hours of life and a maximum of 200 to 250 mL/kg within the first 24 hours, split into four or five feedings
   B. Supplemental immunoglobulin
      1. Bovine or caprine colostrum can be used during the first 24 hours
         a. Colostrum should be from herds that are free from pathogenic disease, such as bovine leukosis virus and caprine arthritis encephalitis virus, that may harm sheep
   C. Vitamin E and selenium supplementation
      1. If ewes have not been supplemented with selenium and are in a selenium-deficient area, lambs should receive selenium
      2. Ewes may be treated during last trimester of pregnancy if using an injectable selenium, to be repeated at intervals of no less than 14 days to a maximum of four treatments
      3. Supplements used in cattle are not recommended for pregnant ewes
      4. Vitamin A and selenium can both be fed to pregnant ewes
   D. Lamb identification
      1. Mark at birth
         a. Methods include ear tagging, paint branding, or spraying the lamb with the litter identification
   E. Contagious ecthyma vaccination
      1. If there is a history of mastitis, lamb losses, and diminished productivity, vaccinate the lambs at birth
      2. Do not vaccinate an unaffected flock or if the disease is only mildly manifested
   F. Tail dock and castration
      1. Tail docking is ideally performed within the first 24 hours in long tail breeds, but only after the lamb has received adequate colostrum
         a. Rubber bands
         b. Electric docker
      2. Dock the tail distal to the tail fold
      3. Castrate lambs up to 7 days of age if using rings or cut-and-pull technique or before 90 days if crushing
      4. Recommend vaccinating lambs with tetanus antitoxin at the time of docking or castration if ewes have inadequate immunity

PORCINE

Puberty

I. Sows
   A. Gilts normally reach puberty around 250 lb (114 kg) or about 200 days (6 to 7 months) in most breeds
II. Boars
   A. Reach puberty about 5 to 7 months
   B. They are mature about 2 years

Breeding Soundness Examination

I. Examination of reproductive tract
  A. Sheath
    1. Should be examined for pus and redness (phimosis) and abscesses, which may be noticed on palpation or observation
  B. Testes and epididymis
    1. Size of the testes is related directly to the ability of the boar to produce sperm
    2. Testes should be of equal size with visible epididymal tails
    3. On palpation, testes should be firm to turgid with no hard areas
    4. Tail and lower body of the epididymis should be palpable with a prominent tail
      a. Cysts can be found in the head and body of the epididymis but might not be easily palpated
        (1) These cysts may cause complete or partial occlusion of the epididymal duct
  C. Penis
    1. Can be examined at the time of semen collection
    2. Check for abnormalities such as persistent frenulum, bite wounds, and, rarely, an amputated penis
II. Libido
  A. In situations where there is hand mating and artificial insemination, boars with low libido are usually detected
    1. Poor libido varies from little to no interest in the sow/gilt in standing heat
III. Semen evaluation
  A. Semen can be collected and evaluated

Semen Collection Techniques and Semen Characteristics

I. Semen collection
  A. Gloved hand technique
    1. Boar is best collected with this technique on a sow in estrus or dummy sow
    2. Sometimes older boars may not collect using hand pressure
    3. Using a sow in heat and letting the boar insert the penis into the vagina until the boar starts to ejaculate will sometimes aid collection
II. Semen characteristics
  A. Volume: 8 to 12 months of age, 150 mL ejaculate
  B. Older boars: 250 mL of ejaculate
  C. Concentration: 150×10^6/mL
  D. Motility: 70% to 90% progressively motile sperm

Estrous Cycle

I. Polyestrus
II. Estrus cycle is approximately 21 days in duration
III. Standing estrus: 48 to 55 hours
IV. Return to estrus: 4 to 7 days after weaning
V. Should be bred 24 hours after the onset of estrus and every 24 hours
VI. Gilts should be bred 12 hours after the onset of estrus and repeated at 12-hour intervals

Signs of Estrus

I. Vulvar swelling
II. Restlessness
III. Alertness
IV. Receptivity to the boar
V. Stationary stance (apply moderate pressure over the loin area with the flat of your hand)

Pregnancy Diagnosis

I. Teasing sow: 18 to 24 days postbreeding
II. Ultrasound: 23 days postbreeding
III. Progesterone assay: 17 to 20 days postbreeding
IV. Estrone sulfate: 25 to 29 days postbreeding

Gestation/Stages of Parturition

I. Gestation: 114 days (3 months, 3 weeks, 3 days)
II. Diffuse placentation
III. Main source of progesterone is from the corpus luteum
IV. Abdominal and mammary development as early as 2.5 months' gestation
V. Stages of parturition
  A. Signs of impending parturition
    1. 24 Hours before parturition: the sow will lie down and rise
    2. 12 Hours before parturition: defecation and urination will increase in frequency
    3. Respiratory rate peaks about 6 hours before birth of the first piglet
    4. 3 to 4 hours before parturition, sows become restless and attempt to nest
      a. Crated animals may chew bars
      b. Sow may then rest and resume these activities up until 15 to 60 minutes before the first piglet is born
  B. Stage 2
    1. Usually lasts 1 to 5 hours
    2. For the delivery of the piglets, the sow usually remains in lateral recumbency, has mild abdominal contractions, passes a small amount of fluid, and wiggles her tail
    3. Time between piglets is 1 minute to 4 hours, but is usually under 15 minutes, depending on the number of piglets
  C. Stage 3

1. Placenta is usually expelled 21 minutes to 12.5 hours later
    a. Placentas may also be expelled between piglets
2. Retained placenta may indicate that additional piglets remain in the uterus

Causes of Dystocia

I. Less than 1% of sows show signs of dystocia
II. Symptoms of dystocia may include
  A. Prolonged gestation
  B. Anorexia and lethargy
  C. Blood-tinged vulvular discharge or the appearance of meconium without the onset of abdominal straining
  D. Abdominal straining and vulvular discharge without the passing of fetuses
  E. Cessation of abdominal straining after the birth of only a few fetuses
  F. Vulvular discharge with a foul smell and discoloration
III. Maternal dystocia
  A. Primary uterine inertia
  B. Secondary uterine inertia
  C. Uterine deviation
    1. Occurs in older sows with an increased number of piglets in the litter
    2. Uterus is pulled ventral to the brim of the pelvis, thereby blocking the passage of piglets
  D. Obstruction of birth canal
    1. Can be caused by constipation, distended bladder, hymen remnant, and swelling of the soft tissues of the birth canal
  E. Oversized piglets
    1. Most common in litters with a small number of piglets
  F. Malpresentations
    1. Account for approximately one third of fetal dystocia
    2. Simultaneous presentation of fetuses in the birth canal or breech presentation is common

Neonatal Care

I. Temperature, 36.8° to 39° C (98° to 102° F); pulse, 200 to 250/min; respiration, 50 to 60/min
II. Piglets should be placed under a heat lamp and kept warm until all piglets are born; then all are placed with the dam to suckle
III. Usually weaned at 3 to 5 weeks of age
IV. Weak, chilled piglets with poor mobility require tube feeding and warming before being placed with their litter
V. Make sure piglets receive colostrum
VI. Administer 1.0 mL injection of iron dextran
VII. Castrate young boars not being retained for breeding
VIII. Piglets are born with a limited supply of energy; therefore must receive food shortly after birth
IX. Not able to maintain deep body temperature if the environmental temperatures are decreased
  A. Area must be draft free and at least 30° C (86° F)
X. Tasks should be performed shortly after birth
  A. Dry piglets to decrease heat loss
  B. Cut umbilical cords approximately 5 cm (2 inches) from the body and dip in a mild disinfectant
  C. Clip needle teeth, notch ears, and dock tails

ACKNOWLEDGMENT

The editors and authors appreciate the original work of Betty Gregan, on which this chapter is based.

Glossary

abdominal ballottement Palpation of the fetal head by pushing the fist or fingertips into the abdominal wall, causing the fetus to move away from and then return to the fist or fingers
adenomyosis Glandular tissue invading the muscle wall of an organ (e.g., uterus)
agouti Brown/gray coat color found in some animals and wolves
allele Alternate form of a gene at the same site on a chromosome that determines different traits in an individual. Alleles may code for the same or for alternate forms of the trait
anasarca Extensive subcutaneous edema found with diseases such as congestive heart failure
ankylosis Abnormal immobilization and solidification of a joint
artificial vagina Device that is used for the collection of semen from male animals, consisting of a solid outer tube and lined by a flexible thin rubber sleeve
ascites Abnormal collection of a serous, edematous fluid in the peritoneal cavity
autosomal Used to describe nonsex chromosomes
back cross Pairing of an F_1 generation hybrid with an organism whose genotype is identical to the parental strain
body condition Examination of a body by comparison to a chart
chorioallantoic membrane Extraembryonic membrane consisting of the chorion and the allantois. In several mammals, it forms the placenta
chromosome Contains DNA (deoxyribonucleic acid), which transfers genetic information
codominance Cross where each allele makes a comparable contribution to the phenotype
colibacillosis Infection with *Escherichia coli*
colostrum Immunoglobulin-rich milk secreted from the mammary gland shortly after parturition: "first milk"

corpus luteum Formed in the ovary after ovulation; produces progesterone
cotyledonary placentation Attachment of fetal membranes to the endometrium occurring only at projections from the endometrium, as in ruminants
cryptorchid Animal with undescended testes
cryptosporidiosis Infection with *Cryptosporidium* spp., causing diarrhea
diffuse placenta When attachment of the fetal membranes of the endometrium is continuous throughout the entire surface of the fetal membrane, as in horse and pig
dihybrid cross Crossing of two traits
diploid Two copies of a chromosome in each cell or nucleus
dominant gene Gene that produces an effect in an organism regardless of the corresponding allele. A dominant gene masks or suppresses the expression of its corresponding allele. The dominant allele is usually written as a capital letter
enterocolitis Inflammation involving the small intestine and colon
entropion Turning inward of the eyelid
epididymitis Inflammation of the epididymis
epistasis Masking of one allele over the genes on another locus
$F_1 F_2$ Family or familial or filial generation
fetal monster Fetus with developmental anomalies to be classified as grotesque and often nonviable
filial Any generation following the parental generation
follicular phase Epithelial lining of the uterus hypertrophies and becomes edematous and congested
footrot Disease involving the foot, mostly caused by bacteria, characterized by dermatitis of the interdigital skin
frenulum Small fold of integuement that limits the movement of a part
freshen Cow or goat that has recently calved and is in its first 2 to 4 weeks of lactation
gene Unit of inheritance
genetics Study of similarities and differences that are passed from parent to offspring
genome All of the genes carried by a gamete (e.g., chromosomal DNA containing a complete set of hereditary factors)
genotype Genetic makeup of an individual
gestation Pregnancy
gilt A female pig used for breeding that has yet to have a litter of piglets
glossal edema Edema involving the tongue
GnRH Gonadotrophin-releasing hormone, a type of hormone that causes gonads to mature to adult state
haploid Having one copy of each chromosome per cell or nucleus
harem mating Mating where one male is mated to five or more females
hCG Human chorionic gonadotrophin, a hormone found in the urine after implantation of the ovum that is used to diagnose pregnancy
heterosis Same as hybrid vigor; a cross performed to produce a better-quality genotype and phenotype
heterozygous Different alleles, for example, Bb
homozygous Identical alleles, for example, BB
hybrid Offspring that are different than the parents
hydrocephalus A condition characterized by an abnormal build up of cerebrospinal fluid in the cerebral ventricular system
IgG Type of antibody in plasma that can cross placental barriers
inbreeding Mating of closely related individuals to produce ever-increasing similarities in the offspring
inbreeding depression Relates to traits of fitness such as early growth, resistance to disease, or fertility, which are multifunctional traits
incomplete dominance Cross in which both genes are expressed equally
inguinal hernia Hernia occurring in the groin area where the thighs meet the folds of abdominal skin
intermediate inheritance Same as incomplete dominance
karyotype Photomicrograph of a single cell in the metaphase stage (meiosis) of division that displays chromosomes in descending order and describes the number and morphology of the chromosomes. It is similar to a blueprint or fingerprint. Karyotype is also called diploid chromosome complement
LH Leutinizing hormone
lethal gene Gene that will cause the death of the embryo or cause serious impairment or death sometime after birth
line breeding Breeding of related individuals to guarantee similar traits in the offspring
lochia Discharge from the vagina occurring the first or second week after parturition
locus Specific site or location of a gene on a chromosome
lordosis Downward curvature of the spine
luteal phase Portion of the estrous cycle in which the effect of the corpus luteum is dominant and the cow is anestrous due to the increased levels of progesterone in the blood
malpresentation Faulty fetal positioning
meconium Yellow-orange gummy material contained in the intestine of a term fetus that constitutes the first stool passed by the newborn
meiosis Sex cell division that results in haploid cells and independent assortment of chromosomes
microcotyledonary placentation Microscopic grouping of villa in the equine placenta where embryo implantation occurs
mitosis Method of cell replication that creates cells identical to the parent cells
monestrus Experiencing one estrus cycle each year
monohybrid cross Crossing of one trait
mummified fetus Conversion of the fetus to a dehydrated state where the soft tissues are reduced in volume, the skin is leather like, and the tissues are deeply stained brown
myometrial contraction Contraction of the smooth muscle coat of the uterus
neonatal Newborn
neonatal isoerythrolysis Condition where there is an immunity to an alloantigen. This occurs when red blood cells from the offspring enter the maternal circulatory system. If the red blood cell antigens are different than that of the dam, this results in the production of antibodies. If there is more offspring of the same mating combination, where the offspring of the same blood type is produced, a hemolytic anemia will occur in the offspring once it has consumed the maternal antibodies contained within the colostrum
omphalitis Inflammation of the umbilicus
orchitis Inflammation of the testicles characterized by inflammation of one or both testes, pain, and sensitivity to touch. Chronic orchitis does not involve pain, but the testes may slowly swell and become hard

outbreeding Same as random breeding; matings to other strains to increase the amount of heterozygous genes
ovulation Release of the egg (ovum) from the ovarian follicle
parturition Act of giving birth
pedigree chart Chart that shows the ancestry of a particular family
penetrance Refers to the appearance in the phenotype of traits determined by the genotype
perosomus elumbus Congenital defect most common in calves and lambs. The vertebral column ends at the caudal thoracic region causing the posterior portion of the body to be joined to the front portion by soft tissue only
phantom mare Dummy mare constructed of a padded, hollow device, about the approximate height and width that would suit the stallion. It is used to collect semen for artificial insemination or semen evaluation
phenotype Physical characteristics of an individual and/or performance of an individual that is expressed
phimosis Condition where the orifice of the prepuce is constricted so that it cannot be pulled back over the glans
pizzle rot Condition, found in castrated male sheep, where there is swelling, scabby ulcerations, and inflammation of the interior/exterior of the prepuce and glans penis
pluriparous Two or more pregnancies that resulted in living offspring
polyestrous More than one estrus cycle in each year
polygenic traits Traits that are due to the interaction of several gene pairs
primary uterine inertia Sluggishness of the uterine contractions during labor due to an overstretching of the uterus, toxemia, or obesity
progesterone Steroid sex hormone that, in pregnancy, protects the embryo and fosters growth of the placenta and, in preparation for lactation, prepares the mammary glands for secretion
puberty Physical stage at which sexual reproduction is possible
Punnett square Chart used by geneticists to show possible outcomes of specific breeding. Also called a checkerboard
recessive gene Gene that produces an effect only when it is inherited from both parents. Usually written in lowercase letters
ringwomb Disease of the ewe where the cervix fails to relax so that there is no outward appearance of lambing. Full-term fetuses may die in utero
schistosomus reflexus Fetus with a cleft abdomen
seasonally polyestrus Occurs in an animal that has several estrous cycles within a breeding season, followed by anestrus until the following breeding season, as in the cat
secondary uterine inertia Sluggishness of uterine contractions during labor due to exhaustion or lack of myometrial contractions
sex chromosomes X and Y chromosomes determine the genetic sex of the individual
sickle hocks Abnormal hock joint where the foot and metatarsus are angled forward
spermatozoa Sperm
tail deflection Deflection of the tail to the side
tail docking Amputation of the tail
test cross Cross performed to determine the genotype of a particular phenotype
tetanus Fatal disease of all animal species caused by the neurotoxin of *Clostridium tetani.* The bacterial spores deposit in the tissue and, under anaerobic conditions, vegetate
transabdominal ultrasound Method of examining abdominal contents by using sound waves or ultrasound
umbilical evisceration Pushing out of the internal organs through the umbilicus
uroperitoneum Condition where the urine is free in the peritoneal cavity
uterine caruncles Fleshy masses located on the walls of the uterus of pregnant ruminants to which the uterus is attached
uterine inertia Sluggishness of uterine contractions during labor
uterine torsion Twisting of the body of the uterus in cows and mares and the uterine horn in sows, resulting in dystocia
variable expressivity Traits that show continuous variation
whelping The birthing process
zonary placentation Fetus is attached to the endometrium by a band that encircles the placenta, as in the dog and cat

Review Questions

1 A hybrid is
 a. An offspring that is different from the parents
 b. An offspring that is identical to the parents
 c. A cross between genetically identical parents
 d. A cross between physically identical parents

2 What is(are) the only accessory gland(s) in a dog?
 a. Bulbourethral glands
 b. Prostate gland
 c. Ampulla
 d. Seminal vesicles

3 The Manx cat is considered to be an example of
 a. Translocation of chromosomes
 b. The expression of a lethal gene
 c. A sex-linked anomaly
 d. A homozygous individual

4 The breeding of related individuals to guarantee similar traits in the offspring is called
 a. Outbreeding
 b. Back cross
 c. Line breeding
 d. Inbreeding

5 A homozygous animal with progressive retinal atrophy is mated to a heterozygote carrier. What is this breeding called?
 a. Inbreeding
 b. Heterosis
 c. Test cross
 d. Back cross

6 On a radiograph, the skeleton of a canine fetus can first be noted at
 a. 45 days' gestation
 b. 30 days' gestation
 c. 10 days' gestation
 d. 62 days' gestation

7 A dominant X-linked gene, B, in the mouse, results in a short, crooked tail; its recessive allele, b, represents a normal tail. If a normal-tailed female is mated to a bent-tailed male, what phenotypic ratio should occur in F_1?
 a. Three bent tail females/one normal tail male
 b. All mice will have a bent tail

c. Two normal tail females/two bent tail males
d. Two bent tail females/two normal tail males

8 Which species has a gestation period of 278 days?
a. Equine
b. Caprine
c. Ovine
d. Bovine

9 Are all genes always expressed?
a. Yes
b. No, the range of penetrance is variable
c. Yes, to some degree
d. No, some traits are polygenic and therefore require specific partners to express a phenotype

10 The three main characteristics of semen evaluation are
a. Volume, mobility, and characteristics
b. Volume, motility, and characteristics
c. Volume, motility, and concentration
d. Volume, parts per million, and concentration

BIBLIOGRAPHY

Blood DC, Studdert VP: *Saunders comprehensive veterinary dictionary,* ed 2, Toronto, 1999, WB Saunders.

Griffiths AJF et al: *An introduction to genetic analysis,* ed 6, New York, 1996, WH Freeman and Company.

Hafez ESE: *Reproduction in farm animals,* ed 5, Philadelphia, 1993, Lea & Febiger.

Lofstedt RM: *Reproductive physiology of the domestic species,* Prince Edward Island, Canada, 1987, University of Prince Edward Island.

Lofstedt RM, Richardson GF: *A manual for theriogenology,* ed 6, Prince Edward Island, Canada, University of Prince Edward Island.

McCurnin DM, Bassert JM: *Clinical textbook for veterinary technicians,* ed 5, Philadelphia, 2002, WB Saunders.

McKinnon V: *Equine reproduction,* Philadelphia, 1993, Lea & Febiger.

Nelson RW: *Canine and feline endocrinology and reproduction,* Toronto, 1987, WB Saunders.

Rose RJ, Hodgson DR: *Manual of equine practice,* Toronto, 1993, WB Saunders.

Sutton T: *Introduction to animal reproduction,* ed 2, Vermilion, Alberta, Canada, 2000, EI Sutton Consulting Ltd.

Tamarin R: *Principles of genetics,* ed 3, Dubuque, IA, 1991, Wm C Brown.

Youngquist RS: *Current therapy in large animal theriogenology,* Toronto, 1997, WB Saunders.

CHAPTER 14

Companion Animal Behavior

Patricia Bonnot

OUTLINE

LEARNING OUTCOMES

After reading this chapter you should be able to:

1. Describe in chronological order the behavioral development of the dog and the cat.
2. Describe the social behavior of the dog and the cat.
3. Describe various methods of preventing behavior problems.
4. Identify intervention techniques that may be used to eliminate or modify abnormal behavior.
5. Describe some common behavior problems in the dog and the cat.
6. Identify abnormal behavior problems.

The study of contemporary animal behavior is based on objective information. The veterinary technician uses a nonverbal, interspecies communication system each time an animal is efficiently manipulated. Accurate knowledge about a species' typical behavior has applications for all animal-related fields.

The primary role of the veterinary technician in behavior counseling is to educate pet owners about normal animal behavior and to provide accurate information about the cause and resolution of behavior problems. The goals of this chapter are to review behavioral theories and to provide some understanding of normal companion animal behavior.

NORMAL CANINE BEHAVIOR

Dogs are highly social animals, and it is well documented that social isolation to varying degrees during critical developmental periods results in various abnormal behavior patterns.

Behavioral Development

I. Characterized by five major phases
   A. Neonate period (0 to 14 days): completely dependent on mother for survival
   B. Transitional period (14 to 21 days): rapid development
   C. Socialization period (3 to 16 weeks): critical period in the formation of social relationships
      1. During weeks 3 to 8, dogs socialize best with other dogs
      2. During weeks 5 to 7 through 12, dogs socialize best with humans
      3. During weeks 5 to 12 through 16, dogs adapt best to novel environments
      4. At approximately 8.5 weeks, substrate preferences for elimination are developed
      5. At 7 to 10 weeks, a fear period is observed where painful or traumatic situations should be avoided
   D. Juvenile period (10 weeks to sexual maturity): learning capacities develop
   E. Adult period (after sexual maturity): continues to learn about environment and add new behaviors

Social Behavior

The domestic dog spends much of its time solely in the company of humans and views its human family as its own pack. Dogs use elements of their normal social behavior to communicate with their pack.

I. A complex social system relies on effective communication through vision, olfaction, auditory means, and physical contact
  A. Visual communication: body postures important (see Figure 14–3)
    1. Dominance gestures: tail held high, head up, ears erect direct eye contact
    2. Subordinate gestures: tail low and wagging, dog rolling on back and presenting inguinal area, nuzzling and licking face of other animal
    3. Display of ritualized gestures: threat, bluff attack, and play-soliciting behavior
  B. Olfactory communication
    1. Via deposition of signals in the environment
      a. Feces and urine or the particular odor of the animal itself
        (1) "Inspection" of the head and anal regions
  C. Vocal communication
    1. Bark (most common): used in defense, in play, as a greeting, or as a general call for attention
    2. Growl: used in defense, warning, or as a threat
    3. Whimpering/whining: used in submission, greeting, or pain
    4. Howl: used primarily when alone—probably for seeking social contact

NORMAL FELINE BEHAVIOR

The domestic cat is a very adaptable, territorial animal that is usually described as asocial. Cats also experience sensitive periods in their development, but these periods are not as well defined as in dogs. Much of a kitten's basic personality is inherited, with a distinct portion influenced by the sire.

Behavioral Development

I. Characterized by five major phases
  A. Neonate period (0 to 14 days): complete dependence on mother for survival
  B. Transitional period (14 to 21 days): increasing independence
  C. Socialization period (3 to 14 weeks): all primary social bonds are formed
    1. During weeks 3 to 5, predatory behavior develops
    2. During weeks 3 to 14, play behavior develops
      a. Locomotory play may be solitary or social, includes running, rolling, jumping, and climbing
      b. Object play may be solitary or social
      c. Social play, with conspecifics, includes wrestling, rolling, and biting
      d. Critical period for socialization to humans begins at 2 to 3 weeks and tapers off by 7 weeks
      e. Critical period for socialization to other cats is 3 to 6 weeks; cats raised in isolation may never adapt to another cat
  D. Juvenile period (14 weeks to sexual maturity): no significant behavioral changes
    1. Improved motor skills and coordination
  E. Adult period (after sexual maturity): behavior can change; may become increasingly independent

Social Behavior

Although the cat may prefer solitude, small social groups may be formed. The social order of cats is influenced by place, time of day, presence of food, and population density. The maintenance of social systems relies on the transmission of information between individuals and groups to minimize close interactions.

I. Vocal communication
  A. Cats can vocalize many sounds and tones
  B. Vocalization is a learned and an instinctive behavior; for example, kittens can hiss before their eyes open
II. Olfactory communication
  A. Provides information regarding individual sexual identity, time spent at location, and reproductive stage
    1. Urine spraying is commonly used for scent marking, particularly by intact males
    2. Feces is seldom used as scent markers; cats often cover feces; however, territorial cats may leave feces uncovered in conspicuous areas
    3. Rubbing behavior: cats may deposit secretions from large sebaceous glands onto objects or individuals
III. Visual communication
  A. Facial features reflect a cat's mood (Figure 14–1)
    1. An undisturbed cat has erect ears, relaxed whiskers in an outward position, normal pupils
    2. A disturbed cat has
      a. Flattened ears
      b. Whiskers flat (defensive) or pulled forward (offensive)

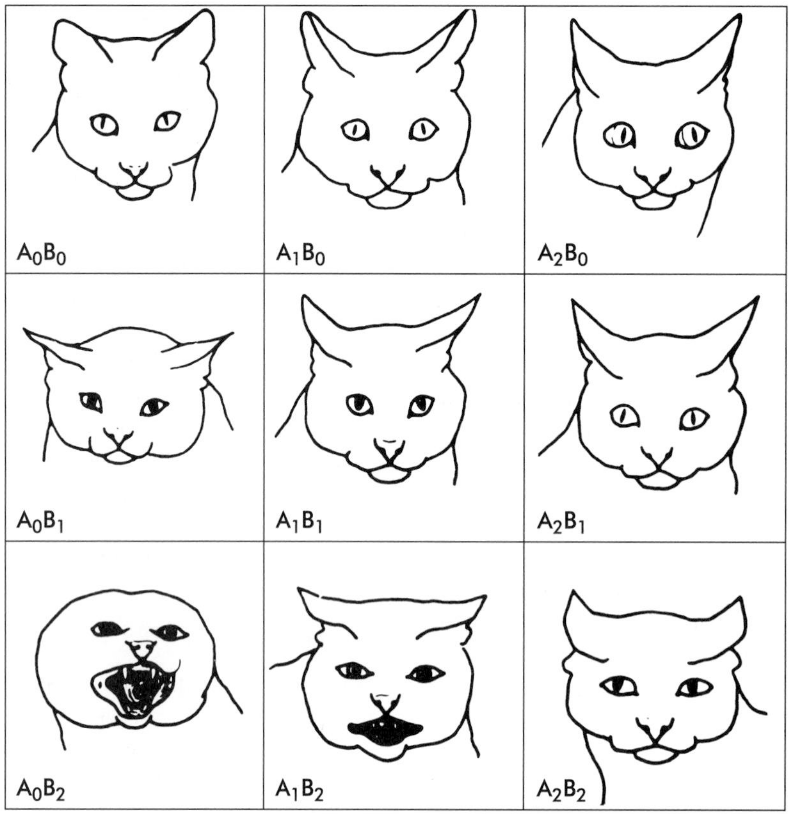

Figure 14-1 Facial expressions of the cat. Aggressiveness is increasing from A0 to A2; fearfulness, from B0 to B2. (From Leyhausen P: *Cat behavior: the predatory and social behavior of domestic and wild cats,* New York, 1979, Garland STPM Press.)

c. Pupils constricted (offensive) or dilated (defensive)
d. Lips pulled back baring the teeth; nose wrinkled

B. Clawing or scratching
   1. Secondary olfactory cues may be left by sweat glands on the paws after scratching objects

C. Body postures also reflect a cat's mood (Figure 14–2)
   1. Friendly cat: carries tail in an upright position
   2. Frightened cat: exhibits a defensive threat posture (body arched laterally, piloerection, and tail held close to body or erect)
   3. Angry cat: exhibits an offensive threat posture (hindquarters elevated, tail held straight out from body then abruptly bending downward, tail tip twitching from side to side)
   4. Play: solicitation postures include rolling over to expose abdominal area, an inverted U-shaped tail position

APPLIED ANIMAL BEHAVIOR

Behavior problems are the biggest threat to the human–animal bond. Most of the behavioral complaints of pet owners are management-related problems that can be prevented or modified by early intervention. Correcting a problem may save an animal's life.

Preventing Behavior Problems

Behavior can be influenced by a multitude of variables: environment, physiology, experience, learning, and genetic predisposition.

I. Pet selection
   A. Many pet owners choose animals that are unsuitable for their lifestyles
   B. Before acquiring a pet, clients should be advised to research species, breed, grooming and exercise needs, required medical care, and reliable sources
   C. Many dog breeders use puppy aptitude (temperament) testing as a general guide for matching pets to people
      1. This test attempts to predict a puppy's future temperament and suitability for a specific task such as obedience trial competition
      2. Because environment has a major role in behavior, the test cannot guarantee that a dog will not develop behavior problems in the future

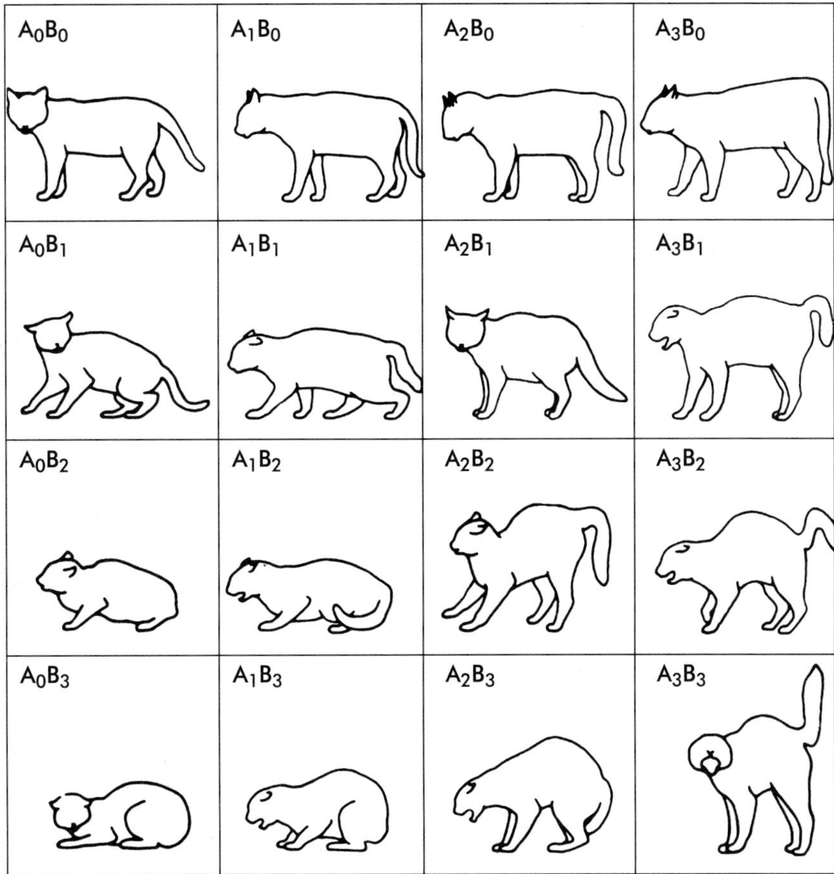

Figure 14-2 Body postures of the cat. Aggressiveness is increasing from A0 to A3; fearfulness, from B0 to B3. (From Leyhausen P: *Cat behavior: the predatory and social behavior of domestic and wild cats,* New York, 1979, Garland STPM Press.)

D. Kittens that come from known sources and have been well socialized by early and extensive handling are more likely to become calm, tractable pets

II. Dog training classes can provide an excellent opportunity for interaction between pet and owner and serve to socialize pets to other dogs
   A. "Puppy class" can start from 8 weeks of age as long as the puppy has received his first vaccination
   B. A good "puppy class" will benefit
      1. Puppies (socialization and learning good manners)
      2. Owners (learning how to prevent behavior problems such as house soiling)
      3. Veterinary clinic (owners will keep their dogs longer because of a sound human-animal bond and less behavior problems)
   C. A qualified instructor teaches owners to implement good manners and basic verbal commands with a positive method and no physical punishment
   D. Owners learn about variability in response to training and may be alerted to a potential behavior problem
   E. Obedience training alone will not remedy all behavioral complaints
   F. A physical method to control a dog is the use of a head halter such as Gentle Leader (Premier Pet Products) or a Promise Collar
      1. This type of behavior suppression provides a calming effect
   G. Other types of training, such as agility, Frisbee, flyball, and skijoring, may help to develop a strong bond between dog and owner as well as improve the physical and mental state of the dog

Intervention Techniques

The veterinary technician must be able to interpret canine and feline behavior and provide pet owners with sound information on the early recognition of potential problem behavior. Patients with extreme behavior problems are best referred to a professional animal behaviorist.

I. Before any intervention for a behavior problem is begun, a thorough behavioral history must be obtained
   A. An exhaustive interview with the owner should be done. The nature, the frequency, and the context must be described as precisely as possible by the owner
II. Possible medical causes of a behavior problem should be evaluated by a veterinarian
III. Major areas of intervention
   A. A combination of techniques is often necessary to solve a problem successfully
      1. Environmental modification
         a. Example: reducing the number of cats in a household may reduce spraying behavior
      2. Physiological intervention
         a. Example: Castration may eliminate roaming, urine marking, and intermale aggression
         b. Drug therapy: rarely curative alone
            (1) Veterinarians have access to a range of drugs to help treat pathological behavior
            (2) Drug therapy must be combined with a behavior modification program to be effective
         c. Disease alters physiological status of animals and consequently effects behavior
            (1) Example: The most sweet and gentle housedog could become aggressive toward children if he is in pain
      3. Behavior modification: through behavior-modification techniques, veterinary technicians can assist pet owners with behavior problems. All techniques use the principles of learning
         a. Operant conditioning (positive reinforcement): a pleasant stimulus (e.g., food) after a behavior; increases the probability of a behavior being repeated
            (1) To be effective, reinforcement must immediately follow the desired behavior
               (a) The timing between the behavior and the reinforcement is critical
            (2) Repetition: response will be stronger if a behavior is reinforced each time
            (3) After a behavior is learned, intermittent reinforcement results in a persistent response
         b. Negative reinforcement: occurs when an animal performs a behavior to avoid an aversive stimulus
            (1) Also serves to increase the probability of that behavior being repeated
         c. Shaping: reinforcement of a sequence of steps (pieces of behavior) that will lead to a complex behavior
            (1) By selectively reinforcing successive approximations of a desired behavior, a new behavior eventually develops
         d. Punishment: application of an aversive stimulus immediately after a behavior serves to decrease the probability the behavior will be repeated
            (1) Most misused behavioral modification technique
            (2) Insufficient by itself because it does not teach appropriate behavior (it only teaches an animal what not to do)
         e. Extinction: withholding or removing reinforcement for a previously reinforced behavior that causes the behavior to cease. It is very difficult to implement because if the behavior is reinforced only once by mistake, it becomes an intermittent reinforcement, which is the most efficient reinforcement technique
         f. Counterconditioning: conditioning an animal to engage in behavior that is incompatible with the undesirable behavior
            (1) Example: teach "sit" to avoid jumping on visitor
         g. Systematic desensitization: process of exposing an animal to a stimulus beginning at an intensity that does not evoke the undesirable response and increasing the intensity in small increments so that the stimulus eventually loses its ability to evoke the undesirable response
            (1) Frequently used to eliminate anxiety or fear response
            (2) Systematic desensitization and counterconditioning (usually implemented simultaneously)
            (3) It is a long, step-by-step process that will not work if a step is skipped
         h. Habituation: when no consequences follow an animal's response to a stimulus, that response habituates or diminishes

COMMON BEHAVIOR PROBLEMS

Canine

Most behavior problems considered undesirable by pet owners are manifestations of normal behavior.

Canine Aggression

Aggression is the most common behavioral complaint of pet owners (Figure 14–3).

I. Aggressive behavior is classified according to the stimulus or circumstances: dominance, possessive, territorial, predatory, play induced, fear induced, pain induced, disease induced, intermale, maternal, learned, irritable, and redirected
II. Factors affecting the development of aggression are inheritability, hormonal, and learning
III. Aggression is not the result of a single cause
IV. Early warning signs usually can be recognizable
V. Not uncommon for a dog to develop more than one type of aggressive behavior problem
VI. Aggression to household members is an extremely common problem
  A. Puppies often show aggression toward their owners
  B. Many dogs that are aggressive often show the signs of conflict behavior
    1. Conflicted body language is usually observed by the owner
      a. After the dog attacks, it may seem remorseful or submissive
  C. Aggressive dogs do not necessarily have a dominant personality
  D. Most aggressive behavior directed toward the owner is based on conflict or fear
VII. Intervention procedures
  A. A thorough background evaluation of the aggression must be performed by the technician or the veterinarian to suggest the right intervention
  B. Castration: especially helpful in intermale dominance and territorial aggression
  C. Rethink dog-owner relationship
    1. Dominating an aggressive dog will not help in most cases
  D. Punishment is contraindicated for aggression
  E. Counterconditioning and desensitization provide the most effective treatment
  F. Drug therapy
  G. Castration and drug therapy: of limited use unless combined with behavioral modification
VIII. Note: problems involving aggression are controlled, never cured

Barking

The most common behavioral complaint of the neighborhood!

I. Remember that barking is a "normal" canine behavior
II. Barking can be initiated by numerous factors
  A. Territorial: e.g., doorbell alarm
  B. Stress: e.g., separation anxiety
  C. Attention: e.g., disruption of household routine or activities
  D. Medical problem (mostly with older dog)
III. Intervention procedures
  A. Counterconditioning and desensitization: most effective
  B. Train to be "quiet" and obedient
  C. Reduce access to windows and doors
  D. Cage training
  E. Antibarking devices: can be effective but BE CAREFUL; it can aggravate the problem if the barking is due to anxiety. The owner should learn proper use by an experienced trainer
  F. Drug therapy (for extreme case of anxiety barking)
  G. Debarking surgery: last alternative if owner is unwilling to apply other techniques

House Soiling

Must differentiate cause with behavioral history.

I. House soiling due to lack of or ineffective house training
  A. Urination and/or defecation usually unrelated to the presence or absence of the owner
  B. Large pools of urine often in one or a few locations
  C. Intervention procedures
    1. Puppies can be housetrained from 4 weeks of age

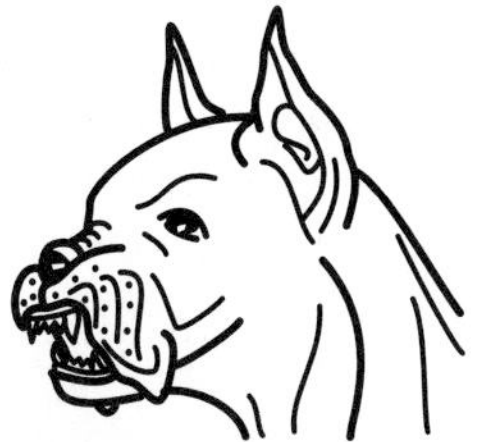
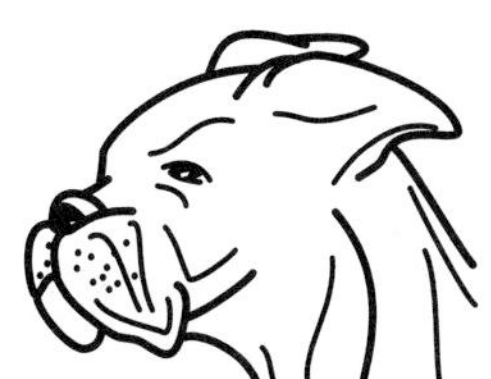
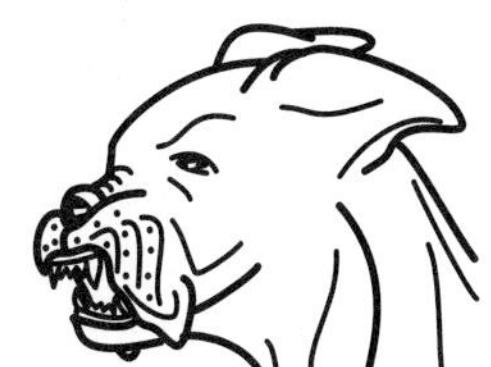

Figure 14–3 A dog's expression at strong aggression *(left)* and pronounced fear *(middle)*, and a mood that contains aggression and fear *(right)*.

2. Dog should be supervised 100% of the time or confined (cage train)
3. Set a regular routine to go outside
   a. After each meal and large drink
   b. After each nap or long period of sleep
   c. After play session or excitement
4. Scolding or rubbing the puppy's nose in excrement is not recommended
5. Reward appropriate behavior immediately when it eliminates outside
6. Owner should learn the body language of the dog before it eliminates

II. House soiling due to territorial marking
   A. Usually male dogs mark their territory after reaching sexual maturity. However, a mature female may also demonstrate the marking of their territory
   B. Unrelated to presence or absence of owner
   C. Small numerous spots of urine are evident
   D. Intervention procedures
      1. Castration
      2. Short-term progestin therapy in conjunction with behavior modification
      3. Punishment may be partially effective (only if caught in act)
      4. Aversive condition: association of an aversive stimulus with a particular location

III. House soiling due to separation anxiety
   A. Urination and/or defecation combined with other behaviors such as vocalization and destruction
   B. Occurs consistently and only when the dog is left alone: usually within 30 minutes after the owner's departure
   C. Factors correlating with the development of the problem
      1. Excessive greeting behaviors
      2. Strong attachment to owner
      3. Change in routine
   D. Intervention procedures
      1. Behavior modification program of counterconditioning and desensitization or habituation techniques to increase the tolerance of the dog to be alone
      2. Antianxiety drug therapy
      3. Cage training will secure the dog. Toys and treats to chew will help to prevent the self-trauma caused by excessive anxiety
      4. Increase in the physical exercise as well as the daily training session (mental exercise) will tire out the dog and decrease the level of anxiety

IV. House soiling due to submissive or excitement-motivated urination
   A. Urination accompanied by excited greeting and submissive body postures
   B. Most often seen in puppies
   C. Intervention procedures
      1. Avoid dominant gestures (e.g., direct eye contact)
      2. Control greeting: keep it low key
      3. Counterconditioning where calm behavior and nonsubmissive postures are rewarded
      4. Punishment will exacerbate the problem
   D. Problem may resolve as puppies mature

V. House soiling due to fear or phobia
   A. Urination or defecation as a consequence of a fear-induced stimulus (e.g., thunderstorm)
   B. Intervention procedures
      1. Source of fear must be identified
      2. Counterconditioning and desensitization program
      3. In some extreme cases, drug therapy could be used

Feline

The most common behavior problem reported by cat owners is elimination: urination or defecation outside the litterbox. This is distinct from spraying, a territorial marking behavior.

Spraying Characteristics

I. Cat assuming standing posture
II. Backing up against a vertical object
III. Releasing urine several inches above the ground
IV. Tail typically may quiver
V. Occurs more frequently in intact males; however, castrated males and spayed females can spray urine
VI. Associated with social conflict and competitive or sexual behavior
VII. Direct relationship exists between the number of cats in a household and the probability of spraying
VIII. May become a habit even if initiating stimulus is no longer present
IX. Intervention procedures
   A. Difficult to resolve because it is difficult to identify the eliciting stimulus
   B. Neutering is always recommended
   C. Modify locations
      1. Make marking areas aversive with unpleasant odors (e.g., muscle rubs) or uncomfortable substrate (e.g., aluminum foil)
      2. Change significance of the area by placement of food, toys, or catnip
      3. Punishment or aversive conditioning may be successful
   D. Resolve conflicts with other cats

1. Increase space available per cat (e.g., cat condos, allowing an indoor cat outdoors)
2. Barricade windows to prevent indoor cats from viewing neighboring cats
3. Antianxiety drug therapy

Elimination Problems

I. Elimination problems can be resolved by changing various components of the litterbox and/or making inappropriate areas less attractive

II. Common causes of elimination outside the litterbox are surface preferences, location preferences, and/or fear associated with the litterbox

III. Intervention procedures

A. Techniques to increase litterbox attractiveness
1. Change style of litterbox (e.g., change covered box to an open box)
2. Keep litterbox clean: remove feces daily
3. Provide at least one litterbox per cat
4. Respect privacy: litterbox should not be in high-traffic, noisy area
5. Odors associated with certain litter may be offensive to cat (e.g., chlorophyll)
6. Changes to litter type, if necessary, should be gradual
7. Plastic litterboxes should be replaced periodically
8. Cats favor fine-ground clumping litters

B. Techniques to decrease elimination at inappropriate locations
1. Clean area and remove odor of elimination
2. Repel cat with aversive odors (e.g., mothballs)
3. Change significance of the area: place food, toys, or catnip in the area

C. Other factors involved in elimination problems
1. Learned preference for scratching on a nonlitter substrate (e.g., carpet under the litterbox)
2. Learned location preferences or aversions
   a. An aversion to the litterbox can develop if pain or something unpleasant is associated with the litterbox
   b. May require a new litterbox, different substrate, a new location, and/or counterconditioning and desensitization techniques
3. Conflict involving another member of the household (animal or human)

Furniture Scratching

I. Scratching is a normal inherited behavior of cats that serves to condition claws

II. It is also a means of visual and olfactory marking and stretching for the front limbs

III. Early learning, genetic variability, and the cat's physical environment have a profound effect on the severity and intensity of scratching behavior within a household

IV. Household scratching can be prevented by providing a suitable scratching post in a prominent location, preferably near the kitten's sleeping area

V. Intervention procedures

A. Minimize damage to furniture by keeping claws trimmed

B. Behavior modification
1. Positive reinforcement (e.g., food, toys, catnip) can make a scratching post more appealing

C. Punishment (e.g., loud noise, water squirt, a tin can filled with rocks and thrown near the cat when caught scratching)

D. Modify environment by moving or covering furniture
1. Place double-sided tape on the specific spot
2. Cats hate the sticky sensation!

E. Restrict access to scratching area

F. Allow cat outdoors

G. Declawing: alternative if owner is unwilling to use retraining techniques

Feline Aggression

I. Intercat

A. Aggression toward other cats
1. Males fighting with other male cats
2. Aggression between cats that have recently been introduced or have known each other since kittenhood
3. Aggression usually occurs when one of the cats becomes socially mature

B. Intervention procedures
1. Neuter all cats and trim nails
2. Separate the cats; the aggressor should be moved to another location
3. Antianxiety drugs may be useful
4. In some cases the removal of one cat from the household may be required

II. Play aggression

A. Play aggression is usually directed toward people
1. It can be associated with early weaning from the mother

B. Intervention techniques
1. Avoid the circumstances that encourage the cat to play in a rough manner
   a. Do not play roughly with the cat at any time
   b. Use a toy to play with instead of your hand

2. Give the cat more toys and acceptable playthings
3. Put a bell on the cat's collar as a early warning system for sneak attacks
4. Trim nails of cat and provide a scratching post
5. If aggressive play behavior persists, ignore the cat
   a. Many times aggressive behavior is attention-getting behavior, ignoring the cat may train the cat to play calmly

III. Redirected aggression
   A. More common in cats than in dogs
      1. Aggressive behavior, which is directed away from the actual stimulus toward another cat or human as a substitution for the stimulus
      2. Many times this behavior is unexpected and inappropriate and produces a fear response in the target substitution
   B. Intervention techniques
      1. Identify the stimulus for aggressive behavior
         a. Example: a cat or bird outside the window
      2. Separate the cats when not supervised
      3. Put a bell on the aggressor as an early warning system
      4. Pay more attention to the victim cat
      5. Startle the aggressor when the first signs of aggression are noticed
         a. Signs include hissing, ears down, piloerection, or aggressive movement toward the victim
      6. Remove aggressor from the household as the last resort

ABNORMAL BEHAVIOR PROBLEMS: OBSESSIVE/COMPULSIVE DISORDERS AND STEREOTYPICAL BEHAVIORS

I. Usually described as maladaptive or inappropriate and sometimes self-destructive

II. Often expressions of normal species—typical behaviors such as grooming, vocalization, and locomotion

III. Etiology
   A. Strong genetic influence
   B. Disease
   C. Conflict induced by environment

IV. Intervention procedures
   A. Environmental management
   B. Environmental enrichment
      1. For cats: box to hide, shelves to climb, food hidden
      2. For dogs: food hidden in toy (Kong, Buster Cube), chewing toys
   C. Increase in the physical exercise as well as the daily training session (mental exercise)
   D. Counterconditioning behavioral therapy
   E. Drug therapy

V. Examples of stereotypical behavior in the dog
   A. Acral-like dermatitis (lick granuloma)
   B. Flank sucking (usually Doberman pinchers)
   C. Tail chasing, circling, and whirling
   D. Fly catching

VI. Examples of stereotypical behavior in the cat
   A. Excessive self-licking and hair chewing
   B. Wool sucking (usually Siamese cats)
   C. Tail biting

ACKNOWLEDGMENT

The editors and author recognize and appreciate the original work of Linda Campbell, on which this chapter is based.

Glossary

aggression Angry and destructive behavior toward another animal or a human

auditory Pertaining to the ear or sense of hearing

aversive Unpleasant

behavior modification Use of various techniques to alter behavior

conspecifics Members of the same species

counterconditioning Technique used to change undesirable behavior by engaging the animal in another behavior that is different from the first behavior

extinction Fading of a conditioned response as a result of nonreinforcement

habituation technique Disappearance of a conditioned reflex by repetition of the conditioned stimulus

negative reinforcement Use of punishment to modify an existing form of a response

olfaction Act of smelling

operant conditioning Type of learning in which a stimulus produces a response and that response is rewarded

piloerection Erection of hair

positive reinforcement Use of a reward to modify an existing form of a response

psychoactive drugs Drugs that modify mental activity

shaping Learning technique in which the animal is rewarded for behavior that resembles the wanted behavior and in gradual succession, is eventually only rewarded for the exaggerated behavior

socialization period Critical age when young animals establish social relationships

stereotypical behavior Anxiety-related disorder such as obsessive-compulsive disorder

successive approximation Consecutively reinforce a close estimate of the desired behavior

systemic desensitization Gradual exposure to stimulus that elicits a response

Review Questions

1 Castration of a male dog will help to eliminate which type of aggressive behavior?
a. Territorial aggression
b. Fear-induced aggression
c. Predatory aggression
d. Redirected aggression

2 Which of the following criteria cannot be modified to affect an animal's behavior?
a. Heritability
b. Physical condition
c. Environment
d. Training

3 In an attempt to shape a new behavior in a dog, which of the following criteria would be least appropriate?
a. Persistence
b. Patience
c. Timing of reward
d. Punishment when dog makes a mistake

4 A 2-year-old dog has developed an intense fear of the vacuum cleaner. Which behavior modification technique would most likely be successful?
a. Punishment
b. Counterconditioning and desensitization
c. Confinement
d. Drug therapy: tranquilize the dog

5 A family wishes to adopt a 4-month-old puppy from a breeder. Which question is least significant?
a. What is the puppy's choice of substance for elimination?
b. Has the puppy been socialized to other dogs and different people?
c. Has the puppy been exposed to novel environments?
d. Do the parents show signs of dominant aggressive behavior?

6 When trying to remove a frightened cat from a kennel, which body postures are you least likely to see?
a. Tail carried upright
b. Pupils dilated
c. Ears flattened against head
d. Crouched position

7 Marking behavior in cats is indicative of
a. Poor nutrition
b. Dirty environment
c. Conflict
d. Lack of attention

8 A young cat that was bottle-fed as an orphan exhibits excessively rough and persistent play with its family. What is a possible developmental cause for this type of play aggression?
a. Lack of socialization to humans
b. Lack of social play
c. Lack of maternal bond
d. Insufficient environmental enrichment

9 A 1-year-old neutered male cat attacks his neutered littermate after watching a strange cat through the window. This is an example of
a. Intermale aggression
b. Territorial aggression
c. Redirected aggression
d. Dominance aggression

10 A 5-year-old spayed dog suddenly starts to urinate on the carpet overnight. The first step an owner should take is to
a. Punish the dog
b. Confine the dog overnight
c. Have the dog examined by a veterinarian
d. Enroll the dog in obedience classes

BIBLIOGRAPHY

Beaver V: *Feline behavior: a guide for veterinarians,* Philadelphia, 1992, WB Saunders.

Borchelt PL: Cat elimination behavior problems. *Vet Clin North Am Small Anim Pract* 21:257, 1991.

Burghardt WF: Behavioral medicine as a part of a comprehensive small animal medical program, *Vet Clin North Am Small Anim Pract* 21:343, 1991.

Campbell WE: *Behavior problems in dogs,* ed 2, Goleta, CA, 1992, American Veterinary Publications, Inc.

Fox MW: *The dog: its domestication and behavior,* Malabar, FL, 1978, Krieger Publishing Company.

Hart BK: *The behavior of domestic animals,* New York, 1985, WH Freeman and Company.

Hetts S: Animal behavior. In McCurnin DM, Bassert JM, editors: *Clinical textbook for veterinary technicians,* ed 5, Philadelphia, 2002, WB Saunders.

Jackson J, Anderson RK: *Early learning for puppies to socialize and promote good behavior,* London, Ontario, 1999, Professional Animal Behavior Associates Inc.

Landsberg GM: Feline scratching and destruction and the effects of declawing, *Vet Clin North Am Small Anim Pract* 21:265, 1991.

Luesher A: *Canine aggression,* London, Ontario, 2001, Professional Animal Behavior Associates.

Luesher WA, McKeown DB, Halip J: Stereotypic or obsessive-compulsive disorders in dogs and cats, *Vet Clin North Am Small Anim Pract* 21:401, 1991.

Overall KL: *Clinical behavioral medicine for small animals,* St Louis, 1997, Mosby.

Pedersen NC: *Feline husbandry, disease and management in the multiple cat environment,* Goleta, CA, 1991, American Veterinary Publications, Inc.

Thorne C, editor: *The Waltham book of dog and cat behavior,* New York, 1992, Pergamon Press.

CHAPTER 15

Small Animal Nutrition

Frances Federbush-Cheslo

OUTLINE

LEARNING OUTCOMES

After reading this chapter you should be able to:

1. Explain the six basic nutrients and their role in supporting life.
2. Understand and calculate a companion animal's maintenance energy requirements based on its particular life stage.
3. Explain why different nutrient levels change with each life stage and what effects excesses or deficiencies may have.
4. Identify key factors that can prevent or help manage FLUTD.
5. Identify, understand, and assist in the management and/or prevention of an obese cat or dog.
6. Understand the role of nutritional management in the aid of the critically ill patient.
7. Identify and describe the various components of a pet food label.
8. Understand the necessary information required to help pet owners make an educated decision of which pet food to feed their animal.
9. Understand a technician's role as a source of information for pet owners about small animal nutrition.

The most commonly asked question of a veterinary technician is "What should I feed my pet?" This chapter will allow a veterinary technician to properly and confidently counsel clients about the dietary requirements of their pets. The importance of small animal nutrition in health management has become increasingly recognized in the past decade. The veterinary technician must be knowledgeable about the commonly used pet foods purchased by the hospital's clients to appropriately respond to questions.

BASIC NUTRITION

To understand what diet is best for a companion animal, one must first understand what nutrients are required by the body for each life stage. A basic understanding of the following six nutrients is essential in discussing small animal nutrition.

ENERGY-PRODUCING NUTRIENTS

Protein

I. Made up of 23 amino acids, the building blocks of proteins
  A. Essential amino acids
    1. Must be present in the diet to manufacture a protein
    2. Cats specifically require taurine in their diet
      a. Taurine deficiency could result in dilated cardiomyopathy, retinal atrophy, or infertility
  B. Nonessential amino acids
    1. Amino acids that the animal can manufacture if not available in the body
    2. Dog can synthesize 10 amino acids; cat can synthesize 11 amino acids

II. Constituent of muscle, hair, blood, organs, etc. and forms hormones and enzymes

III. Excess protein will be burned for energy and can provide 4 kcal/g if energy not obtained from carbohydrates or fat

IV. Only after protein has been used for building body tissues and facilitating certain hormonal processes and other body functions, will it be used for energy
  A. This use of protein for energy is less efficient versus energy derived from fats or carbohydrates

V. Biological value
  A. Evaluates protein usability by the body
  B. Relationship between percent of nutrients digested, absorbed, and retained to the percent of nutrients lost
  C. The greater number of essential amino acids in a protein, the greater its biological value and quality

VI. Animal and plant proteins vary in their composition of essential amino acids
  A. Reciprocally, a combination of both sources of protein in a diet can be complementary and result in a higher biological value

VII. Cats are carnivores and have a higher protein requirement than dogs because they use a certain amount of protein for energy

Carbohydrates

I. Primary function is for energy
  A. Carbohydrates provide 4 kcal/g, same as protein; however, there are no nitrogenous end products as in protein catabolism

II. Made up of carbon, hydrogen, and oxygen chains

III. Two categories, based on digestibility
  A. Soluble: digestible carbohydrates primarily composed of monosaccharides and disaccharides such as glucose and sugar beet
    1. They supply calories to a diet and can be used immediately for energy
  B. Insoluble: indigestible carbohydrates, primarily composed of polysaccharides such as starch, lignin, and peanut hulls (fiber)
    1. The portion of a plant that resists digestion and can provide satiety and bulk to a diet

IV. Digested through the digestive tract
  A. Often used in the management of constipation and diarrhea due to their ability to absorb water, stimulate intestinal contractions, and normalize intestinal transit time

V. Fiber and other insoluble carbohydrates aid in regulating blood glucose levels, which is often recommended in managing diabetes

VI. Fiber is also used in pet foods to increase bulk and promote satiety during periods of weight loss and weight control

VII. Body uses carbohydrates primarily in the form of glucose
  A. If not used, carbohydrates are stored as glycogen in the muscle or liver or as body fat

Fats

I. Provide the most concentrated source of energy at 9 kcal/g of fat

II. Enhance palatability and caloric density of pet foods

III. Required by the fat-soluble vitamins A, D, E, and K for absorption, transportation, and storage

IV. Essential fatty acid (EFA)
  A. Building blocks of fat
  B. Classified as saturated and unsaturated
    1. Saturated: long carbon chains without a double bond
    2. Unsaturated: one or more double bonds
  C. Essential for maintaining skin and coat
  D. Required for the synthesis of cell membranes, prostaglandins, and sex hormones
  E. Three EFAs are required for normal metabolism
    1. Linoleic acid
    2. Arachidonic acid
    3. Linolenic acid
  F. Dogs require linoleic and linolenic acids in their diet. Although one can be reconstructed by the other, the body's ability to facilitate availability is a difficult pathway; therefore, both are deemed as essential
  G. Cats require dietary linoleic and arachidonic acids

V. Important in temperature regulation and protection of internal organs and facilitates immune function

VI. Fatty acid deficiency could result in dermatological problems as well as impair wound healing

VII. Increased dietary fat requirements usually occur during periods of growth, lactation, or increased physical activity

VIII. Excess fat consumption could result in weight gain or obesity if not monitored, as well as diarrhea or steatorrhea (fatty stools) due to the body's inability to digest or absorb excess fat

NON–ENERGY-PRODUCING NUTRIENTS

Water

I. Most essential nutrient required by the body for survival
   A. Needed for almost all body metabolic processes

II. Total daily water requirements equal daily energy requirements in a thermoneutral environment

III. Requirements will vary depending on factors such as environmental temperature, physical activity, metabolism, diet, lactation, and illness

IV. Water comprises approximately 70% of adult body weight

V. Grave illness or death could result if as little as 10% of body water is lost

VI. Essential for absorption of water-soluble vitamins B complex and C

VII. Animals obtain water from metabolic processes or, more important, through ingestion by drinking or eating

VIII. Quantity of water in pet foods varies
   A. Dry kibble: 10% to 12%
   B. Semimoist: 25% to 40%
   C. Canned: 72% to 82%

IX. Animals eating canned food appear to drink less water because they obtain a large portion of daily water requirements from their diet

X. Fresh water must be available at all times
   A. This point must be emphasized to pet owners, especially for dogs housed outside in the winter where there is a risk of water freezing

Minerals

I. Although the total percent of minerals in the body is less than 1%, they are essential for metabolic processes to take place

II. Macrominerals
   A. Dietary requirements expressed in percentages (%)
   B. Examples: calcium, phosphorus, potassium, sodium, magnesium
   C. Aid in maintaining electrolyte and water balance, skeletal integrity, muscle and nerve conduction, and cellular function

III. Microminerals
   A. Dietary requirements expressed in parts per million (ppm)
   B. Also known as trace minerals
   C. Examples: iron, copper, zinc, iodine
   D. Involved in the majority of biochemical reactions in the body

IV. A close interrelationship exists between minerals
   A. Any excess of one or more minerals could result in the deficiency of others, due to lack of absorption or imbalance

V. Mineral supplementation is contraindicated if a high-quality, balanced diet is provided

VI. Minerals have many functions; any deficiencies or excesses could be harmful to an animal, as shown in Table 15-1

Vitamins

I. Function as enzymes, coenzymes, and enzyme precursors

II. Classified by solubility
   A. Water soluble
      1. B complex and C
      2. Not stored in the body at all
      3. Deficiency may occur during periods of excessive water loss such as polyuria, diarrhea, or gastrointestinal disorders that may alter microfloral populations
         a. Supplementation is recommended during these periods
   B. Fat soluble
      1. A, D, E, and K
      2. Stored in fat or liver
      3. Excesses could result in toxicity

III. Cats have specific vitamin requirements that dogs do not
   A. In their diet, they require preformed vitamin A, which is found in the highest constituency in animal tissue
   B. Cats also require the B vitamin niacin because they cannot convert tryptophan, an amino acid, to niacin

IV. Dogs can convert beta-carotene derived from plant sources to vitamin A, which is a characteristic of omnivores; cats cannot

V. Vitamin E also functions as an antioxidant, but the amount decreases as the fat is oxidized

VI. Vitamin functions, deficiencies, and possible toxicities are described in Table 15-2

DAILY ENERGY REQUIREMENTS

How much to feed is as important as what to feed, to ensure that an animal is getting the correct amount and type of food based on its age and lifestyle. Factors that could influence daily energy requirements include growth, lactation, stress, physical exertion, breed, environmental conditions, and age.

Table 15-1 Mineral functions and effects of deficiency and excess

Mineral	Function	Deficiency	Excess
Calcium	Constituent of bone and teeth, blood clotting, myocardial function, nerve transmission, membrane permeability	Decreased growth, decreased appetite, decreased bone mineralization, lameness, spontaneous fractures, loose teeth, tetany, convulsions, rickets (osteomalacia—adults)	Decreased feed efficiency, decreased feed intake, nephrosis, Ca urate stones, lameness, enlarged costochondral junctions
Phosphorus	Constituent of bone and teeth, muscle formation, fat, carbohydrates, and protein metabolism, phospholipids and energy production, reproduction	Diminished appetite, decreased feed efficiency, decreased growth, dull hair coat, decreased fertility, spontaneous fractures, rickets	Bone loss, urinary calculi, decreased weight gain, decreased feed intake, calcification of soft tissues, secondary hyperparathyroidism
Potassium	Muscle contractility, transmission of nerve impulses, acid-base balance, osmotic balance, enzyme cofactor (energy transfer)	Anorexia, decreased growth, lethargy, locomotive problems, hypokalemia, heart and kidney lesions, emaciation	Rare
Sodium and chloride	Osmotic pressure, acid-base balance, transmission of nerve impulses, nutrient uptake, waste excretion, water metabolism	Inability to maintain water balance, decreased growth, anorexia, fatigue, exhaustion, dryness/loss of hair	Occurs only if there is inadequate nonsaline, good quality water available. Causes thirst, pruritus, constipation, seizures, and death. Chronic amounts may induce hypertension resulting in increased heart and renal diseases
Magnesium	Component of bone, intracellular fluids, neuromuscular transmission, active component of several enzymes, carbohydrate and lipid metabolism	Muscular weakness, hyperirritability, convulsions, anorexia, vomiting, decreased mineralization of bone, decreased body weight, calcification of aorta	Urinary calculi
Iron	Enzyme constituent: activation of O_2 (oxidases, oxygenases), O_2 transport (hemoglobin, myoglobin)	Anemia, rough hair coat, listless, decreased growth	Anorexia, weight loss, decreased serum albumin
Zinc	Constituent or activator of 200 known enzymes (nucleic acid metabolism, protein synthesis, carbohydrate metabolism), skin and wound healing, immune response, fetal development, growth rate	Anorexia, decreased growth, alopecia, parakeratosis, impaired reproduction, vomiting, hair depigmentation, conjunctivitis	Relatively atoxic. Reported cases of Zn toxicity from consumption of die-case Zn nuts
Copper	Component of several enzymes (i.e., oxidases), catalyst in hemoglobin formation, cardiac function, cellular respiration, connective tissue development, pigmentation, bone formation, myelin formation, immune function	Anemia, decreased growth, hair depigmentation, bone lesions, neuromuscular, enzootic ataxia, aortic rupture, reproductive failure	Hepatitis, increased liver enzymes
Manganese	Component and activator of enzymes (glycosyl transferases), lipid and carbohydrate metabolism, bone development (organic matrix), reproduction, cell membrane integrity (mitochondria)	Impaired reproduction, perosis (poultry), fatty livers, crooked legs, decreased growth	Relatively atoxic
Selenium	Constituent of glutathione peroxidase and iodothyronine 5′-deiodinase, immune function, reproduction	Muscular dystrophy, reproductive failure, decreased feed intake, subcutaneous edema, renal mineralization	Vomiting, spasms, staggered gait, salivation, decreased appetite, dyspnea, "garlicky" breath
Iodine	Constituent of thyroxine and triiodothyronine	Goiter, fetal resorption, rough hair coat, enlarged thyroid glands, alopecia, apathy, myxedema, lethargy	Similar to deficiency. Decreased appetite, listlessness, rough hair coat, decreased immunity, decreased weight gain, goiter, fever

Continued

Table 15-1 Mineral functions and effects of deficiency and excess—cont'd

Mineral	Function	Deficiency	Excess
Boron	Regulates parathormone action, therefore influences metabolism of Ca, P, Mg, and cholecalciferol	Decreased growth, decreased hematocrit, hemoglobin, and alkaline phosphatase	Similar to deficiency. 150-200 ppm maximum tolerated level
Chromium	Potentiates insulin action, therefore improves glucose tolerance	Impaired glucose tolerance, increased serum triglycerides and cholesterol	1000 mg/day is maximum tolerated level in cats; trivalent form less toxic than hexavalent

Courtesy Dr. Karen Wedekind, Mark Morris Institute.

Table 15-2 Vitamin functions and the effects of deficiency and toxicity

Vitamin	Function	Deficiency	Toxicity
		FAT SOLUBLE	
Vitamin A	Component of visual proteins; differentiation of epithelial cells Spermatogenesis Immune function Bone resorption	Anorexia Retarded growth Poor hair coat Weakness Increased cerebrospinal fluid pressure Aspermatogenesis Fetal resorption Requirement may increase in acute infection due to urine losses (dog)	Cervical spondylosis (cat) Tooth loss (cat) Retarded growth Anorexia Erythema Long bone fractures
Vitamin D	Calcium and phosphorus homeostasis Bone mineralization Bone resorption Insulin synthesis Immune function	Rickets Osteomalacia Osteoporosis	Hypercalcemia Calcinosis Anorexia Lameness
Vitamin E	Biological antioxidant Membrane integrity through free radical scavenging	Sterility (males) Dermatosis Immunodeficiency Anorexia Myopathy	Minimally toxic Increased clotting time: reversed with vitamin K
Vitamin K	Allows blood clotting protein formation	Prolonged clotting time Hypoprothrombinemia Hemorrhage	Minimally toxic Anemia (dog) None described for the cat
		WATER SOLUBLE	
Thiamin (B_1)	Nervous system	Anorexia Weight loss Ataxia Ventral flexion (cat) Paresis (dog) Cardiac hypertrophy (dog) Bradycardia	Decreased blood pressure Bradycardia Respiratory arrhythmia None described for the cat
Riboflavin (B_2)	Electron transport in oxidase and dehydrogenase enzymes	Retarded growth Ataxia Collapse syndrome (dogs) Dermatitis Purulent ocular discharge Vomition Conjunctivitis Coma Corneal vascularization Bradycardia Fatty liver (cat)	Minimally toxic None described for cat and dog

Table 15-2 Vitamin functions and the effects of deficiency and toxicity—cont'd

Vitamin	Function	Deficiency	Toxicity
WATER SOLUBLE			
Niacin (B_3)	Component of energy-producing biochemical reactions	Anorexia Diarrhea Retarded growth Ulceration of soft palate and buccal mucosa Necrosis of the tongue (dog) Reddened ulcerated tongue (cat) Uncontrolled drooling	Low toxicity Bloody feces Convulsions Death None described for the cat
Pyridoxine (B_6)	Neurotransmitter synthesis Niacin synthesis from tryptophan Taurine synthesis Carnitine synthesis	Anorexia Retarded growth Weight loss Microcytic hypochromic anemia Convulsive seizures Renal tubular atrophy, and deposits of calcium oxalate crystals (cat)	Low toxicity Anorexia Ataxia (dog) None described for the cat
Pantothenic acid	Protein, fat, and carbohydrate metabolism in the TCA cycle Cholesterol synthesis Triglyceride synthesis	Emaciation Fatty liver Depressed growth Decreased serum cholesterol and total lipids Tachycardia Coma Lowered antibody response	Toxicity is negligible No toxicity described in dog or cat
Folic acid	Purine synthesis DNA synthesis	Anorexia Weight loss Leukopenia Hypochromic anemia Increased clotting time Elevated plasma iron Megaloblastic anemia (cat) Sulfa drugs interfere with gut synthesis	Nontoxic
Biotin	Component of four carboxylase enzymes	Hyperkeratosis Alopecia (cats) Dry secretions around eyes, nose, and mouth (cat) Hypersalivation Anorexia Bloody diarrhea	No toxicity described in dog or cat
Vitamin C	Synthesized from D-glucose in the liver Synthesis of collagen proteins and carnitine Enhances iron absorption Free radical scavenging Biological antioxidant	Liver synthesis precludes dietary requirement; therefore no deficiency symptoms have been described in normal cat and dog	No toxicity described in dog or cat
Choline	Component membranes and neurotransmitter	Fatty liver (puppies) Thymus atrophy Decreased growth rate Anorexia	No toxicity described for dog and cat
QUASI-VITAMINS			
Carnitine	Transport of long-chain fatty acids into the mitochondria of the cell	Hyperlipidemia Cardiomyopathy Muscle asthenia	No toxicity described for dog and cat

Feeding Methods

I. Free choice
  A. Food is available at all times and the animal determines when and how much to eat
  B. Advantages
    1. Good for pets that will eat to meet their energy requirements and do not overeat
    2. Recommended method during lactation
    3. Most convenient method for pet owners
  C. Disadvantages
    1. Difficult to monitor the pet's consumption, and anorexia may not be noticed immediately
    2. May lead to obesity
    3. Nutritional excesses due to overeating
    4. Economics

II. Time-restricted meal feeding
  A. Unquantified amount of food is available for the pet for a certain period of time, usually anywhere from 10 to 30 minutes
  B. Ideal choice in a multipet household where different diets must be fed
  C. This method can be repeated more than once a day

III. Food-restricted meal feeding
  A. Specific quantity of food offered at specific times during the day
  B. Beneficial for animals that have any type of digestive disorder where small frequent meals are more tolerable
  C. Recommended method for canine breeds prone to gastric dilatation/volvulus (GDV) and for diabetic pets
  D. Can still meet desirable growth with this method
  E. Best feeding method

IV. Maintenance energy requirement (MER) calculations in Table 15-3 are intended for use as a starting point and should be adjusted as necessary based on body condition and lifestyle of the pet
  A. Owners can follow the feeding guidelines on a pet food label as a starting point

Table 15-3 Calculations for maintenance energy requirements

RESTING ENERGY REQUIREMENTS (RER)		
$70 \times \text{Weight (kg)}^{0.75}$ or $30 \times (\text{Weight in kg}) + 70$		
MAINTENANCE ENERGY REQUIREMENTS (MER)		
Canine Feeding Guide		
Puppies	<4 months of age	3 × RER
	>4 months of age	2 × RER
Adult		1.6 × RER
Senior		1.4 × RER
Weight prevention		1.4 × RER
Weight loss		1.0 × RER
Gestation (last 21 days)		3 × RER
Lactation		4 to 8 × RER
Feline Feeding Guide		
Kittens		2.5 × RER
Adult		1.2 × RER
Weight prevention		1.0 × RER
Weight loss		0.8 × RER
Breeding		1.6 × RER
Gestation (gradual increase)		2 × RER
Lactation		2-6 × RER

Courtesy Hill's Pet Nutrition, Inc.

NUTRITIONAL REQUIREMENTS FOR EACH LIFE STAGE OF THE DOG AND CAT

Nutritional requirements vary greatly between each life stages, and proper nutrition will result in a happier, healthier pet over its lifetime.

Gestation and Lactation

I. Nutrition is as important before breeding as it is during gestation and lactation
  A. Poor nutrition could result in low birth weight or increased risk of neonatal mortality

II. Nutritional requirements of a pregnant bitch or queen toward the end of gestation and during lactation are similar to those of a neonate (see Table 15-5 for specific requirements)

III. Period to begin transition to a high-quality, highly digestible growth diet should be during the last 3 to 4 weeks of gestation in the bitch and from the second week of gestation in the queen

IV. It is important to calculate maintenance energy requirements at this stage to ensure that adequate nutrients are being consumed, especially during lactation

V. Cats begin to gain weight in a linear fashion from the beginning of their pregnancy; dogs have the most weight gain during the last 3 to 4 weeks of gestation

VI. Offering small frequent meals is the method of choice for dogs; free-choice feeding is recommended for cats

VII. Due to their ability to store and utilize fat, cats tend to eat less postpartum but soon regain their appetite by the third week

VIII. Fresh water should be available at all times

IX. After weaning has occurred, the cat or dog should be gradually transitioned back to a good-quality, highly digestible maintenance diet

Dogs

Young Dogs

I. Neonates and puppies
  A. Neonates should be encouraged to nurse vigorously after birth to ingest colostrum

Table 15-4 Body condition scoring

Body score 1 Very thin	Ribs are easily palpable with no fat cover. Tailbase* has a prominent raised bony structure with no tissue between skin and bone. Bone prominences are easily felt with no overlying fat. In animals over 6 months, there is a severe abdominal tuck when viewed from the side and an accentuated hourglass shape when viewed from above
Body score 2 Underweight	Ribs are easily palpable with minimal fat cover. Tailbase* has a raised bony structure with little tissue between skin and bone. Bony prominences are easily felt with minimal overlying fat. In animals over 6 months, there is an abdominal tuck when viewed from the side and marked hourglass shape when viewed from above
Body score 3 Ideal	Ribs are palpable with a slight fat cover. Tailbase* has a smooth contour or some thickening and bony structure is palpable under a thin layer of fat between skin and bone. Bony prominences are easily felt with a slight amount of overlying fat. In animals over 6 months, there is an abdominal tuck when viewed from the side and a well-proportioned lumbar waist when viewed from above
Body score 4 Overweight	Ribs are difficult to feel with moderate fat cover. Tailbase* has some thickening with moderate amounts of tissue between skin and bone. Bony structures can still be felt. Bony prominences are covered by a moderate layer of fat. In animals over 6 months, there is little or no abdominal tuck or waist when viewed from the side and the back is slightly broadened when viewed from above. Abdominal fat apron present in cats
Body score 5 Obese	Ribs are difficult to feel under a thick fat cover. Tailbase* appears thickened and is difficult to feel under a prominent layer of fat. Bony prominences are covered by a moderate to thick layer of fat. In animals over 6 months, there is a pendulous ventral bulge and no waist when viewed from the side. The back is markedly broadened when viewed from above. Marked abdominal fat apron present in cats

*Tailbase evaluation is done only in dogs.

B. Colostrum is a special milk produced within the first 24 to 48 hours after parturition that contains maternal antibodies
   1. It is vital for the neonate because it provides a passive immunity
C. After the crucial first 24 to 48 hours, the bitch's milk begins to change and becomes more complete to provide all the nutrients that the growing neonate requires until weaning
D. Nursing should be observed at least four to six times a day
E. Milk provides all the essential nutrients for growth, and the fluids consumed help to increase the body's total circulatory volume
F. Neonates should be weighed daily for the first 2 weeks to ensure adequate growth; normal stool should also be observed
   1. Puppies should gain 2 to 4 g/day/kg or 1 to 2 g/day/lb of anticipated adult body weight. Puppies not achieving this growth curve should be closely monitored
G. Commercial milk replacers are necessary only when supplementing weak or premature neonates, orphans, or large litters or when a dam is unable to produce sufficient milk

II. Weaning
   A. Should begin at approximately 3 weeks of age but can be as early as 10 to 14 days if necessary
   B. Commercially prepared high-quality growth diet should be prepared by blending the diet with water to form a thick soupy gruel-type mixture
      1. This should be offered three or four times a day
   C. Initially, puppies will walk and play in the food, but the nutritive properties will be gained as the pups lick and play with each other
   D. Puppies should be totally weaned and be eating only a moistened dry or canned growth diet by 5 to 7 weeks for large breeds and 6 to 8 weeks for small breeds
   E. Cow's milk should not be offered because the lactose content is greater than the bitch's milk and diarrhea and dehydration could result

III. Growth
   A. Growth diet should be fed from weaning until the puppy achieves skeletal maturity, or about 12 months
   B. Characteristics of a growth diet
      1. Palatable
      2. High digestibility, quality, and increased caloric density (this would decrease dietary consumption and stool volume)
      3. Optimum calcium/phosphorous ratio, approximately 1.2:1
   C. Maintenance energy requirements should be calculated for growth (see Table 15-3)
   D. Puppies should be weighed and evaluated every 2 weeks, using body condition scoring as described in Table 15-4, which is the best

way to determine whether the amount being offered is optimal

1. Pet behavior can also indicate whether more or less food is desired

E. Nutritional characteristics of a growth diet are found in Table 15-5

IV. Feeding large-breed puppies

A. Most common problem is overfeeding and supplementation, which can result in increased incidence of obesity, hip dysplasia, and osteochondrosis

B. Excesses or deficiencies in a diet can affect musculoskeletal development

C. Calcium excesses could result

1. Calcium alone is often the offending mineral and not an imbalance with the calcium/phosphorous ratio
2. In the dog becoming hypophosphatemic as well as hypercalcemic
3. In retarded bone volume, retarded bone modeling, and cartilage maturation

D. Recommended levels of calcium are 1% to 1.6% on a dry matter basis

E. Vitamin D is required in large-breed puppies because

1. It regulates calcium metabolism and aids in the absorption of calcium and phosphorous
2. It increases bone cell activity

F. Food-restricted meal feeding is recommended for large breed puppies based on their MER

G. Feeding a poor-quality, cheaper, lower-caloric-density growth diet, could result in

1. Poor appearance
2. Inferior development
3. Increased incidence of disease
4. Overeating in an effort to meet caloric needs
5. Increase in risk of obesity
6. Higher stool volume

H. Goal of feeding large-breed puppies is to decrease the growth rate but still reach the dog's genetic potential at maturity

Adult Dogs

I. Adult maintenance: lifestyle of the adult dog will determine its nutritional needs

A. Adulthood ranges from approximately 1 to 7 years, depending on size of the dog

1. Smaller breeds mature at an earlier age than larger breeds, but they also age slower

B. Diet and feeding methods should be reviewed with the pet owner; body condition score should be recorded as the dog enters adulthood

C. Supplementing with treats or table scraps should be discouraged, or, if given, they should not exceed 10% of total energy requirements

1. Treats can be made from the regular diet as described in Table 15-6, but the quantity per feeding should be adjusted accordingly

II. Active adult dog

A. Dogs that require increased caloric energy such as hunting, working, show, and guide dogs or toy breeds that eat small amounts of food frequently

B. Increasing a maintenance diet is not always sufficient because caloric needs may surpass ability to consume the appropriate volume of food (known as bulk limiting)

C. Offering a highly digestible, calorically dense food that is higher in fat is recommended

D. If caloric demand is seasonal, such as in hunting or field trial dogs, a transitional period should take place anywhere from 7 days to 3 weeks before the event, with any physical conditioning of the dog

E. Small frequent meals and fresh water should be offered to avoid dehydration, hypoglycemia, and bingeing due to hunger

Geriatric Dogs

I. Small breeds begin their geriatric years at about age 7; large and giant breeds begin around age 5

II. Visual and physiological changes begin to occur

A. Decreased activity level

B. Cataracts

C. Graying muzzle

D. Internally, organs cannot tolerate nutrient excesses or deficiencies as before

III. Reevaluate the dog's diet and lifestyle with the pet owner. It is important that pet owners understand an aging pet's changing nutritional requirements

IV. Maintenance energy requirements should be recalculated for the geriatric patient (see Table 15-3)

V. Characteristics of a geriatric diet should include

A. Reduced fat and calories to avoid weight gain

B. Decreased sodium, protein, and phosphorous, which reduces workload on the cardiovascular system and kidneys

C. Increased EFA and zinc for skin and coat

D. Increased fiber, which slows intestinal transit time, improves nutrient absorption, and regulates bowel movements

E. Increased palatability and digestibility due to decrease in olfactory senses and appetite

VI. Elevated protein quality is crucial when dietary protein restriction is recommended

Table 15-5 Life stage nutritional requirements

	Protein	Fat	Crude fiber	Calcium	Phosphorus	Sodium	Chloride	Potassium	Magnesium	Energy	Vitamin E
DOG FOOD RECOMMENDATIONS											
MMI RECOMMENDATIONS											
Adult maintenance	15-30	10-20	5 max	0.5-1.0	0.4-0.9	0.2-0.4	0.3-0.6	0.4-0.8	0.04-0.15	3.5-4.5	450-1000
Growth (adult BW <25 kg)	22-32	10-25	5 max	0.7-1.7	0.6-1.3	0.3-0.6	0.4-0.8	0.6-0.9	0.04-0.20	3.5-4.5	450-1000
Growth (adult BW >25 kg)	20-32	8-12	10 max	0.7-1.2	0.6-1.1	0.3-0.6	0.4-0.8	0.6-0.9	0.04-0.20	3.0-4.0	450-1000
Older	15-23	7-15	10 max	0.5-1.0	0.25-0.75	0.15-0.35	0.3-0.5	0.4-0.8	0.04-0.15	3.0-4.0	700-1500
Obesity-prone adult	15-30	7-12	5-16	0.5-1.0	0.4-0.9	0.2-0.4	0.3-0.6	0.4-0.8	0.04-0.15	3.0-3.5	450-1000
High energy	22-34	15 min	5 max	0.6-1.0	0.4-0.9	0.2-0.5	0.3-0.6	0.45-0.9	0.05-0.20	>4.5	450-1000
Gestation/lactation	22-35	10-25	5 max	0.75-1.7	0.6-1.3	0.35-0.6	0.5-0.9	0.6-0.9	0.04-0.20	3.5-5.0	450-1000
AAFCO NUTRIENT PROFILES FOR DOG FOODS											
AAFCO growth/reproduction	22 min	8 min	—	1.0-2.5	0.8-1.6	0.3 min	0.45 min	0.6 min	0.04-0.3	3.5-4.0	50-1000
AAFCO maintenance	18 min	5 min	—	0.6-2.5	0.5-1.6	0.06 min	0.09 min	0.6 min	0.04-0.3	3.5-4.0	50-1000
COMMON COMMERCIAL DOG FOODS											
Average moist grocery (30)	41	27	1.8	1.7	1.4	0.9	1.1	1.1	0.11	4.5	na
Average dry grocery (32)	25	12	3.1	1.4	1	0.4	0.7	0.7	0.14	3.9	108
Average dry specialty (93)	28	16	3.3	1.3	1	0.4	0.7	0.7	0.12	4.2	200
Average moist specialty (39)	32	22	2.1	1.2	0.9	0.5	0.9	0.9	0.1	4.4	na
CAT FOOD RECOMMENDATIONS											
MMI RECOMMENDATIONS											
Adult maintenance	30-45	10-30	5 max	0.5-1.0	0.5-0.8	0.2-0.6	0.3 min	0.6-1.0	0.04-0.1	4.0-5.0	550-1000
Growth	35-50	18-35	5 max	0.8-1.6	0.6-1.4	0.3-0.6	0.45 min	0.6-1.2	0.08-0.15	4.0-5.0	550-1000
Obesity-prone adult	30-45	8-17	5-15	0.5-1.0	0.5-0.9	0.2-0.6	0.3 min	0.6-1.0	0.04-0.1	3.3-3.8	550-1000
Older	30-45	10-25	10 max	0.6-1.0	0.5-0.7	0.2-0.5	0.3 min	0.6-1.0	0.05-0.1	3.5-4.5	550-1000
Gestation/lactation	35-50	18-35	5 max	0.5-1.0	0.5-0.9	0.2-0.6	0.45 min	0.6-1.2	0.08-0.15	4.0-5.0	550-1000
AAFCO NUTRIENT PROFILES FOR CAT FOODS											
AAFCO growth/reproduction	30 min	9 min	—	1.0 min	0.8 min	0.2 min	0.3 min	0.6 min	0.08 min	4.0-4.5	30 min
AAFCO maintenance	26 min	9 min	—	0.6 min	0.5 min	0.2 min	0.3 min	0.6 min	0.04 min	4.0-4.5	30 min
COMMON COMMERCIAL CAT FOODS											
Average moist grocery (34)	51	27	1.5	1.8	1.5	0.9	1.3	1.1	0.09	4.3	na
Average dry grocery (26)	35	12	2.2	1.3	1.2	0.4	0.8	0.7	0.12	3.8	102
Average dry specialty (42)	35	18.5	2.4	1.1	0.95	0.5	0.7	0.7	0.09	4.3	249
Average moist specialty (35)	46	28	1.9	1.1	1	0.5	1	0.9	0.1	4.7	na

Nutrients are expressed as percent dry matter. Energy is expressed as kcal ME (metabolizable energy) per gram dry matter. Vitamin E is expressed as IU/kg dry matter.
Nutrient levels of commercial foods are based on averages of manufacturers' published values or analyticals.
AAFCO nutrient profiles presume 3.5 kcal ME/g in dog food and 4.0 kcal/g in cat food. Levels should be corrected for higher energy density.
Courtesy Dr. Philip Roudebush, Mark Morris Institute.

Table 15-6 Homemade treats

CANNED FOOD
1. Cut canned food into bite-sized pieces 2. Place in the microwave on high for 2 to 3 minutes or bake at 350° F for approximately 25 to 30 minutes until desired texture 3. Allow to cool before offering to pet, or refrigerate
DRY FOOD
1. Grind kibbles into a flour 2. Mix enough water to form a dough and shape into cookies 3. Bake at 350° F on cookie sheet for 25 to 30 minutes until crispy 4. Allow to cool; refrigerate unused portion

VII. Owners should be encouraged to continue a daily exercise regimen to maintain muscle tone and circulation

VIII. Avoid supplementing with high sodium treats and high-fat table scraps

IX. Complete physical examination by the veterinarian should be performed, including oral cavity and dental examination, baseline biochemistry panel, and urinalysis to ensure proper functioning of the internal organs

Cats

I. Cats are true carnivores; they possess typical dietary characteristics of other carnivores
   - A. Cats' protein requirements are much higher than those of dogs because cats catabolize protein for energy
     - 1. Dogs (omnivores) primarily use fats or carbohydrates
   - B. Require two amino acids: arginine and taurine
   - C. Require EFA arachidonic acid because, like other carnivores, cats cannot convert it from linoleic acid
   - D. Require vitamins niacin, pyridoxine (vitamin B_6), and preformed vitamin A, of which the two former are found in animal tissue

Kittens

I. Care and management for kittens are similar to the care and management for puppies

II. Kittens should be observed nursing vigorously after birth to ensure they receive colostrum

III. They should be weighed daily for the first 2 weeks of life and should gain approximately 90 to 100 g (3 oz) per week, which basically means doubling their birth weight

IV. Nutrient requirements of the kitten can be reviewed in Table 15-5

V. A good-quality, highly digestible kitten food can be introduced at approximately 3 weeks of age (in the same fashion as for puppies)
   - A. Kittens may not accept the slurry, so offering canned or dry without water is acceptable

VI. Kittens should be free-choice fed during growth

VII. Kittens should be weaned between 8 to 10 weeks of age but not earlier than 6 weeks

Adult Cats

I. Cats by nature are nibblers, but their MER should be calculated and the appropriate amount be left available throughout the day or divided into frequent meals

II. Providing a cat with a premium-quality, highly digestible, calorically dense diet will reduce the risk of disease such as feline lower urinary tract disease (FLUTD)

III. It is important that cat owners understand the phrase "cats aren't born finicky, they are made finicky"

IV. Consistency is important to avoid any type of behavioral problems or to prevent problems with a cat that is a finicky eater

Geriatric Cats

I. Cats enter their senior years at approximately 6 years

II. Less information is available about nutritional and physiological changes that occur in aging cats

III. Geriatric work-up should be done to verify organ function and oral health

IV. Most dietary recommendations for cats are based on research on rats, dogs, or humans

V. Lower urinary tract disease and urolithiasis are uncommon in geriatric cats; however, calcium oxalate urolithiasis is more common in older cats

VI. Nutritional requirements for geriatric felines can be viewed in Table 15-5

FELINE LOWER URINARY TRACT DISEASE (FLUTD)

This disease can be frustrating and potentially devastating for cat owners. Prevention is the most important information a veterinary technician can relay to owners.

I. From 1% to 6% of feline cases seen in a veterinary hospital are reported to be due to FLUTD
   - A. Incidence of new cases is approximately 0.5% to 1.0% per year

II. Exact etiology of FLUTD has not yet been determined
   - A. Cause could be multifactorial but is commonly related to urolithiasis, viral urinary

Table 15-7 Some risk factors reported in cats with lower urinary tract disease

Factor	Comment
Age	Uncommon in cats younger than 1 year. Most common between 1 and 10 years, with peak between 2 and 6 years
Sex	Urethral obstruction most common in males. Males and females have a similar risk for nonobstructive forms of the disease
Neutering	Increased risk of disease in neutered males and females, regardless of age of neutering
Diet	Consumption of an increased proportion of dry food in the daily ration is associated with increased risk of disease
Feeding frequency	Increased frequency of feeding associated with increased risk of disease, regardless of diet
Excessive weight	Obesity associated with increased risk of disease
Water consumption	Decreased daily water consumption associated with increased risk for disease
Sedentary lifestyle	Lazy cats at increased risk of disease
Spring or winter season	Seasonal variation implicated as a risk factor by some investigators, but not others
Indoor lifestyle	Cats using indoor litter boxes for micturation and defecation have increased risk for disease

Courtesy of Williams & Wilkins.

tract infections, or inherited, genital, or acquired disorders

III. Clinical signs often include
   A. Dysuria
   B. Hematuria
   C. Pollakiuria
   D. Urethral obstruction
   E. Inappropriate urination (urinating outside the litterbox)
   F. Frequent squatting in the litterbox
   G. Loss of appetite

IV. Risk factors associated with FLUTD are described in Table 15-7

V. The importance of dietary management with follow-up urinalyses and radiographs must be emphasized to the cat owner to reduce risk of recurrence

VI. Incidence and mineral composition of the most common feline uroliths can be found in Table 15-8

Table 15-8 Mineral composition of 20,343 feline uroliths evaluated by quantitative methods*

Predominant mineral type	No. of uroliths	Percent
Magnesium ammonium phosphate (struvite)	8621	42.4
Magnesium hydrogen phosphate	35	0.2
Magnesium phosphate hydrate	13	0.1
Calcium oxalate	9416	46.3
Calcium phosphate	122	0.6
Uric acid and urates	1136	5.6
Xanthine	11	0.1
Cystine	36	0.2
Silica	3	<0.1
Mixed†	248	1.2
Compound‡	487	2.4
Matrix	220	1.1
Urea	6	<0.1
Drug metabolite	2	<0.1
Total	20,343	100

*Uroliths analyzed by polarizing light microscopy and x-ray diffraction methods. Uroliths composed of 70% to 100% of mineral type listed, no nucleus and shell detected.
†Uroliths did not contain at least 70% of mineral type listed; no nucleus or shell detected.
‡Uroliths contained an identifiable nucleus and one or more surrounding layers of a different mineral type.
Courtesy Carl A. Osborne, Minnesota Urolith Center, University of Minnesota and from Ettinger SJ, Feldman EC: *Textbook of veterinary internal medicine*, ed 5, vol 2, Philadelphia, 2000, WB Saunders.

OBESITY

A veterinary technician has a vital role in helping clients manage and understand obesity in pets. Client education is the key to successful management and, more important, prevention of this condition.

I. Approximately 25% to 44% of companion animals are obese

II. An obese animal is one that weighs more than 15% of its ideal body weight

III. The first objective in helping clients deal with this situation is making the pet owner aware that the dog or cat is obese
   A. Pet owner should also be aware of risk factors involved
      1. Risk factors can include diabetes mellitus, neoplasia, hypertension, dermatosis, and bacterial and viral infections

IV. In cats, obesity can increase the risk of feline hepatic lipidosis

V. The veterinary technician can counsel clients about
   A. Benefits of weight loss, including increased activity, health, longevity, and alertness of their companion animal
   B. Identifying any inappropriate feeding behavior that could have been the cause of obesity

C. Modifying any inappropriate feeding behavior of the pet and the pet owner
D. Obtaining entire household cooperation and understanding of the pet's situation
   1. This should result in a successful weight loss program

VI. Another goal of a weight loss program other than having the pet lose weight is to start the pet on an exercise regimen that will improve cardiovascular conditioning and skeletal support

VII. Goals should be realistic and achievable to be successful
   A. Subgoals are recommended so that pet owners can visualize benefits of their hard work, providing reinforcement to continue until the goal weight is achieved

VIII. Before beginning any weight loss program for a pet, a complete physical examination by the veterinarian should be performed to rule out any medical cause for the obesity
   A. If any illness is identified, it should be treated before a weight loss program is initiated

IX. Determine the ideal weight of the patient and the required kilocalories per day for the patient to achieve that weight. Calorie restriction should be approximately 60% to 70% of the pet's maintenance energy requirements (see Table 15-3)

X. Ideal rate of weight loss
   A. Cats: 0.25 lb/week (115 g)
   B. Small dogs: 0.5 lb/week (230 g)
   C. Medium-size dogs: 1.0 lb/week (500 g)
   D. Large dogs: 1.5 lb/week (750 g)

XI. Charting weight loss is a useful tool for clients to see the success of their efforts

XII. Dogs should be weighed monthly; cats should be weighed bimonthly

XIII. Have scheduled weigh-in periods in your hospital
   A. Post a chart on all patients involved in a "weight loss" program
   B. Plan weekly meetings that allow pet owners to discuss with other owners how their pets are doing
   C. Competition tends to encourage pet owners to stick with the program and your recommendations
   D. Cat owners should be cautioned about too quick a weight loss because cats can develop hepatic lipidosis

XIV. Feeding small, frequent meals throughout the day reduces begging

XV. Acceptable treats while on a reducing diet include ice cubes, ice chips, low-calorie vegetables such as carrots or celery, or taking a portion of the prescribed diet and making homemade treats as described in Table 15-6

XVI. Recording a cat's or dog's body condition score throughout its life is the best way to prevent obesity or to identify it in a new client

CRITICAL CARE NUTRITION

The need for nutritional therapy is emerging as an important factor in treating critically ill patients.

I. Trauma, disease, sepsis, and stress will increase an animal's metabolism, therefore increasing its energy requirements

II. Protein-energy malnutrition may affect depletion of energy stores, wound healing, and pulmonary, cardiovascular, and gastrointestinal function

III. The body eats 24 hours a day whether the gut is fed or not

IV. After a patient is identified as requiring nutritional therapy, the simplest method for administering it should be chosen

Enteral Nutrition

I. Coaxing: warming the food, hand feeding, etc.
II. Appetite stimulants: drugs
III. Force feeding by syringe
IV. Orogastric intubation
V. Nasogastric/nasoesophageal intubation
VI. Esophagostomy tube feeding
VII. Gastrostomy tube feeding
VIII. Enterostomy tube feeding

Parenteral Nutrition

I. Direct intravenous infusion with basic constituents of dextrose, crystalline amino acids, and lipid emulsion

II. Option if enteral nutrition is unsuccessful or contraindicated

III. Calculating illness energy requirements (IER)
   A. MER is rarely met if pet is in a debilitated state
   B. Canine IER = 1.25 to 1.50 × MER
   C. Feline IER = 1.10 to 1.25 × MER

IV. If the diet chosen is tolerated, the product should be introduced gradually
   A. Suggested guidelines
      1. One-third total calories on day 1
      2. Two-thirds of the total on day 2
      3. Total calories on day 3
   B. If human products are used, nutritional supplementation is required

FOOD ALLERGY OR INTOLERANCE

Cats and dogs may exhibit abnormal responses to the food or food additives they ingest. These responses could manifest as gastrointestinal or dermatological signs.

I. Antigenic responses occur at the highest level when food is ingested
II. Clinical cases related to food allergy or food intolerance have been poorly documented or reported
III. Risk factors
    A. Specific foods or ingredients
    B. Proteins that are not easily digested
    C. Any disease that affects intestinal mucosal permeability
    D. Breed
    E. Age: less than 1 year
    F. Concurrent allergic disease
IV. Adverse food reactions could be
    A. Immunological: allergy
    B. Nonimmunological: intolerance
V. Common food allergens reported in North America
    A. For cats: beef, dairy products, fish
    B. For dogs: beef, dairy products, lamb, chicken egg, chicken, soy
VI. Protein (glycoprotein) is often the nutrient of concern in adverse reactions to food
VII. Factors that contribute to a food reaction
    A. Previous exposure to the protein or offending nutrient
    B. Number of different protein sources found in the pet's diet
    C. Digestibility of the protein: poor-quality protein
    D. Protein level
VIII. Identifying the food allergen is key to managing or preventing recurrence
    A. Elimination diet trials can be used for identification of allergens
IX. Trial period should be approximately 4 to 10 weeks
X. A complete diet history, including homemade foods and treats, must be obtained from the pet owner
XI. Ideal elimination diet
    A. Contains a limited number of novel protein sources or a protein hydrolysate
    B. Highly digestible
    C. Avoids protein excess
    D. Avoids additives
    E. Nutritionally balanced for the animal's life stage and body condition score
    F. Avoid treats, supplements, toys, other food sources, chewable medications during trial
    G. Have clients maintain a diet log during the trial, and ensure *everyone* in the household follows the strict regimen
XII. If no clinical improvement is evident after the trial period, then something other than food must be the cause of the animal's clinical signs
XIII. If clinical signs do improve, reintroduce original diet or individual proteins, one at a time, to monitor for a recurrence in the signs
XIV. If a food allergy or intolerance is identified, the veterinary technician can now find a commercially prepared, nutritionally balanced diet that does not contain the offending nutrient or ingredient
XV. Protein hydrolysate diets are an excellent new option as both an elimination diet and a long-term maintenance diet
    A. Potential for an adverse food reaction is significantly reduced because the body's immune system does not recognize the protein as an allergen (if the protein's molecular weight is less than 10,000 Daltons)

HOW TO CHOOSE A PET FOOD

I. Pet owners often seek knowledge and guidance from a member of the veterinary health care team about the best diet for their companion animal
II. It is important to be familiar with premium pet foods sold in the area, as well as products sold or endorsed by the hospital
III. Remember that the pet food label will never give a true reflection of the quality or nutritional value of its contents
IV. Calculating the daily feeding cost (Table 15-9) is beneficial when comparing a poor-quality, low density product with a premium-quality, calorically dense product
    A. Often the cost per day is less for the premium food and the food lasts longer because of the caloric density and digestibility

Table 15-9 Calculating daily feeding costs

Step	Description	Diet A	Diet B
A	Cost per 40 lb bag (640 oz)	$16.00	$31.50
B	Cost per pound of diet (A/40)	$0.40	$0.79
C	Cost per ounce (B/16 oz)	$0.025	$0.49
D	Ounces/cup (by weighing one cup of food)	3.5 oz	3 oz
E	Feeding amounts in ounces/day (based on MER or feeding guide on bag)	17.5 oz (5 cups)	7.5 oz (2.5 cups)
F	Days bag will last (640 oz bag/E)	37	85
G	Cost per day (C × E)	$0.44	$0.37
H	Cost per year (G × 365 days)	$161.00	$135.00

PET FOOD

Pet Food Label

I. A pet food label should include
  A. Product name
  B. Designation: cat or dog food
  C. Net weight
  D. Name and address of manufacturer
  E. Guaranteed analysis
  F. Ingredient panel
  G. Nutritional adequacy statement or purpose of product
  H. Feeding guidelines
  I. Date of manufacture or expiration code

II. In Canada, Consumer Packaging and Labeling Act and Regulations dictate that only product identity, product net quantity, dealer's name, and principal place of business be on the label

III. In the United States, regulation is by the Food and Drug Administration, Department of Agriculture
  A. U.S. law dictates that the following must be on the label: product name, designator, net weight, ingredients, guaranteed analysis, nutritional adequacy statement, feeding guide, and manufacturer or distributor

IV. American Association of Feed Control Officials (AAFCO) is an association established by animal feed control officials as a regulating body to develop standards for uniformity of definitions, policies for manufacturing, labeling, distribution, and sale of animal feeds

V. National Research Council (NRC) is a nonprofit organization that was the recognized authority for substantiation of pet food claims for nutrient requirements before 1990

Guaranteed Analysis (GA)

I. Provides minimum or maximum percentages of certain nutrients that the manufacturer claims the product meets

II. The following nutrients are required to be on the GA. Other nutrients added to the label are at the discretion of the manufacturer
  A. Crude protein: expressed as minimum %
  B. Crude fat: expressed as minimum %
  C. Crude fiber: expressed as maximum %
  D. Moisture: expressed as maximum %

III. Crude: term used to describe the analytical procedure used to estimate the nutrients

IV. Guaranteed analysis should not be used to compare products because values indicated do not reflect exact amounts but only minimums or maximums of a nutrient

V. GA also includes the moisture content of the product; therefore the nutrient value indicated is diluted in moisture, so a canned food may appear to have a lower percent of nutrients than a dry product due to amount of water

VI. Dry weight analysis
  A. Approximate percent of a nutrient based on dry matter of the product
  B. Converting nutrients to dry matter allows for a more accurate comparison of products with different moisture levels (Table 15-10)
  C. Manufacturers should provide nutrients listed on a dry matter basis (DMB) for comparison and accurate values

Ingredient Panel

I. Listed in descending order by weight, beginning with heaviest ingredient

II. Ingredients with a high water content will appear higher on the panel, even if they are of poor nutrient value, than one with less water content

III. Terms used must be common in the feed industry or be assigned by AAFCO

IV. Manufacturers can alter ingredients so that a more desirable ingredient will appear higher on the ingredient panel

V. The same ingredient may be described in various forms, such as wheat being broken down into wheat middling, cracked wheat, whole wheat, and flaked wheat
  A. This can make an ingredient appear to be in smaller quantities in the diet even though, when combined, it forms a large percentage of the diet

VI. AAFCO determines what is meant by terms such as meat byproducts, but it is difficult to know what ingredients were actually used unless one contacts the manufacturer directly
  A. Meat byproduct could be anything, such as liver, lungs, udders, or tongues

VII. Ingredient panel should not be used as a mode of comparison because two ingredient panels could be identical and there is no way to determine the quality or digestibility of the ingredients that each manufacturer uses

Table 15-10 How to calculate the dry weight analysis

Guaranteed analysis from can
  Water 75%
  Protein 10%
  Other dry matter 15%
Calculation of dry weight analysis
  1. Dry matter % = 100% − % moisture
     = 100% − 75% = 25%
  2. % Nutrient ÷ % dry matter × 100
  EXAMPLE: Protein = 10/25 = 0.4 × 100 = 40% protein
Thus dry weight analysis is
  Protein 40%
  Other dry matter 60%

VIII. Formulas can be fixed or variable
   A. Fixed formula: every bag purchased has the same ingredients as the previous
      1. Products in this category tend to be of higher quality and more expensive and have more digestible ingredients
   B. Variable formula: ingredients may change from batch to batch based on ingredient availability and market price

Statement of Nutritional Adequacy

I. AAFCO established guidelines that U.S. manufacturers attempt to meet for nutrient profiles for cats and dogs (see Table 15-5)
II. "Complete and balanced" refers to a diet that contains all essential nutrients in concentrations that are proportional to the energy density of the food
III. Nutritional adequacy statements are based on feeding trials such as that of AAFCO or through a calculation method
IV. Veterinary technicians should recommend products that have undergone feeding trials
V. Statements about "meeting or exceeding" standards without feeding trials are based on a chemical analysis and do not verify the digestibility or true adequacy of a product. Statements help determine if the product is for a specific purpose, as in "Complete and balanced for puppies," or all purpose, as in "Meets the requirements for the life of your cat"
   A. A product with the latter statement on it could have nutrient deficiencies or excesses for a particular life stage because it was formulated for every life stage
VI. Snacks, treats, and therapeutic diets do not require nutritional statements

Glossary

AAFCO American Association of Feeding Control Officials, the regulating body of pet food manufacturers in the United States

aspermatogenesis Inability to form male gametes (sperm)

ataxia Incoordination or wobbliness

carbohydrate Nutrient that provides energy for body tissues

dry matter basis Describes nutrient amounts in percentages as found in the dry weight of a product when the moisture is removed

encephalamalacia Means "softening of the brain"; usually used to denote degenerative brain diseases

enteral Administered through the alimentary canal (mouth, esophagus, stomach, small intestine)

essential amino acids Amino acids the body requires through diet because the body cannot manufacture them

FLUTD Feline Lower Urinary Tract Disease

glycoprotein Class of compounds consisting of a protein conjugated to a carbohydrate

goiter Enlargement of the thyroid gland

guaranteed analysis Describes nutrients in minimum or maximum percentages that a pet food manufacturer claims are met by the product

hepatic lipidosis Another term for fatty liver disease

hydrolysate Compound that is produced through hydrolysis

hydrolysis Breaking of a molecule by the addition of water

hyperkeratosis Increased thickness of the horny layer of the skin

ingredient A raw or processed agricultural product or other element that delivers nutrients to the body

keratomalacia Softening and necrosis of the cornea due to a vitamin A deficiency

MER Maintenance energy requirements; estimated amount of calories required per day for maintenance of a particular life stage

myopathy Inflammation of the muscle

nitrogenous Molecule that contains nitrogen

novel New or not resembling something formerly known

NRC National Research Council

nutrient Food characteristic that provides nourishment to the body

osteomalacia Softening of bones

osteoporosis Condition of marked loss of bone density

parakeratosis Appearance of thickened skin with scale formation and underlying raw red surface, often due to zinc deficiency

parenteral Administered via some other route than the alimentary canal

pollakiuria Abnormally frequent urination

protein Nutrient composed of 23 amino acids

steatitis Inflammation of fatty tissue

taurine Essential amino acid that only cats require in their diet

urolithiasis Formation of urinary stones

Review Questions

1 Energy-producing nutrients are
   a. Protein, fats, water
   b. Carbohydrates, fats, protein
   c. Fats, protein, vitamins
   d. Vitamins, minerals, water

2 Biological value
   a. Pertains to the value of carbohydrates in the diet
   b. Describes the quantity of plant and animal protein sources in a diet
   c. Evaluates protein usability by the body
   d. Pertains to the value of fat in the diet

3 Which nutrient aids in the management of diarrhea and constipation?
   a. Minerals
   b. Fat
   c. Water
   d. Carbohydrates

4 The maintenance energy requirements (MER) for an 8-month-old, 22-kg (48.5 lb) mastiff is

a. 1460 kcal/day
b. 740 kcal/day
c. 2190 kcal/day
d. 3140 kcal/day

5 Characteristics of a canine geriatric diet include
a. Low fiber and sodium and higher fat
b. Decreased sodium and essential fatty acids
c. Restricted protein, phosphorous, and increased fiber
d. Increased fiber, calories, and restricted essential fatty acids

6 Possible clinical signs associated with FLUTD may include
a. Frequent defecation
b. Increased hunger
c. Weight gain
d. Hematuria

7 An animal is considered obese when its weight exceeds what percentage of its ideal weight?
a. 5%
b. 10%
c. 15%
d. 25%

8 Manufacturers are required to include which percentage of the following ingredients in the guaranteed analysis?
a. Maximum crude protein and fat
b. Minimum crude protein and fat
c. Minimum minerals and ash
d. Minimum crude fiber and moisture

9 A pet food claim that is formulated to meet the AAFCO cat food nutrient profile for growth and lactation means that the food
a. Also meets the nutrient profile for adult maintenance
b. Meets NRC standards
c. Has undergone AAFCO feeding trial testing growth and lactation
d. Has been chemically analyzed only to meet the standards

10 The best way to compare the actual nutrients of two pet food labels is by
a. Guaranteed analysis
b. Ingredient panel
c. Nutritional adequacy statement
d. Dry weight analysis

BIBLIOGRAPHY

American Association of Feed Control Officials, Official Publication, Atlanta, GA, 2001.

Case LP, Carey DP, Hirakawa DA: *Canine and feline nutrition, a resource for companion animal professionals,* 2 ed, St Louis, 2001, Mosby.

Colgan M, Brune C: *Hill's healthcare connection,* Topeka, KS, 1999.

Ettinger SJ, Feldman EC: *Textbook of veterinary internal medicine,* 5 ed, Philadelphia, 1996, WB Saunders.

Hand MS et al: *Small animal clinical nutrition,* ed 4, Topeka, KS, 2000, Mark Morris Institute.

McCurnin DM, Bassert JM: *Clinical textbook for veterinary technicians,* ed 5, Philadelphia, 2002, WB Saunders.

Osborne CA et al: Consultations in feline internal medicine. In *Feline lower urinary tract disease: relationships between crystalluria, urinary tract infection, and host factors,* Philadelphia, 2001, WB Saunders.

Osborne CA, Finco DR: *Canine and feline nephrology and urology,* Philadelphia, 1995, Williams & Wilkins.

CHAPTER 16

Large Animal Nutrition and Feeding

James A. Topel

OUTLINE

LEARNING OUTCOMES

After reading this chapter you should be able to:

1. Define the nutrient needs of large animals.
2. Identify the elements that influence nutrient requirements.
3. Identify the parts and functions of large animal digestive systems.
4. Learn of the different feedstuffs in large animal diets.
5. Identify the various life stage nutritional requirements of large animals.
6. Identify the relationship of disease to improper nutrition.

Improper nutrition can be related to as much as 90% of health-related disease in large animals. Reasons for improper nutrition include owners' inadequate training, improper emphasis on prevention and prophylaxis, and lack of consultation. It is advantageous for the veterinary team to combine preventive feeding with herd health. The increased requirements for growth, breeding, and lactation are different from those for maintenance. Ration formulation, a science best left to specially trained individuals in that field, is not covered in this unit.

FEEDING LARGE ANIMALS

Large Animal Nutrition Concepts

I. Livestock nutrition basics
   A. The livestock producer's greatest challenge is producing or purchasing feed that can be consumed by the animal at the least cost, with the best financial return
   B. Nutrients are used for homeostasis, developing body tissues (growth, repair, and finishing), replenishing body tissues (maintenance), reproduction, lactation, and wool and meat production

C. Maintenance nutrient requirements (MNRs) are the levels of nutrients needed in the large animal diet to maintain body weight without a gain or loss
   1. About one half of consumed and absorbed nutrients are needed to meet the MNRs
D. The National Research Council has established feeding standards for the different production or use purposes, for each large animal species

II. Nutrients
A. Protein
   1. Contains nitrogen, sulfur, carbon, hydrogen, and oxygen. Some contain phosphorus
   2. Protein is the main constituent of the soft tissues and organs of the animal body
   3. Amino acids (22 commonly found in proteins) are the building blocks of proteins
   4. Used for growth, reproduction, lactation, repair of body tissues, and the formation of enzymes, antibodies, and certain hormones, as well as for energy
   5. Depending on life stage, protein quality may not be important. However, even though total protein intake may be adequate, digestible protein may be insufficient
      a. Dietary protein requirements are highest in the young growing animal
   6. Protein supplements (soybean meal, cottonseed meal, and linseed meal) are highly digestible protein sources. Common grains (corn, oats, wheat, and barley) and alfalfa hay are good protein sources. Grass hay has the least amount of digestible protein
      a. Highly digestible proteins are considered high in total digestible nutrients (TDNs) and low in fiber
      b. Grass hay is high in fiber but low in TDNs
   7. Nonprotein nitrogen (NPN) (e.g., urea) is a nitrogen source that can be converted to protein by rumen microbes
   8. Deficiencies may result in limited growth, anemia, decreased milk production, infertility, reduced synthesis of certain hormones and enzymes, and possible depressed appetite with weight loss and unthriftiness
   9. Excesses may also affect reproduction
B. Fats
   1. Fats provide dietary energy, source of heat, insulation, and body protection and serves as a carrier for absorption of fat-soluble vitamins
   2. Fat has 2.25 times more energy per gram than carbohydrates or proteins
   3. Fats are classified as
      a. Simple lipids: esters of fatty acids with glycerol or alcohol
      b. Compound lipids: phospholipids, glycolipids, and lipoproteins
      c. Derived lipids: fatty acids and sterols
         (1) Linoleic acid and linolenic acid are essential
         (2) Arachidonic acid is considered essential only if linoleic acid is absent
         (3) Arachidonic acid can be synthesized from linoleic acid
C. Carbohydrates
   1. Carbohydrates are the primary energy source in large animal rations
   2. Carbohydrates are the building blocks for other nutrients (fats)
   3. Carbohydrates are stored in the animal's body by converting to fats
   4. Cereal grains and forages are high in carbohydrate content
   5. Carbohydrates (sugars and starches) are broken down into simple sugars so they can be absorbed from the digestive tract
   6. Microflora in the rumen of ruminants and the cecum of some nonruminants can convert fiber (cellulose, hemicellulose, pectins, and gum) into energy
      a. Lignin is a fiber but is considered to be the indigestible portion found in forages of poor quality
   7. Feed concentrates (grains and high-starch compounds) and forages (grasses and legumes) generally supply all the energy needed in the diet
D. Minerals
   1. Minerals are made of inorganic, solid, and crystalline chemical elements
      a. Total mineral content of animals and plants is called ash
      b. Minerals make up 3% to 5% of the animal body dry weight
   2. A highly complex relationship exists among the minerals
      a. It has been shown that calcium, iron, and copper can interfere with the metabolism of other minerals and nutrients
   3. Minerals that are lacking in the diet can be force fed in supplements combined with common salt
   4. Other than common salt, animals apparently do not have any ability to select needed minerals

a. A mineral block or granular mineral supplement is vitally important for health and should be offered as a free-choice part of the diet

5. Minerals are grouped as macrominerals and trace minerals based on their need in the diet
   a. See Chapter 15 for general mineral functions, deficiencies, excesses. Also see Table 16-1
6. Macrominerals include sodium, chloride, potassium, phosphorus, calcium, magnesium, and sulfur
   a. Calcium and phosphorus
      (1) Make up more than 70% of the minerals in the body
      (2) Generally, a calcium/phosphorus ratio of 1.4 to 2:1 should be provided by the ration
      (3) Common supplements are bone meal, defluorinated phosphates, and dicalcium phosphorus
      (4) Calcium and phosphorus are closely tied to vitamin D and the parathyroid gland
      (5) A large excess of either interferes with absorption of the other, so a balance is necessary
      (6) In Europe, bone meal and other animal-based byproducts have been considered the likely spread of bovine spongiform encephalopathy ("mad cow disease")
   b. Sodium and chlorine
      (1) Hydrochloric acid, a substance rich in chlorine that is obtained from salt, is essential in the digestive processes
      (2) Salt must always be supplied to animals in addition to the amounts contained in the usual well-balanced ration
      (3) Good livestock managers provide free access to salt at all times
      (4) Increased salt intake results in increased water intake
      (5) In severe deficiencies, animals may experience muscle cramps, weight loss, decrease in milk production, and rough hair coat
      (6) Most animals will tolerate large excesses of salt if the water supply is adequate. If the water is contaminated with excess salt, this can cause anorexia, weight loss, and eventually physical collapse (salt toxicosis)
   c. Magnesium
      (1) Magnesium is allied with calcium and phosphorus in the body
      (2) Care must be taken to avoid a magnesium-deficient diet
      (3) Lactating cows are more susceptible, although other stock can be afflicted
      (4) Magnesium-deficient cattle exhibit anorexia and reduced dry matter (DM) digestibility
      (5) Young stock may have defective bones and teeth when deficiencies occur
      (6) Toxicity is rare
   d. Sulfur
      (1) Sulfur is a component of amino acids, biotin, and thiamin
      (2) A deficiency of sulfur leads to reduced growth. Toxicity is unlikely

Table 16-1 Body condition scoring classification for livestock

Body condition scoring scale*		Generalized animal description†	
1.0	1	Emaciated	All bones obviously protruding; no subcutaneous fat is evident
1.5	2	Very thin	Bones visible and easily palpated; minimal subcutaneous fat
2.0	3	Thin	Thin, flat musculature; prominent ribs, pelvic bones, and spinal processes
2.5	4	Moderately thin	Minimal subcutaneous fat; individual ribs not obvious
3.0	5	Moderate	Smooth musculature; bones not visible but palpable
3.5	6	Moderate fleshy	Fat palpable; soft fat over ribs and covering pelvis
4.0	7	Fleshy	Fat visible; ribs difficult to palpate; rounded appearance to pelvis
4.5	8	Fat	Thick neck; ribs difficult to palpate; rounded appearance to pelvis
5.0	9	Grossly obese	Bulging fat all over, patchy pads around tailhead

Reprinted from Grosdidier SR et al: Nutrition. In Pratt PW, ed: *Principles and practice of veterinary technology*, St Louis, 1998, Mosby.

*The body condition scoring scale used depends on the species. Dairy cattle, sheep, pigs, and goats are generally scored on a scale of 1 to 5. Beef cattle and horses are usually scored on a scale of 1 to 9.

†Base the body condition score on the amount or lack of fatty tissue over the neck, ribs, spine, and pelvis without reference to body weight and frame size.

e. Potassium
   (1) Potassium is the major intracellular cation and is involved in osmotic pressure, acid-base balance, and muscle activity
   (2) Deficiencies lead to lethargy, diarrhea, untidy appearance, coma, and even death
   (3) Toxicities can reduce magnesium absorption, which in turn reduces potassium retention

7. Trace minerals include zinc, selenium, manganese, iodine, fluorine, chromium, copper, iron, silicon, molybdenum, and cobalt
   a. Trace minerals and macrominerals have a profound interaction. Deficiencies or toxicities of one may lead to deficiencies or toxicities of another
   b. See Special Nutritional Requirements section for deficiencies and toxicities of trace minerals for each large animal species

E. Vitamins (see Table 15-2 for vitamin function, deficiency, and toxicity)
1. Fat-soluble vitamins are A, D, E, and K
2. Water-soluble vitamins include ascorbic acid (vitamin C) and the B-complex vitamins
3. Ruminants require water-soluble vitamins when they are ill because of a reduced ability to synthesize them
4. Fat-soluble vitamins are stored in the body fat in large amounts; therefore excess in one or more of them can result in a toxic effect
5. Deficiency in any of these vitamins can result in severe health problems
6. Normal, healthy ruminants do not require a dietary source of vitamin B complex, vitamin C, and vitamin K because the rumen microflora or tissues synthesize them
   a. If insufficient vitamin B_1 (thiamin) is produced, polioencephalomalasia will result
7. Vitamin A deficiency may occur if limited or poor-quality forages are fed. Deficiency signs include reproductive failure, night blindness, skin ailments, and weak offspring
8. Vitamin E deficiency along with a selenium deficiency may result in white muscle disease, especially in calves
9. Sun-cured hay is the only natural food with a high vitamin D content: the leafier the better
   a. An hour-a-day exposure to direct sunlight is sufficient to meet daily vitamin D needs

F. Water
1. Adequate water intake is essential for life. Potable water should always be available
2. Water makes up 65% to 85% of an animal's body weight at birth and 45% to 60% of body weight at maturity
3. A loss of 10% of total water content seriously distresses the animal; a loss of more than 12% will lead to shock with death imminent
4. It is essential to dissolve all food before the body may use it
   a. Waste product of the body is removed by water as urine
      (1) Waste of the digestive tract cannot be removed until it has been softened by water
5. Except for very young calves, water should be offered free choice
6. Because of rumen fermentation, cattle need two to three times more water per day than horses

III. Elements that influence nutrient requirements
A. Environment
1. Temperature variations
   a. Cold stress requires more energy
   b. Warmer temperatures decrease appetite
2. Wind, precipitation, and sun exposure
3. Consult district agrologist for specific area requirements

B. Location concerns
1. Soil nutrient leaching and increased animal population leading to overgrazing will affect the quality of the feed that is consumed
   a. Soil and feed tests will provide valuable information
   b. Consult the nutritionist and use services of the district agrologist for specific area requirements

C. Other factors influence nutrient requirements
1. Genetics, body size, gender, breed, reproductive status, health status, stress, exercise, behavior, and availability of nutrients

Ruminant Digestion

Basic Anatomy and Physiology

I. Cattle, sheep, goats, and camelids are ruminants
II. Ruminants are herbivores with a diet composed mainly of plants with high fiber (cellulose) content
III. Ruminants can convert forage unfit for direct human consumption into a consumable product
A. Accomplished through symbiotic relationship with bacteria and protozoa

1. Byproducts of anaerobic fermentation are volatile fatty acids, amino acids, vitamins, methane, and CO_2
   a. Methane and CO_2 are eructated (belched) and the remaining byproducts are used for body maintenance and production

IV. True ruminants, like cattle, have a prehensile tongue for gathering foodstuffs

V. Functional ruminants like llamas use their lips to carefully select the foodstuff and then crop the forage short by shearing the plant stems with their lower incisors and upper dental pad

VI. Stomach of true ruminants is multicompartmented. In cattle, the stomach is composed of four chambers: reticulum, rumen, and omasum, which make up the forestomach, and the abomasum
   A. Reticulum: (honeycomb) forces ingested feed material into the rumen or omasum and regurgitation of ingesta during rumination
   B. Rumen: (paunch) main fermentation vat; the microbial products are available for digestion and absorption
   C. Omasum: (manyplies) filled with muscular laminae or "leaves" to squeeze fluid out of the ingesta
   D. Abomasum (true or glandular stomach)
      1. Corresponds to stomach of monogastrics
      2. Process of peptic digestion of proteins begins here

VII. Functional ruminants, like llamas, have a three-compartment stomach (C-1, C-2, C-3)
   A. Compartments 1 and 2 support microbial anaerobic fermentation (similar to the rumen of cattle)

VIII. Sugars and starches (e.g., concentrates) are fermented more rapidly than cellulose (e.g., forages)

IX. Intraruminal pH is generally between 6.2 and 7.2 depending on the diet
   A. A more acidic rumen is noted in animals fed a high grain diet

X. Conversion of protein, starches, and lipids by microorganisms results in usable nutrients for the host

XI. Microorganisms can use poor-quality protein and NPN compounds (e.g., urea) to make amino acids and energy
   A. Microbial protein passes into the abomasum and is similarly digested to other dietary protein
   B. Microbial protein can form a significant amount of ruminant dietary protein, but the intake of NPN compounds should be carefully monitored
   C. Dietary fiber is required to keep the microbial fermentation chambers active
   D. Microorganisms also synthesize vitamins B and K

XII. To ensure proper microbial population, ruminants require proper feed, appropriate feeding intervals (fermentation is continuous), regurgitation of cud (bolus of food), rechewing (remastication), ensalivation, reswallowing (deglutition), continuous churning, eructation (belching), outflow to the rest of the digestive tract, and sufficient water

XIII. Anatomy and physiology of the small and large intestines in ruminants is similar to those of swine

FEEDING DAIRY AND BEEF CATTLE

Feed Sources (see Boxes 16-1 and 16-2)

I. Roughages or forages include pastures, range plants, plants fed green ("green-chop"), silages and dry forages such as hay (alfalfa, clover, brome, timothy, native grasses, etc.), straw, and chopped corn stalks
   A. Forages generally have large amounts of fiber, low TDNs and energy density, and high bulk (low weight per unit volume)
      1. This is due to the plant cell wall material of cellulose, hemicellulose, lignin, and other compounds
   B. Protein content depends on the type of plant and stage at harvesting
      1. The more mature the plant, the greater is the fiber content but there is less protein, energy, and digestibility

Box 16-1 Typical Roughages Fed to Ruminants

LEGUMES

Alfalfa, red clover, Alsike clover, white clover, sweet clover, birdsfoot trefoil, crown vetch

GRASSES

Kentucky bluegrass, smooth bromegrass, orchard grass, timothy, reed canary grass, tall fescue, redtop, perennial rye grass, southern grasses, Sudan grass, native grasses

Box 16-2 Concentrates Fed to Ruminants

CARBONACEOUS CONCENTRATES

Corn, oats, sorghum, barley, rye, wheat

PROTEINACEOUS CONCENTRATES

Urea, biuret, diammonium phosphate, monoammonium phosphate, ammonium sulfate, soybean meal, cottonseed meal, linseed meal, sunflower meal, safflower meal

C. Hays are divided into legumes (e.g., alfalfa, clover, birdsfoot trefoil) and grasses (e.g., timothy, brome, sorghum, blue grass, and native grasses)
   1. Legumes have higher protein content and a higher protein biological value compared with grass hays
   2. Some legumes such as alfalfa and clover are more likely to cause bloat in cattle
   3. Hay quality is determined by
      a. Mixture of grasses (e.g., brome, alfalfa or bluegrass, and clover)
      b. Stage of maturity when cut (50% bloom, 75% bloom, or full bloom)
      c. Method and speed of harvesting
      d. Spoilage and loss during storage and feeding
D. Silage is roughage that is preserved by ensiling
   1. Most common silages are corn silages and grass or legume silages (also called haylage, which is an example of low-moisture silage)
   2. Silage with a water content of 55% to 75% has the least loss of nutrients from harvesting and storage

II. Concentrates or cereal grains include corn, barley, wheat, oats, and screenings (left over from grain processing)
   A. The way a grain is processed affects its digestibility
   B. Concentrates are fed primarily for energy and/or protein
   C. Grains contain 60% to 80% starch
   D. Fats and oils of plant or animal origin have 2.25 greater energy density than carbohydrates
   E. Corn is the most commonly fed grain
   F. Other than cereal grains, molasses, root crops, and milling byproducts can also be used as energy concentrates

III. Any concentrates that are more than 20% crude protein are classified as protein supplements
   A. Concentrates are classified as carbonaceous (grain) or proteinaceous (processed byproducts)

Special Nutritional Requirements

An adequate diet should include water and feeds containing energy, proteins, minerals, and vitamins.

I. Water
   A. Ad libitum for mature animals
      1. Cattle generally drink 10 to 14 gallons (38 to 53.2 L) per day for a mature nonstressed animal
   B. Dairy cows require 3 to 5 gallons (11.4 to 19 L) of water to produce 1 gallon (3.8 L) of milk
   C. A cow at peak lactation may need up to 45 gallons (171 L) per day, depending on various factors

II. Energy
   A. Energy requirements are greatest during lactation
   B. This requirement must be met with a good grain source and high-quality forage for lactation

III. Protein
   A. Good-quality pasture and forage balanced with grains and topped up high-protein supplements will usually provide adequate protein in the diet during growth and lactation
   B. Maintenance requirements can be supplied with just fair- to good-quality pasture and forage
   C. In cattle, rumen microbes have the ability to convert fair- to poor-quality feedstuff protein sources into a higher-quality protein
   D. In contrast, rumen microbes may actually reduce higher-quality feedstuff proteins through microbial degradation and synthesis of proteins

IV. Minerals
   A. Includes the macrominerals (sodium, chlorine, calcium, phosphorus, magnesium, sulfur, and potassium) and the trace minerals (zinc, selenium, manganese, iodine, fluorine, chromium, copper, iron, silicon, molybdenum, and cobalt). All minerals should be balanced in the diet: neither deficient nor in excess
      1. Sodium and chloride
         a. Best fed free choice in cattle
         b. Salt is important for general thriftiness
      2. Calcium
         a. A deficiency in calcium can occur with high-grain diets
         b. Balance grains with forages. Legumes and high-quality forages are high in calcium
         c. Calcium deficiencies are more rare but can be corrected with the addition of limestone to the feed
         d. Excess calcium during the late dry period may lead to milk fever (parturient paresis)
            (1) Parathyroid gland becomes hyporesponsive and vitamin D is decreased
            (2) Bone calcium reserves are then not readily available at onset of lactation
      3. Phosphorus
         a. Phosphorus availability is influenced by content in the soil

   b. Mature brown summer forage and winter range can be deficient in phosphorus
   c. Phosphorus deficiency results in slow growth, poor appetite, and unthriftiness in young animals. In lactating animals, milk production declines, bones become fragile, and feed intake is poor
   d. Phosphorus deficiencies can be corrected with a phosphorus supplement
4. Iodine
   a. Feeding stabilized iodized salt will prevent deficiencies
   b. Most important in pregnant animals
5. Cobalt
   a. Cobalt is an essential component of vitamin B_{12} (cyanocobalamins)
   b. Feed with the trace mineralized salt
   c. Deficiency develops rapidly because very little is stored
   d. Deficiency shows up as ocular discharge, listlessness, anemia, decreased skin and hair coat quality, abortions, decreased milk production, ketosis, and decreased appetite
   e. Signs of toxicity include decreased growth rates, incoordination, rough hair coat, and elevated hemoglobin and packed cell volume levels
6. Copper
   a. Signs of deficiency include neurological disorders, anemia, lameness, and diarrhea
   b. Signs of toxicity include gastroenteritis, hemorrhagic diarrhea, liver and kidney disease, and increased incidence of respiratory disease in calves
   c. A balance of sulfates and offering trace mineralized salt with copper will generally correct a deficiency
7. Selenium
   a. Growing cattle fed low-protein diets require more selenium and vitamin E in the diet to prevent deficiencies
   b. Cattle fed selenium-deficient diets have increased incidence of reproductive problems, immunosuppression; calves are born weak and have reduced growth weights (white muscle disease)
   c. Levels vary in soil based on region and geological phenomenon
   d. A trace mineralized salt should include selenium and should also supply adequate vitamin E
8. Zinc
   a. Higher levels are required for normal testicular development
   b. High calcium intake increases the need for zinc
   c. Deficiency signs include reduced conception rates, reduction in growth, reduced immune response, decreased appetite, bone irregularities, decreased wound healing, hoof problems, and hair loss
   d. Zinc can be added to trace mineralized salt to prevent deficiencies
   e. Calves are most susceptible to toxicities, with signs including polydipsia, polyuria, diarrhea, pica, anorexia, pneumonia, arrhythmias, and ultimately death
9. Iron
   a. Iron is an essential component of hemoglobin
   b. Deficiencies rarely occur in adults but may be an issue in calves fed an all-milk diet
   c. Treatment for deficiencies includes iron dextran injections in calves and iron sulfate added to a mineral mix in adults

V. Vitamins
   A. Vitamin A
      1. Important for vision, growth, and reproduction
      2. Deficiencies should be addressed immediately by supplementation
   B. Vitamin D
      1. Essential for the absorption of calcium and phosphorus
      2. Deficiency leads to rickets
      3. Deficiency is extremely rare because vitamin D requirements are met by 1 to 2 hours of sunlight a day
   C. Vitamin E
      1. Oxidation rapidly destroys vitamin E
      2. Old hay or ground grains are poor sources
      3. Deficiency is recognized as a common cause of white muscle disease
      4. This vitamin is of practical importance only to the young
      5. Vitamin E interacts with selenium
   D. Vitamin K
      1. Synthesized by rumen microorganisms
   E. B-complex vitamins
      1. Not necessary when the rumen is functioning properly
      2. Milk replacers should be fortified
   F. Vitamin C

1. Not required; ruminants synthesize their own vitamin C

Life Stages

I. Nutrient requirements for maintenance of beef and dairy animals
   A. Maintenance requirements relate to an area where there is no loss or gain in body energy
II. Nutrient requirements of pregnant and lactating beef and dairy animals
   A. Factors to consider before a ration is developed include availability, quality, and cost of feedstuffs
   B. Energy source is the most important part of the ration
      1. Until the energy requirement is met, protein, minerals, and vitamins may not be well used
   C. Cow size does not seem to have much effect on the efficiency of milk production, so it is more important to feed cows on the basis of their potential
      1. Referred to as challenge feeding
   D. Judge individual cow or heifer requirements by body score
      1. A condition score of 3 is desirable before calving to help with the birth and the subsequent rebreeding (see Table 16-1)
   E. It is desirable in the last trimester for the cow to gain an amount of weight equal to what will be lost at calving
   F. An obese animal is as undesirable as an underweight animal because cows may be predisposed to ketosis, along with other problems
   G. Last trimester and lactation are the most important stages, with lactation often exerting the most severe strain
   H. Beef cows can use poor-quality forage fairly well, if they are supplemented to meet nutrient requirements for the stage of pregnancy
      1. In cow/calf management systems, cows produce calves that form part of the breeding herd or are sent to feedlots
         a. They are usually fed forages with supplements as needed
      2. Same considerations apply for pregnant dairy cattle, especially during lactation
         a. Cows in good condition fed good-quality hay or pasture require no extra concentrates until 2 weeks before calving
      3. For lactating cattle, a fully balanced ration with the proper dry matter intake (DMI) is essential for optimum milk production
         a. Concentrates supply the highest level of energy, but a proper proportion is important to prevent obesity, digestive problems, and decreased milk production
         b. Cow's body type and ability to achieve maximum milk production are considered
         c. Generally, dairies use good-quality forages and grains at the correct mixture to achieve the best production that they can without losing body condition on the cow
III. Feeding replacement/breeding animals
   A. Replacement animals are those used in the breeding herd after they come of age
   B. First calf heifers will still be growing at the time of first parturition
   C. Energy intake of breeding animals, males and females, should be controlled so they will not become obese
   D. In calves, adequate colostrum intake is critical within the first 18 hours to ensure maximum absorption of colostral antibodies
      1. Calves should receive 10% to 12% of their body weight in colostrum within the 18 hours, preferably half the total volume within 4 to 6 hours of birth
   E. Beef calves should be "creep fed," which is feeding small amounts of grain in a location to which the dam does not have access
      1. This aids in lowering weaning stress and enables the calves to start to digest foodstuff they will be eating in their postweaning life stage
      2. Beef calves are usually weaned at 6 to 8 months
      3. Creep fed calves will generally show a 50-lb (22.5-kg) weight advantage at weaning
   F. Dairy calves should be pail- or bottle-fed milk until at least 1 month of age
      1. Good-quality calf starter rations and good-quality forages should be fed to encourage rumen development while receiving milk
      2. Longer periods (up to 2 months) of liquid feeding may be beneficial under some conditions because it results in decreased disease and death losses
      3. Proper sanitation of pails and bottles is important to prevent scours
   G. Forages and concentrates should be fed in large enough amounts to ensure continuous growth
IV. Animals fed for consumption
   A. Slaughter usually occurs between 13 and 18 months of age
   B. Beef animals not raised as breeding stock can be fed two ways

1. Weaned calves can be "backgrounded:" the calves are fed sufficient feed to gain between 1 and 1.5 lb (0.45 to 0.68 kg) a day through the winter and fed on pasture through the summer as yearlings
   a. Then they are slowly fed a ration increasing in grain until they reach slaughter weight
2. Weaned calves can also be put directly on a ration increasing in grain until slaughter
   a. This is usually done in a feedlot, although some ranchers keep them on the range
   b. Feedlots usually hire a nutritionist for ration consulting; ranchers will sometimes use whatever feed is readily available and not necessarily in the correct amounts
3. Weather (drought) and availability of feedstuffs are factors to consider in choosing which method is best for feeding beef calves
4. Economics is the overriding factor in this decision

V. Nonbreeding dairy calves
   A. Can be raised as "dairy beef:" usually not pastured and fed a ration in a feedlot to finish operation
   B. Can be fed as veal: fed a total liquid diet to keep the meat low in hemoglobin so that it stays a white color (anemia)

There is no "magic" amount of food that can be calculated to feed each life stage of cattle. Nutritionists factor quality and type of food and available nutrient levels into the ration for each cow in the herd. This has to be done by calculations, using some of the terms listed in the Glossary.

Disease Related to Improper Nutrition

I. Bloat
   A. Bloat is the increase of froth or free gas in the rumen
   B. Allowing cattle to graze on lush (rapidly growing) legume pasture, feeding legume green-chop, or feeding a low-roughage feedlot ration increases the risk
   C. To reduce the risk of bloat, feed cattle dry forages before allowing them to graze on new pasture or consume green-chop

II. Enterotoxemia
   A. Rare in cattle but most commonly caused by overeating of milk, milk replacer, or a high-carbohydrate diet in fast-growing juveniles
   B. *Clostridium perfringens* is the contributing agent, which causes neurological signs and death
   C. To prevent enterotoxemia in cattle, avoid overfeeding and vaccinate for *C. perfringens*

III. Failure of passive transfer (FPT)
   A. FPT occurs when a calf does not receive adequate colostral antibodies
      1. Calves are noted to be less vigorous and are more prone to disease because they do not have the antibodies available to fight disease
   B. Reasons for inadequate colostral antibody absorption include poor-quality colostrum nursed or fed, inadequate colostrum consumed, and first colostrum intake postponed
   C. To prevent FPT, ensure the calf receives adequate high-quality colostrum within the first hours and days of life

IV. Fatty liver disease
   A. Disease occurs when high dietary fat or cholesterol intake is not properly metabolized in the liver or fats are pulled from the adipose tissue in a negative energy state
      1. This leads to an accumulation of lipids in the liver and alters liver function
   B. In a healthy animal, fatty liver disease may be avoided through adequate energy intake

V. Grass tetany (hypomagnesemic tetany)
   A. Most likely to occur in mature cattle and during early lactation in high-producing dairy cattle
   B. Cattle that graze on pastures that are magnesium deficient may become anorexic and may exhibit muscle fasciculations (twitching) or even convulsions
   C. Grass tetany can be prevented by supplementing magnesium in the diet before and into lactation of at-risk animals

VI. Milk fever (parturient paresis)
   A. Milk fever is most often seen after calving in high-producing cows
   B. Decreased blood calcium leads to a decreased appetite; often an animal collapses. These cows are sternally recumbent and turn their head back toward their side
   C. By balancing calcium and phosphorus levels during the "dry period" and avoiding obese animals, milk fever can be prevented

VII. Displaced abomasum (DA)
   A. When the abomasum is filled with gas, it may displace dorsally to either the left (LDA) or right (RDA) side
   B. A cow with a DA will become anorexic, milk production will drop, and on auscultation of the right or left abdomen, an area of resonance (ping) will often be noted

- C. There are many known causes for DAs, but a common thread seems to be the high-producing animal that is fed a high-grain/low-forage diet
- D. Preventive measures include feeding adequate long-stem forages and avoiding moldy feeds

VIII. Ketosis (acetonemia)
- A. Insufficient energy intake in high-producing cattle causes the catabolism of body fats to supply the needed energy. When fat catabolism does not occur properly, ketone levels build up in the bloodstream
- B. Ketosis occurs most often in early lactation and often leads to decreased milk production and appetite
- C. It is confirmed by noting sweet "acetone" breath and testing for urine ketone levels
- D. Ketosis is preventable by maintaining a leaner, healthier animal and by increasing energy intake in early lactation

IX. Thiamin-deficiency polio (polioencephalomalacia)
- A. Polio of ruminants is a noninfectious disease that is characterized by cerebrocorticol necrosis
- B. Cause appears to be thiamin deficiency but has not been completely confirmed. There seems to be an association with animals that are fed imbalanced diets
  1. These imbalances include a high-carbohydrate diet, selenium/cobalt/sulfate imbalances, and evidence of mycotoxins or poisonous plants in the diet
- C. Preventive measures include improving roughage quality, balancing grain intake, and thiamin injections

X. Rickets
- A. Rickets is an imbalance of calcium, phosphorus, and vitamin D in the diet and tends to be more of an issue in young animals
- B. Animals with rickets often have enlarged joints and have difficulty in moving
- C. To prevent rickets in cattle, a proper balance of calcium and phosphorus is critical but should also include the animal having access to direct sunlight and sun-cured hay

XI. Rumen acidosis
- A. Overfeeding of grains may lead to a decrease in rumen pH
- B. Rumen becomes acidic
- C. Rumen function is significantly altered because rumen microbes cannot survive in the lower pH environment
- D. Preventive measures include limiting or balancing concentrate intake with forage intake and if necessary, may require repopulating the ruminal microbes (transfaunation)

XII. Indigestion in calves
- A. Ruminal drinking can cause indigestion in young calves
- B. Cause of this indigestion is due to insufficient closure of the reticular groove, which allows milk to pool in the undeveloped rumen and not bypass directly to the abomasum
  1. Affected calves become unthrifty
- C. Affected calves can be treated by allowing them to suck on the herdsman's fingers before feeding to facilitate the closure of the reticular groove

XIII. Urea toxicity
- A. Overconsumption of urea leads to toxic levels of ammonia in the bloodstream, which can make cattle sick or result in death
- B. Be sure to balance NPN intake with conventional high-protein concentrates

XIV. Water belly
- A. Urinary tract obstruction from urinary calculi leads to rupture of the urethra or urinary bladder
- B. Castrated males are most susceptible
- C. Carbonate calculi are most common
- D. Cattle on high-grain diets develop struvite crystals
- E. Silicate calculi may be seen in animals out on open range in certain geographical areas
- F. Preventive measures are limited to economically feasible feed management practice changes when an increased incidence of urethral obstructions occurs in an individual herd

XV. White muscle disease
- A. White muscle disease is a polysystemic disease caused by vitamin E and selenium deficiencies
- B. Juvenile cattle are the most susceptible
- C. Clinical signs in ruminants include swollen painful muscles, stiffness, and muscle weakness
- D. Preventive measures include supplementing vitamin E and selenium in the late gestation cow

FEEDING SHEEP AND GOATS

The numbers of veterinarians in sheep practice are few; there are fewer sheep than cattle, and their value is considerably less. Goats are becoming more popular as a source of meat and milk. Sheep raised for wool and meat goats are managed similarly to beef cattle. Dairy goats are managed more intensely because of high nutritional requirements for milk production.

I. Adequate nutrition is important for the economical soundness of sheep and goat rearing. As with cattle, definitions for nutritional requirements in all life stages can be difficult because of the wide variety of environmental conditions in which sheep and goats are maintained
   A. Different stages include
      1. Increased lamb and kid crop
      2. Continuous and rapid growth of lambs and kids
      3. Heavy weaning weights
      4. Heavy fleece weights
      5. Milk production

Feed Sources (see Boxes 16-1 and 16-2)

I. Good hay is a highly productive feed; poor hay, no matter how much is available, is suitable only for maintenance

II. Grains/concentrates can include barley, oats, wheat, bran, beet pulp, soybeans, and corn

III. Goats must be allowed to consume "browse" (brushy plants) and "forbs" (leafy plants)

Special Nutritional Requirements

An adequate diet should include water and feeds containing energy, proteins, minerals, and vitamins.

I. Water
   A. Ad libitum for mature animals
      1. Generally drink 1 to 1.5 gallons (4.5 to 6 L) per day
   B. One-half gallon (2 L) per day for fattening lambs and kids

II. Energy
   A. Maintenance energy requirements can be met by feeding good-quality forages with access to browse and forbs
   B. Energy requirements are greater 8 to 10 weeks after start of lactation
      1. This requirement must be met with a good grain source and high-quality forage for lactation

III. Protein
   A. Good-quality pasture and forage will usually provide adequate protein
   B. Sheep digest poor-quality proteins as well as or better than cattle
   C. Sometimes a supplement is indicated. Concentrates or NPN may be an option

IV. Minerals
   A. Include sodium, chlorine, calcium, phosphorus, magnesium, sulfur, potassium, and the trace minerals (cobalt, copper, iodine, iron, manganese, molybdenum, zinc, and selenium)
      1. Salt
         a. Best fed free choice
         b. Adults will consume 10 g of salt daily
         c. Salt is important for general thriftiness
      2. Calcium
         a. Legumes and high-quality forage are high in calcium
         b. A deficiency in calcium can occur on high-grain diets (e.g., corn silage)
         c. Calcium deficiencies are more rare but can be corrected with the addition of limestone to the feed
      3. Phosphorus
         a. Phosphorus availability is influenced by content in the soil
         b. Mature brown summer forage and winter range can be deficient in phosphorus
         c. Phosphorus deficiency results in slow growth, poor appetite, and unthriftiness in young animals. In lactating animals, milk production declines, bones become fragile, and feed intake is poor
         d. Phosphorus deficiencies can be corrected with a phosphorus supplement
      4. Iodine
         a. Deficiencies can be prevented by feeding stabilized iodized salt
         b. Most important in pregnant animals
      5. Cobalt
         a. Feed with the trace mineralized salt
         b. Deficiency develops rapidly because very little is stored
         c. Deficiency shows up as anemia, loss of appetite, retarded growth, general emaciation, rough hair coat, and a loss of milk production
      6. Copper
         a. Pregnant animals require 5 mg of copper daily
         b. Molybdenum and inorganic sulfates can affect copper absorption
         c. Signs of deficiency include anemia, brittle or fragile bones, and loss of wool or hair pigment
         d. A balance of sulfates will usually correct a deficiency problem
         e. Copper can be added to the trace mineralized salt
         f. Sheep are susceptible to copper toxicity
            (1) With acute toxicity, a severe gastroenteritis develops with hemorrhagic diarrhea as the typical sign
            (2) Chronic toxicity leads to liver and kidney disease, resulting in death

7. Selenium
   a. Levels vary in soil
   b. Supplementation can be provided by injections, oral feeding, or addition of trace mineralized salt
   c. Deficiency can cause nutritional muscular dystrophy, white muscle disease in lambs, and periodontal disease of the molars
   d. Toxicity results in loss of appetite, loss of hair, sloughing of hoofs, and eventual death
8. Zinc
   a. Higher levels are required for normal testicular development
   b. High calcium intake increases the need for zinc
   c. Signs of deficiency include slipping of wool, swelling and lesions around hooves and eyes, excessive salivation, anorexia, wool eating, general listlessness, reduced food consumption, reproductive problems, and reduction of growth
   d. Zinc can be added to trace mineralized salt

V. Vitamins
   A. Vitamin A
      1. Very low levels are present at birth
      2. If dams are deficient, young may be born dead or so weak they die within a few days; females may abort during the latter stage of pregnancy
      3. Injury to the optic nerve may occur in growing animals, cerebrospinal fluid pressure is elevated, and a staggering gait may develop
      4. Immediate action is required in the form of vitamin A injections and a corrective diet
   B. Vitamin D
      1. Essential for the absorption of calcium and phosphorus
      2. Deficiency leads to swollen leg joints and beaded ribs (rickets)
      3. Deficiency is extremely rare because vitamin D requirements are met by 1 to 2 hours of sunlight a day
   C. Vitamin E
      1. Oxidation rapidly destroys vitamin E
      2. Old hay or ground grains are poor sources
      3. Deficiency is recognized as a common cause of white muscle disease
      4. This vitamin is of practical importance only to the young
      5. Vitamin E has a direct relationship with selenium
   D. Vitamin K
      1. Synthesized by rumen bacteria
      2. Becomes toxic in moldy sweet clover
   E. B-complex vitamins
      1. Milk replacers should be fortified
      2. Deficiency may result if animal goes "off feed" for a long period of time
         a. Death will likely occur if deficiencies are not corrected
   F. Vitamin C
      1. Not required; ruminants synthesize their own vitamin C

Life Stages

I. Breeding and pregnant animals
   A. Period of weaning to breeding is critical because a high rate of twinning and milk production is desired
   B. Females should not be allowed to become excessively fat
   C. There should be a slight daily weight gain from weaning to breeding
   D. After mating, females can be maintained on good pasture
   E. During the last 6 to 8 weeks of pregnancy, growth of the fetus is rapid; therefore nutrition should be increased gradually. This can be achieved by the addition of supplements

II. Lactating animals
   A. Good pasture is fine for grazers (sheep)
      1. Dairy goats are browsers and should be offered high-quality hay and a complete grain ration to maximize milk production
   B. If it is winter and the animal is confined, a good grain and forage ration with the addition of trace mineralized salts should be fed

III. Feeding lambs and kids
   A. Newborns should nurse within several hours of birth to ensure colostrum intake. Neonates can then nurse or be fed milk or milk replacer for approximately 2 months
   B. At 2 weeks of age, they should have free access to creep feed (ground coarse or rolled grain and hay)
   C. They should be creep fed until pasture comes available
   D. If they are not to be pastured, they should be finished in a dry lot
   E. Slowly convert to whole grain in small amounts at first, then increase until the animal is on full feed

F. In addition to grain, the animal is fed a complete diet of hay with a supplement
G. Market weight is reached in 3½ to 4 months of age

IV. Orphaned young
A. Orphans should be raised on extra milk or milk replacers
B. Ensure they receive adequate colostrum
1. Keep an extra supply of frozen colostrum for orphans
C. Give water to drink in addition to the milk when they are put on creep at 9 to 10 days of age
D. They can be weaned at four to five weeks of age if consumption of creep feed is at a reasonable level

Disease Related to Improper Nutrition

I. Bloat
A. Disease similar to that in cattle
B. Sheep and goats fed on mature pasture with available browse are unlikely to bloat

II. Enterotoxemia
A. Disease similar to that in cattle except it is more common in sheep and goats
B. Preventive measures are similar to cattle; other measures in lambs include vaccination with *C. perfringens* type D and types C and D in breeding ewes
C. If an outbreak occurs in lambs, an enterotoxemia antiserum may also be administered

III. FPT
A. Similar to that in cattle

IV. Grass tetany
A. Disease similar to that in cattle

V. Ketosis (lambing paralysis)
A. Seen most commonly in ewes (during the last trimester) carrying twins or triplets
B. Preventive measures include feeding the ewe a higher-energy diet supplied through increased grain intake

VI. Thiamin-deficiency polio
A. Disease similar to that in cattle
B. Goats (doe) may be affected while nursing the kids

VII. Rickets
A. Disease similar to that in cattle

VIII. Rumen acidosis
A. Disease similar to that in cattle

IX. Urea toxicity
A. Disease similar to that in cattle

X. Water belly
A. Disease similar to that in cattle
B. Most common in castrated pygmy goats, although there is an increased incidence in all males
C. Other preventive measures in sheep and goats include increasing salt availability and avoiding vitamin A deficiency

XI. White muscle disease
A. Disease similar to that in cattle
B. White muscle disease is most common in the rapidly growing individuals of a flock

Raising sheep and goats can be a relatively low maintenance operation if done properly; however, it is important to find the best feedstuff available in your area. Keep in mind that because of the size and constitutions of sheep and goats, deficiencies or toxicities can develop rather quickly; death rates can be high as a result.

FEEDING CAMELIDS

Llamas, alpacas, vicunas, and guanacos are part of the group known as South American Camelids. Camelids are not classified taxonomically as ruminants but are considered to be functional ruminants. Functional ruminants, like true ruminants, have the ability to convert roughage to usable nutrients. Camelids consume both grass and legume forages and browse and forbs with equal relish. In South America, camelids never need concentrates or supplements and are rarely fed cured hay because they thrive well on the native grasses and forbs. This section on camelid nutrition discusses the feeding and nutrition of camelids in North America to maintain proper health.

Feed Sources

I. Forages
A. Although camelids are native to South America and thus have evolved to thrive on forages of that region, they still have the ability to thrive on native grasses of North America
B. Typical grasses and legumes grown in North America that are fed to true ruminants can be fed to camelids
1. Camelids are extremely efficient in their ability to convert forages to energy
a. Obesity is a concern in overfed camelids
2. Camelids do best when they are allowed to graze on pasture
C. Feed consumption is based on a percentage of body weight and is higher in the smaller animal and lower in the larger animal
1. A 50-kg (110-lb) camelid will consume feed at 1.4% of its body weight on an "as-fed" basis

2. A 150-kg (330-lb) camelid will consume feed at 1.1% of its body weight on an "as-fed" basis

II. Browse and forbs
   A. Browse and forbs are an extremely important part of the camelids' diet. Camelids are selective consumers of shrubs and leaves. Camelids should be allowed free access to these food sources when available

III. Concentrates
   A. Because camelids are such efficient converters of forage to usable nutrients, concentrates are rarely, if ever, needed
   B. Concentrates may be useful in cases where increased energy and protein are necessary
   C. Mixtures of grains and protein supplements can be used as concentrates

IV. Supplements
   A. Minerals and vitamins can be supplied in block or granular form if the extra nutrients are needed in the diet
      1. Llamas prefer to chew on salt blocks instead of licking them

Special Nutritional Requirements

I. Water
   A. Camelids should have access to and be allowed to consume clean water at libitum
      1. Camelids are less likely to consume contaminated water compared with other animals
   B. If water intake is restricted, feed consumption will be decreased, lactation will be decreased or may cease, and in some extreme cases the camelid may become hyperthermic
   C. Camelids' erythrocytes may be more resistant to osmotic pressure changes when the animal consumes large volumes of water. This is a characteristic of camels due to the ability of the oval erythrocyte to swell up to 240% of normal size without rupturing
      1. In other species, the round erythrocytes can swell to only 150% of normal size before rupturing
   D. Water requirements of camelids are approximately 9% to 13% of body weight (kg) when on pasture
   E. Camelids living in cold climates need to have a heated waterer because they will not break through the ice to get water
   F. Trail llamas frequently do not drink during the day even if they have access to water

II. Energy
   A. Camelids may be able to convert fiber to energy more efficiently than other ruminants
   B. In comparison to cattle, camelids have a lower metabolizable energy (ME) requirement
   C. Like other ruminants, energy sources include forages and the grains/concentrates that are consumed

III. Protein
   A. Protein requirements are directly related to energy requirements and similar to those of sheep and goats
      1. Protein requirements are 31 g protein per Mcal DE
   B. Camelids can convert poor-quality low-level protein as efficiently as can sheep
   C. Crude protein intake of 10% is adequate for maintenance, and crude protein intake of 16% is required for growth, lactation, and late pregnancy
      1. Crude protein requirements are calculated on a 100% DM basis

IV. Minerals
   A. Calcium and phosphorus
      1. A camelid's final diet should contain more than 0.3% calcium on a DM basis
      2. Calcium/phosphorus ratio should not be less than 1.2:1
      3. Calcium and phosphorus levels are rarely deficient in temperate climate pasture, but tropical climate pastures may be deficient in phosphorus
   B. Sodium and chloride
      1. Camelids should have free access to a mineral block
   C. Cobalt
      1. Need for cobalt is similar to that of other domestic large animals
      2. A deficiency of cobalt eventually leads to thiamin and ascorbic acid deficiency and reduced glucose and ATP levels
         a. Signs of deficiency include ocular discharge, lethargy, weakness, poor weight gain, anemia, ketosis, rough hair coat, and decreased conception rates
      3. Signs of toxicity are similar to those of deficiencies
   D. Copper
      1. Signs of deficiency and toxicity similar to those of cattle and sheep
         a. Camelids are quite sensitive to copper toxicity
      2. Llamas and alpacas fed side-by-side with sheep in copper-deficient areas did not develop deficiencies
   E. Iron
      1. Iron deficiency in llamas and alpacas is thought to be a factor in the failure to thrive syndrome seen in the cria (neonate)

a. Camelid milk contains little iron, much like other domestic large animals

2. Signs of deficiency and treatment methods are similar to those of other domestic large animals

F. Selenium

1. As in other animals, selenium and vitamin E must be balanced
2. Signs of deficiency are similar to signs in cattle and sheep
3. Selenium supplementation is best offered in a grain mix or as part of a trace mineralized salt block

G. Zinc

1. Zinc has close interactions with calcium, copper, iron, and vitamin A
2. Zinc deficiency in llamas and alpacas may present as a dermatitis
3. Signs of toxicities have not been observed or reported in llamas and alpacas
4. Zinc should be incorporated into trace mineral mixes to prevent deficiencies

H. Iodine

1. Llamas and alpacas are at risk when raised in iodine-deficient areas in North America
2. Prevention of deficiencies is easily accomplished through iodine supplementation in the mineral mix or grain mix
3. Iodine toxicity is rare but is readily prevented by avoiding excessive therapy with iodine-containing medications and preventing overconsumption of iodized salts

V. Vitamins

A. Microbes in the first compartment of camelids synthesize B-complex vitamins, vitamin C, and vitamin K

1. Deficiencies occur when first compartment microbial activity is altered
2. Importance of vitamins B complex, C, and K is similar to that for other ruminants

B. Species-specific data for vitamins A, D, and E are limited in camelid medicine

1. Signs of deficiency/toxicity and treatment methods are best taken from other ruminant species data and applied to camelids
2. Importance of vitamins A, D, and E is similar to that for other ruminants

Life Stages

Although specific life stage nutrition resources are not available, a practical guide to each stage can be extrapolated from those for other large animal species. These guidelines include the following.

I. Ensure the cria (neonate) receives adequate colostrum from the dam within the first 18 to 24 hours after birth

II. Juveniles will need extra energy and a high-quality protein source for growth. A balanced source of minerals and vitamins will also be important in growth

III. The adult should be fed for maintenance to avoid issues with obesity

IV. Pregnant dam will need more energy and protein in the last trimester for growth of the fetus

V. Lactating dam will need higher energy and protein levels to nurse the cria

Disease Related to Improper Nutrition

I. FPT

A. Similar to cattle

II. Failure to thrive/wasting syndrome

A. Some llamas have been observed to become anorectic, lose weight, and die

B. This condition is a complex syndrome that may be caused by many factors but certainly may be in part due to poor nutrition

C. Proper nutrition plays a major role in prevention of this syndrome

III. Metabolic bone disease (rickets)

A. As seen in other mammals, metabolic bone disease is caused by inadequate levels of calcium, phosphorus, and vitamin D

1. Other factors that may cause this disease include protein deficiency and primary diseases of the kidney, liver, and intestine

B. In addition to these factors, some camelid owners suspect the high calcium content in alfalfa disrupts the absorption of phosphorus, thus leading to rickets

C. Clinical signs and preventive measures are the same as those in other animals

IV. Obesity

A. Overfeeding of concentrates leading to obesity is a frequent problem

B. Feeding camelids to excess is not only costly but also leads to health problems such as infertility and hyperthermia

C. All nutritional requirements should be balanced to fit the individual animal

1. Feed more energy to underweight animals and decrease energy in overweight animals

V. Starvation/inanition

A. Underweight camelids due to starvation may be a common problem among inexperienced owners

1. Other factors that should be considered in underweight animals are infectious and parasitic diseases

B. Identifying marked weight loss in camelids may be difficult for the owner because the thick fiber coat of camelids obscures the view of the backbone
   1. Camelid owners should be instructed to evaluate body weight and body condition by
      a. Weighing and recording body weights on a regular basis
      b. Performing a body score on the animal (see Table 16-1 as a guide)
         (1) Locations for evaluating body conditions on camelids are over the withers, the fiberless area behind the elbow, between the rear legs, the chest between the front legs, and the perineum

C. Prevention of starvation is more a management issue that is simply addressed by frequently observing and weighing animals and feeding an adequate well-balanced diet

Monogastric Digestion

BASIC ANATOMY AND PHYSIOLOGY

I. Mouth and esophagus
   A. Tongue, teeth, and salivary glands are important for proper prehension, mastication, mixing, and deglutition
      1. Lips of horses are important in prehension of foodstuffs
      2. Swine saliva acts as a lubricant and as a buffer to regulate stomach pH and contains salivary amylase to break down carbohydrates
      3. Equine saliva contains no enzymes
      4. Horses cannot regurgitate because of one-way esophageal peristalsis

II. Stomach
   A. Stomach of swine is a muscular organ that causes the physical breakdown of food through powerful contractions
      1. Hydrochloric acid, pepsin, and rennin are the digestive enzymes secreted by the stomach
      2. Swine stomachs maintain a pH of 2 and have a strong bactericidal effect on ingested microorganisms
   B. Equine stomach is smaller relative to that of other animal species
      1. Horses should be fed small portions more frequently per day
      2. Equine stomach does not mix foodstuffs well, so digestive disorders often originate in the stomach

III. Small intestine
   A. Small intestine of swine and horses is divided into the duodenum, jejunum, and ileum, like all monogastric animals
   B. Small intestine is important because digestive enzymes are mixed with chyme (food mixture from the stomach), digestion continues, and nutrients are absorbed
   C. A unique characteristic of horses is that they have no gallbladder so constantly secrete bile into the duodenum

IV. Large intestine
   A. Cecum
      1. Cecum of swine has minimal function in digestion
      2. Cecum of horses, however, is quite large (up to 15-gallon [4-L] capacity in mature animals) and serves to break down cellulose and synthesize nutrients via microbial fermentation much like the rumen of cattle
   B. Colon
      1. Function of the colon in swine and horses is resorption of water, bacterial fermentation of vitamins B and K, synthesis of protein, some break down of fiber, and limited nutrient absorption
      2. Water is absorbed primarily from the small colon in horses
   C. Rectum
      1. Serves to store waste before defecation

FEEDING SWINE

I. Swine are omnivores and as such can accommodate some dietary fiber

II. Swine exhibit a better rate of gain from concentrates, which are fortified with energy, protein, and mineral and vitamin supplements to form the normal diet

III. Advanced technology is highly evident in many swine operations today
   A. Formulation of diets is more precise and economical, with synthetic nutrients, high-quality byproducts, and new feeds
   B. Swine operations use the technology of their feed supplier to meet the nutritional needs of all pigs in the herd
   C. Feeding a premix in their regular grain ration will meet nutritional needs
   D. Nutrient deficiencies of these grains are corrected by the premix
   E. All life stages are met with different premix formulations

Feed Sources, Preparation and Feeding of Grains

I. Improvements in gain and feed efficiency can be expected from grinding grain, but if grain is ground too fine, digestive problems can be created

II. Grain should be reduced to a medium-fine particle size
III. Common grains are corn, oats, wheat, barley, and sorghum

Special Nutritional Requirements

I. Water
   A. Best given free choice with easy access
II. Energy (chiefly carbohydrates and fat)
   A. Energy content in a diet controls the amount eaten
   B. Fiber corresponds directly to fat
   C. High-energy diets are fed during lactation
III. Protein and amino acids
   A. Amino acids are essential for maintenance, growth, gestation, and lactation
   B. Amino acids indispensable for growing pigs are arginine, histidine, isoleucine, leucine, lysine, methionine, phenylalanine, threonine, tryptophan, and valine
      1. Three of greatest importance are lysine, tryptophan, and threonine
IV. Minerals
   A. Calcium and phosphorus
      1. Primarily for skeletal growth
      2. Play important metabolic roles in the body
      3. Adequacy is essential to gestation and lactation
      4. Easily supplied by use of tankage, meat meal, meat and bone and fish meal, limestone, and oyster shell
   B. Sodium chloride
      1. Recommended salt allowance is 0.25% of the total diet
      2. Supplied by animal and fish byproducts in the diet
   C. Iodine
      1. Used by the thyroid gland to produce thyroxine
      2. Supplied as iodized salt
   D. Iron and copper
      1. Necessary for hemoglobin formation and to prevent nutritional anemia
      2. Sow's milk is severely deficient in iron
      3. Feeding lactating sows increased levels of iron does not seem to pass sufficiently high levels to piglets
   E. Cobalt
      1. Present in the B_{12} molecule
   F. Manganese
      1. Essential for normal reproduction and growth
   G. Potassium
      1. Requirements are met in the feedstuffs
   H. Magnesium
      1. Essential for growing swine
   I. Zinc
      1. In swine nutrition, zinc is interrelated with calcium
      2. Supplemented zinc is recommended to prevent parakeratosis
   J. Selenium
      1. Vitamin E is interrelated with selenium
      2. Selenium requirement depends on soil conditions where crop for feed is grown. Most swine today are raised in total confinement
V. Vitamins
   A. Vitamin A
      1. Use of stabilized vitamin A is common
      2. Natural vitamin A tends to get destroyed under normal environmental conditions
   B. Vitamin D
      1. Necessary for proper bone growth and ossification
      2. Vitamin D needs can be met by exposing pigs to direct sunlight for a short period of time each day
      3. Sources: irradiated yeast, sun-cured hays, activated plant or animal sterols, fish oils, and vitamin A and D concentrates
   C. Vitamin E (tocopherol)
      1. Required by swine of all ages
      2. Interrelated with selenium
      3. Green forage, legume hays, and cereal grains all contain appreciable amounts of vitamin E
   D. Vitamin K
      1. A fat-soluble vitamin, necessary for blood clotting to convert fibrinogen to fibrin
      2. Supplement vitamin K for added insurance
   E. Thiamin, riboflavin, and niacin
      1. Thiamin is not of practical importance in the diet
      2. Riboflavin is a requirement of breeding stock and lightweight pigs
         a. Crystalline form of riboflavin (and niacin) is added to premixes
      3. Riboflavin is naturally found in green forage, milk byproducts, and brewer's yeast
      4. Natural sources of niacin include fish and animal byproducts
   F. Pantothenic acid
      1. Especially important for female (reproduction)
      2. Crystalline form is added in premixes
      3. Natural sources include green forage, legume meals, milk products, and brewer's yeast
   G. Pyridoxine (vitamin B_6)
      1. Present in plentiful quantities in feed ingredients usually fed to swine

H. Choline
   1. Essential for normal functioning of liver and kidneys
   2. Supplementing choline has shown to increase litter size
   3. Naturally found in fish solubles, fish meal, and soybean meal

I. Vitamin B_{12}
   1. Required by the young pig for growth and normal hemopoiesis
   2. Present in animal, marine, and milk products
   3. Crystalline form is added to premixes

J. Biotin, folic acid, and ascorbic acid
   1. Biotin and folic acid are essential for growth
   2. There is no evidence to indicate the need to supplement

Life Stages

I. Management of breeding sows and litters
   A. Breeding sows are limit fed from breeding up to the last trimester
      1. Sows are fed 4 to 6 lb (1.8 to 2.7 kg) of a complete ration supplying 6000 to 7000 kcal ME
   B. In the last trimester, feed is increased to get additional energy to the rapidly growing fetuses
      1. Sows are fed a complete ration that supplies 9000 to 10,000 kcal ME per day
      2. Care should be taken not to overfeed the sow because this will directly affect milk production during lactation
      3. The more vigorous a baby pig is, the better is its chance for survival. To produce healthy pigs, the gestation diets must be adequate in all nutrients
   C. During lactation, energy intake will be increased to 15,000 to 20,000 kcal ME per day
      1. Fat may be added to the diet to improve feed palatability and energy density

II. Management of piglets
   A. Care should be taken to ensure that each piglet has nursed regularly
      1. Keep the sow's teat line clean so the piglets are less likely to develop scours
         a. Scouring leads to poor gains or even death
   B. An anemia prevention program should be in place
      1. Injection or oral iron dextran should be given within 3 days of birth
   C. A palatable pig starter diet should be available from 2 weeks of age until weaning

III. Starter pigs
   A. Piglets are weaned at 3 to 5 weeks of age and are fed as starters until they weigh 40 to 50 lb (18 to 22.7 kg)
      1. Starter pigs are fed ad libitum
   B. Starter rations are high in protein (20% to 24%), nutrient dense, supplied as a pellet, and often purchased from a commercial feed supplier because of the feed complexity
   C. Starter ration is eventually changed to a ground feed in the last couple weeks of the starter period

IV. Management of growing/finishing market hogs
   A. For today's market hog, higher levels of protein and less energy are fed to develop the leanest animal
      1. Feeds are evaluated on their amino acid content
      2. Protein sources supplied in the growing/finishing ration are usually soybean meal, meat and bone meal, and synthetic amino acids
         a. Synthetic amino acids are lysine, methionine, threonine, and tryptophan
   B. Grower/finishers are fed ground cereal grains (corn, wheat, sorghum, and barley), which make up to 85% of a typical ration
   C. Growing/finishing rations are fortified with numerous minerals and vitamins
      1. Calcium and phosphorus is balanced at a 1 to 2:1 during this period
   D. Housing and space are very important aspects in growing/finishing swine

A veterinary technician's role in a swine facility involves herd health and piglet care. Nutritional needs and problems are met by the feed supplier with premixes and rations tailored to each individual operation and life stage of the pig.

Disease Related to Improper Nutrition

I. Anemia
   A. Anemia is a regularly diagnosed problem in baby pigs
   B. Baby pigs should be given iron dextran by injection (150 to 200 mg) or as an oral solution
   C. Iron can also be supplied in the prestarter ration of piglets that are creep feeding
   D. Vitamin E should be given just before the iron injection to prevent iron toxicity

II. FPT
   A. Similar to that of other livestock
   B. Runt piglets within a litter fail to thrive and may need special attention

III. Parakeratosis
   A. Metabolic disturbance due to a deficiency of zinc and an excess of calcium in the diet

B. Disease is characterized by changes in the skin, mainly skin lesions. The skin lesions are areas of excessive growth and keratinization of the skin epithelium

C. Parakeratosis is prevented and treated by balancing zinc and calcium in the diet

FEEDING HORSES

Horses are herbivores and are classified as hindgut fermenters. The stomach has a relatively small capacity (5 to 15 L) and contributes little to the digestion of the feed. Horses must eat frequently. Enzymatic digestion similar to that of dogs and cats occurs in the small intestine. Any ingested food that reaches the cecum and large intestine undergoes microbial fermentation. There is no gallbladder for storage, and bile is excreted continuously.

Feed Sources

I. Horse consumes most of its nutritional requirements in the form of forages such as hay and pasture
   A. Quality of dry roughage depends greatly on the stage of maturation at harvesting and weather conditions during harvest
   B. Soil quality also has an effect on forage quality
   C. Ensiled forage is not generally fed because of the sensitivity of horses to molds and mycotoxins that may be in silage

II. Ideal forages include grass hay (brome grass, orchard grass, Bermuda grass, and timothy), legume hay (alfalfa and clover), and grazing pastures
   A. Straw and corn stalks are not recommended as a feed because of the low nutritional value and the risk of compaction if too much is consumed
   B. Hay and grasses contain varying amounts of cellulose and starch, depending on their maturity
   C. It is important for horses that all forages are clean and dry with no mold or dust present. Forages should be leafy, have a green color, and be harvested earlier so plant fiber can be easily digested

III. Grains are used as a supplement to any forage feeding program
   A. Amount of grain will be indicated by horse's life stage and/or workload
   B. Corn, barley, wheat, and oats are common grain supplements
   C. Protein supplements such as linseed meal, soybean meal, and milk protein (foal diet) can be offered to improve feed protein values
   D. Horses should be fed forages before grains to ensure proper and complete digestion of the grain
      1. If grains are fed before or with forages, the grains are passed in the feces before they are adequately digested
   E. Fat and vegetable oil supplementation has been suggested to provide energy for growing, lactating, and working horses
   F. Fermentable fiber byproducts such as rice, wheat bran, and beet pulp are becoming more popular
      1. Wheat bran is often used in conjunction with psyllium to improve fiber bulk to prevent or treat sand colic in horses

IV. Horses should be kept free from disease and dewormed on a regular basis to fully benefit from good nutritional practices

Special Nutritional Requirements

I. Carbohydrates supply 80% to 90% of dietary energy for horses and are available in the forms of grains, forages, and supplements. The interaction of minerals and vitamins and their availability in the grains and grasses grown can be complex

II. Minerals and vitamins
   A. Amount required for all minerals vary according to age, weight, and work of the horse
   B. Minerals and vitamins for the horse are essentially the same as for cattle (see earlier section)
   C. If feedstuff is deficient in minerals, a mineral supplement may be fed free choice
      1. If a mineral deficiency is suspected, do not overlook the resources of the local diagnostic laboratory
      2. Any deficiency is often the result of anorexia or poor-quality feed
   D. Over supplementation generally occurs inadvertently by well-meaning owners
   E. For ease of definition for horse feeding, minerals can be divided into two groups: macrominerals and microminerals
      1. Macrominerals
         a. Macrominerals are constituents of bones and structural proteins
         b. Expressed as parts per hundred
         c. Potassium: most forages have this available
         d. Calcium and phosphorus: for bone and cell function
            (1) Ratio is about 1.7:1 in foals and 1 to 1.3:1 in adults
            (2) Deficiency can cause abnormal bone growth and thin weak bones. Mild deficiencies may cause subtle lameness
            (3) Excess calcium may impair trace mineral and phosphorus absorption.

Excess phosphorus can cause a secondary nutritional hyperparathyroidism

e. Magnesium
   (1) Deficiency is very uncommon but if present will cause staggering, nervousness, and convulsions

f. Sodium chloride (salt) is necessary for cell function and water balance
   (1) Salt is typically fed in a block
   (2) Horses lose 30 grains of salt in every lb of perspiration; working horses require additional salt in their grain rations
   (3) Salt added to a ration does not take care of the other minerals if the forage and grain are deficient

2. Microminerals
   a. Referred to as trace minerals; only small amounts needed by the horse
   b. Measured as parts per million (mg/kg)
   c. Iodine
      (1) Produces the hormone thyroxine, which is needed in fetal development
      (2) Deficiencies can cause serious fetal abnormalities
      (3) Foals will be born weak and prone to infections and may not suckle or stand; thyroid glands can be enlarged
      (4) Mares may have goiter, a longer gestation, and retained placenta
      (5) Excess can cause same symptoms as deficiency
   d. Copper
      (1) Important for cartilage, bone, and pigment formation and for utilization of iron
   e. Iron
      (1) Necessary to form hemoglobin
      (2) Deficiency causes anemia
      (3) Overuse of injectable iron can cause iron toxicity
   f. Manganese and zinc
      (1) Zinc deficiency may cause hair loss and poor wound healing
      (2) Zinc excess can cause bone problems and lameness
   g. Selenium
      (1) Needed with vitamin E
      (2) Deficiency causes white muscle disease. Foals are born weak and unable to stand, suckle, or breathe normally. Mares have reduced fertility and increased incidence of retained placentas
      (3) Excess causes serious health problems. Overdose can cause sudden excitability and difficulty breathing. Chronic high intakes cause lameness, loss of mane or tail hair, and hoof deformity

III. Protein
   A. Feeding excess protein is wasteful. A strong ammonia odor exists in stables where horses are fed excess protein
      1. Alfalfa hay will cause stronger ammonia smell than grass hay due to increased nitrogen
   B. Protein-deficient diets are very harmful
      1. Signs can be low weight gains or weight loss and skeletal stunting in young horses

IV. Water
   A. Water is vital
   B. Horse's body is made up of 70% water
   C. Horses drink 2 to 4 L water/kg DM feed eaten (1 gallon/2 lb of dry feed). A 1000-lb (455-kg) horse fed hay will drink about 40 to 50 L (10.5 to 13 gallons) daily
   D. Intake also depends on size of horse, amount and type of diet fed, outdoor temperature, and amount of work being done

Life Stages

I. Feeding programs are based on the following
   A. Age (weanling, yearling, 2-year-old, mature adult, senior)
   B. Current weight and ideal for age
   C. Function: idle, working, or breeding
   D. Feeds available in the area
   E. Management, including housing conditions and overcrowding

II. Feed consumption
   A. A proper horse-feeding program provides adequate water and energy to ensure proper body condition (see Table 16-1)
   B. Calculations are generally based on a horse's weight and the amount of feed required per 100 lb (45 kg) of horse
      1. Adult at maintenance requires about 1.2% to 1.5% of body weight of forage DM per day
         a. Example: A 1000-lb (450-kg) horse requiring 1.5% dietary forage would receive 15 lb (7 kg) of hay per day or, in practical terms, three 5-lb (2.3-kg) "flakes" of hay per day
      2. Energy levels need to be increased when exercise or work increases and is generally supplied by grains and concentrates

3. Pregnancy demands an increase in energy of 20% to 30%, depending on the stage
4. Peak lactation may need 75% increase in energy
5. Ribs should be felt but not seen in young horses

III. Feeding the horse
   A. Feeding suckling foals and weanlings
      1. Suckling foals
         a. Ensure the foal stands within 2 hours of birth and begins nursing. Adequate colostrum intake is critical within the first 18 hours to ensure maximum absorption of colostral antibodies
            (1) Healthy foal will nurse from the mare 25 to 30 times per day and ingest 20% or more of their body weight in milk
         b. Foal will obtain the majority of its nutrients from nursing for the first several months of life
            (1) Make sure the mare is fed adequate amounts of high-quality feedstuffs while nursing the foal
         c. Offer small amounts of creep feeds and high-quality forages beginning as early as 1 to 2 weeks of age
            (1) Commercial concentrate mixtures (sweet feed) supplying 16% crude protein are recommended
            (2) Young foals may be offered creep feeds top dressed with milk protein/milk replacer if they are not gaining weight adequately
         d. Starting at 2 to 3 months of age, feed 1 lb of grain (0.45 kg) concentrate per day and increase to 1 additional lb of grain concentrate for every month of age through weaning, with a maximum of 7 to 9 lb (3.2 to 4 kg) of grain concentrate
         e. Start deworming foals at 2 to 3 months of age
            (1) Continue a deworming schedule of every 30 to 60 days throughout life
      2. Weanlings
         a. Weanlings should be fed 6 to 8 lb (2.7 to 3.6 kg) of concentrate per day and at least 1 lb of high-quality forage for every 100 lb (45 kg) of body weight through 12 months of age
         b. DM intake should equal 3% of body weight
   B. Feeding yearlings and 2-year-olds
      1. Yearlings can be fed free choice high-quality hay and pasture at this stage
      2. Yearlings and 2-year-olds should still be receiving an adequate supply of protein, vitamins, and minerals to ensure proper growth and development of the body tissues and skeleton
         a. Trace mineralized salt blocks should be made available
      3. A 13% crude protein concentrate can be fed at this stage
      4. DM intake should equal 2.5% of body weight
   C. Feeding the mature horse, dry mare, and gelding
      1. A mature animal that is idle or ridden or worked infrequently can be maintained on hay or pasture alone
         a. DM intake should equal about 1.75% of body weight
      2. A calcium/phosphorus and salt supplement should be offered to these animals
      3. Concentrates can always be offered in small amounts or can be increased based on the amount of work. Make changes in diet slowly, preferably over 7 to 10 days
         a. Concentrate protein levels may be fed at 8.5% to 10% crude protein
   D. Feeding for reproduction
      1. Gestation
         a. A mare can be fed at maintenance levels until the last 90 days of gestation
         b. During late pregnancy, the mare needs 20% more energy and an increase to an 11% crude protein level
         c. During the last 3 weeks of gestation the mare needs 30% more energy, more calcium and phosphorus, and 1.75 to 2.0 lb (0.7 to 0.9 kg) of legume hay per 100 lb (45 kg) of body weight
            (1) If nutrient intake was adequate during gestation, the mare should have gained an extra 10% body weight
            (2) Lactation
               (a) Same ration type fed to yearlings can be used for the lactating mare
               (b) Bring the mare to a full feed regimen providing 1 to 1.5 lb (0.45 to 0.7 kg) of concentrate per 100 lb of body weight within 7 to 10 days postpartum
               (c) If rebreeding the mare while she is still lactating, be sure to consider the total energy requirements needed for maintenance, lactation, and rebreeding. Offer additional amounts of feed to

allow the mare to gain weight to get her in breeding condition

E. Feeding the working or performance horse
   1. Exercise increases a horse's need for energy, not necessarily the protein and mineral requirements
   2. A hard working horse may require more concentrate than forage to supply the needed energy
      a. Be sure to feed at least 1 lb (0.45 kg) forage per 100 lb (45 kg) of body weight to minimize digestive disturbances
      b. A light working horse on 8.5% crude protein concentrate needs 0.5 to 1.5 lb (0.2 to 0.7 kg) of grain per hour of activity per day
      c. A moderate working horse on 8.5% to 10% crude protein concentrate needs 2 to 3 lb (0.9 to 1.4 kg) of grain per hour of activity per day
      d. A heavy working horse on 8.5% to 10% crude protein concentrate needs at least 4 lb (≥1.8 kg) of grain per hour of activity per day
   3. After heavy exercise, be sure to cool the horse down before allowing the horse to drink. A hot horse is more likely to have digestive disturbances and to founder if allowed to drink immediately after exercise

F. Feeding stallions
   1. Feed stallions at maintenance levels when not used for breeding
   2. Offer some additional grain during the breeding season to keep the stallion in good breeding condition

G. Feeding hospitalized horses
   1. A sick horse has the same nutritional deficits, stresses, and catabolic wasting problems that small animals have when they are sick. Major gastrointestinal disturbances (e.g., colic and colitis), including decreased gastrointestinal motility, often lead to an animal that is unwilling to eat
   2. It may be necessary to administer a slurry of feedstuffs by a nasogastric tube to ensure the animal receives some nutrients until it is ready to eat on its own

Disease Related to Improper Nutrition

I. Rhabdomyolysis (myositis, azoturia, Monday morning sickness)
   A. Acute inflammatory disease of muscle
      1. Clinical signs of disease include excessive sweating, nervousness, abdominal distress, reluctance to walk or move, stiff gait, and coffee-colored urine (myoglobinuria)
   B. True cause of rhabdomyolysis is unclear, but it is associated with a high-grain or -concentrate diet throughout the week and then rest for 1 to 2 days; this is when they develop clinical signs
   C. Preventive measures include reducing feed intake when a horse is not working and exercising the animal during the rest period

II. Colic
   A. Many different causes of colic exist. Potential nutritional issues include inadequate water intake, overfeeding, overeating on new pasture, and improper feeding
   B. Preventive measures for colic include proper feeding and deworming practices, free access to salt to encourage adequate water intake, and limiting exposure to new pasture

III. Choke
   A. Choke is not considered a true nutritional disease but can be attributed to improper feeding practices
   B. Most common causes of choke are inadequate water intake, feedstuffs that are fed too dry, feedstuff particle sizes that are too large, and a horse that is a greedy eater
   C. Preventive measures include encouraging adequate water intake, soaking feedstuffs before feeding (e.g., beet pulp and alfalfa cubes), and using hay nets or restrictive muzzles to slow feed intake of greedy eaters

IV. Diarrhea (colitis)
   A. Nutritional diarrhea is uncommon in the equine foal or adult, and not all cases can be associated with some specific disease or nutritional imbalance
   B. Any change in feed or feeding regimen and nutritional imbalances could change the gastrointestinal environment and lead to diarrhea
   C. It is best to offer only good-quality feedstuffs and balanced diets and to change feeds or feeding regimens slowly over a 7- to 10-day period

V. FPT
   A. Similar to that in livestock
   B. Foals nursing mares that came into milk early and were leaking colostrum and foals later diagnosed with neonatal maladjustment syndrome ("dumby-foal") tend to be at the greatest risk
   C. Prevention is similar to that in livestock. Taking a proactive role in ensuring the foal stands and nurses within the first few hours of life is critical

VI. Heaves

Table 16-2 Relative nutrient content of various feedstuffs for livestock

	Relative nutrient content						
			Minerals		Vitamins		
Feedstuff group	Protein	Energy	Macro	Micro	Fat-Sol.	B-complex	Fiber
High quality roughage	+++	++	++	++	+++	+	+++
Low quality roughage	+	+	+	+	−	−	++++
Cereal grains	++	+++	+	+	+	+	+
Grain millfeeds	++	++	++	++	+	++	++
Fats and oils	−	++++	−	−	−	−	−
Molasses	+	+++	++	++	−	+	−
Fermentation products	+++	++	+	++	−	++++	±
Oil seed proteins	+++	+++	++	++	+	++	+
Animal proteins	++++	+++	+++	+++	++	+++	+

Reprinted from Grosdidier SR et al: Nutrition. In Pratt PW, ed: *Principles and practice of veterinary technology*, St Louis, 1998, Mosby.

A. Essential cause of heaves is unknown, but it is associated with the consumption of moldy feeds or dusty feeds at times of challenge (e.g., upper respiratory disease, pneumonia)
B. Incidence of heaves may be decreased by feeding good-quality dust-free feedstuffs or by moistening dusty feeds

VII. Laminitis and chronic founder
A. Laminitis is often associated with consumption of excess grain, lush pasture, or water
B. By providing a proper ration and monitoring consumption of feedstuffs, most instances of nutritionally induced laminitis and chronic founder can be prevented

VIII. Moonblindness (periodic ophthalmia, equine recurrent uveitis)
A. Occurrence of moonblindness appears to be associated with a lack of riboflavin and with bacterial or viral disease
B. By feeding rations that contain at least 40 mg of riboflavin per day (green grass and green leafy hay), incidences of moonblindness may be reduced

IX. Rickets
A. As in other large animals, rickets is associated with imbalances of calcium, phosphorus, and/or vitamin D
B. By balancing the minerals and vitamins in the ration, rickets can be prevented

X. Water belly
A. As in other large animal species, males are most often affected
B. Clinical signs, cause, and prevention of water belly are similar to those of other large animal species

Consult the district agrologist for types of feeds and nutrient levels in your area. There are usually pamphlets available on the care and feeding of horses that pertains to the climate and area in which you are situated. All horses are individuals, and feeding programs should stress that. The diet must be balanced for proteins, minerals, and vitamins.

Ruminant, swine, and equine feeding is a science that should be practically met whenever possible in agricultural operations. Large animal veterinarians who have a herd health practice will rely heavily on nutritional diagnosis. The importance of the technician is to be able to take accurate descriptions of feeding programs, know where discrepancies may occur, and know what mineral and vitamin deficiencies occur in the area. A technician in a large animal practice will have to answer questions regarding feeding programs, and it helps to have some common knowledge of basic nutrition (Table 16-2).

ACKNOWLEDGEMENT

The author and editors recognize and appreciate the original work of Sandy Hass, on which this chapter is based.

Glossary

additive Ingredient or combination of ingredients added to the basic feed to fulfill a specific need

ad libitum Means "as needed"; also thought of as free choice

background Feed a calf to gain 1 to 1.5 lb (0.45 to 0.7 kg) of body weight a day

biological value Percentage of true absorbed protein that is available for productive body functions

bloom Stage of flowering in legumes. Usually classified as early, 50% bloom, 75% bloom, or full bloom

browse Brushy plant, a shrub, a bush, or a tree of small stature

carbonaceous High in energy; some feedstuffs are naturally high in energy

choke Obstruction of the esophagus with feedstuffs or foreign bodies. Seen most often in the horse and cattle

colostrum First milk from postparturient animal that is high in antibodies and is nutrient rich

concentrates Classification of a feedstuff. Concentrate feeds include corn, milo, cottonseeds, barley, wheat, etc. Concentrates are feeds that are low in fiber. A concentrate is divided into two categories: protein or energy
cria Neonatal llama and alpaca
deglutition Act of swallowing
digestible energy (DE) Gross energy of a food minus the energy lost in the feces. This measurement can have a tendency to overestimate the available energy of high-fiber feedstuffs
digestion Process of protein, carbohydrate, and fat break down into absorbable nutrients
dry matter intake (DMI) Percentage of dry matter that an animal consumes. A very important criterion for formulating rations
ensiling Harvesting process by which a forage is chopped and placed in a storage unit (e.g., silo) that excludes oxygen. Through fermenting, lactic acid is produced
eructation "Belching" of rumen gas
feedlot Where a beef or dairy animal is fed to slaughter. Feed resources must be known to calculate a balanced ration
feedstuff Also called feed; any dietary component that provides some essential nutrient
forbs Leafy plant
founder Inflammation of the tissue that attaches the hoof to the foot, also called laminitis. Founder is considered to be a more chronic condition, whereas laminitis is either acute or chronic
gross energy (GE) Related to chemical composition. It has no real value in assessing feed but has to be used in determining the energy value of feedstuffs
haylage Ensiled chopped alfalfa
herbivore Species of animal that depends entirely on plants for food
legumes Leafy hay such as alfalfa, red and white clover, birdsfoot trefoil, and vetch
maintenance nutrient requirements (MNRs) Levels of nutrients needed to sustain body weight without gain or loss
mastication Reduction in feed particle size by chewing
Mcal Megacalorie; 1 Mcal is equal to 1000 kcal
metabolizable energy (ME) Measure of the dietary energy available for metabolism after energy losses that occur in the urine (UE) and the combustible gases are subtracted from digestible energy. DE and ME are correlated
NPN Nonprotein nitrogen includes compounds (e.g., urea and biurates) that are not true protein in nature but contain nitrogen and can be converted to protein through bacterial action in the rumen of livestock
nutrient Substance that can be used as food
parakeratosis In swine, it is caused by a zinc deficiency and is characterized by excessive growth and keratinization of the skin
potable water Clean, fresh water suitable for drinking
premix Total ration mixed with various feedstuffs at the feed mill
proteinaceous High in protein value. Some feedstuffs have a naturally high protein value
ration Amount of total feed provided to one animal during a 24-hour period for the desired productive purpose
regurgitation Casting up of undigested material (cud); cud is remasticated and reswallowed
replacement heifer Female calf placed in the breeding herd at 24 to 30 months of age, when she has her first parturition
rhabdomyolysis Severe muscle damage that can occur when horses are fed a high-grain or -concentrate diet throughout the week and then are rested for 1 to 2 days. They develop clinical signs that include myoglobinemia and myoglobinuria (coffee-colored urine)
roughages or forages Consist of most or all of the plant, such as pasture and hay
scours Neonatal diarrhea
silage Ensiled chopped corn
springing heifer Pregnant (first calf) heifer
tankage Act or process of storing or putting in a tank; animal residues left after rendering fat in a slaughter house used for fertilizer or feed
tocopherol Vitamin E
total digestible nutrients (TDNs) Attempts to measure digestible energy in weight units. The basis is rather simple: every feed has a total energy. After it has been through the animal, measure what comes out. What is left over is the TDN
total mixed ration (TMR) Practice of weighing and blending all feedstuffs into a complete ration
transfaunation Repopulation of healthy ruminant rumen microbes into another ruminant with poor rumen function or decreased rumen microbial population. This is most often accomplished through siphoning the healthy rumen microbes from a donor animal (microbe-rich liquid or transfaunate) via a stomach tube and then placing an orogastic tube in the recipient's distal esophagus or rumen and administering the transfaunate

Review Questions

1 Geographical factors that affect nutrition and feeding in large animals are
   a. Environment
   b. Temperature variations
   c. Wind, precipitation, sun exposure
   d. All of the above

2 The "fermentation vat" in ruminants is the
   a. Omasum
   b. Abomasum
   c. Rumen and reticulum
   d. None of the above

3 Proteins are important for all of the following except
   a. Growth and reproduction
   b. Lactation
   c. Prevention of digestive problems
   d. Repair of body tissues

4 The purpose of creep feeding is to
   a. Allow young access to grain that the dams are denied
   b. Allow dams access to grain that the young are denied
   c. Increase ovulation before breeding
   d. Improve lactation capacity of dairy cattle

5 Vitamin A deficiency in cattle results in all except
   a. Rickets
   b. Reproductive failure

c. Night blindness
d. Poor hair coat

6 A mineral that should be provided as free access for ruminants and cattle is
a. Copper
b. Calcium/phosphorus combination
c. Salt
d. Manganese

7 The greatest energy demand for most species occurs during
a. First trimester of pregnancy
b. Last trimester of pregnancy
c. Peak lactation
d. Growth as a yearling

8 Ruminants do not require
a. Vitamins B, C, and K
b. Vitamins A, D, E, and K
c. Vitamins A, B, and C
d. A source of protein

9 An injection given routinely to piglets at birth is
a. Seven-way clostridial injection
b. Iron
c. Vitamins A, D, and E
d. Selenium

10 Suitable feed sources for horses are
a. NPN source of protein
b. Hay and grasses
c. Barley
d. Molasses

BIBLIOGRAPHY

Aiello SE et al: *The Merck veterinary manual,* ed 8, Rahway, NJ, 1986, Merck & Co, Inc.

Aiello SE et al: *The Merck veterinary manual,* ed 8, Rahway, NJ, 1998, Merck & Co, Inc.

Church D, Kellems R: *Livestock feeds and feeding,* ed 5, Portland, OR, 2001, Prentice-Hall Career & Technology.

Fowler ME: *Medicine and surgery of South American camelids,* ed 2, Ames, 1998, Iowa State University Press.

Grosdidier SR et al: Nutrition. In Pratt PW, editor: *Principles and practices of veterinary technology,* St Louis, 1998, Mosby.

Jurgens MH: *Animal feeding and nutrition,* ed 8, 1997, Dubuque, IA Kendall/Hunt.

McCurnin D: *Clinical textbook for veterinary technicians,* Philadelphia, 2002, WB Saunders.

National Research Council: *Nutrient requirements of beef cattle,* ed 7, Washington, DC, 1996, National Academy Press.

National Research Council: *Nutrient requirements of dairy cattle,* ed 6, Washington, DC, 1988, National Academy Press.

National Research Council: *Nutrient requirements of goats: angora, dairy, and meat goats in temperate and tropical countries,* ed 5, Washington, DC, 1996, National Academy Press.

National Research Council: *Nutrient requirements of horses,* ed 5, Washington, DC, 1996, National Academy Press.

National Research Council: *Nutrient requirements of sheep,* ed 6, Washington, DC, 1985, National Academy Press.

National Research Council: *Nutrient requirements of swine,* ed 9, Washington, DC, 1988, National Academy Press.

Naylor J, Ralston S: *Large animal clinical nutrition,* St Louis, 1991, Mosby.

Radostits et al: *Veterinary medicine: a textbook of the diseases of cattle, sheep, pigs, goats, and horses,* ed 9, Philadelphia, 2000, WB Saunders.

CHAPTER 17

Laboratory Animal and Pocket Pet Medicine

Mary Martini

OUTLINE

LEARNING OUTCOMES

After reading this chapter you should be able to:

1. List the research uses and behavioral characteristics of mice, rats, hamsters, gerbils, rabbits, guinea pigs, chinchillas, hedgehogs, and degus.
2. Describe the handling and breeding consideration, signs of pain and distress, and health conditions of the above species.
3. List suggested sites and volumes for injection and sampling.
4. Suggest appropriate housing conditions for each species.
5. Discuss zoonotic diseases and their effect on research and personnel.
6. Discuss laboratory animal allergens and their affect on personnel.

Laboratory animals have been used in research for many years. In the past couple of decades, growing concern from the public over the use of animals in research has led to the establishment of guidelines to promote better care and responsible use of laboratory animals. The information provided in this section is also useful in a clinical setting when dealing with these species as pet animals. In addition to the information provided in this text, an excellent reference handbook for laboratory animals is *Formulary for Laboratory Animals,* 2nd Edition, 1999, by C. T. Hawk and S. L. Leary in association with the American College of Laboratory Animal Medicine, Iowa State University Press. This formulary covers analgesics, sedatives, anesthetics, anti-infectives, and parasiticides and is an invaluable resource.

MOUSE *(MUS MUSCULUS)*

Origin and Uses in Research

I. The laboratory mouse today is purposely bred for research
II. The different strains of mice in laboratories are defined by ecological and genetic characteristics
III. Outbred, inbred, and congenic stock are strains defined by genetic characteristics
  A. Outbred strains are the result of random mating to achieve genetic variations. An example of an outbred mouse is the CD-1. Outbred mice are considered to express heterozygosity and to represent the diversity of the human population
  B. Inbred strains are the result of brother/sister, father/daughter, mother/son matings for a minimum of 20 consecutive generations. An example of an inbred mouse is the Balb/C. Inbred mice are genetically homozygous and therefore are very useful in transplantation research
  C. Congenic strains are animals that genetically differ at one particular locus
  D. Transgenic strains are the result of microinjection of DNA into mouse eggs for the production of very specific disease models; particularly useful in studying some forms of cancer
IV. The strains of mice defined by ecological characteristics can be divided into axenic, gnotobiotic, specific pathogen free, barrier sustained, and conventional
  A. Axenic, or germ-free, animals are hysterectomy derived, free from any microorganisms, and maintained in a germ-free isolation-type housing system
  B. Gnotobiotic mice are germ-free mice that have been introduced to one or more known nonpathogenic microorganisms. They are housed in isolators or barrier units
  C. Specific pathogen–free (SPF) and viral antibody–free (VAF) animals are those free from specific pathogenic organisms
  D. Barrier-sustained animals are gnotobiotic animals maintained under sterile conditions in a barrier unit. All air, bedding, and water must be sterilized; staff usually shower and aseptically scrub and dress before entering
  E. Conventional animals are those housed with no special precautions. They are typically SPF/VAF in origin
  F. In both a barrier-sustained and conventional housing facility, sentinel animals are used to ensure that the animals maintain their expected health status
V. Mice are the most widely used vertebrate in toxicology studies and biomedical research

Characteristics: Behavioral and Physiological

I. Mice are social animals and can usually be housed in small groups if they are compatible
II. Males that have reached puberty may fight
III. Occasionally the dominant mouse in a group will remove the facial hair from all the other mice in the cage. This is called barbering and can be a source of stress to the submissive mice, so the "barber" should be removed from the cage
IV. Mice are nocturnal animals
V. A unique anatomical feature of mice is the bone marrow of the long bones, which is functional throughout their lives
VI. Mice have a highly developed sense of smell and an acutely sensitive sense of hearing. They can respond to a range of ultrasonic frequencies and are more

likely to be disturbed by high-pitched sounds and ultrasounds than by lower frequencies

VII. Mice have an expected life span of 1 to 2 years

VIII. Rectal temperature: 36.5° to 38.0° C (97.5° to 100.5° F)

Handling and Restraint

I. Mice should be picked up by the base of the tail. Never pick up a mouse by the middle or tip of the tail because you may cause degloving or sloughing of the outside of the tail

II. For assistance in restraining a mouse, the mouse can be placed on a wire grid, such as the cage lid, so that its front feet grip the bars. The handler should then carefully grasp the loose skin on either side of the neck and over the back with the thumb and forefinger. The body of the mouse is laid across the palm of the hand and the tail is restrained under the little finger

III. Tubular restraining devices can be used for blood collection and other procedures

IV. The best methods of permanent identification of mice are ear punching, tail tattooing, and the insertion of a microchip that can be scanned for identification, along with cage card identification. For all of these procedures, consideration must be made for the pain level involved; anesthesia may be appropriate for tattooing and microchip insertion; for ear punching, use of a topical analgesic such as Emla cream is recommended

Breeding Considerations

See Table 17-1 for reproductive data.

I. If a group of female mice are exposed to a male mouse, the majority of these female mice will be in estrus the third night. This is known as the Whitten effect

II. The Bruce effect is a pregnancy block that occurs when a pregnant female is exposed to a strange male within 48 hours of copulation. The female will return to estrus in 4 or 5 days

III. From 12 to 36 hours after mating, a waxy postcopulatory plug can be found in the vagina

IV. Postpartum estrus occurs within 24 hours of parturition

V. The female will build a small shallow nest a couple of days before parturition

VI. Typically the female will have her pups during the dark hours. She will walk around the cage during labor and delivery and then retrieve the pup to the nest

Sampling

For injection routes, sites, needle sizes, and volumes, see Table 17-2.

Table 17-1 Reproductive data

Species	Litter size	Weight at birth (gauge)	Weaning age (days)	Puberty	Breeding age	Estrus cycle	Mating	Gestation
Mouse	6-12	1	21 days	4-6 wk	6 wk	4-5 days, Whitten and Bruce effects	Harem 1:4	19-21 days
Rat	7-14	5-6	21 days	4-6 wk	10-12 wk	4-5 days, Whitten and Bruce effects	Harem 1:6	20-22 days
Guinea pig	2-6	60-200	21 days	3-4 wk	12 wk	16 days, polyestrus	Harem 1:5-10	63 days
Hamster	4-12	1-2	21 days	4-6 wk	6-7 wk	4 days, polyestrus, F will exhibit lordosis	Monogamous or harem 1:4	16 days
Gerbil	4-5	3-4	21-28 days	10 wk	10-12 wk	4-6 days, polyestrus	Monogamous (mate for life) or harem 1:3	24-26 days
Rabbit	6-10	40	6-8 wk	5-9 mo	6-9 mo	Induced polyestrus	Hand mating, 1:10-15	28-34 days
Hedgehog	3-4	15	5-6 wk	6 mo Can become sexually active as early as 7 wk	5-12 mo	Biannual	Harem 1:3	31-35 days
Chinchilla	1-2	30-60	6-8 wk	8 mo	8 mo	38 days, polyestrus, vaginal closure membrane	Harem 1:12	111 days
Degu	5-6	15-30	4-5	45 days	6 mo	Induced polyestrus	Monogamous or harem 1:5	90 days

Table 17-2 Recommended needle sizes and sites and maximum volumes for injection/sampling

Species	SQ	IM	IP	IV	Sampling (nonlethal)*
Mouse	<23 Gauge 2-3 mL Scruff	25 Gauge 0.05 mL/site Quadriceps, posterior thigh	25 Gauge <3 mL Lower right quadrant	<25 Gauge 0.2 mL Lateral tail vein, saphenous	Saphenous vein, lateral tail vein, jugular, retro-orbital sinus†: 100 μL Cardiac†: 1-2 mL Tail nick: 50 μL, DO NOT REMOVE VERTEBRAE
Rat	<23 Gauge 5-10 mL Scruff, back	23-25 Gauge 0.3 mL/site Quadriceps, posterior thigh	22-23 Gauge 5-10 mL Lower left quadrant	<23 Gauge 0.5 mL Lateral tail vein, saphenous vein, dorsal penis vein, sublingual	Saphenous vein, lateral tail vein or artery, retro-orbital sinus†: 1 mL Cardiac†: 3-5 mL Jugular vein†: 2-3 mL
Hamster	23 Gauge 3-5 mL Scruff	23 or 25 Gauge 0.1 mL/site Quadriceps, posterior thigh	23 Gauge 3-4 mL Lower right quadrant	25 Gauge 0.3 mL Difficult, cut down to jugular, cephalic, tarsal, lingual	Retro-orbital sinus†: 0.5 mL Jugular cut-down†: <2 mL, 23 Gauge Cephalic, tarsal, lingual: 0.5 mL, 25 Gauge Cardiac†: <2 mL, 23 Gauge
Guinea pig	<21 Gauge 5-10 mL Scruff, back *Tough skin	23-25 Gauge 0.3 mL/site Quadriceps, posterior thigh	<21 Gauge 10-15 mL Lower abdominal quadrant	<23 Gauge 0.5 ml slowly Marginal ear vein, saphenous, penile	23 Gauge Anterior vena cava: 2-3 mL Ear vein: 0.5 mL Cardiac†: 0.5 mL Penile, saphenous, jugular: 2-3 mL
Rabbit	21-23 Gauge 30-50 mL Scruff, flank	<21 Gauge 0.5-1.0 mL/site Lumbar, quadriceps	(Not recommended) 21 Gauge 50-100 mL	23 Gauge 1-5 mL, slowly Marginal ear vein, saphenaus	21 Gauge Marginal ear vein, 2-3 mL Central ear artery: 30 mL Cardiac†: use only for terminal bleeds, 100+ mL
Gerbils	23 Gauge 2-3 mL Scruff	25 Gauge 0.1 mL/site Quadriceps, posterior thigh	23 Gauge 2-3 mL Lower abdominal quadrant *See notes in text	25 Gauge 0.2-0.3 mL Lateral tail vein	23-25 Gauge Lateral tail vein, saphenous, retro-orbital sinus†: 0.2-0.4 mL Cardiac†: 1 mL
Chinchilla	<21 Gauge 5-10 mL Scruff, back	23-25 Gauge 0.3 mL/site Quadriceps, posterior thigh	<21 Gauge 10-15 mL Lower abdominal quadrant	25 Gauge 1 mL slowly Saphenous, cephalic	<23 Gauge Jugular: 2-3 mL Cranial vena cava: 2-3 mL Cephalic, saphenous: 1 mL
Hedgehog	21 Gauge × 3.5 inch spinal 5-10 mL Mantle, back	21 Gauge × 3.5 inch spinal 0.3 mL/site Mantle, back	Not recommended, but could follow GP guidelines	25 Gauge 0.5-1.0 mL Saphenous, cephalic	23-25 Gauge Saphenous, cephalic: 0.5 mL Jugular: 1 mL
Degu	23 Gauge 2-3 mL Scruff	25 Gauge 0.1 mL/site Quadriceps, posterior thigh	23 Gauge 2-3 mL, Lower abdominal quadrant	25 Gauge 0.2-0.3 mL Lateral tail vein, saphenous	23-25 Gauge Lateral tail vein, saphenous: 0.5 mL Cardiac†: 1-2 mL

*Before collecting any blood sample, always calculate the amount that can be safely drawn based on body weight and blood volume for that particular species and the health status of the animal. Generally, 4% to 7% of blood volume, dependent on species, can be safely drawn. Consider replacing equal amounts of fluid (i.e., physiological saline).

†Cardiac and jugular cut-down bleeding must be done under anesthesia. Because of the risk of postprocedural complications, cardiac puncture is generally only used for a terminal procedure. Retro-orbital sinus bleeding must be done under anesthesia or sedation.

I. Gastric gavage can be done by placing a bulbed, curved dosing needle over the tongue, into the esophagus, and then into the stomach
II. Simple blood sampling procedures (e.g., saphenous) can be done on awake but restrained mice
III. To perform retro-orbital sinus or cardiac puncture sampling, anesthesia must be used
IV. Cardiac puncture is generally considered a terminal procedure due to potential complications
V. Before blood collection, always calculate the maximum safe volume that can be withdrawn
   A. Mice have approximately 70 to 80 mL/kg total blood volume
      1. Of this, 10% to 15% can be safely withdrawn every 2 to 3 weeks
VI. Collection of urine and feces can be done by placing the animal in a metabolic cage or by collecting the samples as the animal is restrained because it will often urinate and defecate. A hematocrit tube can be used to collect the urine

Signs of Pain and Distress

I. The following are signs of pain and distress in mice
   A. Weight loss, dehydration, sunken eyes, and change in urine and fecal output and consistency due to decreased food and water intake
   B. Hunched posture
   C. Lethargy, depression, and withdrawal from the group
   D. Change in locomotion
   E. Decreased grooming and ruffled hair coat
   F. Ocular and nasal discharge may be seen along with increased and labored breathing
   G. Change in behavior, particularly when handled or manipulated. May vocalize or try to bite handler
   H. Scratching excessively, licking, or biting at painful areas, which may lead to self-mutilation
II. Analgesics, such as buprenorphine and butorphanol, are appropriate to administer to a mouse in pain

Health Conditions

I. Respiratory disease
   A. Sendai virus causes pneumonia, is often latent and becomes apparent in young weanling, stressed mice, or in combination with bacterial infections. It is self-limiting in immunocompetent mice
   B. Bacteria that may contribute to respiratory infections include *Pasteurella pneumotropica, Klebsiella pneumoniae, Mycoplasma pulmonis,* and *Corynebacterium kutscheri*
   C. Clinical signs are: weight loss, ruffled hair coat, hunched posture, anorexia, dyspnea, chattering, and sudden death
   D. Treatment with antibiotics (e.g., tetracycline in drinking water) for secondary bacterial infections
II. Mouse hepatitis virus
   A. Caused by a coronavirus. It is often a latent infection that can lead to encephalitis and/or hepatitis in mice
   B. Causes wasting disease in immunosuppressed animals such as SCID mice
   C. Clinical signs include dehydration, weight loss, diarrhea, and sudden death
   D. To control disease in a colony, breeding should cease, consider hysterectomy derivation, and place filter tops on cages
III. Tyzzer's disease
   A. *Clostridium piliformis* is the bacterium involved
   B. Most commonly affects immunosuppressed animals and those kept in poor housing
   C. Causes dehydration, weight loss, diarrhea, and sudden death
   D. These bacteria are spore formers that are highly infectious to a number of laboratory animals. Isolation is imperative; culling or hysterectomy derivation of the colony should be considered
IV. Epizootic diarrhea of infant mice (EDIM)
   A. A disease caused by a rotavirus that affects suckling mice
   B. Clinical signs include soft yellow feces or fecal staining of the anogenital area in mice less than 2 weeks of age
   C. Filter top cages should be used to prevent the spread of this disease
   D. Cull-affected litters
V. Pinworm
   A Two strains: *Aspicularis tetraptera* and *Syphacia obvelata*
   B. Both strains can be observed on fecal floatation, but *S. obvelata* can also be detected by making a cellophane tape impression of the perineal area
   C. Use anthelmintic such as ivermectin or pyrantel palmate and carefully sanitize the environment because these eggs are "sticky"
   D. Unapparent infection, but may decrease growth rate
VI. Mites
   A. Several different species of mites can affect mice, including *Myobia musculi* and *Myocoptes musculinus*
   B. The most obvious signs of mite infection are alopecia, pruritus, and dermatitis

C. Mites can be diagnosed by close examination for mites in the fur; pluck or scrape and examine findings under magnification
D. Easiest and most economical control of mites is through exposure to the vapors from pest strips (dichlorvis)

RAT *(RATTUS NORVEGICUS)*

Origin and Uses in Research

I. The rat is a rodent of the family Muridae
II. Rats were being used as experimental animals by the early 1800s
III. Uses in biomedical research include cardiovascular disease, metabolic disorders such as diabetes mellitus, organ transplantation, toxicology, neurobehavioral studies, cancer susceptibility, and renal disease studies
IV. Rats are raised and maintained in ecological classes similar to mice
V. Common outbred strains include the Wistar, Sprague-Dawley, Long Evans, Kyoto, and Wistar-Kyoto
VI. Through selective breeding and mutations, more defined and inbred strains can be produced to suit a specific study
Examples:
A. CAR/CAS: caries resistant/susceptible
B. BB: spontaneous diabetics
C. Brattleboro: diabetes insipidus
D. Zucker: obesity

Characteristics: Behavioral and Physiological

I. Rats are generally docile and may become tame and easily trained if handled frequently
II. Rats can be communally housed and may share raising of their young
III. Rats are omnivorous, feed primarily at night, and are generally fed a commercially prepared laboratory rodent diet
IV. Rats have a life expectancy of 2.5 to 3 years; a restricted protein and fat diet will extend life expectancy for months
V. They display a range of behavioral traits and are intelligent, making them suitable for behavioral studies
VI. Rats do not have a gallbladder
VII. Rats, like other rodents, have a layer of brown fat distributed over their back and neck. In a young rat this plays a role in thermoregulation, but its significance decreases with age
VIII. Rats have continually erupting incisors, called hypsodontic
IX. The harderian gland is a lacrimal gland located behind the rat's eyeball that secretes a lipid- and protein-rich secretion that lubricates the eye. In some disease conditions and in times of stress, these red secretions will overflow the eye and stain the face
X. Albino rats have very poor vision and rely on their facial whisker and their sense of smell for orientation
XI. Rats will practice coprophagy
XII. Rectal temperature: 35.9° to 37.5° C (96.6° to 99.5° F)

Handling and Restraint

I. Rats should not be picked up by their tail because it could result in degloving of the tail, exposing the coccygeal vertebrae
II. Two commonly used methods of picking up and restraining a rat
A. Place hand over the shoulder and back area, with the mandibles just in front of the thumb and forefinger
B. Place hand over the shoulder and back area with the head between the first two fingers and the thumb behind the rat's foreleg
C. With both of these restraint techniques, it is important to use your other hand to secure the hind limbs and tail (base of tail can be held in these secure positions)
III. Rats can be identified by using cage cards, coat color, and/or placement of markings or tattooing the tail or ear pinna (under anesthesia)

Breeding Considerations

See Table 17-1 for reproductive data.

I. Female rats are polyestrous and can breed year round
II. The Whitten effect (see Mouse) is less pronounced in rats than in mice. The Bruce effect (see Mouse) does not affect rats as it does mice. Pseudopregnancy in rats is rare
III. A white, waxy, postcopulatory plug is present in the vagina for 12 to 24 hours after mating
IV. Females have a postpartum estrus cycle within 48 hours. Because of this, usually the male is removed just before parturition and placed back in with the female(s) after weaning

Sampling

For injection routes, sites, needle sizes, and volumes, see Table 17-2.

I. Gastric gavage can be performed by placing a ball-tipped, curved dosing needle over the tongue, into the esophagus, and then into the stomach
II. For blood collection, oral dosing, physical examinations, and injections, it is important to have one person restrain the rat while the other performs the technical procedure

III. Before blood collection, always calculate the maximum safe volume that can be withdrawn. Rats have approximately 50 to 65 mL/kg total blood volume. Of this, 10% to 15% can be safely withdrawn every 2 to 3 weeks

Signs of Pain and Distress

See Mouse. Clinical signs are similar. Rats in pain should also be provided with analgesia through administration of analgesics, such as butorphanol and buprenorphine.

Health Conditions

I. Parvovirus
   A. Three main serogroups include rat virus (RV), H-1 virus, and rat parvovirus (RPV)
   B. Can cause a wide range of symptoms varying with the viral strain and the age and immune status of the rat. Young rats can display tremors, ataxia, jaundice, stunted growth, and oily hair coats. Mature rats tend to have asymptomatic latent infections and can exhibit signs of paralysis, scrotal cyanosis, and hemorrhage in times of stress or if they become immunocompromised
   C. Because these viruses are shed in urine, feces, saliva, and milk and are vertically transmitted through direct contact and fomites, it is highly contagious. It has severe potential to interfere with research

II. Coronaviruses
   A. Although there are several coronaviruses that affect rats, the primary three are considered to be sialodacryoadenitis virus (SDAV), rat coronavirus (RCV), and the causative agent of rat sialoadenitis virus (CARS)
   B. Intramandibular and/or ventral cervical swelling is a common clinical sign, as well as red porphyrin staining of the face and paws, sneezing, anorexia, photophobia, bilateral or unilateral suborbital or periorbital swelling, squinting, blinking, bulging eyes, and occasional self-mutilation of the eyes
   C. Disease is self-limiting with high morbidity and low mortality rates but has the potential to interfere with research
   D. These viruses are highly contagious via respiratory aerosol or direct contact

III. Sendai virus
   A. An RNA virus of the family Paramyxovirus (parainfluenza virus type 1)
   B. Usually asymptomatic relative to the host's immune status, age, etc. High morbidity and low mortality rates
   C. Clinical signs include respiratory difficulty, chattering, wheezing, weight loss, decreased breeding efficiency, and anorexia
   D. Can have a dramatic effect on research, particularly reproductive, respiratory, and nutritional studies

IV. Murine mycoplasmosis
   A. Disease caused by *Mycoplasma pulmonis*
   B. Very common in pet and conventionally housed rats
   C. Carried in the upper respiratory tract and transmitted via aerosol, direct contact, and in utero transfer, making it a highly contagious disease; affected animals should be quarantined away from others
   D. There are two major areas that can be affected by an infection with *M. pulmonis*
      1. The respiratory system clinical signs include sniffling, moist rales, sneezing, chattering, weight loss, rough hair coat, and torticollis (head tilt)
      2. The genital infection will cause breeding inefficiencies and infertility
   E. Tetracycline hydrochloride in the drinking water will suppress clinical signs

V. Mammary tumors
   A. Neoplasms in the mammary tissue are common in most strains of rats
   B. Tumors can be large but rarely metastasize
   C. They may be surgically removed but often grow back

VI. Endoparasite and ectoparasite (see Mouse)

SYRIAN HAMSTER *(MESOCRICETUS AURATUS)*

Origin and Uses in Research

I. The Syrian (or golden) hamster is a rodent of the family Cricetidae. The origin of the golden hamster is the Middle East, where, unfortunately, the natural habitat is being destroyed

II. The Syrian hamster is popular as both a pet and a research model

III. The hamster has a unique evertable pouch used to transport food but also very useful for research on tumor induction and transplant and studies on microcirculation

IV. Hamsters are also of use in hypothermia studies because they possess the ability to go into short periods of pseudohibernation when temperatures are under 48° F (10° C) and daylight hours shorten

V. Inbred strains of hamsters have been produced as animal models of epilepsy, muscular dystrophy, and heart failure

Characteristics: Behavioral and Physiological

I. Female hamsters are generally larger, stronger, and more aggressive than males

II. Hamsters are burrowers and like to hoard their food

III. They are solitary animals under natural conditions and are best kept separate
IV. They are expert escape artists; cages should not be made out of wood, aluminum, or soft plastic and must have a tight fitting lid
V. Flank glands are sebaceous glands used to mark territory. Although both males and females have them, they are quite prominent in the males
VI. Hamsters are omnivores; diets can be supplemented with fresh fruit and vegetables
VII. They are nocturnal animals that will put many kilometers on a running wheel through the course of one night
VIII. Hamsters will choose different areas of their cage for food storage, nesting, defecation, and urination
IX. Urine has a high pH of 8, which is full of crystals, giving it a turbid, milky appearance
X. Hamsters have a life expectancy of about 2 years
XI. Rectal temperature, 37.0° to 38.0° C (98.6° to 100.4° F)

Handling and Restraint

I. Hamsters are extremely deep sleepers and can be aggressive if woken up and startled, so it is important to awaken the hamster before handling
II. Hamsters can be gently scooped up in the palm of the hand or in a plastic/metal container
   A. To restrain for a physical examination or technical procedure, they can be grasped by the loose skin over the neck and shoulder area using the whole hand (hamster should appear to be smiling when effectively restrained)

Breeding Considerations

See Table 17-1 for reproductive data.

I. During the winter months, hamsters will exhibit a normal decrease in fecundity and mortality in litters increases; this effect can be only partially reduced by keeping the temperatures between 22° and 24° C (71° to 75° F) and on a 12- to 14-hour light cycle
II. Monogamous pairs are frequently established before sexual maturity to avoid the possible fighting that can occur when a male is placed in a cage with a strange female
III. In a harem set-up, bring the male to the receptive female, 1 hour before the dark light cycle, observe them closely for fighting, and separate if this occurs. Separate also after breeding has occurred to avoid injury to the male
IV. The estrous cycles last about 4 days; on the second day of estrous the female has a vaginal discharge that has a distinctive pungent odor that attracts the male. The female will usually approach the male for breeding within 3 days of this postovulatory discharge
V. The gestation period for the hamster is only 16 days. It is advisable to not disturb the female and her litter until at least 7 days postpartum or she may cannibalize her offspring

Sampling

For injection routes, sites, needle sizes, and volumes, see Table 17-2.

I. The hamster has few accessible veins for blood collection and injection. The cephalic vein, tarsal vein, lingual vein (requires anesthesia), or jugular vein (requires anesthesia and surgical cutdown) can be used
II. Most of the techniques for injection and gavage are the same as in the rat and mouse
III. Oral medication can be placed in the cheek pouch
IV. Collection of urine and feces can be done by placing the hamster in a metabolic cage; often when restrained, they will urinate or defecate
V. Before blood collection, always calculate the maximum safe volume that can be withdrawn. Hamsters have approximately 65 to 80 mL/kg total blood volume. Of this, 10% to 15% can be safely withdrawn every 2 to 3 weeks

Signs of Pain and Distress

The hamster is usually a healthy and hardy animal. Clinical signs of pain are the same as those listed for the mouse.

I. Ocular discharge is commonly associated with stress and may be accompanied by an increase in respiratory rate
II. It is unusual for a hamster to be constipated. Diarrhea, when it occurs, is profuse liquid, staining the perineal area
III. Lateral recumbency is unusual and indicative of an unwell hamster

Analgesics are appropriate to administer to a hamster in pain; the selection and use of these agents should be in consultation with a veterinarian.

Health Conditions

I. Wet tail (proliferative ileitis or transmissible ileal hyperplasia)
   A. The exact causative agent is unknown, but several types of bacteria have been cultured from hamsters with proliferative ileitis, including *Campylobacter* spp., *Campylobacter*-like organisms, *Escherichia coli,* and a *Lawsonia intracelluaris*–like organism
   B. Clinical signs include profuse watery diarrhea, lethargy, weight loss, severe depression, irritability, anorexia, and sudden death within 3 days of clinical signs

C. May be predisposed by stresses of confinement and weaning with highest mortality in nursing or newly weaned animals between 3 to 8 weeks of age
D. Erythromycin in the drinking water has been shown to effectively decrease the mortality rate
E. Best method of control is prevention through a high level of hygiene and avoidance of stress

II. Tyzzer's disease *(Clostridium piliformis)*
A. Not commonly seen in hamsters, but this may be due to lack of diagnosis because the clinical signs are similar to those of wet tail and the causative organism is difficult to culture
B. Treatment for Tyzzer's disease with tetracycline has been successful in other rodents
C. *C. piliformis* is a spore-forming bacteria; thorough decontamination of the housing facility is imperative after an outbreak to prevent reinfection

III. *Salmonella* spp.
A. Hamsters may be more susceptible to *Salmonella* spp. than other rodents
B. Clinical signs include lethargy, rough hair coat, weight loss, distended abdomen, and increased respiratory rate
C. Zoonotic disease; strict hygiene protocols should be adhered to when working with suspect animals

IV. Lymphocytic choriomeningitis virus (LCM)
A. LCM is a zoonotic disease that causes meningitis in humans
B. Clinical signs of the disease in hamsters are difficult to detect because they usually are asymptomatic
C. May present as a chronic wasting disease
D. Virus is shed in the urine

V. Antibiotic sensitivity
A. Hamsters have predominantly gram-positive intestinal flora and tend to develop a fatal gram-negative enterotoxemia when given certain antibiotics

VI. Pneumonia
A. This is a relatively common health concern with hamsters
B. Commonly associated with *Pasteurella pneumotropica*
1. Clinical signs include respiratory distress and ocular discharge
C. Sendai virus may produce pneumonia in suckling hamsters. Hamsters have shown to be susceptible to the pneumonia virus in mice

VII. Endoparasites and ectoparasites
A. Pinworms and mites can affect hamsters similarly to other rodents (see Mouse)

MONGOLIAN GERBIL *(MERIONES UNGUICULATUS)*

Origin and Uses in Research

I. Gerbils are desert dwellers and can be found in northern Africa, India, Mongolia, northern China, and some sections of eastern Europe

II. The gerbil is a rodent of the Cricetidae family. Although the Mongolian gerbil is by far the most commonly used research and pet strain, there are many variations of gerbils with a wide range of sizes and colors

III. Gerbils are useful in radiation studies because they are more resistant to radiation than other common laboratory animals. They are also used in studies relating to epilepsy, infectious disease, endocrinology, and lipid metabolism

Characteristics: Behavioral and Physiological

I. Gerbils are gentle and friendly. They are curious animals that will explore all new environmental enrichment thoroughly, particularly tubes and other devices that mimic their natural burrowing behavior

II. Gerbils are active throughout the day with their peak of activity occurring during the dark hours

III. They are incredibly driven to burrow and will occasionally damage caging and cause self-mutilation with their intense burrowing activities

IV. Some strains can be susceptible to epileptiform seizures after excitement, stress, sudden noises, etc., with spontaneous recovery and no noted ill effects

V. Gerbils have a great capacity for temperature regulation and can tolerate temperatures between 0° and 32° C (32° and 92° F) in comparison with most laboratory animals

VI. Relative humidity should be lower for these animals (30% to 50%) in comparison with most laboratory animals
A. When the humidity is over 50%, the fur will stand away from the body and appear to be matted, as opposed to the sleek, smooth appearance

VII. Gerbils are herbivorous and grainivorous. Care should be exercised when feeding seeds because gerbils are extremely fond of sunflower seeds and will eat them to the exclusion of all other foods. Standard laboratory rodent diet should be fed
A. Gerbils hoard food, with the female exhibiting this behavior more than the male

VIII. Feces are tubular, dry, and almost black in color

IX. Gerbils have a low to moderate requirement for dietary water (but must always be supplied with clean, fresh water) and in turn put out very little urine, keeping odors down in comparison with other laboratory animals

X. Gerbils tend to nonaggression and can be group housed in large numbers (in accordance with housing density standards) by sex, at weaning

XI. Like rats, gerbils have a harderian gland in the orbit of the eye
 A. Red coloring may appear around the eyes and neck if excessive secretion occurs

XII. Like most laboratory rodents, gerbils have a sensitivity to cedar bedding that is enzyme induced

XIII. Average life expectancy in the gerbil is 3 years

XIV. Rectal temperature, 37.0° to 38.5° C (98.6° to 101.3° F)

Handling and Restraint

I. Gerbils tolerate handling well, and there are generally no problems associated with the handling of young litters and newborn pups

II. To move a gerbil from cage to cage, scoop the gerbil up gently with both hands, ensuring that it cannot jump out of your hand. They can also be transferred by securing one hand over the back, with the gerbil's head between the first two fingers

III. To restrain a gerbil for a physical examination or technical procedure, grip the base of the tail with one hand and the loose skin around the neck and shoulder area with the other hand
 A. Extreme care should be taken to avoid grasping the tail away from the base because this could cause degloving of the tail
 B. Gerbils do not tolerate being turned on their backs; they will struggle

Breeding Considerations

See Table 17-1 for reproductive data.

I. Gerbils are monogamous and will mate for life. Care should be taken if introducing a new mate because this quite often results in severe fighting

II. Male gerbils will aid in the care of the young, but if separated to avoid postpartum mating he should be returned to his mate within 2 weeks of separation

III. Harem mating systems can be set up in production facilities with one male to two or three females

IV. The estrous cycle lasts about 4 to 6 days with spontaneous ovulation

V. Matings tend to occur during the dark hours

Sampling

For injection routes, sites, needle sizes, and volumes, see Table 17-2.

I. Sampling procedures are similar to those performed in mice and rats

II. Because gerbils dislike being placed on their backs, the intraperitoneal injections are given with the animal carefully restrained (described earlier) but held vertically, with head slightly declined, while the needle is placed into the lower left or right abdominal quadrant

III. Before blood collection, always calculate the maximum safe volume that can be withdrawn. Gerbils have approximately 65 to 85 mL/kg total blood volume. Of this, 10% to 15% can be safely withdrawn every 2 to 3 weeks

Signs of Pain and Distress

The clinical signs of pain and distress in the mouse apply to gerbils.

I. Gerbils are normally extremely active and nervous and under severe stress may temporarily collapse

Analgesics are appropriate to administer to a gerbil in pain; the selection and use of these agents should be in consultation with a veterinarian.

Health Conditions

I. Tyzzer's disease *(Clostridium piliforme)*
 A. Gerbils are highly susceptible to infection by *C. piliforme* and are commonly used in laboratories as sentinels for this organism because transmission readily occurs through contact with soiled bedding
 B. The disease causes high morbidity and mortality rates in weanling-age gerbils
 C. *C. piliforme* is a spore-forming bacterium that can be spread to other animals in a research facility. Thorough decontamination must occur after an outbreak of this disease
 D. Clinical signs of Tyzzer's disease include acute death, lethargy, rough hair coat, and diarrhea
 E. Treatment may be successful with the addition of oxytetracycline in the drinking water and fluid therapy for dehydrated individuals

II. Nasal dermatitis, or "sore nose"
 A. This disease is seen to be a byproduct of stress and anxiety. In high-stress situations, gerbils will attempt to alleviate their stress by excessive burrowing. Porphyrins secreted during stress-induced chromodacryorrhea may be irritating to the skin. The lesions resulting are commonly contaminated with *Staphylococcus aureus* and/or *S. xylosus,* which is considered an opportunistic pathogen
 B. Clinical signs include facial or nasal dermatitis that can progress into chronic moist dermatitis. In very severe cases, and where the underlying cause has not been rectified, the disease can lead to wasting, anorexia, and possibly death

C. Treatment must address evaluating and eliminating the cause of the stress. The lesions can be cleaned and then topically treated with appropriate antibiotic ointments. Clay bedding material can be used instead of shavings or chips

III. Salmonella
   A. Outbreaks cause diarrhea, perineal staining, anorexia weight loss, and sudden death
   B. Typically, animals will recover after a short bout of diarrhea
   C. Zoonotic potential; when dealing with these animals, exercise good personal hygiene

IV. Malocclusion and overgrowth of incisors are fairly common and require regular trimming of the teeth

V. Gerbils over the age of 2 show a high incidence of tumors
   A. Malignancies appear as spontaneous neoplasms involving the ovaries, ventral sebaceous glands, kidney, adrenal gland, and skin

VI. Although dehydration is uncommon, if gerbils do not have access to fresh water (due to blocked sipper tube, immature animals that cannot reach the sipper tube, etc.), this could lead to lower fertility rates, decreased body weights, and possibly death

RABBIT *(ORYCTOLAGUS CUNICULUS)*

Origin and Uses in Research

I. The rabbit is a lagomorph of the family Leporidae

II. Present breeds are derived from the wild European rabbit. These wild rabbits still exist today in northwestern Africa and Europe

III. Breeds of rabbit are divided by size, shape, and color variations
   A. Large breeds (6.4 to 7.3 kg, or 14 to 16 lb) include the Giant Chinchilla and the Flemish Giant
   B. Medium breeds (1.8 to 7.3 kg, or 1 to 14 lb) include the New Zealand White and Californian
   C. Small breed (0.9 to 1.8 kg, or 2 to 4 lb) include the Dutch and Polish

IV. The New Zealand White is the most common specific pathogen–free (SPF) rabbit produced commercially for research

V. Rabbits are useful in biomedical research for alimentary, aging, cancer, cardiovascular, genetic, immunology, virology, and toxicology studies, as well as many other areas. Rabbits are quite commonly used to produce antibodies

Characteristics: Behavioral and Physiological

I. Rabbits are docile, alert, gregarious burrowers
   A. They are generally a social animal but may be housed singly in a laboratory situation to avoid fighting and to prevent ovulation and pseudopregnancy in females

II. Rabbits are crepuscular

III. Aggressive or nervous rabbits may stomp their hind feet and may spray urine
   A. If they panic or are handled roughly, they may scream

IV. Rabbits are herbivorous. They should be fed a commercially prepared, pelleted, high fiber rabbit diet and supplemented with good quality grass hay and fresh vegetables; fruits can be given as treats

V. Rabbits have a higher requirement for fiber than other species; a high-fiber diet will decrease the incidence of hairballs

VI. Rabbits have highly vascularized ears, allowing for easy intravenous and intraarterial access; they serve as the rabbit's heat regulatory organ

VII. Rabbits have two pairs of upper incisors; a smaller pair (peg teeth) are found behind the larger pair
   A. Both pairs grow continuously (open rooted) and may need to be trimmed if not naturally worn down, otherwise leading to health conditions such as malocclusion
   B. Enamel is found on the entire tooth surface

VIII. Rabbits have a chin gland, which is more obvious in males

IX. Rabbit urine is unlike other species in that it is quite thick and cloudy and contains crystalline material
   A. Suckling babies and fasting adults have clear, crystal-free urine

X. Daytime feces are usually hard and dark-green, round pellets. Rabbits tend to eat most of their food at dusk; the first 4 hours after eating goes toward the production of these fecal pellets
   A. Night feces (cecotroph) are moist, stronger in odor, brighter green, and mucus covered
      1. Coprophagy of these cecotrophs, directly from the anus, is normal behavior in rabbits and helps increase the digestibility of proteins and maintain adequate nutrition and intestinal flora
      2. These pellets are formed in the 4 hours after the day pellets are formed

XI. Average life expectancy of a rabbit is 5 to 6 years

XII. Rectal temperature: 38.5° to 40.0° C (101.3° to 104° F)

Handling and Restraint

I. Approach rabbits slowly and talk to them softly to avoid startling them

II. Rabbits can be picked up

   A. By grasping the loose skin over the neck area with one hand and supporting the hind limbs with the other, taking care that the nails do not get caught in the caging
   B. To transport the rabbit, place the rabbit on your forearm with its head tucked in your elbow and your same hand supporting the hind limbs. The other hand should be over the rabbit's shoulder, being prepared to grasp this skin again in case it struggles
   C. Rabbits must never be picked up by their ears

III. To handle rabbits for physical examination or technical procedure
   A. Place the rabbit on a nonslip surface (examination table with a mat) and carefully restrain with both hands to prevent it from jumping off the table. If possible (i.e., during ear bleeds), wrap the rabbit in a towel or laboratory coat to comfort and protect it from hurting itself
   B. Rabbits can be carefully laid on their backs, on the handler's lap
      1. Start by sitting on a stool or on the floor with rabbit on your lap with its head toward your abdomen
      2. Cover the rabbit's eyes with one hand and hold the scruff of skin over the shoulders with the other
      3. Gently roll the rabbit so that its feet are closely tucked into your abdomen and its head rests near your knees; if the rabbit struggles, make sure that your hand is still covering its eyes. Once it has quieted, resume slowly

IV. When placed back in the cage, it should go in back end first so it does not jump in, which risks breaking its back

V. Rabbits are generally easy to handle, with training, but be aware that they have powerful bites and can charge and scratch

Breeding Considerations

See Table 17-1 for reproductive data.

I. Rabbits are induced ovulators and do not have an estrous cycle but do have a period of receptivity that lasts between 7 and 10 days

II. Pregnant does need to be provided with a clean, dry, well-bedded nest. They will also hair pluck to line the nest

III. Does will not retrieve kits that leave the nest. If kits are found outside the nest, they will need to be warmed immediately

IV. Do not disturb the doe during parturition

V. Cannibalism is rare in rabbits

VI. Cross-fostering works well with rabbits, so large litters should be decreased in size by cross-fostering to another doe with a similar age litter

VII. As in rodents, thermoregulation is regulated by brown fat in young rabbits

Sampling

For injection routes, sites, needle sizes, and volumes, see Table 17-2.

I. Collection of feces and urine can be done by placing the rabbit in a metabolic cage

II. Liquid oral medications can be given by introducing the dosing syringe into the interdental space and pointing the tip toward the back of the mouth. Pills can also be given by pushing them through the interdental space and back toward the molars

III. If nasogastric tubes are necessary, it is recommended to obtain a radiograph of the rabbit after placement because rabbits will not cough when saline is introduced directly into the lungs

IV. Before blood collection, always calculate the maximum safe volume that can be withdrawn. Rabbits have approximately 57 to 65 mL/kg total blood volume. Of this, 10% to 15% can be safely withdrawn every 2 to 3 weeks

Signs of Pain and Distress

I. Difficult to identify signs of pain because rabbits often hide their symptoms

II. Rabbits that appear to be unwell should have a full physical examination that includes temperature, respiration rate, heart rate, and body weight
   A. Careful examination of the animal may find decreased muscle mass, dehydration, ocular discharge, debris in ears, nictitating membranes, inappetance, staining of perineal area, lesions, limited movement, and other signs
   B. Careful examination of the cage will be helpful in determining if the rabbit is unwell
      1. Look for leftover feed, diarrhea, uneaten cecotrophs, lack of feces, unconsumed water (sipper tube may be faulty)

III. Rabbits in pain may be lethargic, remain at the back of the cage, and face away from sources of light

Analgesics are appropriate to administer to a rabbit in pain; the selection and use of these agents should be in consultation with a veterinarian.

Health Conditions

I. Pasteurellosis: *Pasteurella multocida*
   A. Rabbits under stress (such as during and after shipping) and in poor health conditions are more susceptible
   B. The major causative agent is "snuffles," or upper respiratory tract infections in rabbits. The other organisms that are cultured include

Bordetella bronchiseptica and *Moraxella catarrhalis*

C. Rabbits with pasteurellosis could have the following on clinical presentation: upper respiratory tract infection, otitis, pleuropneumonia, bacteremia, and abscesses
   1. Clinical signs include nasal discharge, ocular discharge, dermatitis, torticollis, vaginal discharge, and abscess formation

D. Antibiotic therapy is indicated as treatment, but watch for gastrointestinal upset
   1. In cases of torticollis, it may also be appropriate to administer analgesics, corticosteroids, and an antinausea/vertigo drug
   2. Abscesses may require lancing and then flushing

E. Pasteurellosis is quite contagious, through direct and indirect transmission; sick animals must be isolated or culled

II. Trichobezoars (hairballs)

A. This disease is associated with feeding a diet that is low in fiber

B. Suspect a hairball in an anorectic rabbit

C. The hairball can sometimes be palpated, or radiography can assist in diagnosis

D. Nonsurgical treatment should be attempted first. Force feeding a slurry of high-fiber chow, offering free choice hay and fresh vegetables, and giving the proteolytic enzymes bromelin and papain

III. Coccidiosis

A. Rabbits can be infected with hepatic coccidia *(Emeria stieda)* or intestinal coccidia (several different types)

B. Clinical signs of intestinal coccidiosis include diarrhea and possibly death in cases of heavy infections

C. Clinical signs of hepatic coccidiosis include diarrhea, abdominal swelling, weight loss, anorexia, icterus, and sudden death

D. Diagnosis through identification of oocysts on fecal examination

E. Prevention must consist of isolation of infected rabbits and a thorough clean up of the environment daily to remove sporulated oocysts
   1. Treatment with sulfonamides have proved effective to control heavy infections

IV. Dermatitis/alopecia

A. Can be caused by a number of agents, including fur and ear mites, dermatophytes, malocclusion, and possibly barbering
   1. Mites can be confirmed through skin scraping/fur plucking or careful examination of the ear
   2. Dermatophytosis causes alopecia and will require a culture for fungal organisms to diagnose
   3. Malocclusion can cause scalding around the mouth and chin due to excess salivation; teeth will need to be trimmed regularly using a dental unit or a Dremmel tool or the incisors can be permanently removed
   4. Barbering usually occurs due to lack of dietary fiber: increase fiber in diet and provide rabbit with chewing material such as branches and wood blocks

GUINEA PIG (*CAVIA PORCELLUS* [CAVY])

Origin and Uses in Research

I. Wild Caviae still exist in Peru, Argentina, Brazil, and Uruguay

II. Member of the rodentia suborder Hystricomorpha; other rodents in this suborder include the chinchilla and the porcupine

III. The most common strains of guinea pig used in research today include the Duncan-Hartley, Hartley, and inbred strains 2 and 13

IV. The most common pet strains include the Peruvian (long haired), Abyssinian (short haired with rosettes), and the English (short haired)

V. Primarily used in genetics, anaphylaxis, microbiology, immunology, nutrition, and audiology studies. Diagnostic tests to diagnose infectious diseases use guinea pig serum

Characteristics: Behavioral and Physiological

I. Nervous but tame and easily handled

II. They may freeze at unexpected sounds or stampede at unexpected movements

III. Group-housed guinea pigs rarely fight except when overcrowded or if strange males are in the presence of a female in estrous

IV. Have poor jumping/climbing abilities and may be housed in low-walled, open-topped pens

V. Guinea pigs have constantly erupting (hypsodontic) teeth, which may lead to malocclusion and "slobbers" (see Health Conditions)

VI. Guinea pigs lack the L-gluconolactone oxidase enzyme, involved in the synthesis of ascorbic acid (vitamin C) from glucose; therefore it is of extreme importance that sufficient amounts be provided in the diet (also see Scurvy, Health Conditions)

A. Commercially prepared laboratory guinea pig diets contain a form of vitamin C that is stable for approximately 90 days (or longer; see product information

B. Guinea pig food available in pet stores is notoriously deficient; guinea pigs fed this diet will need to be provided with supplemental ascorbic acid at a rate of 5 mg/kg daily for a mature adult and 30 mg/kg daily for pregnant and immature animals

C. Guinea pigs are monogastric herbivores and cecal fermenters. In addition to their pelleted diet, they should be offered free choice hay and some fresh vegetables and fruit (but not more than 10% to 15% of the weight of the pelleted food) as treats

D. Guinea pigs respond poorly to diet change. They tend to establish their eating preferences early in life and will chose not to eat as opposed to eating new food. Introduction of novel feedstuffs early in life diminishes this response

VII. Guinea pigs respond poorly to stress and antibiotic therapy

VIII. Both males and females have two nipples. Females have no difficulty raising litters of more than four offspring

IX. Guinea pigs are considered to be quite messy and often play with the sipper tubes of their water bottles and drain the bottle

X. They are coprophagic, eating cecotrophs throughout the day

XI. Average life span is 2 to 4 years

XII. Rectal temperature: 37.2° to 39.5° C (99° to 103.1° F)

Handling and Restraint

I. Lift by grasping firmly and gently over their shoulders, with two fingers behind and two fingers in front of the forelimbs. The rump must always be supported with the other hand

A. It is important for the safety of the guinea pig that all technical procedures are performed with one person holding the animal while the other performs the task

Breeding Considerations

See Table 17-1 for reproductive data.

I. Females should be bred before the age of 6 months (preferably between 2.5 and 3 months) because of the risk of fusion of the pubic symphysis, leading to failure of the fetus to pass and thus dystocia

II. Guinea pigs can be successfully mated monogamously or as a harem

A. They are spontaneous ovulators; ovulation occurs 10 hours after estrus and 2 to 3 hours postpartum

III. Guinea pigs have a vaginal closure membrane that closes over the vagina when the sow is not in estrus

A. Closes after estrus or copulation and the expulsion of the vaginal plug and ruptures shortly before parturition

IV. During the latter stages of pregnancy, the sow becomes extremely heavy. Care must be taken to provide adequate support when handling and to ensure easy access to food and water

V. Sows do not build nests

VI. Newborn guinea pigs are precocious and relatively mature with hair, erupted teeth, and open eyes

Sampling

For injection routes, doses, needles sizes, and blood volumes, see Table 17-2.

I. Accessing veins for injections or bleeding tend to require sedation or anesthesia

II. Oral dosing can be achieved using a ball-tipped dosing needle

III. Urine and fecal samples can be obtained by placing the guinea pig in a metabolic cage

IV. Before blood collection, always calculate the maximum safe volume that can be withdrawn. Guinea pigs have approximately 65 to 90 mL/kg total blood volume. Of this, 10% to 15% can be safely withdrawn every 2 to 3 weeks

Signs of Pain and Distress

I. Key signs of pain and distress include withdrawal, vocalization, rough coat, and unresponsiveness

II. Acceptance to capture and restraint

III. Lethargy

IV. Sunken dull eyes, dehydration

V. Increased, and possibly labored, respiratory rate

VI. Weight loss, diarrhea, decreased food and water consumption

VII. Tendency toward barbering under dietary stress, hair loss, scaly skin

VIII. Group aggression

IX. Excessive salivation

X. Change in locomotion, lameness, careful gait

Health Conditions

I. Scurvy (hypovitaminosis C)

A. Clinical signs include lameness, lethargy, weakness, anorexia, rough hair coat, diarrhea, weight loss, change in teeth and gums, nasal and ocular discharge. The limb joints are often affected and may be enlarged and painful to the touch

B. Treatment should include daily dosing with ascorbic acid (5 to 10 mg/kg for maintenance) in the food, water, per os or parenteral injection. This should reverse the effect of deficiencies

C. Prevention is key. Always provide fresh (within 90 days of milling) pellets that have been stored in an air-tight container in a cool, dark storage area. Supplement feed with vitamin C–rich fruits and vegetables such as oranges, kale, red pepper, or cabbage

II. Antibiotic-associated enterotoxemia
  A. Intestinal flora in guinea pigs is predominantly gram positive, and when treated with antibiotics that act on gram-positive organisms (penicillin, ampicillin, chlortetracycline, lincomycin, erythromycin, tylosin), the intestinal flora will be drastically altered, leading to an overgrowth of gram-negative organisms
  B. Clinical signs include diarrhea, dehydration, hypothermia, and anorexia
  C. Treat symptomatically and with supportive care. Fluids should be administered; *Lactobacillus* sp. can be useful to reestablish normal flora
  D. Prevention through use of appropriate antibiotics. Guinea pigs seem to tolerate trimethoprim-sulfa, chloramphenicol, and enrofloxacin (Baytril) well

III. Malocclusion
  A. Guinea pigs have open-rooted incisors, premolars, and molars
  B. Clinical signs include anorexia, weight loss, and excess salivation ("slobbers") that can lead to dermatitis. Thorough examination of the entire mouth is necessary; use of a vaginal speculum or otoscope and sedation or anesthesia may be helpful to observe the molars and oral mucosa
  C. Trim teeth with a dental tool, Dremmel tool, or rongeurs
  D. As with most animals that are prone to malocclusion, there is a genetic predisposition and therefore all animals with this problem should not be selected as breeders

IV. Cervical lymphadenitis
  A. "Lumps" is a disease caused by *Streptococcus zooepidemicus* and occasionally *Streptobacillus moniliformis,* bacteria normally found in the conjunctiva and nasal cavity that enter the bloodstream through abrasions in the oral mucosa
  B. This disease is easily recognizable; the guinea pig will present with cervical masses that contain pus
  C. Treatment includes surgical excision of the affected cervical lymph nodes or draining and flushing abscess followed by systemic antibiotic treatment
  D. Because guinea pigs seem to be more prone to this disease in a stressful environment, prevention includes removal of overt sources of stress and a healthy balanced diet

V. Bacterial pneumonia
  A. Commonly caused by *Bordetella bronchiseptica* and *Streptococcus pneumoniae*
  B. Clinical signs include depression, anorexia, nasal and ocular discharge, and dyspnea
  C. Diagnosis may be made on clinical signs, radiography, and culture and sensitivity of nasal exudates. It is difficult to collect blood from guinea pigs without causing stress, but a complete blood cell count could also help in the diagnosis
  D. Treatment options include fluid and antibiotic therapy

VI. Salmonella
  A. Was once the most frequently reported bacterial infection in guinea pigs; common serotypes include *S. typhimurium* and *S. enteriditis*
  B. Clinical signs include anorexia, dull and ruffled hair coat, lethargy, and sudden death
  C. Diagnosis through blood culture or culture of spleen
  D. Antibiotic treatment will eliminate clinical signs but will not eliminate *Salmonella* sp. from the colony. Prevention includes thorough hand washing and ensuring that all vegetables and fruit are properly washed before feeding
  E. This organism has zoonotic potential

VII. Anesthetic complications/considerations
  A. Subcutaneous ketamine must be given as a deep muscular injection because it will cause sloughing of the tissue
  B. Important to use atropine
  C. Muscular movement may occur during surgical anesthesia

VIII. Dermatitis and alopecia (see Rabbit, Health Conditions)

CHINCHILLA (*CHINCHILLA LANGIER*)

Origin and Uses in Research

I. Chinchillas are in the same family as guinea pigs; they are both hystricomorph rodents from South America. The chinchilla is a native of Peru, Bolivia, Chile, and Argentina

II. Hunted for their prized pelts in the early 1900s, they are very rare in the wild and may actually be extinct

III. Used almost exclusively for hearing research

Characteristics: Behavioral and Physiological

I. Chinchilla are easy to handle and curious and have a curled and tufted tail that is carried high
II. They are monogastric herbivores and cecal fermenters
III. Chinchillas and guinea pigs are very similar in their anatomic and physiological characteristics, but unlike the guinea pigs, chinchillas do not require a dietary source of ascorbic acid
IV. Chinchillas require a dust bath frequently (daily to every other day is optimal)
  A. One recommendation is to make your own using 9 parts silver sand with 1 part Fuller's earth, or it can be purchased commercially. Do not use playground sand
  B. A round fishbowl makes an excellent dust bath container because it retains the sand
  C. They will dust bathe for up to 1 hour. Afterwards, remove dust bathe from cage to keep cage clean
V. Chinchilla teeth, like those of the guinea pig, are all open rooted and continually erupt
  A. They are naturally yellow in color
  B. To help avoid malocclusions, provide with chew toys, pieces of clean wood, fruit tree branches (unsprayed, of course), and porous rock to gnaw
VI. They should be fed a commercially prepared chinchilla diet and free choice high-quality grass hay
  A. Alfalfa hay can be used short term but is not preferable because it is very rich and could cause digestive disturbance
  B. Hay is important as it provides them with the chewing that they need, it reduces their stress, and it provides them with a low-energy roughage that will not promote obesity
  C. Fresh, clean fruits and vegetables can also be given as treats. They love raisins, but too many have been reported to cause dental caries
VII. Their coat is extremely luxurious and contains more fur per square inch than any other animal
VIII. They are virtually odorless
IX. They love to climb and jump; caging should provide areas in which to hide and to climb
X. In nature they tend to be most active around dawn and dusk, but in a home or research environment they are active throughout the day
XI. They have four toes on front and rear feet
XII. They are coprophagic and tend to consume their cecotrophs in the morning and early afternoon
XIII. Expected life span is 10 years
XIV. They can be quite comfortable in cool temperatures but do not tolerate temperatures over 26° C (79° F) and high humidity
XV. Rectal temperature: 38.0° to 39.0° C (100.4° to 102.2° F)

Handling and Restraint

I. If the chinchilla has been hand raised, it will probably come out of the cage quite willingly and onto your open hands
II. If you must remove it from its cage, the chinchilla can be grasped around the scruff of the neck/shoulders with one hand and the base of the tail with the other
  A. Rough or inexperienced handling could frighten the chinchilla and cause fur slip (loss of a large patch of fur)
  B. If the tail is grasped anywhere but the base, it might slough off
III. It is appropriate, and safer for the chinchilla, to have one person restrain while the other person performs the technical procedure or physical examination

Breeding Considerations

See Table 17-2 for reproductive data.

I. Females have a vaginal closure membrane, similar to that of guinea pigs, that is open only during estrus and parturition
II. They have three pairs of mammary glands
III. Like guinea pigs, they are placentophagic
IV. Females do not nest build but will use a nesting box, which can help keep the kits warm
V. Young are born precocious with teeth and open eyes and ears
VI. Can set up polygamous or monogamous matings. In commercial chinchilla farms, the male will be permitted to access a number of females' cages by a back runway to which only he has access. The females wear collars to prevent them from leaving their cage
VII. Cross-fostering and hand raising are usually successful

Sampling

For injection routes, doses, needles sizes, and blood volumes, see Table 17-2.

I. Can be very sensitive to injectable medications; whenever possible, give medications orally
  A. Chinchillas will often take pills and chew them up
  B. Medications can be given in raisins or on bread or by crushing and adding to food

Signs of Pain and Distress

I. Indifference to human attention, lethargy
II. Dull hair coat and eyes
III. Perineal staining
IV. Weight loss
V. Change in locomotion
VI. Anorexia
VII. Excess salivation

Health Conditions

Although chinchillas have been used in research and raised as pets and for their fur, there is not a lot of reference material pertaining to their disease problems. One thing to keep in mind is that they are similar in many aspects, including health concerns, to the guinea pig. Fortunately there is an abundance of reference material pertaining to guinea pig diseases and this can be followed when trying to diagnose, treat, and prevent diseases in the chinchilla.

I. Malocclusion (see Guinea Pig Health Concerns)
II. Choke and bloat
  A. Chinchillas cannot vomit
  B. Clinical signs of choke include retching, drooling, dyspnea, and anorexia. Animals that are bloated will lie on their sides with swollen abdomens
  C. Important to decompress the abdomen by passing a gastric tube or inserting a needle or trocar
  D. Similar to rabbits, chinchillas can also get trichobezoars; cause and treatment are basically the same as for the rabbit
III. Constipation
  A. Due to feeding a diet that is too rich in concentrated food and not enough roughage
  B. Clinical sign of constipation is straining to defecate and small, dry fecal pellets
IV. Fur ring and paraphimosis
  A. Caused by a ring of fur around the penis that eventually stops the penis from retracting into the prepuce
  B. Clinical signs include excessive grooming, straining to urinate, passing only small volumes of urine, and an engorged penis resulting in paraphimosis
  C. Ring will need to be cut or rolled (lubricate first) off the penis
  D. All males should be checked on a regular basis (weekly)
V. Alopecia
  A. Can be caused by *Trichophyton mentagrophytes* (ringworm), particularly if seen on the nose or front feet or behind the ears
  B. Diagnosis and treatment similar to those for other species
  C. Zoonotic potential

HEDGEHOGS *(ATELERIX ALBIVENTRIS)*

Origin and Uses in Research

I. Hedgehogs are small, insectivores native to England, parts of Europe, Africa, and Asia
  A. The type of hedgehog that is typically kept as a pet in North America is the African pygmy hedgehog, native to equatorial and central Africa
II. From the insectivore family Erinaceidae
III. Share a lipoprotein identical to those found in human blood, contributing to the formation of clots; therefore used for cardiovascular research

Characteristics: Behavioral and Physiological

I. Hedgehogs are nocturnal animals
II. The hedgehog will roll into a protective ball when it hears a loud noise or is touched by an unfamiliar person
III. Generally a solitary creature
IV. Hedgehogs can occasionally be seen "self-anointing," which is triggered by a novel scent. The hedgehog will lick at the novel item and produce large amounts of saliva, which it will spread over its back and flank with its tongue
V. Can be trained to use a litterbox but avoid using clumping cat litter as it will stick to the anus and cause impactions
VI. Hedgehogs should be provided with a running wheel for exercise. Be prepared because they will defecate in this wheel, so ensure that it is easily cleanable
  A. Caging should have a solid bottom; they tend to get their feet caught in wire bottoms
  B. Hedgehogs need to be housed in a warm (24° to 30° C or 75° to 85° F), draft-free area
    1. Supplemental heat in the form of a heat lamp may be required
  C. If caging is large enough, a warm water swimming area could be added
VII. Hedgehogs need to be fed a commercially prepared hedgehog diet that is relatively high in protein and low in fat. Hedgehogs that are fed just cat food tend to develop cystitis or urolithiasis
  A. Be careful not to overfeed as they can become obese. Because they are nocturnal, feed them at night and remove any uneaten feed in the morning
  B. Crickets and mealworms can be given as treats (a couple every other day is plenty)
VIII. Toenails need to be trimmed on a regular basis
IX. Expected life span of 6 to 8 years
X. Rectal temperature: 35.3° to 35.9° C (95.5° to 96.6° F)

Handling and Restraint

I. Basically, these animals will roll into a tight ball as soon as you need to have a look at them; for a detailed examination, the animal may need to be anesthetized or sedated with isoflurane. This technique is probably less stressful than trying to get them to uncurl

II. Sometimes getting them to walk into a clear plastic tube will allow you to have a general look at them

III. There are a few methods that have been documented to uncurl and restrain a hedgehog

  A. With an assistant holding a towel directly below the table edge, push the hedgehog toward the edge of the table. It will probably uncurl to protect itself from falling over the edge; when it does, quickly grasp it by the hind legs

  B. Placing the hedgehog in a pan of shallow water (about 1 inch) will usually entice it to uncurl; then grasp the hind legs

  C. Hedgehog can be placed on its back on the examination table; wait until it tries to right itself and then grasp the hind legs

IV. Once you have the hedgehog uncurled, you can "mantle scruff" it with a gloved hand. One person should scruff while the other performs the procedure

Breeding Considerations

See Table 17-1 for reproductive data.

I. It is quite common for hedgehogs to cannibalize their young, especially if they are disturbed. Do not handle the sow or the litter for at least the first 7 to 10 days

  A. Once the young have left the nest at about 21 days, they are ready to be habituated to humans and should be handled daily

II. Females can conceive as young as 8 weeks of age but should not be bred until they are at least 6 months. They will be healthily productive until about 2.5 years of age

III. Move the female to the male's cage; otherwise she might be territorial and attack him. Watch carefully for fighting and remove her if this occurs. She should be left for at least 3 days

IV. Young are born blind with a membrane covering their spines

Sampling

I. Intramuscular and subcutaneous injections can be given into the mantle using a 3.5-inch spinal needle

II. The saphenous, jugular, and cephalic veins are accessible

III. Fecal and urine samples can be collected using a metabolic cage for a brief period of time

Signs of Pain and Distress

I. Weight loss, sunken sides

II. Lethargy: for example, lack of wheel running, if this was normal

III. Change is consistency of fecal pellets

IV. Decreased appetite

V. Change in locomotion

VI. Dyspnea, nasal discharge, increased lung sounds, coughing, wheezing

Health Conditions

I. Respiratory disease

  A. Bacterial causative agents include *Bordetella bronchiseptica, Mycoplasma* spp., and possibly *Pasteurella multocida.* Can also be caused by lungworm (if allowed to eat slugs or snails because they are the intermediate host), lung threadworm, neoplasia, and environmental stress such as chilling

  B. Clinical signs include coughing, wheezing, lethargy, dyspnea, increased lung sounds, inappetance, and nasal discharge

  C. Diagnosis by culture, radiography, auscultation, endoscopy, and cytology

  D. Treatment depends on outcome of examination, but basics include

    1. Increase temperature to 27° to 30° C or 80° to 85° F and administer oxygen (incubator could be used)

    2. Administer, in the least stressful method possible, antibiotics, bronchodilators, anthelmintics, etc.

II. Dermatitis and alopecia

  A. Hedgehogs can get fleas, ticks, mite infestations, and dermatophyte infections. Mites commonly seen include psoroptes, sarcopties, and demodex

  B. Clinical signs include cutaneous lesions particularly around the head, scratching, anemia, loss of spines (denuding), and visualization of the ectoparasite

  C. Diagnosis is made by microscopic examination of skin scrapings and/or skin biopsy if mites are suspected; culture of skin scraping if ringworm is suspected; or visually inspecting the entire animal if fleas or ticks are suspected

  D. Treat according to diagnosis. Ivermectin (at 200 to 500 μg/kg) has been used successfully in hedgehogs to eliminate mites

III. Additional miscellaneous diseases

  A. Hedgehogs have been found to carry *Salmonella* organisms, a zoonotic potential

B. Obesity is quite common and can be controlled by restricted feeding and increased exercise (most hedgehogs are fed ad libitum and housed in cages that are too small to allow for behaviors such as digging, foraging, and wheel running that would assist in burning calories
C. Wide range of internal parasites, including *Crenosoma striatum* (lungworm) and *Capillaria* sp. (threadworms)
D. Human herpes simplex virus 1 can cause chronic hepatitis

DEGU *(OCTODON DEGUS)*

Origin and Uses in Research

I. The degu is a rodent of the Octodontidae family
II. A native of Chile, it ranges the western slopes of the Andes
III. Has been referred to as the "trumpet-tailed rat" or "brush tail rat"
IV. Uses in research include studies on diabetes mellitus, reproduction, thymus in immune function, and genetic variation in enzymes

Characteristics: Behavioral and Physiological

I. Very social animals. In nature they live in large colonies very similar to the prairie dog; like the prairie dog, they are also considered to be agricultural pests
II. They are diurnal and active throughout the year
III. Degus are herbivorous and grainivorous and thrive on commercially prepared laboratory rodent diet
  A. Degus lack the ability to properly digest sugars; avoid feeding them fruits of any sort and any vegetable that is high in sugar, such as carrots. Examples of vegetables that can be given to degus as a treat are beet greens, sweet potatoes, turnips, brussels sprouts, bok choy, and kale
  B. Avoid giving them too many raw peanuts and sunflower seeds as this has been reported to cause fatty liver disease
  C. Diet should be supplemented with free choice high-quality grass hay
IV. Degus can be intensively active for short periods of time. They have the ability to climb trees. For these reasons, the ideal cage will allow enough space for rambunctious play, social interactions, a running wheel, and climbing areas
V. They tend to sleep in short cycles of about 20 minutes in duration
VI. Probably due to their social structure, degus make a wide variety of vocalizations, specific to certain stimulus or behaviors
VII. Like chinchillas, degus need to have access to a dust bath (see Chinchilla for details)
VIII. Also like chinchillas, degus have orange, open-rooted teeth
IX. Degus quite openly acknowledge familiar people and other degus. When someone they recognize enters the room, they will stand up on their hind legs and squeak quite loudly
X. Average life span is 5 to 7 years in captivity

Handling and Restraint

I. Hand-tamed degus can be picked up by presenting an open hand and allowing them to walk on. Once they are on your hand, use both hands to secure them. Useful when transferring to a clean cage
II. To restrain a degu for a physical examination or technical procedure
  A. Grip the base of the tail with one hand and the scruff (the loose skin around the neck and shoulder area) with the other hand, similar to a gerbil
    1. Or place fingers on both sides of the head behind the mandibles, similar to a rat
  B. Extreme care should be taken to avoid grasping the tail away from the base as this could cause degloving of the tail
  C. Two people should be involved in technical procedures
III. Degus rarely bite, but they will if they are frightened or startled. They tend to emit a loud squeak when handled improperly or frightened: take this sound as a warning

Breeding Considerations

See Table 17-1 for reproductive data.

I. Females have four pair of teats (eight mammae)
II. Males do not have a true scrotum (like chinchillas); the testes are contained within the inguinal canal or abdomen
III. The relatively long gestation period (90 days) means that newborn degus are fairly well formed. They are born fully furred and with open eyes
IV. The male will assist in caring for the young and, whenever possible, should be left with the female
V. Young degus can be handled after 7 days of age; early habituation has a positive impact on handling by humans in the future
VI. Degus are thought to be induced ovulators

Sampling

I. Techniques used in other members of the rodent family are applicable to degus

Signs of Pain and Distress

I. Isolation from the group, lack of interest in socializing with familiar people, lethargy
II. Change in consistency of fecal pellets

III. Weight loss, inappetance
IV. Polyuria/polydipsia
V. Alopecia/dermatitis
VI. Lameness

Health Conditions

There seems to be a profound lack of scientific documentation on health conditions in degus. This is apparently due to the fact that few infectious lesions have been noted in this animal. Reported naturally occurring infections include *Echinococcus granulosus* (tapeworm) and *Trypanosoma cruzi* (protozoa). Lesions that are commonly seen that are associated with diabetes mellitus include cataracts, amyloidosis, and hyperplasia of the islets of Langerhans.

Clinical signs of disease should be followed up and treated similarly to those in other rodents.

GENERAL CAGING AND HOUSING

I. Select the size of cage appropriate to the species; see Table 17-3

Table 17-3 Housing data

Species	Temperature* (°C, / °F)	Relative humidity† (%)	Ventilation (air changes/hr)‡	Lights (hr)	Caging	Other conditions§
Mouse	22-25/72-78	50-70	8-12	12-14 nocturnal	Shoebox or suspended mesh	Can be group housed in same-sex groups, occasionally males of certain strains will fight and need to be separated. Barbers should be removed. Provide nesting material and places to hide such as plastic pipe sections.
Rat	20-25/68-76	50-55	10-20	12-15 nocturnal	Shoebox or suspended mesh	Can be group housed in same-sex groups. Provide nesting material; places to hide, such as cardboard boxes; exercise wheels.
Guinea pig	18-22/66-72	50-60	4-8	12-15 crepuscular	Shoebox, floor pens or stalls, suspended mesh	Light changes should be gradual. Not necessary to have a lid on cages that are greater than 40 cm in height. Group house females.
Hamster	21-24/70-78	45-65	6-10	12 nocturnal	Shoebox	House in groups if raised and weaned together, otherwise separate at puberty. Hibernation brought on by decrease in temperature and light hours.
Gerbil	15-24/60-78	40-50	8-10	12-14 nocturnal/ diurnal	Shoebox	Burrowers, produce less urine (therefore less ammonia) and have dry fecal pellets.
Rabbit	16-20/62-70	40-50	10-20	12-14 crepuscular	Floor pens or stalls, suspended mesh	Group house compatible females, mature males will fight. Provide raised platforms for resting on or hiding under.
Hedgehog	22-27/70-80	45-65	8-10	12-14 crepuscular, hibernate	Aquariums or shoebox	Bedding should be deep and dry; use hide box, exercise wheel, litter pan.
Chinchilla	15-22/60-70	40-70	8-10	12-14 nocturnal	Solid bottom or suspended mesh	Important to allow dust bathing at least twice per week. Provide chewing devices or wood.
Degu	20-24/65-78	40-50	8-10	12-14 diurnal, active throughout year	Solid bottom or suspended mesh	Provide hiding spaces and deep bedding for burrowing. Can climb so provide sticks and platforms.

Information from Canadian Council on Animal Care (CCAC): *Guide to the Care and Use of Experimental Animals, Volume 1,* Ottawa, Canada, 1993.
*Information from National Research Council: *Guide for the Care and Use of Laboratory Animals.* Institute of Laboratory Animal Resources, National Academy Press, 1996 (suggests that the range of temperature for all listed species is between 64° to 79° F and 18° to 26° C).
†The range of humidity for each is 30% to 70%.
‡The CCAC is gradually increasing their expectations regarding ventilation for most laboratory animals to 15 to 20 air changes/hr.
§Noise greater than 50 dB or ammonia levels greater than 22 ppm are detrimental to most laboratory animals.

Table 17-4 Zoonoses

Diseases	Causative organism/ distribution	Laboratory species	Means of spread, vectors	Outcome of infection, to humans
Salmonellosis	Bacteria Worldwide	Mice, rats, guinea pigs, hedgehogs, chinchilla	Ingestion, inhalation, contact	Gastroenteritis (vomiting, diarrhea), headache, and fever
Campylobacter	Bacteria Worldwide	Hamsters	Ingestion	Abdominal pain and severe diarrhea
Lymphocytic choriomeningitis	Arena virus Worldwide	Hamsters, rodents	Contact, inhalation, congenital transmission, tissue culture transmission	Aseptic meningitis, encephalitis or meningoencephalitis: temporary illness with nervous symptoms or permanent disability associated with the central nervous system
Ringworm	Fungus: *Microsporum, Trichophyton* Worldwide	Guinea pigs, rodents, rabbits, chinchilla	Direct contact, soil may be a reservoir	Progressively itchy, weeping, chronic dermatitis
Tularemia/ rabbit fever	*Francisella tularesis* Circumpolar in northern hemisphere	Rabbits, rodents	Inhalation, contact, tick and insect bites, ingestion of contaminated food and water	Without antibiotic treatment, fatal in 5% of cases; diagnosis by antibody identification via blood testing; signs are fever, lethargy, anorexia, coughing, diarrhea
Plague	*Yersinia pestis* Western United States, South America, Asia, Africa	Rodents	Flea bites, inhalation	Fever, shivering, severe headaches, swollen lymph glands Pneumonic plague may be a complication; coughing produces bloody frothy sputum, labored breathing
Pseudotuberculosis (yersiniosis)	*Yersinia pseudotuberculosis* Northern Hemisphere	Rodents	Contact, contaminated food and water, ingestion	Coughing, chest pain, shortness of breath, fever, sweating, poor appetite, weight loss
Rat bite fever	*Streptobacillus* and *Spirillum minus* Worldwide	Rodents	Rodent bites, ingestion	Inflammation at site of bite, swollen iymph nodes, bouts of fever, rash, painful joints
Leptospirosis (Weil's diease)	*Leptospira* spp. Worldwide	Rodents	Contact, urine contaminated soil and water	Fever, chills, headache, muscle aches, eye inflammation, skin rash
Hantavirus	Hantavirus	Mice	Contact, inhalation	Fever and muscle aches (1 to 5 wk postexposure), shortness of breath, coughing

II. Animals should be confined securely and comfort and safety ensured, permitting normal postural and behavioral adjustments

III. Environmental enrichment should be provided for social and behavioral needs

IV. Animals that are social in nature should not be housed singly unless necessary for research protocol and approved by the appropriate body (animal care committee). When social animals must be housed singly, they should be able to see, hear, and smell their conspecific

V. Provide adequate ventilation, viewing, and easy access to animal

VI. Food and water delivery systems
   A. Must provide easy access to all age and size of animals within the microenvironment
   B. Must not be contaminated with excrement
   C. Must be thoroughly cleanable, and in some cases they must be able to withstand sterilization in an autoclave
   D. Degus often play with their watering systems, which may flood the cage

VII. Housing design and material must facilitate cleaning and disinfection. Although ease of cleaning is important, this should not be the factor that determines which style of housing is used. For example: wire-bottom cages with excreta pans for rabbits are perhaps easier to clean than when rabbits are housed on solid-bottom pens on shavings, but the floor pens are preferable for many other reasons and are cleanable, too, with a bit more effort

VIII. Consider light intensity, noise level, ventilation, and temperature effects on the animal's microenvironment and ensure that they are within recognized guidelines

IX. All ceiling, wall, and floor surfaces in a laboratory animal facility must be made of a sealed, nonporous material to facilitate thorough disinfection

ZOONOSIS

From an occupational health standpoint, as well as for animal colony management, it is important to be aware of the diseases that can be transmitted from one species to another, including humans (Table 17-4).

LABORATORY ANIMAL ALLERGY

I. Laboratory animal allergy (LAA) is the most common health condition that affects people working in a research animal facility
   A. At risk are the technicians, investigators and their staff, and facility support staff such as front office administrative personnel
   B. From 10% to 30% of people working in this field will develop allergic symptoms

II. LAA is a hypersensitivity to certain substances, such as the proteins found in dander, urine, serum, and saliva
   A. Does not cause a reaction in a nonallergenic person
   B. The immune system produces antibodies to the specific proteins, and this results in observable signs

III. Observable symptoms
   A. Rhinitis
   B. Conjunctivitis
   C. Contact urticaria (hives)
   D. Asthma
   E. Anaphylaxis

IV. Risk of exposure should be assessed; there are certain tasks, such as cage cleaning, cage changing, handling the animals, and sweeping that increase exposure. Once the risk of the task has been assessed, the appropriate control method should be chosen
   A. Engineering controls: these are the most appropriate controls in the long term
      1. Consider substituting bedding for less dust, providing better localized ventilation, and using HEPA vacuums
   B. Administrative controls: switching jobs within the facility, cross-training
      1. Improve personnel hygiene
      2. Medical surveillance program
   C. Personal protective equipment: respirators (must be fit tested), facility-specific clothing, eye protection
      1. Do not wear street clothes into the animal facility because allergens can be carried home on clothing. Also, avoid taking facility clothing home because this exposes members of your family to allergens
      2. Avoid wearing soiled clothing into the common facility areas such as the lunch room; this will decrease the exposure of the administrative staff

ACKNOWLEDGMENT

The editors and author recognize and appreciate the original work of Amanda Hathaway and Jodilynn Pitcher, on which this chapter is based.

Glossary

axenic Also referred to as germ free; these animals are hysterectomy derived, free from any microorganisms and maintained in a germ free isolation type housing

barbering Occurs when one animal clips or chews the fur of another, usually around the muzzle or head to show dominance

barrier sustained Gnotobiotic animals that are maintained under sterile conditions in a barrier unit

Bruce effect Pregnancy block that occurs when a pregnant female is exposed to a strange male within 48 hours of copulation

cecotrophs Soft night and early morning fecal pellets ingested directly from the anus

chromodacryorrhea Secretion of dark red fluid from the harderian gland

congenic Animals that genetically differ at one particular locus; having similar genotypes

conspecific Member of the same species

coprophagia Eating of one's stools or feces

crepuscular Becoming active at twilight or just before sunrise

degloving Removal of the skin from its underlying structures

denuding Stripping or laying bare of any part

diurnal Becoming active through the day

fecundity Able to produce offspring frequently and in large numbers

gavage Force feeding/medicating usually through a tube passed into the stomach

gnotobiotic Germ-free animals that have been introduced to one or two known nonpathogenic microorganisms

harderian gland Lacrimal gland located behind the rat's eyeball that secretes a lipid- and protein-rich secretion that lubricates the eye

harem mating Mating one male with two or more females

high-efficiency particulate air (HEPA filter) Used in clean rooms, biological safety cabinets, laminar flow units, etc., to filter out contaminating particles as small as 0.3 μm in diameter

hypsodontic Teeth that continuously erupt

immunosuppressed Diminished immune response

inbred Inbreeding resulting from mating between closely related animals for at least 20 generations

latent infection Condition or infection that may not be clinically noted in the animal, but under stress or poor health conditions it develops into a recognizable disease state

lordosis Abnormal curvature of the spine; may be shown by a female as a sign of receptiveness to a male

malocclusion Genetic or dietary related condition in which the apposing teeth do not meet when the jaw is closed

mantle Thick muscle layer running along the back and supporting the spine

microenvironment Isolated habitat, usually within a cage

monogastric Refers to having a single-chambered stomach

nocturnal Becoming active at night

outbred Result of random breeding to achieve genetic diversity

paraphimosis Inability to retract penis due to swelling

phenotype Outward visible expression of the hereditary constitution of an organism

placentophagia Animals that consume their placenta

sentinel An animal used to monitor disease in other animals

SPF Specific pathogen free

transgenic animals Animals whose hereditary DNA has been augmented by the addition of DNA from a source other than parental germplasm, usually from another animal or a human, using recombinant DNA techniques

trichobezoars Mass of hair found in the gastrointestinal tract, caused from animals licking themselves. Often called a hairball

VAF Viral antibody free

Whitten effect Majority of a group of female mice when exposed to a male mouse will be in estrus the third night

Review Questions

1 Which two types of animals require dust baths?
   a. Rabbit and chinchilla
   b. Chinchilla and degu
   c. Degu and gerbil
   d. Degu and hedgehog

2 Which species does not practice coprophagy as a necessary nutritional supplement?
   a. Mouse
   b. Chinchilla
   c. Guinea pig
   d. Rat

3 Which species is unable to synthesize vitamin C?
   a. Rabbit
   b. Degu
   c. Guinea pig
   d. Hamster

4 Which of the following are zoonotic diseases?
   a. Salmonella, ringworm, lymphocytic choriomeningitis
   b. Salmonella, ringworm, chromodacryorrhea
   c. Ringworm, chromodacryorrhea, lymphocytic choriomeningitis
   d. Ringworm, scurvy, chromodacryorrhea

5 Inbred strains are the result of at least how many generations of bother × sister mating?
   a. 10
   b. 20
   c. 30
   d. 40

6 Which species is known to go into pseudo-hibernation if housing temperatures are decreased?
   a. Hamster
   b. Hedgehog
   c. Gerbil
   d. Degu

7 Intramandibulary swelling and red porphyrin staining on face and paws of a rat could indicate signs of what disease?
   a. Mite infestation
   b. Sialodacryoadenitis virus
   c. Sendai virus
   d. *Mycoplasma pulmonis*

8 Chromodacryorrhea is commonly referred to as red tears and is
   a. A zoonotic viral condition
   b. A bacterial condition
   c. Caused by porphyrin secretions from the Harderian gland
   d. Caused by a secretion from the hibernating gland

9 Which animal is an insectivore?
   a. Chinchilla
   b. Hedgehog
   c. Gerbil
   d. Degu

10 A rabbit presents with torticollis. What could be causing this?
   a. A hairball
   b. May have been improperly handled and has now fractured its vertebrae
   c. An infection caused by *Pasteurella multocida*
   d. Malocclusion

BIBLIOGRAPHY

Animals for Research Act, 1983, Government of Ontario.

Bell JC, Palmer SR, Payne JM: *The zoonoses: infections transmitted from animals to man,* London, 1988, Edward Arnold, 1988.

Brown SA: *Rabbit medicine,* Proceedings of the 21st Waltham's/Oklahoma State University Symposium, Oklahoma.

Buckland MD et al: *A guide to laboratory animal technology,* London, 1981, William Heinemann Medical Books Limited.

Canadian Association for Laboratory Animal Science, *CALAS training manual,* Ottawa, Canada, 1995, CALAS.

Canadian Council on Animal Care: *Guide to the care and use of experimental animals, vol 1,* Ottawa, Canada, 1993, CCAC.

Canadian Council on Animal Care: *Guide to the care and use of experimental animals, vol 2,* Ottawa, Canada, 1980-1984, CCAC.

Field KJ, Sibold AL: *The laboratory hamster and gerbil,* Boca Raton, FL, 1999, CRC Press.

Fine J, Quimby FW, Greenhouse DD: Annotated bibliography on uncommonly used laboratory animals: mammals, *ILAR News* XXIX:4, 1986.

Flecknell PA: *Laboratory animal anaesthesia,* ed 2, San Diego, 1996, Academic Press.

Harkness JE, Wagner JE: *The biology and medicine of rabbits and rodents,* ed 4, Philadelphia, 1995, Lea & Febiger.

Harris JC: *Chinchillas: a complete introduction,* Neptune City, NJ, 1987, TFH Publications Inc.

Harrison DJ: *Innovative methods for controlling exposure to laboratory animal allergens.* Notes from workshop presented at the American Association for Laboratory Animal Science

Conference, Baltimore, MD, October 2001.

Hawk CT, Leary SL: *Formulary for laboratory animals,* ed 2, Ames, 1999, Iowa State University Press.

Hillyer EV, Quesenberry KE: *Ferrets, rabbits and rodents: clinical medicine and surgery,* Philadelphia, 1997, WB Saunders.

Hrapkiewicz K, Medina L, Holmes DD: *Clinical laboratory animal medicine: an introduction,* ed 2, Ames, 1998, Iowa State University Press.

Johnson-Delaney C: Notes from the Internet, *African pygmy hedgehogs,* http://www.whh.org/help/africa/africa22.htm

Kraft H: *Diseases of chinchillas,* Neptune City, NJ, 1959, TFH Publications.

Krinke GJ: *The laboratory rat,* San Diego, CA, 2000, Academic Press.

Laber-Laird K, Swindle M, Flecknell P, editors: *Handbook of rodent and rabbit medicine,* Tarrytown, NY, 1996, Pergamon Press.

Maronpot RR: *Pathology of the mouse,* Vienna, IL, 1999, Cache River Press.

National Research Council, Committee on Rodents, Institute of Laboratory Animal Resources: *Rodents,* Washington, DC, 1996, National Academy Press.

National Research Council, Institute of Laboratory Animal Resources: *Guide for the care and use of laboratory animals,* Washington, DC, 1996, National Academy Press.

National Research Council: *Occupational health and safety in the care and use of research animals,* Washington, DC, 1997, National Academy Press.

Plunkett SJ: *Emergency procedures for the small animal veterinarian,* ed 2, Spain, 2001, Harcourt Publishers Ltd.

Poole et al: *The UFAW handbook on the care and management of laboratory animals, vol 1, terrestrial vertebrates,* ed 7, New York, 1999, Blackwell Science.

Wagner JE, Manning PJ: *The biology of the guinea pig,* New York, 1976, Academic Press.

Waynforth HB, Flecknell PA: *Experimental and surgical technique in the rat,* ed 2, London/Toronto, 1992, Academic Press.

Wrobel D, Brown SA: *The hedgehog: an owner's guide to a happy healthy hedgehog,* New York, 1997, Howell Book House.

CHAPTER 18

Exotic Animal Medicine

Rebecca M. Atkinson

OUTLINE

LEARNING OUTCOMES

After reading this chapter you should be able to:

1. Describe the anatomical and physiological differences in avian and reptilian species compared with mammals.
2. Describe optimum housing and husbandry for reptilian and avian species.
3. Describe restraint and handling for reptilian and avian species.
4. Describe nursing care and procedures for reptilian and avian species.
5. List optimum nutritional requirements for various avian and reptilian species.
6. Identify common clinical conditions and infectious diseases by describing their etiology, clinical signs, and pathology.
7. Describe ectoparasitic and endoparasitic diseases in reptilian and avian species.

Avian Medicine

CLASSIFICATION

I. Class Aves
   A. Order Psittaformes (psittacines: parrots, cockatoos, macaws, budgies, cockatiels)
   B. Order Passeriformes (songbirds: finches, canaries)
   C. Order Anseriformes (waterfowl: ducks, geese, swans)
   D. Ciconiformes (waterbirds: cranes, herons)
   E. Falconiformes (raptors: falcons, hawks, eagles, owls)
   F. Galliformes (fowl: poultry, pheasants, peafowl)

ANATOMICAL AND PHYSIOLOGICAL COMPARISON OF AVIANS AND MAMMALS

There is a reduction and modification of organs and organ systems to obtain the capacity for flight. Lack of teeth, hollowing of bones, shortened gastrointestinal tract, presence of air sacs, higher rate of metabolism, oviparity, and feathers are all adaptations for weight reduction and flight ability.

I. Integument
   A. Thinner and more delicate than in mammals
   B. Consists of the epidermis, dermis, and subcutaneous layers
   C. Modifications may include the legs, feet, beak, cere, or cheek patches
   D. The ventral surface of the female bird can modify during breeding season to form a brood patch
   E. The dermal layer contains the feather follicles arranged in rows, called pterylae, separated by featherless rows called apteriae
   F. Smooth muscles attach to the follicles and are responsible for feather fluffing to conserve heat (similar to piloerection of hair in mammals)
   G. Deficient of glands with the exception of the meibomian glands of the eyelid, uropygial gland above the tail base, and the holocrine gland of the external ear canal
   H. Feathers are epidermal structures analagous to mammalian hair and serve in insulation, thermoregulation, courtship displays, and flight
   I. Feather types
      1. Contour (e.g., body and flight feathers)
      2. Plume (e.g., down and powder down)
      3. Semiplume (e.g., bristles and hairs)
   J. Molting is the process of shedding and the regrowth of feathers, influenced by season, temperature, nutrition, stress, species, and sex. Molting occurs at least yearly, systematically and gradually, never leaving the bird featherless. In pet birds, heavy molting may occur twice yearly
II. Sensory: senses of smell and taste are poorly developed; visual senses are extremely well developed
   A. Color vision: rods and cones are present, the numbers dependent on diurnal or nocturnal habits
   B. Three functional eyelids: upper, lower, and nictitating
   C. Eyeballs are fixed in their sockets; however, the bird is able to rotate its head almost 360 degrees
   D. Movement of one eye is independent of the other (no consensual reflex)
   E. Sclerotic ring is the bony ring around the eye, where the cornea joins the sclera
   F. Pecten: a brown vascular fringe that projects from the lower medial wall of the eye toward the lens; assumed to provide nutrients to the avascular retina
III. Skeleton: extreme adaptations for flight
   A. Bones are pneumatic (hollow): lightweight
   B. Some of the air sacs are in direct communication with the proximal bones (e.g., the interclavicular with the humerus)
   C. Fusion of bones: carpometacarpus, tarsometatarsus, and the pelvic girdle (synsacrum)
   D. Pectoral girdle consists of a tripod of bones: clavicle, coracoid, and scapula
IV. Digestive system varies with gross anatomical differences and short transit time (3 to 12 hours)
   A. Galliformes and psittacines possess a true crop
   B. Falconiformes have a poorly developed crop, the owls lack a crop entirely
   C. Ciconiformes and other fish-eating birds lack a crop
   D. Beak is epidermal tissue: its characteristics vary based on the species feeding habits
   E. Oral cavity is made up of the tongue, glottis (no epiglottis), and pharynx
   F. Proximal esophagus leads to crop, distal esophagus lead to stomach (proventriculus and ventriculus)
   G. Associated organs: liver and spleen
   H. Small intestine; duodenum, jejunum, and ileum
   I. Pancreas and gallbladder (absent in most psittacines) empty into the terminal segment of the duodenal loop (rather than the proximal segment as in mammals)
   J. Large intestine; paired caeca (absent in psittacines), rectum, and cloaca
   K. Cloaca; coprodeum (digestive), urodeum (urinary), and proctodeum (collection chamber)
V. Respiratory: unique anatomy
   A. No diaphragm
   B. Larynx: at anterior end of the trachea, complete rings, not sound producing
   C. Syrinx: at base of the trachea, sound producing
   D. Bronchi to lungs
   E. Lungs: the most efficient gas exchange system among the vertebrates
      1. Compressed dorsally against the ribs, fixed, and do not expand during inspiration
      2. Unidirectional flow through the lungs
      3. Cross-current relationship between the parabronchial gas and blood
      4. Countercurrent relationship between the blood and capillaries
      5. Increased diffusing capacity for oxygen
   F. Air sacs
      1. Nine pair (based on the chicken as a model): single interclavicular, cervical, anterior thoracic, posterior thoracic, abdominal

B. If the quick of the nail is cut, it will cause the nail to bleed
   1. Silver nitrate or hemostatic powder can be used to stop the bleeding
   2. Any blood loss in birds is considered serious; therefore each nail should be examined after trimming

IV. Wing clipping
   A. Wing clipping is used to limit the bird's flying ability and as an aid in training and taming
      1. The wing trim should only allow the bird to glide a short distance off the floor
      2. There are several types of wing trims
         a. The most common is where all of the primary feathers are trimmed
         b. Only the tips of the primaries are trimmed (for larger birds)
         c. Trimming the first six primary feathers on each wing for smaller birds
      3. During the wing trim the underside of the wing should be examined for immature or growing blood feathers
         a. If a blood feather is accidentally cut, the feather will bleed and must be pulled out immediately to prevent blood loss
      4. A newly wing trimmed bird should be placed on the floor so that it does not attempt to soar and it can become aware of the change in its flying ability

V. Blood collection
   A. Sites
      1. Right jugular (the right is slightly larger than the left)
      2. Brachioulnar or cutaneous ulnar (wing vein)
      3. Medial tibiotarsal or medial metatarsal (leg vein)
      4. Toenail clipping is not recommended
   B. Blood is collected using a 23- or 25-gauge needle
      1. A sample can be collected in a heparinized syringe and transferred to a microhematocrit tube
      2. Pressure should be applied directly to the site of the collection after removal of the needle
      3. The site should be evaluated for bleeding before releasing the bird

VI. Blood analysis: Coulter counter cannot be used for avian blood due to the nucleated red blood cells; complete blood cell count can be obtained by combining the Unopette system and hemocytometer count, which give an absolute heterophil and eosinophil count, with a differential count from a smear

VII. Intraosseous catheter placement is in the proximal tibia or distal ulna

VIII. Intramuscular injections are generally performed in the pectoral muscle (renal portal system and possible nephrotoxicity if leg is used)
   A. The feathers may be wet down with water before inserting the needle in the thickest part of the breast muscle
      1. The plunger should be pulled back to detect the aspiration of blood into the hub of the needle
      2. If blood is present, the needle should be removed and placed in a new site
      3. Pressure should be applied to the site and the site should be examined for visible blood

IX. Subcutaneous injections are not often used due to leakage at the site
   A. For subcutaneous medications, the dorsal scapular area and the ventrolateral abdomen may be used

X. Oral administration/tube feeding is performed using a metal or plastic feeding tube (metal for psittacines) inserted gently down the esophagus into the crop
   A. The bird must be in an upright position with the neck extended
   B. The tube is inserted between the beaks, over the tongue, and into the esophagus and then into the crop
      1. Inject the medication slowly; if the bird shows any signs of coughing, remove the tube and restart the procedure

NUTRITION: DIETS AND PROBLEMS

I. Proper psittacine diet
   A. Pelleted or extruded "complete" psittacine diet: 18% to 20% protein for an adult, 20% to 25% protein for a juvenile
   B. Seeds should be restricted due to the high fat component
   C. Budgies do not synthesize iodine and thus require iodine in their diet
   D. Grit is not necessary as a supplement

II. Waterfowl diet: commercially available

III. Poultry diet: commercially available

IV. Circoniformes are carnivorous: feed fish and frogs

V. Raptorial species are carnivorous: feed mice, rats, quail, and chicks

VI. Dietary problems
   A. Hypovitaminosis A: unhealthy mucous membranes and epithelium, red tears caused by ruptured ocular blood vessels seen in African gray parrots

B. Hypocalcemia: "metabolic bone disease" and nutritional hypoparathyroidism, leading to hypocalcemic tetany observed in psittacines
C. Calcium/phosphorous imbalance: normal ratio is 1.5:1 (e.g., sunflower seed has a calcium/phosphorous ratio of 8:1)
D. Thiamine deficiency: stargazing and opisthotonos
E. Hypovitaminosis E and selenium deficiency: cause degeneration of skeletal muscles, referred to as white muscle disease

NONINFECTIOUS DISEASES AND CONDITIONS

I. Predisposing factors such as immunosuppression, dehydration, malnutrition, starvation, poor hygiene, below optimal environmental conditions, chilling, and stress can leave the bird susceptible to disease
II. Trauma: dislocations, fractures, soft tissue damage, and pododermatitis
III. Feather conditions may occur from boredom ("feather-picking"), hypoparathyroidism, stress, improper molting, skin allergies, or ectoparasites (the later being uncommon)
IV. Egg-binding and chronic egg-laying: abdominal distention, dyspnea, and hypocalcemic seizures
V. Regurgitation/vomiting; normal courtship behavior, lead poisoning, foreign body, or a gastrointestinal problem
VI. Toxins
  A. Inhalents from household products, paints, pesticides
  B. Toxic plants
  C. Lead toxicity
    1. Clinical signs of lethargy, depression, green diarrhea, paresis, paralysis and convulsions
    2. Pet bird sources include stained glass, old paint, soldering, wine foil, galvanized wire, batteries, pellets, antique jewelry
    3. Waterfowl ingest cast lead shot from the bottom of ponds
    4. Raptorial species ingest waterfowl with lead shot in their muscle (secondary lead toxicity)
    5. Treatment includes chelation therapy with calcium disodium versonate and supportive care (removal of the object is often difficult)

INFECTIOUS DISEASES

Bacterial Diseases

I. Normal gastrointestinal flora of psittacines are predominately gram positive
II. Normal gastrointestinal flora for raptors and other carnivorous species are predominately gram negative
III. Common diseases in psittacines, poultry, raptors, and waterfowl
  A. Chlamydiosis (psittacosis, ornithocosis)
    1. Cause: *Chlamydiophila psittaci*
    2. Clinical signs: include green diarrhea, pneumonia, nasal and ocular discharge, lethargy, or totally asymptomatic
    3. Lesions include splenomegaly, hepatomegaly, pericarditis, air sacculitis, and pneumonia
    4. Zoonotic: causes flulike symptoms in people
    5. Diagnosis: polymerase chain reaction on feces and blood
    6. Treatment: tetracycline, doxycycline, or azithromycin, and supportive care
  B. Avian tuberculosis
    1. Cause: *Mycobacterium avium*
    2. Clinical signs: chronic weight loss and lethargy
    3. Diagnosis by acid-fast test on feces or biopsy of the infected liver or intestinal mucosa
    4. Treatment: long-term combined antibiotic therapy
    5. Zoonotic potential for immunosuppressed humans
  C. Coryza: upper respiratory disease
    1. Cause: *Haemophilus* and *Mycoplasma*
    2. Clinical signs: rhinitis, sinusitis, and upper respiratory signs
    3. Diagnosis: culture and sensitivity
  D. Pneumonia and air sacculitis: lower respiratory tract infections
    1. Cause: several bacteria, including *Pasteurella, Yersinia* (pseudotuberculosis), *Streptococcus,* and *Staphylococcus*
    2. Clinical signs: hyperpnea, dyspnea, abdominal breathing, and cyanosis
    3. Diagnosis: culture and sensitivity
  E. Avian cholera or pasteurellosis
    1. Cause: *Pasteurella multocida*
    2. Clinical signs: diarrhea, ataxia, septicemia, and sudden death, or asymptomatic
  F. Bacterial enteritis
    1. Cause: various bacteria, including *Clostridium*
    2. Botulism occurs when spoiled food and algae bloom undergo anaerobic conditions
    3. Clinical signs in waterfowl: weakness, "limberneck," paresis, paralysis, and death
    4. Treatment: supportive care and antitoxin (for botulism)

Viral Diseases

The following viral diseases occur in psittacines, poultry, raptors, and waterfowl unless otherwise stated.

Disease	Etiology	Clinical signs/occurrence
Avian influenza	Orthomyxovirus	Congestion, sneezing, rhinitis, and pneumonia
Avian pox	Various pox strains, each species specific	Crusty, raised, pox lesions round the eyes, beak, and feet
Hemorrhagic viral enteritis	Adenovirus	Occurs commonly in turkeys and poultry, also reported in budgies and lovebirds
Newcastle's disease (PMV)	Paramyxovirus (nine virus types are currently identified)	Ataxia, opisthotonos, and seizures
Marek's disease	Herpesvirus	Necropsy lesions are gray or white neoplastic lesions on various organs, especially liver Common problem in poultry
Pacheco's disease	Herpesvirus	Anorexia and sudden death Occurs in outbreak conditions in psittacines
Duck plague	Herpesvirus	Diarrhea and sudden death Common problem in waterfowl
Budgie fledgling disease (BFD)	Polyomavirus	Abdominal distention, hepatomegaly, and dystrophic feather formation Occurs in young budgies and other psittacines
Psittacine beak and feather disease (PFBD)	Circovirus	Clubbing of feather shafts, feather atypia, beak lesions, or feather loss Diagnosed by a feather biopsy and histology
Proventricular dilation disease (PDS)	Considered to be caused by a virus yet unidentified	Continual weight loss, neurological signs, and death Diagnosis may be made on history, clinical signs, fluoroscopic examination, and crop biopsy. Definitive diagnosis is only on necropsy due to the segmental nature of the virus and difficulty in locating the lesion on a biopsy

Mycotic Diseases

I. Aspergillosis
  A. Cause: *Aspergillosis fumigatus*
  B. Clinical signs: lethargy, droopy wings, anorexia, respiratory distress
  C. Common in stressed or weak patients, primarily a secondary disease
II. Candidiasis
  A. Cause: *Candida albicans,* an opportunistic yeast
  B. Clinical signs: gray to white plaque lesions in the oral cavity, esophagus, and crop
  C. Common in pigeons, raptors, and psittacines

PARASITES

Ectoparasites

I. Biting lice (Mallophaga) only
II. Mites
  A. Scaly leg and face mites: *Knemidocoptes*
    1. Common in budgies and other psittacines
    2. Lesions on the beak, eyelids, and legs
  B. Tracheal mites: *Sternostoma tracheacolum*
    1. Common in finches, canaries, budgies, and poultry
    2. Clinical signs: sneezing, open-mouth breathing, dyspnea, and loss of voice
III. Ticks
IV. Hippoboscid flies are seen on raptorial birds
V. Most ectoparasites are easily treated with ivermectin or dilute carbaryl dusting powders

Endoparasites

I. Nematodes
  A. Ascarids
  B. Microfilaria
  C. Gapeworm (*Syngamus tracheae* in galliformes and *Cyathostoma* sp. in waterfowl)
  D. Several species of *Capillaria*
II. Cestodes: uncommon
III. Trematodes: uncommon
IV. Protozoa
  A. Coccidiosis
    1. Cause: *Eimeria*
    2. Occurs in finches, poultry, waterfowl, and raptors
    3. Clinical signs: anorexia, lethargy, diarrhea, and wasting
  B. Histomoniasis
    1. Cause: *Histomonas*
    2. Clinical signs: "blackhead" in turkeys
  C. Trichomoniasis
    1. Cause: *Trichomonas*
    2. Clinical signs: oral plaques similar to *Candida* and *Capillaria*
  D. Hemosporidia

1. Cause: blood protozoans *Hemoproteus, Leucocytozoan,* and *Plasmodium*
2. Common in low densities in wild caught psittacines and most waterfowl and raptors
3. Problem occurs only at high densities or under stress

E. Giardiasis
1. Cause: *Giardia*
2. Zoonotic disease
3. Clinical signs: soft, green mucoid feces and diarrhea

Reptilian Medicine

CLASSIFICATION

I. Class: Reptilia
- A. Order: Chelonia (turtles and tortoise)
- B. Order: Crocodilia (crocodiles, alligators, and caimans)
- C. Order: Rhyncocephalia (tuatara)
- D. Order: Squamata
  1. Suborder: Serpentes (snakes)
  2. Suborder: Sauria (lizards)

ANATOMICAL AND PHYSIOLOGICAL COMPARISON OF REPTILES AND MAMMALS

I. Lifestyle
- A. Terrestrial
- B. Aquatic (freshwater)
- C. Marine
- D. Arboreal

II. Life span: wide range among species
- A. Seven years in a red-eared slider
- B. One hundred fifty years in a Galapagos tortoise

III. Growth and metabolism
- A. Slow metabolic rate
- B. Continual growth; growth rate slows nearing maturity

IV. Integument
- A. Scales or scutes
- B. Chelonians have a superficial layer of keratin shields, which make up the carapace dorsally and the plastron ventrally
- C. Lizards have bony plates in the dermis called osteoderms
- D. The skin is made up of the dermis and epidermis
- E. Healing is much slower than mammals due to the decreased metabolic rate
- F. Periods of ecdysis (shedding of the skin)
- G. Autonomy: the ability of a lizard to shed its tail when captured, the new tail will lack vertebrae

V. Sensory
- A. The eye in lizards has a movable eyelid but the nictitating membrane is reduced and nonfunctional
- B. The eye in snakes has no moveable eyelid or nictitating membrane; instead there is a spectacle covering the eye that maintains moisture and is shed during ecdysis

VI. Skeletal
- A. Appendages as limbs (most species)
- B. Appendages modified as flippers (aquatic turtles)
- C. Appendages entirely lacking (snakes)
- D. Pythons and boas possess vestiges of hind limbs evident as spurs on either side of the cloaca
- E. Chelonians have their entire limb girdles housed within their ribcage (shell)
- F. Snakes and lizards have articulation of the upper jaw via the presence of a joint between the ptyeroid and the cranium, permitting the swallowing of large prey
- G. Six rows of teeth, which are continually replaced
- H. Lizards and snakes have external ears
- I. Snakes use heat sensitive pits in their snout (pythons, vipers, rattlesnakes) and the tongue as ears

VII. Digestive
- A. Well-developed epiglottis
- B. Glottis is located anterior to allow breathing while ingesting prey
- C. Esophagus, stomach, small intestine, large intestine, cloaca
- D. Cloaca is common opening for urogenital and digestive tract

VIII. Respiratory
- A. Diaphragm absent
- B. Lizards and snakes: respiration controlled by movement of intercostal muscles
- C. Turtles: respiration controlled by alternating body cavity pressure during locomotion and pharyngeal pumping
- D. Left lung in snakes is reduced or absent
- E. Lizards have two saccular lungs; some species have air sacs similar to birds
- F. Turtles have two saccular lungs compressed dorsally against the carapace
- G. Turtles have a membranous structure that divides the pleural and peritoneal cavities
- H. Tolerate higher levels of carbon dioxide and are capable of long periods of breathe holding, making inhalation of anesthetics difficult

IX. Thermoregulation

A. Ectothermic: rely on environmental temperature to maintain their own body temperature and metabolic processes

X. Circulatory
   A. The crocodile is the first vertebrate to develop the complete interventricular septum and therefore a four-chambered heart
   B. All other reptiles have a three-chambered heart
      1. Two atria
      2. One ventricle
      3. Incomplete interventricular septum prevents the mixing of blood by current flows
   C. Blood cells
      1. Nucleated red blood cells
      2. Thrombocytes (similar to mammalian platelets)
      3. Heterophils (analogous to mammalian neutrophils)
      4. Eosinophils
      5. Basophils
      6. Lymphocytes
      7. Monocytes
      8. Azurophils: unique to reptiles; function may be similar to heterophils but unknown

XI. Urogenital
   A. Metanephric kidneys
   B. Some species possess a bladder
   C. Terrestrial species excrete uric acid
   D. Aquatic species excrete urea and ammonia
   E. Renal portal system present, allows blood from the caudal portion of the body to pass through the kidneys before entering the main vascular system
   F. Turtles have single extrudible penis
   G. Lizards and snakes have two hemipenes
   H. Reproduction by oviparity in caiman, alligators, turtles, lizards, and snakes
   I. Reproduction by viviparity or ovoviviparity in lizards and snakes

HOUSING

I. Clinic housing
   A. Incubators
   B. Stainless steel dog kennels

II. "At home" housing
   A. Controlled temperature and humidity
   B. Aquarium
   C. Terrarium
   D. Custom-made cage
   E. Each species has its own preferred optimal temperature ("POT"): range from 12° to 21° C (53° to 69° F) for temperate species to 26° to 39° C (75° to 103° F) for tropical species
   F. Aquatic turtles should have an aquarium filter flow and a water temperature of 21° to 26° C (70° to 80° F)
   G. The common green iguana's "POT" is 29° to 39° C (85° to 102° F)
   H. Consider normal activity for the species (i.e., arboreal species need climbing trees, burrowing species need deep litter, shy and nocturnal species need a hide box)
   I. Basking area or "hot spot" where temperature is higher with direct light source (heat lamp)
   J. Substrate can be newspaper, aquarium gravel, corncob bedding, or sand litter
   K. Clean, shallow water dish
   L. Chameleons will not drink from a water dish; use a dripping water bottle
   M. Ultraviolet light source is necessary: activates vitamin D for calcium absorption
   N. In warm climates or during the summer months, some reptiles may be housed outdoors to obtain natural ultraviolet radiation
   O. Heated rocks are not recommended (thermal injury)
   P. Humidity is an important factor, 50% to 70% the optimum for most species
   Q. Photoperiod of 12 hours daylight is suitable for all reptiles
   R. Reptiles hibernate near 5° C (40° F): causes anorexia and other stress-related diseases

RESTRAINT AND HANDLING

I. Restraint
   A. Venomous snakes: should be restrained only by experienced herpetological personnel
   B. Nonvenomous snakes: restrain behind the head and support the body
   C. Large constrictors: should be handled by two people
   D. Lizards: grasp behind the head and hold the pelvis and tail in the other hand; caution against claws and tail lashing in defense (trimming the toenails first is a good idea)
   E. Restraint for radiographs: in some lizards by applying mild digital pressure to the eyes, causing a quiescent state that lasts for a few minutes (vagovagal response)
   F. Turtles: restrain by carapace, anterior to the hind legs

II. Temperature, pulse, and respirations
   A. Temperature values are not useful: reptiles are ectothermic
   B. Respirations: ranges from 4 to 30 breaths per minute
      1. A pediatric stethoscope can be used to evaluate the cardiac and respiratory systems

C. Heart rate: ranges from 40 to 100 beats per minute

NURSING CARE

I. Physical Examination
   A. Reptiles and amphibians require at least an annual physical examination to record baseline values
   B. Patient's history should include previous medical history, weight, sex, age, diet, husbandry, and length of ownership
      1. Species and the origin of the animal should also be noted
   C. A fecal analysis should be conducted for prophylactic deworming
   D. A thorough examination of body structures should be conducted checking for lesions, discharge, and bleeding
      1. Behavior and temperament of the animal should also be noted
II. Blood collection
   A. Ventral tail vein (lizards, turtles)
      1. Animal can be in either dorsal recumbency with the ventral aspect of the tail facing up, or the animal can be in ventral recumbency with the tail hanging off the end of the table
      2. Needle is usually held vertical to the tail, and the puncture is made along the midline of the tail
   B. Dorsal and ventral buccal veins of the mouth (snakes)
   C. Right jugular vein (turtles)
      1. Needle should be introduced in a cranial to caudal direction, while a restrainer is holding the head
   D. Dorsal venous sinus (turtles)
   E. Nail clip is not recommended
III. Blood analysis: Coulter counter cannot be used due to nucleated red blood cells; complete blood cell count can be obtained by combining the Unopette system and hemocytometer count, with a differential count from a smear
IV. Intraosseous catheterization
   A. Site: proximal tibia (trochanteric fossa) or femur
   B. Materials needed include local anesthetic, suture material, adhesive tape, 18- to 25-gauge needle, bandaging material
   C. Procedure
      1. Use anesthesia if necessary, if the animal is very ill, only local anesthesia may be needed
      2. Aseptically prepare the site for surgery
      3. If needed, local anesthetic can be infiltrated around the site
      4. Use a twisting motion while advancing the needle into the bone
      5. To check for proper placement, inject a small amount of heparinized saline into the bone. The saline should flow freely
      6. Inject the fluid or drugs (most drugs licensed for intravenous administration can be infused safely into the bone marrow; check the drug insert for verification)
      7. Suture the catheter in place by making tape wings for handling. Apply antibiotic cream and a light bandage to the area
      8. The catheter should be flushed every 6 to 8 hours with heparinized saline
      9. Removal of catheter is usually after 48 to 72 hours
V. Intramuscular injection
   A. Dorsal portion of the body in snakes and the front leg in lizards and turtles
   B. Injections should not be given in the rear leg because of the potential for nephrotoxicity due to the renal portal system
VI. Subcutaneous fluids: similar to mammals
VII. Fluids may be given intracoelomically to turtles, which is similar to intraperitoneal administration in reptiles and amphibians
VIII. Oral administration/tube feeding via plastic feeding tube
   A. Forced feeding for nutritional supplementation is often required for animals that are not eating
   B. The procedure is quite easily performed because there is very little danger of administering the slurry of food into the trachea in most reptiles
      1. Glottis in reptiles is cranial (at the base of the tongue) and is easily visualized when the mouth is opened with a speculum

NUTRITION: DIETS AND PROBLEMS

Snakes

I. All snakes are carnivorous; diet preference is species dependent
   A. Rats
   B. Mice
   C. Gerbils
   D. Chicks
   E. Fish
II. Feed once weekly up to once monthly, depending on body size and species

Turtles

I. Turtles may be carnivorous, omnivorous, or herbivorous
   A. Carnivorous: trout chow, fish, or pinkie mice

B. Omnivorous: a mix of the two diets
C. Herbivorous: salad of leafy greens, especially calcium and vitamin A–rich foods

II. Feed daily for most species

Lizards

I. Insectivorous species (geckos, chameleons, anoles, and skinks): crickets and mealworms supplemented with calcium powder; feed daily
II. Carnivorous species (monitors): whole prey diet; feed a few times weekly
III. Omnivorous species: vegetables, fruit, crickets, mealworms; feed daily
IV. Herbivorous species (green iguana): calcium-rich vegetables (broccoli, squash), leafy greens (escarole, endive); feed daily
V. May need to use a calcium and vitamin supplement

CLINICAL CONDITIONS AND DISEASES

I. Poor management: temperature, humidity, or housing
  A. Anorexia
  B. Hypothermia
  C. Trauma
  D. Rodent bites
  E. Dysecdysis (improper shedding)
II. Nutritional problems
  A. Herbivorous and insectivorous species commonly have dietary problems
  B. Metabolic bone disease or hypocalcemia
    1. Common in green iguana
    2. Occurs when the ratio of calcium and phosphorous is reversed (normal is 1.5:1)
    3. Clinical signs may include pathological fractures of the long bones; osteodystrophia fibrosa; swollen, soft, poorly mineralized bones; swollen jaw; and undefined bone cortices on radiographs
    4. Treatment: calcium therapy, ultraviolet light supplementation, and diet correction
  C. Hypovitaminosis A
    1. Common in turtles
    2. Clinical signs: palpebral edema, swollen eyes, edematous bulge in the inguinal skin, anorexia
    3. Treatment: vitamin A injection initially, then diet correction
    4. Therapy for a secondary bacterial infection may also be required
  D. Hypovitaminosis E or steatitis: occurs when rodents for food are stored too long

INFECTIOUS DISEASES

Bacterial Diseases

The bacterial diseases are listed by clinical problem rather than by specific pathogen.

I. Stomatitis or mouth rot
  A. Cause: suboptimal temperatures, unhygienic environment, malnutrition, trauma
  B. Common bacteria isolated include *Pseudomonas* and *Aeromonas*
  C. Begins as edema of the gums; may progress to osteomyelitis of the jaw if left untreated
II. Pneumonia
  A. Cause: suboptimal temperatures and low humidity
  B. Common bacterial isolates: *Aeromonas* and *Klebsiella*
III. Septicemia
  A. Cause: a variety of bacteria; common bacteria isolated: *Pseudomonas* and *Aeromonas*
  B. Clinical signs include pinpoint focal necrosis of the skin, small lumps or abscesses along the body or tail, and lethargy
IV. Septicemic cutaneous ulcer disease
  A. Identified in aquatic turtles
  B. Caused by *Citrobacter*
V. Salmonellosis
  A. Important zoonotic disease; causes bloody diarrhea and severe enteritis in humans
  B. Cause: *Salmonella;* normal bacterial flora of many reptiles, especially aquatic turtles

Viral Diseases

Viral diseases are uncommon.

I. Paramyxovirus in snakes
II. Viral encephalitis in snakes
III. Herpesvirus in iguanas and turtles

Protozoal Diseases

I. Cryptosporidium
  A. Problem in snakes causing regurgitation, anorexia, and death
  B. A zoonotic disease causing diarrhea and lethargy in humans

Mycotic Diseases

I. Pneumonia caused by *Aspergillosis, Beauvaria,* and *Cladosporium*

PARASITES

Ectoparasites

I. Ticks: common on snakes
II. Mites: common on snakes and iguanas

Endoparasites

I. Coccidia
II. Entamoeba
III. Cestodes
IV. Trematodes
V. Nematodes

A. Cestodes, trematodes, and nematodes may affect the oral, respiratory, gastrointestinal, and circulatory systems

Glossary

apteriae Featherless area on a bird
arboreal Living in trees
autonomy Ability of a lizard to shed its tail when captured
carapace Dorsal shell of chelonians
carnivorous Eats primary flesh
cere Area at the base of a bird's beak
chelation therapy Substance is combined with a metallic ion to produce an inert chelate
clubbing of feathers Feathers have a coiled structure due to improper eruption from the feather sheath
dysecdysis Improper shedding in reptiles
ecdysis Shedding of the external skin in reptiles
ectothermal Animal relies on the environmental temperature to maintain their own body temperature and metabolic rate
hemipenes Two vascular sacs, which act as a penis in snake and lizards
herbivorous Eats on plants and plant products
herpetology Branch of zoology dealing with reptiles
holocrine Type of secretion that is formed by the entire gland
intracoelomic Into the body cavity or coelom
intraosseus Into bone
limberneck Paralysis of the neck
meibomian gland Sebaceous follicle between the cartilage and conjunctiva of the eyelids
metanephric Embryo-like kidney
nictitating Third eyelid in animals; a fold of conjunctiva attached at the medial canthus of the eye
omnivorous Eating any sort of food
opisthotonos Form of spasm in which the body is bowed downwards and the head and tail are bowed upwards
osteodystrophia fibrosa Clinical condition in which fibrous tissue replaces bone (also called fibrous osteodystrophy)
osteomyelitis Inflammation of the bone usually due to a pyogenic infection
oviparous Producing eggs in which the embryo matures outside of the maternal body
ovoviviparous Producing live young that hatch from eggs inside the maternal body
parabronchial Tertiary branch in the avian lungs
paresis Slight or incomplete paralysis
phallic organ Pertaining to the penis
piloerection Erection of the hair
plastron Ventral shell of chelonians
pododermatitis Inflammation of the skin of the foot
ptyerylae Feather tracts on birds
spectacle A round lens. Snakes lack movable eyelids and their corneas are protected by a spectacle which is shed and renewed after each shed
steatitis Inflammation of the fatty tissue
stomatitis Inflammation of the mucosa of the mouth
tetany Continuous spasm of a muscle; steady contraction of a muscle without twitching
uropygial Gland located laterally to the tail that secretes oil to aid in waterproofing of feathers
vagovagal response Arising as a result of efferent and afferent impulses through the vagus nerve
viviparous Bearing live young

Review Questions

1 The digestive system in the bird includes the following anatomical structures, beginning cranial to caudal
a. Crop, glottis, proventriculus, gizzard
b. Beak, glottis, crop, proventriculus, gizzard
c. Crop, ventriculus, gizzard
d. Beak, glottis, esophagus, crop, gizzard

2 The bird has _______ pairs of air sacs that make up the respiratory system.
a. 4
b. 6
c. 9
d. 13

3 The heterophil can be compared with a (an) _______ in mammals.
a. Eosinophil
b. Neutrophil
c. Lymphocyte
d. Monocyte

4 Female birds have only one functional _______ and a slightly larger _______ vein.
a. Left ovary and oviduct; right jugular
b. Right ovary and oviduct; left jugular
c. Right kidney; left medial tibiotarsal vein
d. Left kidney; right medial tibiotarsal vein

5 Blood analysis in avian and reptilian species cannot be run on a Coulter counter due to
a. Presence of nucleated red blood cells
b. Small size of the cells
c. Presence of heterophils
d. Large size of the cells

6 Avian and reptilian species have a renal portal system; therefore
a. Nephrotoxic drugs should not be given in the back legs
b. Nephrotoxic drugs should be injected only in the back limbs for a 24-hour period after injections in the front limbs
c. Any drug injected will be excreted rapidly
d. Any nephrotoxic drug will be absorbed and slowly excreted from the animal

7 Some lizards may be restrained for radiography by
a. Manual restraint
b. Pressure on their eyes
c. Holding their tail in position
d. Inhalation anesthetic only

8 Vitamin D and calcium absorption in reptiles depends on
a. Optimum temperatures
b. An ultraviolet light source
c. A heating pad or hot rock under the substrate
d. Optimum humidity in the enclosure

9 Reptiles are sometimes difficult to anesthetize due to
   a. Their size
   b. The fact that they can tolerate high levels of carbon dioxide and can hold their breath for long periods of time
   c. Their integument structure and cell formation
   d. The fact that they are ectothermic and therefore require high temperatures before induction

10 Birds and terrestrial species of reptiles excrete
   a. Urine
   b. Ammonia
   c. Urea
   d. Uric acid

BIBLIOGRAPHY

Avian

Altman R: Perching birds, parrots, cockatoos, and macaws (psittacines and passerines). In Fowler ME, editor: *Zoo and wildlife medicine,* Toronto, 1978, WB Saunders.

Cooper JE: *Veterinary aspects of captive birds of prey,* ed 2, Gloucestershire, 1978, Standfast Press.

Harrison GJ, Harrison LR: *Clinical avian medicine and surgery,* Toronto, 1986, WB Saunders.

Humphreys PN: Waterbirds. In Cooper JE et al, editor: *Manual of exotic pets,* Gloucestershire, 1985, British Small Animal Veterinary Association.

McCurnin DM, Bassert JM: *Clinical textbook for veterinary technicians,* ed 5, WB Saunders, 2002.

McDonald SE: Anatomical and physiological characteristics of birds and how they differ from mammals, *Proc Assoc Avian Vet* 372, 1990.

Pettingal OS: *Ornithology in laboratory and field,* ed 4, Minneapolis, 1970, Burgess Publishing Co.

Pratt PW: *Principles and practice of veterinary technology,* St Louis, 1998, Mosby.

Stunkard JA: *Diagnosis, treatment and husbandry of pet birds,* ed 2, Edgewater, 1984, Stunkard Publishing.

Taylor M: Companion bird management and nutrition, *Proc Assoc Avian Vet* 409-431, 1990.

Turner T: Cagebirds. In Cooper JE et al, editors: *Manual of exotic pets,* Gloucestershire, 1985, British Small Animal Veterinary Association.

Reptile

Evans HE: Reptiles, introduction and anatomy. In Fowler ME, editor: *Zoo and wildlife medicine,* Toronto, 1978, WB Saunders.

Frye FL: *Biomedical and surgical aspects of captive reptile husbandry,* Lenexa, KS, 1981, Veterinary Medicine Publishing Co.

Jackson OF, Lawrence K: Chelonians. In Cooper JE et al, editors: *Manual of exotic pets,* Gloucestershire, 1985, British Small Animal Veterinary Association.

Jacobsen ER: Diseases in reptiles. In Johnston DE, editor: *Exotic animal medicine in practice,* the Compendium Collection, Newark, NJ, 1986, Veterinary Learning Systems Co Inc.

Jacobsen ER, Kolias GV: *Exotic animals,* New York, 1988, Churchill Livingstone.

Lawrence K: *Lizards, addendum and snakes.* In Cooper JE et al, editors: *Manual of exotic pets,* Gloucestershire, 1985, British Small Animal Veterinary Association.

Marcus LC: *Veterinary biology and medicine of captive amphibians and reptiles,* London, 1981, Lea & Febiger.

Murphy JB, Collins JT: *A review of the diseases and treatments of captive turtles,* Kansas, 1983, AMS Publishing.

Pratt PW: *Principles and practice of veterinary technology,* St Louis, 1998, Mosby.

PART IV

Anesthesia and Pharmacology

CHAPTER 19

Anesthesia

Kathleen Alston

OUTLINE

Preanesthetic Medication
- Advantages
- Disadvantages
- Examples

Injectable Anesthetic Medication
- Barbiturates
- Propofol
- Cyclohexamines
- Etomidate
- Guaifenesin
- Fentanyl

Inhalation Anesthetic Medication
- General Considerations
- Advantages
- Examples

Parts of an Anesthetic Machine
- Maintenance and Environmental Concerns

Breathing Systems
- Rebreathing System
- Nonrebreathing System

Breathing Circuits
- Circle System
- Universal F-Circuit
- Bain System (Coaxial)

Vaporizers
- Classification

Monitoring
- Eye
- Pedal Reflex
- Jaw Tone
- Cardiovascular System
- Respiratory System
- Capillary Refill Time
- Mucous Membrane Color
- Temperature

Stages of Anesthesia

Analgesia

Muscle Relaxants

Ventilation

Fluid Therapy
- Fluid Characteristics
- Fluid Calculation

Blood Loss

Acid-Base Balance

Oxygenation and Anesthetic Equipment Problems

LEARNING OUTCOMES

After reading this chapter you should be able to:

1. Understand the indications, advantages, disadvantages, effects on the body, and the associated adverse side effects of the commonly used preanesthetic.
2. Explain the rationale, effects on the body, and advantages and disadvantages of the commonly used intravenous, intramuscular, and inhalation anesthetic agents.
3. Identify or describe the components of general anesthesia, including the various stages and planes.
4. Define the rationale for and the various parameters that should be monitored during anesthesia, and describe why blood pressure is important to monitor.
5. Understand the differences between advantages and disadvantages of rebreathing and nonrebreathing systems.
6. Be familiar with the various parts of the anesthetic machine.
7. Differentiate between a precision and a nonprecision vaporizer, and recognize the advantages and disadvantages of each.
8. Understand the important concepts of analgesics and muscle relaxants.
9. Understand the techniques of assisted and controlled ventilation.
10. Understand the principles involved with providing proper fluid therapy and for maintaining the acid-base balance.
11. Identify oxygenation problems that might occur.

Anesthesia is a broad subject and could involve extensive reading. This chapter condenses the information by discussing the commonly used anesthetic agents, equipment, and procedures. Although much of this chapter could pertain to any species, the emphasis is on domestic dogs and cats.

PREANESTHETIC MEDICATION

Advantages

I. Advantages will vary with different drugs but may include
   A. Reduced stress to the animal
   B. Smoother induction and recovery
   C. Decreased amount of induction and possibly maintenance agent required
   D. Analgesia intraoperatively and postoperatively
   E. Reduced secretions
   F. Reduced autonomic reflexes
   G. Handler safety

Disadvantages

I. Disadvantages are minimal
   A. Cost is a common concern
      1. The higher cost can be offset by the use of decreased amounts of induction and maintenance agents
   B. Time factor
      1. Premedication given subcutaneously usually takes 20 minutes to reach peak effect but can last up to 2 hours
      2. If time is an issue, most premedication can be given intramuscularly (IM) or even intravenously (IV) (with caution)
   C. Some (e.g., xylazine, acepromazine, opioids, and diazepam) have been associated with temporary behavior and personality changes

Examples

I. Anticholinergics (parasympatholytics): for example, atropine, glycopyrrolate (Robinul-V)
   A. Exerts effect by blocking the actions of the parasympathetic neurotransmitter acetylcholine at the muscarinic receptors
      1. Reverses the parasympathetic effects
   B. Indications and effects
      1. To prevent or treat bradycardia by suppressing stimulation of the vagal nerve
      2. In combination with opioids
      3. To reduce salivary and tear secretions
      4. Promotes bronchodilation
      5. Blocks the stimulation of the vagus nerve preventing bradycardia and reduced cardiac output
      6. Dilate pupils (mydriatic)
      7. Thicker mucus secretions in the airway may occur, especially in the cat and horse
      8. Reduces gastrointestinal activity by inhibiting peristalsis
   C. Contraindications
      1. Tachycardiac patients
      2. Possibly with geriatrics or with other conditions such as congestive heart failure that could not handle a potential tachycardia
      3. Conditions such as constipation or ileus, which would further reduce peristaltic action of the intestine (i.e., endoscopic procedures)
   D. Glycopyrrolate and atropine produce basically the same effect
      1. Glycopyrrolate has a slower onset of action and generally has less potential for producing a tachycardia or cardiac arrhythmia
      2. Atropine is more potent and faster acting
      3. Salivation is also more effectively suppressed with glycopyrrolate

II. Phenothiazines (tranquilizers): for example, acepromazine, chlorpromazine
   A. Indications
      1. Good sedation for healthy animals undergoing elective procedures
      2. Antiemetic
   B. Contraindications
      1. Convulsing/epileptic patients, seizure history, head trauma
         a. Acepromazine may reduce the seizure threshold of the animal
      2. Shock (hypovolemic) and hypothermia because of peripheral vasodilation that can lead to hypotension
      3. Depressed patients
      4. Caution with geriatrics and pediatrics; use a lower dose or consider alternative agents such as benzodiazepines
      5. Liver or kidney disease
      6. Allergy testing because of antihistamine effect
   C. Other effects
      1. Antiarrhythmic effect
      2. May cause excitement rather than sedation
      3. Personality changes that usually subside within 48 hours

III. Benzodiazepines (tranquilizers): for example, diazepam (Valium), zolazepam, midazolam (Versed), and lorazepam (Ativan)
   A. Indications
      1. Convulsing/epileptic patients, seizure history, cerebrospinal fluid tap and/or myelogram
      2. Minimal cardiovascular or respiratory depression so useful in geriatric and pediatric animals and other moderate- or high-risk patients
      3. Ideal for older, depressed, or anxious patients

4. It also works effectively as an induction agent when used with ketamine

B. Contraindications
   1. Normal, excitable, healthy animal (may cause excitement in some dogs, cats, and horses)
      a. Does not sedate or tranquilize animals but has antianxiety and calming effects that may make animal more difficult to control when inhibitions and anxieties are removed
   2. Neonatal animals and animals with poor hepatic dysfunction because of poor metabolism

C. Diazepam injectable is soluted with propylene glycol, because of its solubility in oil, not water
   1. May precipitate with other drugs
   2. It stings and does not work well if given via routes other than IV

D. Midazolam is water soluble and readily combines with opioids such as butorphanol and oxymorphone

E. Reversed with flumazenil if adverse effects seen

IV. α_2-Agonists (thiazine derivative): for example, xylazine (Rompun, Anased), romifidine, detomidine (Dormosedan), and medetomidine (Domitor)

A. Stimulates the α_2-adrenoceptors, causing a decrease in the release of norepinephrine

B. Indications
   1. Potential side effects limit use to sedation only, not for preanesthetic medication
   2. Can use to sedate a vicious animal before euthanasia
   3. Have some short (16 to 20 minutes) analgesic effects
   4. Will cause vomiting in up to 50% of dogs and 90% of cats
   5. Xylazine and detomidine are used most frequently in horses
   6. Xylazine is also used in ruminants, but in much lower doses

C. Contraindications and other effects
   1. Considerable potential for side effects, especially if given IV
   2. Profound cardiovascular effects include bradycardia, profound hypotension, decreased contractility and stroke volume, and second-degree heart block
   3. Also when concerned about respiratory depression, hepatic and renal function, and if prone to gastric dilation and torsion
   4. Associated with temporary behavior and personality changes
   5. Reduces pancreatic secretions causing transient hyperglycemia, which may be harmful in dehydrated patients
   6. Opioids will exacerbate these effects

D. Medetomidine has greater potency and fewer adverse side effects than xylazine
   1. Greater affinity for the α_2-adrenoceptors (mediates the sedation effects) and less for the α_1-adrenoceptors

E. Reversal
   1. Yohimbine (Yobine) and tolazoline can reverse the effects of xylazine
   2. Atipamezole (Antisedan) is specific to medetomidine

F. Xylazine can be absorbed through skin abrasions or mucous membranes
   1. Wash any drug spilled on human or animal skin immediately

V. Opioid: commonly used opioids are morphine, oxymorphone (Numorphan), butorphanol (Torbugesic, Torbutrol), hydromorphone, meperidine (Demerol, Pethidine), and fentanyl

A. Act by reversible combination with one or more specific receptors in the brain and spinal cord
   1. Produces a variety of effects such as analgesia, sedation, dysphoria, euphoria, and excitement
   2. May act as an agonist (stimulating agent) or antagonist (blocking agent) at each type of receptor
      a. Pure agonists stimulate all receptors—morphine, fentanyl, and oxymorphone
      b. Mixed agonists/antagonists block one type of receptor and stimulate another—butorphanol
      c. Pure antagonists such as naloxone will reverse the effects of pure and mixed agonists with very little clinical effect on their own
   3. Also classified according to the analgesic activity or addiction potential
      a. Pure agonists are more effective for severe pain
      b. In order of decreasing potency, they are
         (1) Fentanyl, oxymorphone, buprenorphine, butorphanol, meperidine, and pentazocine

B. Commonly used as an analgesic in premedication, as induction agent, or postoperatively for balanced anesthesia and preemptive pain control
   1. Provide some sedation and may potentiate the action of the sedative that it is given with (synergistic effect)

2. Fentanyl, sufentanil, and oxymorphone are often part of a balanced anesthetic regimen
   a. Fentanyl is available as a transdermal patch in various sizes for long-term analgesia
      (1) Takes 8 to 12 hours to become effective but lasts up to several days
      (2) Very few cardiovascular effects and does not significantly contribute to vasodilation or hypotension
      (3) Heating pads can increase transdermal uptake
         (a) Use caution when placing fentanyl patches in areas that may come in contact with heat; accidental overdose can occur
   b. Used as neuroleptanalgesia in combination with tranquilizer
   c. Morphine can be injected epidurally or subarachnoidally for regional analgesia

C. Reversible by use of pure antagonists agent such as naloxone or nalmefene
   1. Compete with the opioids for the specific receptor sites
   2. Possible to titrate the naloxone dose so as to remove side effects yet keep the analgesic properties

D. Other effects in addition to analgesia include
   1. Either stimulate or depress the central nervous system
      a. Depends on the dose, species, and opioid agent
         (1) Excitement occurs if given IV rapidly
         (2) Horse and cat are particularly susceptible to the excitatory effects
            (a) Thus give morphine at very low doses in cat
         (3) Dogs generally show sedation although hypnosis can be seen at higher doses in sick animals
         (4) Dogs that are not in pain may show excitement especially if given without any other agents
   2. Cardiopulmonary effects include bradycardia, possible hypotension with release of histamine especially if given IV (morphine and meperidine), and increased muscle contraction (inotropic effect) in low doses (morphine)
   3. Respiratory depression is dose dependent
   4. Gastrointestinal effects depend on the agent and may initially include diarrhea, vomiting, and flatulence
      a. Constipation may occur as the result of prolonged gastrointestinal stasis
   5. Addiction
   6. Body temperature decreases and panting in dogs because of resetting of the thermoregulatory center in the brain
   7. Miosis in dog and pig and mydriasis in cat and horse
   8. Increased responsiveness to noise
   9. Cough suppression
   10. Excessive salivation
   11. Sweating, particularly in horse

E. Contraindications
   1. Previous history of opioid excitement
   2. Morphine has a higher incidence of producing vomiting (depending on the dose)
      a. Avoid with cases of gastrointestinal obstruction, diaphragmatic hernia

F. Classified as narcotic in Canada and Schedule II in the United States with strict regulations

VI. Phencyclidines (cyclohexamine): for example, ketamine (Ketaset, Ketalean, Vetalar) and tiletamine hydrochloride (in combination with zolazepam [Telazol])
   A. Produces cardiovascular stimulation
   B. Increases muscular rigidity
   C. Causes salivation
   D. Indications
      1. Immobilization of patient
      2. Mucous membrane application via the mouth is effective
   E. Contraindications
      1. Never use alone except in cat
      2. Avoid as a preanesthetic medication in dog
      3. Avoid in animals with seizure history
         a. Can cause convulsions with high doses
            (1) More likely to occur with dog
            (2) Can be minimized by combining with a tranquilizer
      4. Produces poor visceral analgesia, but fair to good peripheral analgesia
      5. Increases cranial pressure; do not use in neurological cases that may have a possibility of brain herniation
      6. Increases ocular pressure; do not use in cases where a perforation of the eye chamber is suspected
      7. Prolonged, unreliable recoveries

VII. Neuroleptanalgesics
   A. Any combination of an analgesic and a tranquilizer (i.e., oxymorphone and acepromazine)
   B. Indications
      1. Heavier sedation (depending on dose) for short procedures (i.e., wound suturing, porcupine quill removal)

2. Cardiac or shock cases
C. Contraindications
1. Animal will become hyperactive to auditory stimulus
2. May defecate or vomit
3. May pant
4. May cause bradycardia

INJECTABLE ANESTHETIC MEDICATION

Barbiturates

I. Classification
A. Oxybarbiturates: for example, phenobarbital (considered as an anticonvulsant, not an anesthetic) and pentobarbital (Nembutal or Somnotol)
B. Thiobarbiturate: for example, thiopental (Pentothal)
C. Methylated oxybarbiturates: methohexital (Brevital)
II. Also classified by speed of onset of action
A. Long acting (e.g., phenobarbital): 8 to 12 hours
B. Short acting (e.g., pentobarbital): 45 to 90 minutes
C. Ultrashort acting (e.g., thiopental): 5 to 15 minutes
D. Methylated oxybarbiturate
III. Barbiturates in general can be used for sedation, anticonvulsants, and general anesthesia
A. Commonly used as induction agents to allow endotracheal intubation followed by maintenance with an inhalant anesthetic such as halothane or isoflurane
IV. Causes unconsciousness at an adequate dose
V. Depresses respiration and cardiovascular system to varying extents
A. Give to effect (amount necessary to induce anesthesia)
B. Give as a bolus (usually one third to one half of the calculated dose given rapidly)
VI. Nonreversible
VII. Protein binding
A. Level of plasma protein can alter rate and amount of absorption of the barbiturates
B. Barbiturates will bind to protein
1. The amount of barbiturate free in the circulation and not bound to protein will increase if the patient is hypoproteinemic
a. More barbiturate will thus be available to penetrate the central nervous system and cause unconsciousness
VIII. Lipid solubility increases in the barbiturates from the long acting to the ultrashort acting
A. There is quicker onset of action with the shorter acting barbiturates because they cross the blood-brain barrier faster
B. This also accounts for the quicker recovery of the shorter-acting barbiturate
C. Recovery from these drugs depends on a combination of redistribution (to muscle and fat) and hepatic metabolism
1. If a drug has low lipid solubility, there is little or no redistribution and recovery depends mostly on metabolism (a slow process)
2. If a drug has high lipid solubility, it is readily redistributed from the blood to the muscle and fat tissue, where it is not available to act on the brain
a. Recovery from a highly lipid-soluble drug is thus faster
D. As the blood levels decline because of metabolism, small quantities of the redistributed drug reenter the circulatory system from muscle and fat and are also metabolized
E. The low levels that arise from the muscle and fat stores are not sufficient to clinically alter the level of consciousness
F. Eliminated from the body by liver metabolism and excretion of metabolites from urine
IX. Examples of barbiturates
A. Phenobarbital
1. Used mostly as a sedative for excitable dogs or as an anticonvulsant for epileptic-type seizures
2. Sedation can last up to 24 hours, depending on the dose
B. Pentobarbital
1. Once used commonly for anesthetic inductions, it now has been replaced mostly by the ultrashort-acting barbiturates
2. It can also be used to control seizures (although electroencephalographic seizure activity may persist)
3. It can be administered intramuscularly for sedation, without tissue reaction
4. With IV induction there is significant effect at 1 minute after injection
a. Maximum effect is in 5 minutes
5. Recovery by metabolism is slow and rough in all animals except in sheep, where recovery is smoother and faster
C. Thiopental
1. Found as crystalline powder in multidose vials that can be made in various concentrations
a. Limited stability once reconstituted
b. Avoid injecting air that may cause premature precipitation
2. Has a high lipid solubility
a. Enters the brain rapidly

b. Redistribution from the brain to other tissues
    (1) Therefore initial recovery is fairly quick
c. It is redistributed to muscle and fat tissue and metabolized very slowly
d. Avoid in sight hounds because of prolonged recovery

3. Problems with recovery will occur if subsequent doses have been given for maintenance of anesthesia and if the muscle and fat tissues are saturated
    a. Cumulative effect with repeated administration
    b. Recovery will be slow and possibly rough
    c. Best to use for induction only or a maximum maintenance of 30 minutes
4. Significant effect is noted 30 to 60 seconds after injection
5. There is a transient arrhythmogenic potential with this drug, especially if given rapidly
6. Transient apnea may also be noted if given rapidly
7. If given perivascular at a concentration of greater than 2.5% (25 mg/mL), it can cause extreme irritation of surrounding tissues and may lead to sloughing of the tissues
    a. If this accidentally occurs, DILUTE the perivascular thiopental by injecting small amounts with normal saline around the site
8. Poor relaxation and analgesia when used alone
9. Can be used in combination with propofol for induction

D. Methohexital
1. Highly lipid soluble and rapidly metabolized
    a. It has the quickest onset, shortest duration, and quickest recovery (even if used for long-term maintenance)
2. Good choice of barbiturates for sight hounds or other patients of excessive lean body
    a. These patients seem to be extremely sensitive to barbiturates (because of poor ability to metabolize and a lack of fat storage), and they have prolonged recoveries
3. Liver metabolism is more rapid; therefore additional administration is not cumulative
4. Good choice for brachycephalics to obtain quick and smooth intubation and rapid recoveries without "hangover" effects
5. Induction effect is noted 15 to 60 seconds after injection
6. Induction and/or recoveries may be rough and accompanied by convulsions
    a. Effect minimized if good sedation given
7. Lethal dose is only two to three times the anesthetic dose
8. Methohexital can cause profound respiratory depression

Propofol (Diprivan, Rapinovet)

I. Used for sedation, induction, and/or anesthesia maintenance by repeated bolus injections or continuous infusion

II. Rapid acting with smooth, excitement-free induction

III. Rapid smooth recovery because of redistribution and rapid metabolism because of redistribution to vessel-rich areas such as brain rather than to muscle or fat

IV. More easily and rapidly biotransformed by the liver than barbiturates
    A. Much less or possibly no "hangover" effect

V. First choice for induction in sight hounds and other lean body patients
    A. If unavailable, use methohexital

VI. Ideal for injectable maintenance of anesthesia because there is no accumulation

VII. Minimal cardiovascular effects but may cause tachycardia, bradycardia, transient arterial and venous dilation, and depressed cardiac contractility
    A. Still considered safe on most cardiac patients

VIII. Contraindications and cautions
    A. Transient apnea has been reported after rapid IV injection
        1. Apnea is very dependent on how quickly the drug is given, and has caused respiratory arrest in some cases
    B. Avoid in animals that are hypotensive such as in blood loss, dehydration, recent trauma, or severe illness
    C. May see transient excitement and muscle tremors

IX. Good anticonvulsant

X. Nonirritating with incidental perivascular injection

XI. Some muscle relaxation occurs but analgesia is poor

XII. Will support bacterial growth because of soy content
    A. Opened vials should be discarded within 6 hours to avoid contamination

Cyclohexamines

I. Classified as dissociative anesthetic

II. Examples include ketamine and tiletamine

III. Produces catalepsy, amnesia, and questionable analgesia
IV. Inhibits *N*-methyl-D-aspartate (NMDA), resulting in analgesia
  A. Selective superficial analgesia
  B. Visceral pain not abolished
V. Pharyngolaryngeal reflexes are partially intact
VI. Excessive skeletal muscle tone, which can be minimized by prior administration of tranquilizers, sedatives, or benzodiazepine
VII. Mild cardiac stimulation (increased blood pressure, decreased cardiac contractility, and increased heart rate)
  A. May induce pulmonary edema or acute heart failure in animals with preexisting heart conditions
VIII. Apneustic breathing, rate may increase, may be decreased in arterial P_{CO_2} especially after IV administration
IX. Hyperresponsive and ataxic during recovery
X. Small percentage of cats will show convulsive behavior, especially with large doses
XI. Minimally sensitizes the heart to catecholamine-induced arrhythmias
XII. Other side effects include
  A. Tissue irritation
  B. Increased salivation and lacrimation
  C. Increase in cerebrospinal fluid pressure
  D. Open eyes with central dilated pupil
  E. Nystagmus (repetitive side-to-side motion of the eyeball)
  F. An increase in intraocular pressure
  G. Temporary personality changes
  H. Excitement on recovery
XIII. Effects partially reversed by adrenergic and cholinergic blockade
XIV. Dogs are more likely to seizure and therefore ketamine should be combined with a tranquilizer (i.e., acepromazine or diazepam when used with dogs)
XV. Metabolized by the liver and excreted somewhat in an unchanged form through kidneys in dog
  A. Excreted primarily by the kidneys in cat
  B. Use with caution in animals with hepatic or renal disease
  C. Can be used in cats in urethral obstruction, provided that renal disease is absent and the obstruction has been eliminated
XVI. Use with caution in seizure disorders or those undergoing neurological system procedures
XVII. Ketamine
  A. Ketamine is commonly combined with diazepam or other benzodiazepines as an induction agent
  B. This provides muscle relaxation and smoother recoveries than with ketamine alone
  C. In species where IV administration is not possible or easily accessible, ketamine can be combined with midazolam and given IM
XVIII. Tiletamine
  A. Tiletamine and zolazepam (benzodiazepine) are combined commercially in Telazol for use in all animal species
  B. Same action as ketamine/diazepam but can be given IM or subcutaneous (SQ); therefore
    1. Good for exotics and aggressive animals

Etomidate (Amidate)

I. Very safe, rapid-acting, ultrashort-acting, rapidly distributing, noncumulative induction agent
II. Interacts with $GABA_A$ receptors as with barbiturates
III. Very popular for animals with cardiac disease, as it has little to no effect on cardiac output, respiratory rate, and blood pressures
IV. Can be given as repeated bolus or continuous infusion
V. Occasionally may cause vomiting, diarrhea, excitement, apnea on induction and post-anesthesia
  A. Can be inhibited with proper preanesthetic
VI. Is a mild respiratory depressant
VII. Does not produce a histamine release
VIII. Produces excessive muscle rigidity and seizures in horse and cattle
IX. Rapidly metabolized in the liver
X. Does cross placental barrier, but effects are minimal because of rapid clearance
XI. IV injection may be painful and my cause phlebitis, especially in the smaller veins

Guaifenesin (glycerol guaiacolate)

I. Available as a white powder, to be mixed usually with warm sterile water or dextrose
II. This is a common decongestant and antitussive, and is commonly used for its effect as a central muscle relaxant, mostly in large animals
  A. Minimal effects of the diaphragm at relaxant dosages
III. Induction and recovery are excitement free
IV. Minimal respiratory and cardiac effect
V. Does cross placental barrier, but effects on fetus are minimal

Fentanyl

I. Although considered primarily an analgesic, it can produce unconsciousness and is used as an injectable induction agent, often in combination with a tranquilizer, sedative, or benzodiazepine

A. Referred to as neuroleptanalgesia

II. It is very safe for high-risk patients because it does not cause apnea and does not affect contractility or cardiac output

INHALATION ANESTHETIC MEDICATION

General Considerations

I. Are vapors or gases that are directly absorbed into the system through the lungs

II. Are absorbed from the alveoli to the brain relatively rapidly

III. Primarily eliminated unchanged by the lungs

A. Biotransformation of inhalation anesthetics to metabolites does occur to some degree

1. Metabolism is generally by hepatic microsomal enzymes

IV. Factors that affect the brain concentrations of volatile anesthetic include

A. Delivery of suitable concentrations of agent, which depend on the vapor pressure, boiling point, and anesthetic system

B. Factors responsible for delivering the anesthetic from the lungs, which include the alveolar partial pressure of the anesthetic, the inspired concentration, and the alveolar concentration

C. Factors that affect the lung, brain, and tissue uptake such as solubility, tissue and arterial blood flow, anesthetic concentration, type of tissue, and its blood supply, among other factors

1. Increased solubility leads to slow induction and slow recovery

a. There is a relatively high blood-gas partition coefficient

(1) Is the solubility of an inhalant anesthetic between the blood and gas

(2) The higher the number, the greater is the solubility of the anesthetic

(3) Larger amount of anesthetic has to be taken in before anesthesia results

V. Potency of inhalation anesthetics often expressed as MAC

A. This is the minimum alveolar concentration of an anesthetic that produces no response in 50% of patients exposed to painful stimulus

B. The lower the MAC, the more potent is the anesthetic

1. A lower concentration is thus required to maintain a similar anesthetic depth

C. Values vary among species and are affected by age, temperature, disease, other central nervous system–depressant drugs, and pregnancy

VI. See Tables 19-1 and 19-2 for physical and pharmacological properties of selected inhalation agents

Advantages

I. Advantages over injectable anesthesia

A. Easier to control and change depths of anesthesia

B. Excreted mainly by respiration; therefore recovery is fairly rapid and there is little metabolism

C. Requires administration of oxygen (O_2) to the patient, which provides a patent airway if an endotracheal tube is used

D. Respiratory and cardiovascular depression is minimal at safe concentrations

E. Provides some analgesia and muscle relaxation

F. Less accumulation, and recoveries are rapid

Examples

I. Examples of inhalation agents

A. Methoxyflurane: MAC 0.23% (minimal alveolar concentration)

Table 19-1 Physical properties of the common inhalation anesthetics

	Nitrous oxide	Halothane	Methoxyflurane	Isoflurane	Sevoflurane
Formula	N_2O	$CF_3CHClBr$	$CH_3OCF_2CHCl_2$	$CF_3CHClOCHF_2$	$CFH_2COCF_3CF_3$
Molecular weight	44	197	165	184	200
Date of first clinical use	1845	1956	1959	1981	
Trade name	–	Fluothane	Metofane Penthrane	Forane Aerrane	SevoFlo
Saturated vapor pressure (mm Hg)	800 (p.s.i)	243	22.5	261	160
Solubility					
Blood	0.47	2.4	13	1.4	0.6
Oil	1.4	224	825	60	53
Rubber	1.2	120	635	62	
MAC in dogs (%)	188	0.87	0.23	1.2	2.1-2.3

Modified from Warren RG: *Small animal anesthesia*, St Louis, 1989, Mosby.

Table 19-2 Pharmacological properties of selected agents

Property	Methoxyflurane	Halothane	Isoflurane	Sevoflurane
Muscle relaxation	Excellent	Fair	Good	
Effect on nondepolarizing muscle relaxants	None	Increased	Greatly increased	Probably increased
Analgesia	Excellent	Slight	Slight	Slight
Effect on respiration	Marked depression of rate and depth	Some depression	Depression	Depression
Effect on heart	Mild depression	Severe depression	Slight	Slight
Potential for causing cardiac arrhythmias	Some	Very common	None reported	None reported
Effect on blood pressure	May decrease	Decreases	Decreases	Decreases
Elimination from the body	Metabolism 50% Respiration 50%	Metabolism 20% Respiration 80%	Respiration 99%	Respiration 97%
Effect on the liver	Rare toxicity reported in humans	May rarely cause hepatitis in humans	None reported	
Effect on the kidneys	Toxicity reported in humans and animals	None reported	None reported	Possible risk of toxicity
Lipid solubility	High	Moderate	Low	Low
Maintenance range	0.25% to 1%	0.5% to 2%	1% to 3%	

Modified from McKelvey D: Halothane, isoflurane and methoxyflurane, *Vet Tech* 12(1):25, 1991.

1. Most potent inhalation anesthetic
2. Advantages
   a. Good analgesia and muscle relaxation
   b. Minimal arrhythmogenicity
   c. Low vapor pressure: can use with a precision or nonprecision vaporizer
   d. Slow plane changes reduces chance of sudden overdose
3. Disadvantages
   a. Increased solubility so slower induction and recovery
   b. Possible renal toxicity (environmental pollution concerns)
   c. Respiratory depression at deep surgical planes
   d. Slow response to changes in concentration, which may be a concern if surgical bleeding occurs
   e. Not suitable for mask induction because of excitement that may occur
4. Due to concerns over safety of personnel administering methoxyflurane, as well as documented increase in birth defects and impairment of kidney and liver function, this is no longer a commonly used inhalation agent
5. If used, an ACTIVE scavenger system must be in place, systems should be leak tested and maintained meticulously, and all reasonable precautions taken to avoid inhalation by personnel

B. Halothane: MAC 0.8%
1. Advantages
   a. Less respiratory depression
   b. Lower solubility than methoxyflurane; therefore faster induction and recoveries and faster response to changes in concentration
   c. Not nephrotoxic
   d. Can mask induce
2. Disadvantages
   a. Higher vapor pressure requires an out-of-circle precision vaporizer for maximum safety
   b. Arrhythmogenic potentials
   c. Cardiac depression resulting in hypotension (dose related)
   d. Little analgesia
   e. Hepatotoxic

C. Isoflurane: MAC 1.2% in dog, 1.6% in cat
1. Advantages
   a. Cardiovascularly safer with reduced arrhythmogenicity and better cardiac output
   b. Minimal liver metabolism
   c. Lower solubility and therefore faster induction and recoveries and a faster response to changes in concentration (faster than halothane)
2. Disadvantages
   a. Respiratory depression
   b. Occasional stormy recoveries
   c. More expensive
   d. Similar higher vapor pressure as halothane, therefore requires an out-of-circle precision vaporizer
   e. Vasodilation results in similar blood pressure as with halothane (dose related)

D. Sevoflurane MAC 2.4%
   1. Advantages
      a. Low solubility; therefore extremely rapid induction and recoveries
      b. Nonpungent
      c. Produces good muscle relaxation and analgesia
      d. Nonarrhythmogenic
   2. Disadvantages
      a. Respiratory depression similar to that of isoflurane
      b. Rapidly crosses placenta and will cause fetal depression
      c. Much more expensive than halothane or isoflurane
   3. Although it has not been documented, it is commonly held that Sevoflurane is superior to other inhalants for most avian species
      a. The smooth rapid induction and recovery minimize stress on these delicate patients
   4. Slight "hangover" that is present with other inhalants is lessened or absent with Sevoflurane
E. Desflurane MAC 7.2%
   1. Advantages
      a. Extremely low solubility, thus extremely rapid induction and recovery
      b. No hepatotoxicity or nephrotoxicity
   2. Disadvantages
      a. Requires a special, electrically heated vaporizer, which is extremely expensive
      b. Pungent and produces airway irritation, which provokes coughing and breath holding
         (1) Mask induction is very difficult
      c. Can cause malignant hyperthermia in some species
      d. Recovery may be too rapid and may cause unpleasant recoveries, requiring resedation
F. Nitrous oxide (N_2O)
   1. Advantages
      a. Can be used to speed inhalation induction by the second gas effect
      b. N_2O initially passes from the alveoli into the blood in large volumes
      c. The inhalant agent and O_2 are at a lower percentage
         (1) This difference effectively increases the concentrations of the inhalant agent and O_2 in the alveoli
      d. Availability to the blood is affected
      e. Provides additional analgesia (species variable)
      f. When used during anesthesia maintenance, it reduces the amount of other anesthetic agents required
         (1) Reduces the percent of halothane or isoflurane
      g. Minimal cardiovascular and respiratory effects
      h. No metabolism
         (1) Rapid effects
   2. Disadvantages
      a. Cannot be used alone (MAC >100%)
      b. Danger of hypoxia if not used properly
      c. Because use of N_2O reduces inspired O_2 levels to 33%, there is a danger of hypoxia if used with patients with respiratory problems
         (1) These problems include pneumonia, lung tumors, pulmonary edema, diaphragmatic hernia, or other conditions compromising the patient's ability to oxygenate
      d. Cannot be used with animals with gas-occupying cavities (i.e., gastric dilation, intestinal obstruction, pneumothorax)
         (1) N_2O has an increased partial pressure and low solubility in blood
            (a) Therefore nitrous oxide will diffuse into gas-occupying cavities faster than the rate at which resident gases leave
            (b) This causes an increased pressure in these cavities
   3. Method of use
      a. For mask induction
         (1) Initially use 100% O_2 with gradual increases in percentage of inhalant anesthetic agent
         (2) When high levels of inhalant agent are reached, turn on N_2O at an $N_2O:O_2$ ratio of 2:1 to continue induction
            (a) This provides 66% N_2O/33% O_2
      b. If you plan to use N_2O as part of your anesthetic maintenance, continue with the 2:1 ratio
         (1) To ensure adequate oxygenation of the patient
            (a) Never have O_2 levels below 500 mL/min (flowmeters may not be accurate below this)
            (b) Never have O_2 levels below 30 mL/kg/min (three times metabolic requirements) to ensure adequate oxygenation of the patient

c. When using N_2O with a partial rebreathing or nonrebreathing system (i.e., Bain), make sure total fresh gas flow (N_2O and O_2 combined) is at least 130 mL/kg/min, of which 33% should be O_2 (see section on breathing systems)
d. If the patient's O_2 saturation or mucous membrane color deteriorates (gray, cyanotic) at any time throughout the procedure, it is best to discontinue N_2O use in case hypoxia is impending
e. When the procedure is complete
   (1) Turn off the N_2O at the same time as the inhalant anesthetic
   (2) If N_2O is turned off too soon, you may be withdrawing a necessary analgesic source and therefore will have to increase the inhalant anesthetic agent to continue the procedure
f. Increase the O_2 flow rate to 100 mL/kg/min with a rebreathing system or 300 mL/kg/min with a nonrebreathing system
g. Keep patient on this increased O_2 flow rate for at least 5 minutes to prevent diffusion hypoxia
   (1) When N_2O is turned off, there is a flood of N_2O from the blood back into the alveoli
      (a) This displaces the O_2 in the lower respiratory tract and limits the O_2 available to the patient
h. Observe the patient for at least 5 minutes after O_2 source is removed to ensure that the patient is oxygenating well on room air
   (1) Especially note mucous membrane color and capillary refill time
   (2) Supplemental O_2 by a face mask should be used if needed

PARTS OF AN ANESTHETIC MACHINE

I. Best understood by following the flow of O_2 from the tank through the tank to the patient and back to the machine again
II. Gas cylinders
   A. Oxygen and nitrous oxide are contained in compressed gas metal cylinders
   B. Found as E cylinders that are usually attached to the machine via yokes that are equipped with a specific pin system
      1. Tanks also come in large G or H cylinders
   C. Pressure gauge attached to the cylinder indicates the pressure of the gas in the tank
      1. The pressure in a full O_2 cylinder is about 2200 pounds per square inch (p.s.i.) or 15,000 kilopascals (kPa)
      2. Oxygen tanks should be changed when pressure drops below 100 to 200 p.s.i. (680 to 1360 kPa)
      3. The volume of O_2 in an E tank can be calculated by multiplying the p.s.i. by 0.3
         a. A full tank of 2200 p.s.i. (15,000 kPa) will contain 660 L of O_2 (2200×0.3)
   D. Nitrous tanks are stored at lower pressure
      1. A full tank is 770 p.s.i. (5170 kPa)
      2. Nitrous tanks should be changed when pressure gauge drops to less than 500 p.s.i. (3400 kPa)
         a. Both liquid and gas states are present, but the gauge reads only the gas state
         b. Liquid evaporates to more gas as soon as the gas leaves the tank so that the pressure in the tank will not change until all of the liquid has evaporated
III. Pressure-reducing valve (or regulator)
   A. Reduces the high pressure of the O_2 or nitrous oxide leaving the tank to a low pressure of 50 p.s.i. (340 kPa)
IV. Flowmeter
   A. Measures O_2 or nitrous oxide in L/min
   B. Allows the anesthetist to set the O_2 or nitrous oxide flow rates that will be delivered to the animal
   C. Newer machines have a low flowmeter (<1 L) and a high flowmeter (0 to 5 L) for O_2
      1. This ensures greater accuracy
   D. As the gas passes through the flowmeter, gas pressure is reduced further from 50 p.s.i. (340 kPa) to 15 p.s.i. (100 kPa)
V. Vaporizer
   A. Converts the liquid anesthetic into a gas state and controls the amount of vaporized anesthetic to the carrier gases
VI. Inhalation/exhalation flutter valves or check valves
   A. Ensures a unidirectional flow of gas to and from the animal when delivering via a circle system
VII. Y-connector
   A. Connects the endotracheal tube to the inspiratory and expiratory tubes of a circle system
VIII. Rebreathing bag or reservoir bag
   A. Allows the animal to breathe easier from a reservoir of gas
   B. The reservoir bag can also be used to deliver O_2 (with or without anesthetic gas) and manually assist respirations, which is commonly called bagging

C. Bags should have a minimum volume of 60 mL/kg of patient weight

IX. Carbon dioxide (CO_2) absorber/soda lime canister
   A. Used in rebreathing systems to remove CO_2 from the expired gases
   B. Exhaust gases enter a canister containing soda lime or barium hydroxide
      1. Na^+, K^+, Ca^{2+}, and Ba^{2+} hydroxide reacts with the exhaled CO_2 and water to form carbonate
         a. Heat is liberated and the pH decreases
   C. A pH color indicator turns blue on consumption
      1. When the soda lime or barium hydroxide granules turn color or the granules become hard instead of crumbly, they are saturated with CO_2 and should be replaced
      2. When in use, granules will produce heat and condensation inside the canister
      3. The color reaction is time limited so exhausted crystals should be removed immediately and replaced with new granules
   D. Should be changed after 6 to 8 hours of use depending on the size of the animal and the gas flow rate
   E. If machines are left standing for longer than 30 days, granules should be replaced before using machine

X. Exhaust valve
   A. Also called "pop-off" valve, or pressure relief valve
   B. Exhaust gases leave the system via the exhaust valve entering the scavenger system
   C. Valve can be fully or partially open when a patient is using the machine
   D. Valve is closed for leak tests or when filling the reservoir bag for assisted respirations

XI. Manometer
   A. Measures the pressure in the system in mm Hg or cm H_2O
      1. Generally calibrated from −30 to +50 cm H_2O
   B. Gauge thus reflects the pressure of gas in the animal's airways and lungs
   C. The pressure should be at 0 and never more than 15 cm H_2O (11 mm Hg)
   D. When providing positive assisted ventilation, the pressure should not exceed 15 to 20 cm H_2O (11 to 15 mm Hg)

XII. Oxygen flush valve
   A. O_2 bypasses vaporizer, delivering 100% O_2 to breathing system
   B. Enables the anesthetist to flush the system with pure O_2
   C. Fills the reservoir bag and system for leak tests
   D. Also flushes anesthetic gases out of the circuit and replace gases with 100% O_2
   E. Never use O_2 flush with Bain system attached to a small animal because it produces too much pressure

XIII. Scavenger system
   A. Attached to the exhaust valve
   B. A basic scavenger system consists of tubing that collects waste gases and directs them outside of the building or to a charcoal canister that absorbs waste anesthetic gases
   C. Scavengers can be active systems (e.g., vacuum pump or a fan) or passive systems (e.g., tubing to a hole in an exterior wall of the building)

XIV. Negative pressure relief valve
   A. Some newer machines have this safety valve
   B. If negative pressure is created in the system, the valve will open and allow room air into the circuit
   C. Negative pressure could be because of an active scavenger system or a low to nil O_2 supply

Maintenance and Environmental Concerns

I. Oxygen tanks must be turned off to prevent excess pressure on the regulator
   A. Flush remaining O_2 to minimize damage to pressure gauge and reducing valves
   B. Turn flowmeter off to prevent sudden rush of O_2 into the flowmeter when O_2 is turned back on
      1. Do not overtighten because the knobs can be twisted off

II. After each anesthesia induction, removable machine parts and anesthetic equipment that have come in contact with the animal should be washed in a mild soapy solution, soaked in a cold disinfectant, thoroughly rinsed, and air dried
   A. The dome valves and absorbent canister should be occasionally disassembled and wiped dry
      1. Flutter valves need periodic removal and cleaning with a disinfectant to prevent adherence to the machine housing

III. Vaporizers should be turned off when not in use and periodically emptied to prevent buildup of the preservative and other residue
   A. Best to clean and recalibrate by authorized personnel every 6 to 12 months
   B. Isoflurane does not contain a preservative

IV. Barium hydroxide or soda lime granules found in the CO_2 absorbers need replacing when the granules have changed color or cannot be easily crumbled

A. Do not tightly pack and leave about 1 cm (½ inch) of air space
B. Avoid having dust enter tubing or hoses of the machine

V. Rubber items will likely need to be replaced after prolonged use

VI. Environmental pollution can be minimized through proper equipment use and scavenging of the gases

A. Safe exposure limit for inhalant anesthetic agents has been set at 2 parts per million (p.p.m.) in room air
   1. Everyone, especially pregnant women, should avoid high levels of waste anesthetic gases
   2. Much of the anesthetic levels are because of leaks in anesthetic machines
B. Vaporizers and CO_2 absorbers should be filled with minimal personnel in the room and in a well-ventilated area, while wearing masks and gloves
C. Do not turn the vaporizer on and off until the patient is connected to the machine
D. During recovery, keep patient in a well-ventilated area and on the machine until expired gases are scavenged
E. Use active scavenging whenever possible to ensure waste gases are drawn out of the area
   1. If passive scavenging is used, keep the hose as short as possible and have it travel downward toward the exhaust
   2. If it is not possible to install scavengers in all rooms where machines are used, either use an activated charcoal cartridge that must be replaced after 12 hours or substitute injectable anesthetics
F. Before anesthesia, the machine should be checked for both high- and low-pressure leaks
   1. Leakage of nitrous is the major environmental concern
   2. A high-pressure system test monitors NO_2 and O_2 leakage
      a. Leaks occur between the tank and flowmeter
      b. Can be checked by turning on the tank, noting the tank pressure gauge reading and turning the tank off again
         (1) The flowmeter should be set at zero so that there is no line evacuation of the gas
         (2) In 1 hour, the tank pressure gauge should still have the same reading
      c. Can also be checked by putting 100% detergent solution on any tank connections or joints
         (1) Bubble formations will indicate a leak
   3. A low-pressure system leak is in the anesthetic machine itself
      a. It occurs between the flowmeter and patient
      b. To check, turn the tank on, close the pop-off valve, and occlude the end of the hose so the gas should have nowhere to escape
         (1) Adjust the flowmeter to at least 2 L/min of O_2, allowing the bag to fill gradually and then turn off the flowmeter
         (2) If there is no escape of air when the inflated bag is gently squeezed, then there is no low-pressure system leakage
      c. The system can also be checked by occluding as above and using the flowmeter to allow the system to pressure at 30 cm H_2O
         (1) Turn off the flowmeter
            (a) The pressure should be maintained for 10 seconds
      d. One can also listen for the hiss of escaping air or use a detergent solution, as described earlier

BREATHING SYSTEMS

Rebreathing System

I. Rebreathing systems (e.g., circle systems)

A. Rebreathing refers to breathing a mixture of expired gases and fresh gases
B. The amount of CO_2 in inhaled gases depends on
   1. Whether the breathing system has a CO_2 absorber
   2. The flow rate of fresh gases (the higher the fresh gas flow rate, the more expired gas is pushed out the scavenger and not rebreathed)
C. Depending on the flow rate of fresh gas, the system is classified as a closed system (total rebreathing of expired gases) or a semiclosed system (partial rebreathing of expired gases)
D. Closed system
   1. With closed systems the fresh gas flow rate does not exceed the patient's metabolic O_2 consumption of 5 to 10 mL/kg/min
   2. The system may be used with a closed pop-off valve and a fresh gas flow of 5 to 10 mL/kg/min

3. Expired gases are recirculated (after CO_2 removal) with incoming fresh gases
4. Danger of increased CO_2 accumulation if CO_2 absorber not working efficiently
5. It is economical and there is minimal pollution
6. It takes longer to change planes of anesthesia
7. O_2 depletion and N_2O buildup are common, so do not use N_2O with this system
8. This system requires constant monitoring to ensure pressures do not build up in the system if the O_2 flow delivered exceeds the metabolic requirement
9. It is the author's belief that unless uninterrupted observation of this system is permitted, it can be dangerous to run a rebreathing system with the pop-off valve closed, if the pop-off valve has no safety release at high pressures
   a. It is recommended to leave the pop-off valve slightly open to prevent increases in pressure in the system and to adjust the O_2 flow rate accordingly to prevent the rebreathing bag from collapsing
      (1) If the bag does not collapse, you can be confident you are delivering sufficient O_2 to meet the patient's metabolic requirement

E. Semiclosed or partial rebreathing system
   1. With semiclosed systems, the fresh gas is delivered in excess of metabolic consumption at 25 to 50 mL/kg/min (suggested economical flow)
   2. The gas escapes through the pop-off valve to the scavenger or after having the CO_2 removed by the soda lime and then recirculates with the fresh gases
      a. Higher flows can be used; then less rebreathing will occur

F. N_2O buildup is less of a concern with higher flow rates
   1. Important to flush the system to prevent nitrogen buildup from the expired gases

Nonrebreathing System

I. There is no mixing of inhaled and exhaled gases and no rebreathing of expired gases; all expired gas goes to the scavenger
II. CO_2 absorber not required
III. Fresh gas flow rates required at 200 to 300 mL/kg/min
IV. Fresh gas flow rate of 130 to 200 mL/kg/min with the Bain system
   A. May be some rebreathing of exhaled gases if a reservoir bag and low flow rate

BREATHING CIRCUITS

There are many kinds of breathing circuits available. The most common in veterinary medicine are circle systems, universal F-circuits, and Bain systems.

Circle System

I. Consists of a CO_2 absorber (i.e., soda lime canister) with inspiratory and expiratory unidirectional valves (check valves or flutter valves), two breathing hoses connected with a Y piece to the patient, rebreathing bag, and pop-off valve (exhaust valve) and scavenger
II. Can be used as a nonrebreathing system (200 mL/kg/min), partial rebreathing system (25 to 50 mL/kg/min), or total rebreathing system (5 to 10 mL/kg/min)
III. An advantage is the mixture of expired gases with incoming gases, which humidifies and warms the incoming gases
IV. The main disadvantages of the circle system occur with smaller patients
   A. Excess weight and bulk of the hoses
   B. Excess dead space
   C. The resistance to breathing through unidirectional valves

Universal F-Circuit

I. Basically a modified circle system where the inspiratory hose is placed within the expiratory hose
II. Still requires a CO_2 absorber, rebreathing bag, unidirectional valves, pop-off valve, and scavenger
III. Incoming fresh gas is warmed also by expired gases
IV. The advantage is lighter weight and less bulk
V. A disadvantage is that if the circuit is stretched when in use, the end of the inspiratory hose pulls away from the end of the expiratory hose
   A. This is considered a safety feature to prevent breakage of hoses, but it increases the amount of dead space
   B. When not stretched, the dead space is at least comparable to the circle system

Bain System (Coaxial)

I. Consists of one tube inside another tube
   A. Fresh gases flow through the inner tube, and the unused fresh gases and exhaled gases flow through the outer tube
   B. There also is a rebreathing bag with a clip on the tubing between the reservoir bag and scavenger connection but no CO_2 absorber

II. Between breaths, the fresh gases flow through the inner tube toward the patient and then back through the outer tube toward the scavenger

III. When the patient inspires, the gases are drawn from the inner tube, which will be 100% fresh gases or a mixture of fresh gases and expired gases, depending on the fresh gas flow rate

IV. This system can be used as a nonrebreathing system with a fresh gas flow rate of 200 to 300 mL/kg/min
   A. The high flow rate pushes exhaled gases away down the outer tube, so there is no rebreathing of exhaled gases

V. This system can also be used as a partial rebreathing system with a flow rate of 130 to 200 mL/kg/min
   A. Flow rate pushes most of the exhaled gases away but there is partial rebreathing of some exhaled gases

VI. Bain system is ideal for small patients (<7 kg [15 lb])
   A. Lightweight
   B. Minimal dead space
   C. Little resistance to breathing

VII. This system is good for all small animals in general but is not economical when patient is more than 10 kg (22 lb)

VIII. Limiting factor is the size of patient
   A. The O_2 flowmeter must provide flow rates required for a partial or nonrebreathing system (130 to 300 mL/kg/min)
   B. Total volume of the Bain hose must be greater than the tidal volume of respiration of the patient to effectively prevent rebreathing

IX. Good for procedures involving the head (less tubing in the way)

X. Good for procedures with much manipulation (i.e., radiography, because there is less weight pulling on the animal)

XI. Warming and humidification are minimal with partial rebreathing

XII. Requires a precision vaporizer

VAPORIZERS

Vapor pressure is characterized by the amount of vapor related to its liquid in a closed container; the pressure exerted by the gas is called the vapor pressure and will increase with increases in temperature. Because most anesthetics vaporize at a concentration higher than necessary for clinical anesthesia, a vaporizer is used to deliver diluted anesthetics to patients.

Classification

I. Accuracy
   A. Precision vaporizer
      1. Enables delivery of controlled concentrations of anesthetic vapor independent of time, temperature, and fresh gas flow rate
         a. Temperature and flow rate are compensated for by the vaporizer or manually by the anesthetist
      2. Percentage of anesthetic is determined by dial, chart, or mathematical calculation
      3. Because of internal resistance, precision vaporizers must always be placed out-of-circle because the patient cannot physically draw gases through them
      4. A disadvantage is that they are more complex and therefore more expensive and require more servicing
   B. Nonprecision vaporizer
      1. Do not deliver a constant percentage because of changes in temperature, fresh gas flow rates, ventilation changes, liquid and wick surfaces, and the amount of liquid anesthetic in vaporizer
      2. Percentage of anesthetic delivered cannot be calculated
      3. Little internal resistance, therefore can be used in-the-circle
      4. Although they can be used out-of-circle, the nonlinear concentrations delivered make anesthesia depth hard to control
      5. Vaporizers are simple and less expensive and require less servicing

II. Location
   A. VOC (vaporizer out-of-circle)
      1. Vaporizer is added to the system between the O_2 flowmeter and the circle (circle consisting of inspiratory and expiratory valves, breathing hoses, CO_2 absorber, pop-off valve, scavenger, and rebreathing bag)
   B. VIC (vaporizer in-the-circle)
      1. Vaporizer is placed inside the breathing system, usually between the inspiratory valve and the patient
      2. VICs are always nonprecision
      3. The carrier gas (i.e., O_2) passes over the surface of the anesthetic liquid or past a wick
      4. Incoming gases mix with warmed exhaled gases in the system
      5. Better vaporization of liquid is obtained when low fresh gas flows are used
         a. High flows cool liquid and reduce vaporization
      6. These vaporizers are also safest when used with agents with low vapor pressure (e.g., methoxyflurane)

MONITORING

The signs you observe from monitoring may differ depending on the species and the anesthetic agents being used. The following signs are general for domestic small animals (i.e., cat and dog).

Eye

I. Position
   A. Eye will rotate ventral-medially during stage III, plane 2 of anesthesia
   B. Eye will return to central when the patient is too light or too deep
II. Palpebral reflex (blink)
   A. Stimulated by lightly touching the medial or lateral canthus of the eyelids
   B. Lateral palpebral reflex is eliminated before the medial palpebral reflex as the patient becomes deeper
   C. Reflex will become slow, weak, and then absent in stage III, plane 2 with most inhalant agents
   D. If an analgesic has been given or injectable anesthesia alone or methoxyflurane is used, then a mild medial palpebral reflex is acceptable
III. Corneal reflex
   A. Stimulated by lightly touching the cornea of the eye
   B. This reflex should be present under anesthesia
   C. Absence of this reflex indicates anesthesia overdose
   D. Considering the potential damage that can be inflicted on the cornea and the wide range of other monitoring options available, this reflex should not be tested unless necessary
IV. Pupil size
   A. Generally dilated when in a light, nonsurgical plane
   B. Constricted in a light surgical plane
   C. Dilated in a deep plane
   D. Note that sympathetic responses such as pain or certain drugs (e.g., atropine) will dilate the pupils

Pedal Reflex (Pain Response)

I. Stimulated by pinching the skin between the toes
II. Normal response is to withdraw the leg
III. This response should become slower and weaker to absent as the anesthetic plane becomes deeper, being completely eliminated by a light surgical plane

Jaw Tone (Muscle Tone)

I. Stimulated by attempting to spread the jaws apart two to three times
II. Normal response is to resist
III. A good reflex to check before intubation
IV. This response should become weaker as the anesthetic plane becomes deeper and should be absent in a light surgical plane
V. If a good analgesic or methoxyflurane has been used, mild jaw tone can remain if all other monitoring signs indicate an appropriate plane of anesthesia
VI. Some breeds will appear to have increased jaw tone because of increased muscle mass in this area (e.g., Rottweiler)

Cardiovascular System

I. Heart rate
   A. Most accurately measured with a stethoscope
   B. Can also be measured by digital readout of mechanical monitoring equipment
   C. Normal rate under anesthetic is 70 to 140 beats per minute for dog and 110 to 140 beats per minute for cat
      1. Minimal acceptable heart rate in anesthetized dogs is generally 60 beats per minute
   D. Heart rate may decrease with deepening anesthetic plane but may also stay constant or increase with a dangerously deep plane and/or with hypotension
   E. Bradycardia (decreased heart rate) is not always a sign of deep anesthesia. Heart rate may decrease with
      1. Certain drugs prone to producing bradycardia
      2. End stage hypoxia (e.g., because of respiratory obstruction)
      3. Vagal nerve stimulation (e.g., pressure on the eyes, manipulation of abdominal contents, pressure during intubation)
II. Pulse rate
   A. Measure by palpation of an artery
   B. Pulse deficits (difference between heart rate and pulse rate) should be noted
III. Rhythm
   A. Arrhythmias can be monitored by arterial palpation but are more accurately monitored with an electrocardiogram
IV. Blood pressure
   A. Palpation of a peripheral pulse can indicate drastic increases or decreases in blood pressure but not actual values
   B. Blood pressure is more accurately measured by an indirect or direct arterial blood pressure monitoring system
      1. There are many commercially available monitoring devices. Most will measure

systolic, diastolic, and mean pressures and can be set to read at regular timed intervals

a. Commonly, pressures are read every 60 to 120 seconds
b. Direct blood pressures can be monitored through placement of arterial line and provide a constant reading
c. Superior to indirect monitoring but may not be practical in regular practice because of specialized equipment (i.e., transducers) that is necessary for this type of monitoring
d. Doppler is affordable and, when used in conjunction with a blood pressure cuff and sphygmomanometer, can give a fairly accurate systolic pressure, as well as a good heart rate and sound
   (1) Doppler sensor is placed over a peripheral pulse, usually on the dorsal pedal artery
   (2) Cuff is placed proximally to the probe
   (3) Cuff is then inflated until the pulse is no longer audible
   (4) Be careful to inflate carefully, or you could dislodge your cuff
   (5) Slowly release the inflation, until the first "swish" or beat is heard
   (6) This is the systolic pressure
   (7) Diastolic pressure is not easily heard using this method, so often only systolic pressure is monitored
   (8) Minimally acceptable systolic pressures are 80 mm Hg in dog and 90 mm Hg in cat
   (9) Do not tape the cuff in place; this will distort the reading
   (10) Also, using an inappropriate-size cuff on any method will give you distorted readings, so ensure you have a proper cuff size for the patient
      (a) A cuff that is too big will give lower readings; conversely, one that is too small will give higher readings

C. Normal blood pressures
   1. Systolic: 100 to 160 mm Hg
   2. Mean arterial: 80 to 120 mm Hg
   3. Diastolic: 60 to 100 mm Hg

D. Generally blood pressure will decrease as the anesthetic plane deepens. Mean blood pressure in dogs should not be allowed to drop under 60 mm Hg
   1. Kidneys will become inadequately perfused below this level and this may result in renal impairment after anesthesia

E. Hypovolemia will reduce blood pressure
   1. Can counteract by giving small boluses of IV fluids in 10- to 50-mL increments depending on size (10 for cats, 50 for average 20-kg [45-lb] dog)

F. Hypercapnia will increase blood pressure

Respiratory System

I. Monitor rate and depth (character) of the ventilation

II. Under anesthesia normal rate is 8 to 20 breaths per minute and normal tidal volume is 10 to 15 mL/kg

III. All induction drugs have the potential to cause a transitory apnea. One must monitor the patient's respiratory rate and O_2 saturation carefully, immediately on induction to ensure smooth transition to stage 3

IV. In a very light plane of anesthesia, the ventilation will be irregular in depth and rate in response to stimulation

V. In a surgical plane, the rate and depth are generally regular

VI. In a deep plane of anesthesia, breathing may become shallow and rapid or both the rate and depth may decrease

VII. As the plane gets deeper, there will be some thoracic muscle paralysis producing paradoxical breathing (abdomen rises and chest falls during an inspiration)

VIII. Blood gas levels can also be monitored
   A. O_2 levels will define the patient's oxygenating ability
   B. CO_2 levels will define the ventilation status
   C. Hypoventilation is indicated by increased CO_2 levels (respiratory acidosis)
   D. Hyperventilation is indicated by decreased CO_2 levels (respiratory alkalosis)

IX. Monitoring of O_2 levels may be performed with a pulse oximeter. Keep in mind, however, that this will display only O_2 saturation, and not CO_2 levels

Capillary Refill Time

I. Acquired through digital compression on any unpigmented mucous membrane
   A. Time between release of pressure and return of blood flow to the area

II. A normal capillary refill time (CRT) is less than 2 seconds

III. Good indication of how well cardiac output is affecting peripheral perfusion
   A. It is important to monitor this in conjunction with blood pressure

IV. CRT will generally become longer with deepening anesthetic planes and hypovolemia

Mucous Membrane Color

I. Generally pink in unpigmented areas
II. Mucous membranes may change color to a gray tinge or blue with decreased O_2 levels in the blood; however, this change may be delayed and is not considered a good forewarning
III. High CO_2 because of hypoventilation may produce a very bright pink, vasodilated, mucous membrane color
IV. Pale mucous membranes may occur with anemia, hypothermia, or with light planes of anesthesia when pain is occurring

Temperature

I. Decreases in body temperature and slow metabolism can reduce the amount of anesthetic agent required
II. It is important to monitor and support body temperature from the time of sedation through recovery
III. Monitor rectal or axilla peripheral temperature with a digital thermometer, or monitor core temperature with an esophageal temperature probe
IV. Hypothermic patients should be actively rewarmed to 37.5° C (99° F), after which heat sources should be removed to prevent hyperthermia
    A. It is very important in nursing care to fully recover your patient with SAFE warming tools (i.e., hot water bottles, BAIR hugger machines)
        1. Placing a recovering animal on a heating pad unattended is not recommended
        2. To prevent burning of the patient, any heat source used should not produce heat over 42.0° C (107.6° F)
        3. Physical sources of heat should be wrapped in a towel before placement against the patient
        4. Postoperative monitoring of the patient should include a hands-on examination of the placement of heat sources to ensure they are adequate and not becoming too cold

STAGES OF ANESTHESIA (DEPTHS)

I. Stage 1
    A. Induction stage, stage of analgesia, and altered consciousness
    B. From beginning to loss of consciousness
    C. Sensations become dull
    D. Loss of pain
    E. Pupils are normal in size, then begin to dilate when entering stage 2
    F. Blood pressure may be elevated
    G. Respiration rate is generally increased, may be irregular
    H. Vomiting, retching, and coughing may occur
II. Stage 2
    A. Stage of delirium or excitement, loss of consciousness
    B. Excitement and involuntary muscular movement. May appear to "struggle"
    C. Eyes closed, jaw set. Reflexes present, may be exaggerated
    D. Pupils dilated, light reflex still present
    E. Respiration irregular. Panting or breath holding is common
    F. Vomiting may occur
III. Stage 3
    A. Stage of surgical anesthesia
    B. Respiration full and regular
    C. Pupils begin to constrict
    D. Palpebral blink is absent (or minimal with methoxyflurane)
    E. Four subplanes
        1. Subplane I
            a. Eyeball begins to rove, pupil is light responsive, and medial palpebral still present
            b. Muscle tone still present
            c. Pain reaction still present
            d. Respiration is one-half thoracic and one-half abdominal
            e. Blood pressure and heart rate are normal
        2. Subplane II
            a. Ideal surgical plane
            b. Respiration becomes deep and regular
            c. Fixed eyeball, often rotated ventrally. Sluggish pupillary response
            d. Increase in heart and respiratory rate is mild in response to surgical pain
            e. Peripheral reflexes (i.e., pedal, palpebral) are absent
        3. Subplane III
            a. Increased abdominal respiration, delayed thoracic inspiratory effect (intercostal paralysis)
            b. Respiration rate decreases, breaths are no longer deep and regular
            c. Eyeballs fixed and usually centrally rotated
            d. Pupils begin to dilate
            e. Pulse fast and feeble
            f. Blood pressure decreased. Fails to respond to surgical pain stimulation
        4. Subplane IV

a. Progressive respiratory paralysis
b. Tidal volume decreased
c. Palpebral and corneal reflexes absent
d. Pupils dilated and not light responsive
e. Heart rate decreased, blood pressure significantly low
f. Apnea or jerky inspirations
g. Pale mucous membranes and prolonged CRTs

IV. Stage 4
A. Stage of medullary paralysis
B. Apnea
C. Cardiac arrest

V. Ideally, a smooth induction goes from stage 1 to stage 3, quickly bypassing stage 2

ANALGESIA

I. Depending on the individual patient and the procedure, consider
A. Which agent to use
B. Timing (preprocedure, intraprocedure, or postprocedure) of administration
C. Length of analgesia required
D. Choice of route of administration (e.g., systemic [SQ, IM, IV], local, regional, or epidural)

II. If the patient is in pain, analgesics should be provided in the preanesthetic medication to help alleviate pain and anxiety and provide for a smoother induction

III. Administration of analgesics preoperatively and intraoperatively will allow reduction of induction and/or maintenance anesthetic agent required by the patient and maintain a level plane of anesthesia with proper analgesia

IV. Analgesics should be provided during and/or after any surgical or otherwise painful procedure before recovery from anesthesia
A. Timing is important, because if given postoperatively before swallowing reflex is present, extubation may be prolonged significantly

V. Application of analgesia before conscious awareness of pain will have a positive influence on the effect of the analgesia
A. It has been proven that pain is much easier to prevent if given after surgical procedures than to wait until the animal is showing signs of pain
B. "Chasing" the pain should be avoided at all times because it is not ideal patient care and in some cases can be borderline unethical

VI. By decreasing pain on recovery, stress of the patient is decreased and therefore a quicker, more successful recovery is promoted

VII. Some examples of choices of analgesic agents
A. Nonsteroidal anti-inflammatory drugs (NSAIDs), for systemic use
1. These include aspirin, acetaminophen, carprofen, ketoprofen, and, more recently, meloxicam
2. They appear to be excellent for use in musculoskeletal pain
3. They are commonly used in conjunction with opioids, as it is safe to do so
4. Acetaminophen must never be used in cats and is rarely used in dogs
5. Ketoprofen and carprofen are excellent, especially for immediate postoperative use in orthopedic procedures, and provide strong safe analgesia in degloving injuries
6. Long-term use of these drugs for arthritis and other joint diseases is common, but care must be taken to monitor kidney function regularly, as they can be nephrotoxic
7. Meloxicam is less nephrotoxic and is better tolerated for long-term use

B. Opioids for systemic and epidural use
1. See information contained in section on premedication for opioids

C. Local anesthetics for systemic, local, regional, or epidural use
1. Lidocaine or lidocaine 2% (with epinephrine) is commonly used for local anesthesia
a. Indicated for procedures that are minimally invasive and short in duration and cover a small surface area
b. Lidocaine is infiltrated around the site via needle and syringe
c. It has immediate onset, but some practitioners like to give the drug a chance to spread through the tissues and will allow 5 or so minutes for it to "take"
d. Effective for up to 2 hours, but variable with each animal
e. There is no sedation with this type of drug, and no analgesia once the numbness wears off
(1) Important from a restraint and analgesia point of view
2. Epidurals are commonly given in orthopedic procedures to lessen the amount of maintenance anesthesia used and to provide comfort analgesia to the patient intraoperatively

a. It also tends to increase chances for a smooth, stress-free, nonpainful recovery
b. Common epidural drugs include procaine, lidocaine, and bupivacaine
c. Morphine is often added for stifle procedures (i.e., cruciate ligament surgery)

MUSCLE RELAXANTS

I. Neuromuscular blocking agents are used to
  A. Relax skeletal muscles for better manipulation of joints and bones
  B. Obtain better surgical exposure
  C. Control ventilation
  D. Assist in tracheal intubation
  E. Immobilize the eyes for ocular surgery (very common use)
  F. Reduce amount of anesthetic agent used when deep anesthesia will not be tolerated by the patient
II. Requires ventilation of the animal at all times
III. Requires some form of additional analgesia
IV. Requires close monitoring for depth of anesthesia because several monitoring signs will be eliminated
  A. Eliminated signs include jaw tone, eye position, palpebral blink, spontaneous breathing
  B. Blood pressure monitoring via direct (arterial) monitoring is recommended
V. Nerve stimulators are an asset
  A. Aid in the assessment of effect of the neuromuscular block
  B. Indicate time to give subsequent doses
  C. Indicate when to reverse
VI. Some examples of neuromuscular blocking agents: succinylcholine, gallamine, pancuronium, atracurium, and vecuronium
  A. Doses, length of effect, side effects, and reversal agents differ

VENTILATION

I. Assisted (occasional sigh or additional breaths) or controlled (intermittent positive pressure ventilation [IPPV])
II. Manual or mechanical
III. Goal is to maintain near normal acid-base status and oxygenation and to counteract CO_2 retention
IV. In some cases only assistance is needed (e.g., obese patient, patient in head-down recumbency, hypothermia, pulmonary disease)
  A. Occasional "sighing" or "bagging" the patient (e.g., once or twice a minute) may achieve these goals
    1. To properly bag an animal, close the popoff valve, apply steady pressure to the bag, release, and IMMEDIATELY reopen the pop-off valve
    2. When squeezing the bag, it is important to make sure that the manometer reading stays below 20 mm Hg
V. In many cases it is necessary to control the ventilation (IPPV) (i.e., when using neuromuscular blocking agents; with thoracic surgery, diaphragmatic hernia, or gastric torsion; or with any patient that is obviously hypoventilating)
VI. Observe guidelines and reassess results continually
  A. Rate: 8 to 12 breaths per minute
  B. Inspiration-to-expiration ratio: 1:2
  C. Tidal volume: 15 to 20 mL/kg (30 mL/kg for open chest)
    1. 12 mL/kg if greater than 40 kg (84 lb)
    2. 20 mL/kg if less than 10 kg (22 lb)
  D. Inspiratory pressure: 12 to 20 cm H_2O (30 cm H_2O with open chest)
VII. The goal of using these parameters is to decrease CO_2 levels slightly below normal, thereby eliminating spontaneous breathing and allowing control of ventilation
  A. Therefore in most cases it is not necessary to use a neuromuscular blocking agent to perform IPPV
  B. A CO_2 monitor is a useful device
    1. Normal reading should be between 35 and 55 cm H_2O
      a. CO_2 should never be allowed to go beyond 60 cm H_2O
    2. Hyperventilation of cases involving possible brain herniation should be adjusted so that readings are 29 cm H_2O
VIII. Double-check all ventilation with visualization for "normal" chest movement; reassess other parameters of the patient (mucous membrane color, CRT, heart rate, pulse strength, and blood gases when available)
IX. Concerns
  A. Generally decrease percentage of inhalant anesthetic delivered to the patient because you will be ventilating better for the patient than if it were spontaneous; therefore more anesthetic will be delivered
  B. If the patient breathes spontaneously while IPPV is performed, it is an indication of
    1. Underventilation
      a. An indication for you to increase the minute volume by increasing the rate and/or volume of breaths
      b. Patient is in pain
        (1) Increase level of inhalant anesthetic if possible
        (2) Add nitrous oxide
        (3) Give intraoperative opioids

c. Patient is at a light anesthetic plane

C. If you are ventilating adequately, the patient will not attempt to breathe spontaneously

D. Overventilation
   1. Overventilation has potential to damage an animal's lungs
      a. Rupture of alveoli, leading to pneumothorax or mediastinal emphysema
   2. Decreased cardiac output and venous return
   3. Excessive CO_2, leading to respiratory alkalosis

E. With pneumothorax, ventilate with caution and be prepared for the possibility of a tension pneumothorax
   1. It is best to manually ventilate these cases so you can evaluate the ease of the resistance to the rebreathing bag
   2. There will be difficulty squeezing the rebreathing bag or an increased pressure will register on the pressure gauge of the ventilator or anesthetic machine with chest expansion

F. When removing the patient from the ventilator, continue to ventilate for several minutes after discontinuing inhalant anesthetic; this will help eliminate the inhalant from the patient's system and speed recovery
   1. Decrease the minute volume (rate and/or volume) to allow CO_2 levels to increase slightly in the patient's system to stimulate the patient to breath spontaneously

FLUID THERAPY

If time allows, the patient should be stabilized for fluid imbalances, electrolyte imbalances, anemia, and hypoproteinemia before proceeding with anesthesia.

Fluid Characteristics

I. Most stable anesthetic cases are maintained on an IV replacement crystalloid such as Normosol R or Plasmalyte 148 as opposed to a maintenance crystalloid such as Normosol M or Plasmalyte 56

II. Replacement crystalloids should have high sodium and chloride levels and a low potassium level, similar to plasma

III. Replacement crystalloids are administered at 5 to 10 mL/kg/hr for routine, healthy anesthesia or surgery

IV. It is common to run long procedures at 10 mL/kg/hr for the first hour, decreasing to 5 mL/kg/hr for subsequent hours

V. Having the patient on IV fluids allows you to
   A. Replace fluid loss because of preoperative water and/or food restriction, evaporation from open body cavities, and/or breathing dry gases
   B. Maintain hydration, tissue perfusion, and organ function (especially renal)
      1. This is monitored by keeping blood pressure values within normal ranges as laid out previously
   C. Replace some blood loss
   D. Maintain patent IV access in the case of an emergency

Fluid Calculation

I. For dehydrated patients, if time does not allow hydration status to be fully stabilized before anesthesia, 50% of the fluid deficit can be replaced IV over the 20 to 30 minutes required for effective premedication

II. Total volume to treat dehydration is calculated as

$$\frac{\%\ \text{Dehydration}}{100} \times \text{weight (kg)} \times 1000 = \text{mL to give}$$

   A. Example: dog that is 7% dehydrated

$$\frac{7}{100} \times 20 \times 1000 = 1400\ \text{mL}$$

III. Give 700 mL 20 to 30 minutes before anesthesia induction
   A. Recognizing that instability may persist until the entire deficit is replaced, continue at an increased fluid administration rate of 20 to 90 mL/kg/hr during the remainder of anesthesia or until the deficit is replaced to maintain good blood pressure

IV. A maximum fluid rate of 60 (cats and older dogs) to 90 (other dogs) mL/kg/hr to replace the calculated fluid loss is a safe rapid administration rate in awake and anesthetized patients

V. Other abnormal losses, such as surgical bleeding, are also replaced

BLOOD LOSS

I. Anemia from acute blood loss is more critical

II. Patients with chronic anemia will tend to compensate and may tolerate a lower packed cell volume (PCV)
   A. If PCV is less than 25% in dogs or 20% in cats, whole blood or packed red blood cells (colloids) should replace the surgical fluids and be started before anesthesia if possible
      1. Oxyglobin may also be used when available
   B. If PCV is normal but total protein (TP) is less than 3.5 g/dL plasma, dextrans or hetastarch should replace surgical fluids (artificial colloids)

III. Total volume to improve PCV or TP is calculated as follows

$$\frac{\text{Desired PCV (TP)} - \text{recipient PCV (TP)}}{\text{Donor PCV (TP)}} \times \text{wt (kg)} \times 50 = \text{mL (vol)}$$

IV. When blood or plasma is used to correct anemia or hypoproteinemia during surgery, the rate of administration is 3 to 10 mL/kg/hr
   A. Blood should be given slowly for the first 5 to 10 minutes to observe for transfusion reactions
   B. Observe for reaction signs: hypotension, tachypnea, tachycardia, poor CRT, vomiting (if awake), pallor, and urticaria

V. When blood, plasma, or artificial colloids are given to treat chronic anemia, the rate of administration should not exceed 20 (cats and older dogs) to 30 (other dogs) mL/kg/hr

VI. For acute intraoperative blood loss, 10% to 15% of the total body blood volume can be replaced with replacement crystalloid fluids, provided the PCV and TP were normal to begin with
   A. To calculate the volume lost, consider that the total body blood volume is approximately 100 mL/kg in dogs and 75 mL/kg in cats; for example
      1. For a 10-kg dog
      2. 10 kg × 100 mL/kg = 1000 mL total blood volume
      3. 10% blood loss = 100 mL
   B. When replacing a 10% to 15% blood loss with crystalloids, replace at two to three times the volume lost (in addition to the surgical fluid rate)
      1. Only one third of the crystalloid volume will stay in the vascular compartment
      2. The remaining two thirds of the crystalloid volume will move into the interstitial space (e.g., for the same 10-kg dog with a 10% blood loss, replace with a total of 200 to 300 mL of crystalloids)
   C. If greater than 15% blood loss is replaced with crystalloids, there is a risk of hemodilution
      1. Any blood loss over 15% of the total body blood volume may require replacement with whole blood or packed red blood cells
      2. Unlike crystalloids, the whole volume of colloids administered will remain in the vascular compartment; therefore the volume of colloid administered will be equal to the volume of blood loss
      3. If the condition of the patient allows, begin with an initial slow drip rate for 5 minutes to watch for transfusion reaction, then continue administration of the remainder of the colloid as fast as the loss occurs
   D. In an emergency situation, the slow initial administration may not be possible; the need for fast administration of blood may outweigh the risk of a transfusion reaction
   E. In cases where acute ischemia is present (i.e., GDV or equine colic) where blood supply to important structures is impaired or occluded, Oxyglobin is indicated to replace blood loss and combat hypovolemia and shock
      1. It has much smaller molecules than regular blood so it can oxygenate these areas when regular blood cannot
      2. Oxyglobin is very valuable in cases such as these; however, it is extremely expensive and hard to obtain

ACID-BASE BALANCE

Defined by pH, which is the result of processes in the body tending toward acidosis or alkalosis.

I. Mechanisms that regulate pH are respiratory or metabolic in nature and are maintained by three systems
   A. Chemical buffers
      1. Bicarbonate (carbonic acid)
      2. Phosphate (red blood cells, kidneys)
      3. Hemoglobin
   B. Respiratory
      1. By breathing and alteration of CO_2 the lungs can regulate the concentration of carbonic acid
   C. Kidney
      1. Elimination of excess acid or bases: carbonic acid—CO_2 equilibrium

$$CO_2 + H_2O = H_2CO_3 = H^+ + HCO_3^- \text{ (respiratory) (metabolic)}$$

II. Disturbances in acid-base balance can be found in one of four categories
   A. Respiratory acidosis
      1. CO_2 production is greater than CO_2 excretion
      2. Indicated on blood gas analysis by an increase in CO_2 levels
      3. Caused by anything that depresses ventilation (hypoventilation) and impairs excretion of CO_2 (i.e., deep anesthesia, pulmonary disease, respiratory obstruction)
      4. May also be caused by increased CO_2 production with malignant hyperthermia
      5. Increase in CO_2 causes a gain in acids, therefore the pH decreases
      6. Other signs: increased cardiac output (hypertension), vasodilation, and ventricular arrhythmias
      7. Natural compensation of the body with time through the kidneys (although chronic hypercapnia is rare)

8. Respiratory acidosis can be treated by
   a. Ventilating the patient with a higher minute volume (increase the tidal volume and/or respiration rate) than what the patient was breathing spontaneously to help remove some of the CO_2
   b. Treatment of the underlying disease (i.e., pneumonia)

B. Respiratory alkalosis
1. CO_2 excretion is greater than CO_2 production
2. Indicated on blood gas analysis by a decrease in CO_2 levels
3. Caused by excessive controlled ventilation (IPPV) or anything that stimulates spontaneous hyperventilation and therefore removal of CO_2 such as pain and excitement
4. Causes excess loss of H^+ and gain in bases
5. Other signs: may produce tachycardia and electrocardiographic changes
6. Natural compensation of the body with time through the kidneys, although chronic hypocapnia is rare; therefore compensation is seldom seen
7. Respiratory alkalosis can be treated by
   a. Decreasing the minute volume if the patient is being ventilated
   b. If the patient is breathing spontaneously and hyperventilating, assess and treat the cause of hyperventilation such as light anesthesia, pain

C. Metabolic acidosis
1. Indicated on blood gas analysis by low adjusted base excess (ABE) or low HCO_3^-
2. Common causes are lactic acid gain (commonly caused by decreased tissue perfusion), renal failure, body secretions rich in HCO_3^- that are lost and not reabsorbed (i.e., diarrhea)
3. Causes loss of HCO_3^-, which means an H^+ gain
4. Natural compensation by rapid response of respiratory system by hyperventilating
5. Metabolic acidosis can be treated
   a. For a mild imbalance, give an alkalinizing IV solution (containing lactate, gluconate, acetate)
   b. For more severe imbalances, treat with sodium bicarbonate
      (1) Dose is calculated as follows: ½ ABE × wt (kg) × 0.3 = mEq of sodium bicarbonate
      (2) This volume should be given slowly IV (over 15 to 30 minutes)
      (3) Deaths have occurred during fast administration of sodium bicarbonate in dehydrated animals
         (a) HCO_3^- combines with H^+ to produce CO_2 and H_2O
         (b) CO_2 will rapidly enter the brain; HCO_3^- will take longer to enter cells
         (c) Excess CO_2 in the brain will drop the pH of the central nervous system further, resulting in coma and death: paradoxical central nervous system acidosis

D. Metabolic alkalosis
1. Indicated on blood gas analysis by high ABE or high HCO_3^-
2. Caused by stomach vomiting (loss of H^+), hypochloremia (increased renal absorption of HCO_3^-)
3. Natural compensation through the respiratory system by hypoventilation resulting in a mild respiratory acidosis
4. Metabolic alkalosis can be treated, if severe, by replacing the lacking element
   a. Potassium may be necessary if hypokalemic
   b. Chloride may be necessary in the vomiting patient

III. Interpretation of blood gas results

A. Normal values

pH:	7.35 to 7.45
Po_2:	400 to 500 mm Hg (arterial, 100% inspired O_2)
	150 to 250 mm Hg (arterial, N_2O/O_2 mix inspired)
	90 to 100 mm Hg (arterial, room air inspired)
	50 to 200 mm Hg (venous, 100% inspired O_2)
	30 to 60 mm Hg (venous, room air inspired)
Pco_2:	35 to 45 mm Hg (arterial, will increase by 6 mm Hg with venous sample)
HCO_3^-:	20 to 24 mEq
ABE:	−4 to +4

B. When interpreting values of blood gas there may be two disorders: a primary disorder and a secondary (compensating) disorder
1. First look at the pH
   a. pH less than 7.35: acidosis
   b. pH greater than 7.45: alkalosis
2. Then look at the Pco_2 and ABE to determine respiratory and metabolic conditions respectively
3. Generally the pH will vary in the direction of the primary disorder
4. Generally the component with the greatest change is the primary disorder
   a. Natural compensation is usually not 100% and seldom will there be an overcompensation

(1) P_{CO_2} greater than 45: respiratory acidosis
(2) P_{CO_2} less than 35: respiratory alkalosis
(3) ABE less than –4: metabolic acidosis
(4) ABE greater than +4: metabolic alkalosis

IV. ABE considers any alteration in P_{CO_2} and adjusts, so even if the CO_2 is abnormal, the ABE can be relied on to determine the metabolic state

V. HCO_3^- can be used as an indication of metabolic state if the CO_2 is normal
  A. HCO_3^- less than 20: metabolic acidosis
  B. HCO_3^- greater than 26: metabolic alkalosis

OXYGENATION AND ANESTHETIC EQUIPMENT PROBLEMS

I. If patient seems to be poorly oxygenating, it may be because of something as simple as a mechanical problem such as a detached endotracheal tube, disconnected or leaking rebreathing bag, or a kinked or blocked breathing hose or endotracheal tube
  A. The correction for such problems is obvious once the problem is isolated
  B. If the rebreathing bag is empty, the flow rate could be too low or the flowmeter is off
    1. An overdistended bag could be because of a pop-off valve that was inadvertently closed, a flow rate that was too high, or poor scavenging
  C. A leak in the system may be because of a hole in the rebreathing bag or tubing, disconnected or leaking tubes or rebreathing bags, or a problem with the scavenging system

II. If a patient seems "light," the problems may be because of one of the following
  A. An empty vaporizer, one that is not working properly or an inadequate setting
  B. Hoses or attachments that are not properly placed
  C. There may be excessive CO_2 buildup because of an exhausted CO_2 absorbent or sticky unidirectional valves
  D. If the nitrous oxide is set too high relative to the O_2 flow, the patient may be receiving a hypoxic mixture

III. If a patient seems "deep"
  A. The vaporizer may be set too high or not working properly
  B. Patient may be severely hypercapnic or hypoxic or may be hypotensive

IV. Other problems may be clinical problems such as pneumonia, lung pathology, diaphragmatic hernia, and pulmonary edema
  A. These cases may best be handled anesthetically with a neuroleptanalgesic, in which case supplemental O_2 is required, through either a nasal catheter or face mask
  B. If a general anesthetic is used on these cases, oxygenation may be improved by assisting or controlling the ventilation

ACKNOWLEDGMENT

The author and editors recognize and appreciate the original work of Cynthia Stoate, on which this chapter is based.

Glossary

acidosis Increase in acid pH in blood and body tissue
adjusted base excess (ABE) Measures the change in HCO_3^- when the effects of CO_2 are eliminated
agonist Drug that has an affinity for a receptor, thereby producing an effect
alkalosis Increase in base pH in blood and body tissue
analgesia Relief of pain
anemia Decrease in erythrocytes
antagonist Substance that blocks a specific action by binding with the receptor so that the agonist cannot do so
antisialogogic Drug that prevents salivation
apnea Cessation of breathing
arrhythmia Any variation from the normal rhythm of the heartbeat
brachycephalic Breeds with short, wide heads
bradycardia Decreased heart rate
bronchodilators Agents that cause dilatation of the lungs
catalepsy Rigidity of muscles
dysphoria Disquiet, restlessness, or malaise
epidural anesthesia Injection of local anesthetic into the epidural space of the spinal cord
euphoria Exaggerated sense of well-being, absence of pain or stress
hypercapnia Excess of CO_2 in the blood
hypertension Increased arterial blood pressure
hyperventilation Increased rate and/or depth of ventilation leading to a decreased CO_2 level
hypnotic Agent that induces sleep or hypnosis
hypotension Decreased blood pressure
hypoventilation Decreased rate and/or depth of ventilation leading to an increased CO_2 level
hypovolemia Decreased volume of plasma in the body
hypoxia Low O_2 levels in the blood
inotropic Agent that affects the force of cardiac muscular contractions
IPPV Intermittent positive pressure ventilation
minimal alveolar concentration (MAC) Concentration that prevents 50% of patients from responding to painful stimulus
miosis Decreased pupil size
mydriasis Increased pupil size
preemptive Often used in relation to analgesia whereby an agent is given before the procedure to minimize pain and discomfort

subarachnoid Space between the arachnoid and the pia mater. Blocks are produced by injecting local anesthetic into this space around the spinal cord

synergist Agent that acts with or enhances the activity of another

tachycardia Increased heart rate

tachypnea Increased respiration, usually shallow and rapid

urticaria Vascular reaction in the skin resulting in red, slightly raised patches

vasodilation Dilation of a vessel

Review Questions

1 Acepromazine is contraindicated in epileptics because it can
a. Cause hypotension
b. Lower the seizure threshold
c. Not be combined with anticonvulsants
d. Cause catatonia

2 Injectable diazepam is soluted with
a. Hydrogen peroxide
b. Calcium carbonate
c. Propylene glycol
d. Ethyl alcohol

3 If propofol is given to a patient too rapidly, it may cause
a. Profound transient apnea
b. Irritation of the vein
c. A long-lasting excitement phase
d. Seizures

4 A popular induction drug for patients with cardiac disease is
a. Thiopental
b. Lidocaine
c. Innovar-vet
d. Etomidate

5 This inhalant agent requires a special, electrically heated vaporizer.
a. Halothane
b. Isoflurane
c. Sevoflurane
d. Desflurane

6 Nitrous oxide is contraindicated in
a. Orthopedic procedures
b. Painful procedures
c. Pneumothorax
d. Exotics

7 Flowmeters on newer machines have
a. Numbers in imperial and metric
b. A pop-off valve attached to the flowmeter
c. Low and high flowmeters for greater accuracy
d. Alarms for hypoxia

8 Minimally acceptable systolic pressures are
a. 80 mm Hg in dogs and 90 mm Hg in cats
b. 60 mm Hg in dogs and 120 mm Hg in cats
c. 40 mm Hg in dogs and 80 mm Hg in cats
d. 120 mm Hg in dogs and 60 mm Hg in cats

9 Ideally, a smooth induction should bypass
a. Stage 1
b. Stage 2
c. Stage 3
d. Stage 4

10 Which of the following is NOT true of a Doppler?
a. Affordable
b. Can measure systolic pressure
c. Can measure direct arterial pressure
d. Can provide accurate heart rate

BIBLIOGRAPHY

Kirk RW, Bistner SI: *Handbook of veterinary procedures and emergency treatment,* ed 6, Philadelphia, 1995, WB Saunders.

Lumb WV, Jones EW: *Veterinary anesthesia,* ed 3, Baltimore, 1996, Williams & Wilkins.

McCurnin D: *Clinical textbook for veterinary technicians,* 5th ed, Philadelphia, 2002, WB Saunders.

McKelvey D, Hollingshead KW: *Small animal anesthesia and analgesia,* 2nd ed, St Louis, 2000, Mosby.

Muir WW, Hubbell JAE: *Handbook of veterinary anesthesia,* 3rd ed, St Louis, 2000, Mosby.

Sawyer DC et al: *Anesthetic principles and techniques,* 6th ed, East Lansing, 1981, Michigan State University Press.

Short CE: *Principles and practice of veterinary anesthesia,* Baltimore, 1987, Williams & Wilkins.

CHAPTER 20

Pharmacology

Elizabeth Warren

OUTLINE

LEARNING OUTCOMES

After reading this chapter you should be able to:

1. Understand basic classifications of drugs and general characteristics of each type.
2. Understand the importance of proper drug administration and problems associated with incorrect administration.
3. Be aware of common, yet potentially serious, adverse effects that can occur with certain drugs.
4. Explain the processes of drug absorption, distribution, metabolism, and excretion.
5. Be aware of potential human health hazards associated with the handling of certain drugs.

Pharmacology is a science that deals with the origin, nature, chemistry, effects, and uses of drugs. This chapter will review the basic concepts of pharmacology by exploring definitions, pharmacokinetics, and distinctive characteristics of common drugs.

Although veterinary technicians do not, by law, prescribe drugs, they are often responsible for the administration of drugs to animals in the hospital and for dispensing drugs per the veterinarian's prescription. In the hospital ward, the veterinary technician is often the person calculating the amount of drug to give, preparing the dosage, administering the drug, and observing its effects. In the exam room, the veterinary technician often has the first and last contact with the client and patient and should therefore be a source of current drug information.

The tables in this chapter contain examples of common drugs in use in veterinary practice at the time of publishing. For supplementary information, consult a formulary, which contains complete lists of drugs, their major effects, indications, contraindications, and dosages.

DEFINITIONS AND BASIC TERMINOLOGY

I. A drug is "any chemical compound that may be used on or administered to humans or animals as an aid in diagnosis, treatment, or prevention of disease or other abnormal conditions, for the relief of pain or suffering, or to control or improve any physiologic or pathologic condition"[1]

II. A poison is "a substance that, on ingestion, inhalation, absorption, application, injection, or development within the body, in relatively small amounts, may cause structural damage or functional disturbance"[2]
   A. The drugs we use in veterinary medicine to help our patients could very easily become poisons if used inappropriately. All drugs are potential poisons

III. Drugs have a generic name usually derived from the chemical structure of the drug. A single generic drug can have several trade or proprietary names

A. For example, the drug neomycin is the active ingredient in the brand name products Bio-sol, Tritop, Panalog, and Tresaderm

IV. In the United States, drugs are approved by regulatory agencies after rigorous testing and development
   A. Approval is given for the specific doses, indications, and species that are tested
   B. Using a drug in any way other than the approved way is called extra-label use
      1. Veterinarians must often resort to extra-label use when there is no drug available that is specifically labeled to treat the condition diagnosed in a particular patient
   C. The Animal Medicinal Drug Use Clarification Act of 1994 (AMDUCA) provides legal guidelines to veterinarians for extra-label drug use and the American Veterinary Medical Association (AVMA) has produced a brochure explaining those guidelines

V. Drugs are manufactured in many dosage forms
   A. Capsules, tablets, solutions, suspensions, ointments, semisolids, and extracts are all examples of dosage forms
   B. Some drugs, particularly suspensions, are labeled "shake well" because of the likelihood of particulate settling out of solution during storage
      1. In general, it is a good idea to gently mix all solutions by rotating and rocking before administration to ensure proper distribution of the drug particles unless otherwise specified by the manufacturer

VI. Drugs stored in the veterinary hospital must be maintained and handled correctly to ensure their safety and efficacy as well as the safety of staff working with them
   A. Drugs must be stored according to the environmental conditions (temperature, humidity, light exposure), expiration date, and reconstitution recommendations on the label or package insert
   B. A Material Safety Data Sheet (MSDS) must be on file in the hospital for every chemical used in the facility
      1. Some drugs are considered hazardous and have special handling procedures proscribed by the Occupational Safety and Health Administration (OSHA). There are numerous sources for obtaining information about the correct storage, use, and disposal of hazardous drugs

VII. Drugs that have the potential to be abused are called controlled drugs and are under both Food and Drug Administration (FDA) and Drug Enforcement Agency (DEA) regulation
   A. These drugs are classified by the DEA according to their abuse potential and are denoted by the symbols C-I (most abuse potential) through C-V (least abuse potential). Schedule I drugs have no current acceptable medical use and will not be found in veterinary practices
   B. Schedule II drugs are highly regulated drugs that have restricted medical uses, stringent record keeping standards, and specific storage requirements
      1. C-III-V drugs are generally treated in the same way in terms of required record keeping and storage facilities
   C. Canadian Food and Drug Act Schedules specify which drugs are over-the-counter (OTC), prescription, control, and narcotic
      1. Medications requiring prescriptions fall under three Federal Drug Schedules: F (part 1), G (controlled substances), and N (narcotics)

VIII. Drug withdrawal times are important in food animal medicine
   A. Any drug given to a food animal can potentially be transferred to people through ingestion of animal products
   B. Drugs dispensed for food animals have the withdrawal time listed on the label
   C. Many books listing withdrawal times are available to the practitioner
   D. Rules regarding extra-label use of drugs in food animals are more stringent than in companion animals because of withdrawal time regulations

IX. Important information that can be obtained from the package insert or other drug references include
   A. Indications: the approved uses of the drug
   B. Precautions: usually mild side effects or adverse effects (any effect other than the intended effect) that may occur with normal usage
   C. Contraindications: situations in which the drug should NOT be used
   D. Overdose: this section will describe the toxic effects which can occur when too much drug is given or when drug accumulates in the body
   E. Dosage and administration: the recommended amount and route by which the drug should be given

PHARMACOKINETICS

I. A drug must reach its target tissue in the correct amount (within the therapeutic range), which must be maintained for the correct amount of time, to exert the desired effect

II. Proper administration of a drug is critical and must include administering the right drug, at the right time, by the right route, in the right amount, to the right patient. These "five rights" should be verified whenever a drug is administered or dispensed[3]

A. If at any time the medication orders are unclear, double-check them with the attending veterinarian
B. Vials and containers of different drugs and different concentrations of the same drug may have a similar label design. It is best to use the "three checks" system when preparing drugs
   1. Look at the drug name and concentration as you pull the bottle off the shelf
   2. Look again as you are preparing the dose
   3. Check a third time as you are returning the drug to the shelf
C. Watch concentrations carefully. Many drugs come in small animal and large animal concentrations
   1. Administering the correct amount of the incorrect concentration of drug could be a fatal mistake
D. Drugs must be administered at specific time intervals that may vary by route of administration to maintain a therapeutic level
   1. For example, ingesta interferes with the absorption of some drugs so timing doses around mealtimes becomes important
E. Drugs labeled for one route of administration may not be absorbed, and may be dangerous, if administered via other routes
   1. Never give a drug intravenously (IV) unless it is specifically labeled for IV use or the attending veterinarian has verified that route of administration
   2. Drugs are generally administered either orally (PO), by injection (subcutaneous [SQ], intramuscular [IM], and intravenously IV most commonly), topically (skin, eye, ear), or by inhalation

III. Therapeutic index (TI) is "the relationship between a drug's ability to achieve the desired effect compared with its tendency to produce toxic effects"[3]
A. TI is the comparison between a drug's ability to reach the desired effect and its tendency to produce toxic effects
   1. TI is expressed as a ratio between the LD_{50} (dose of a drug that is lethal in 50% of the animals in a trial) and the ED_{50} (dose of a drug that is effective in 50% of the animals in a trial): $TI = LD_{50}/ED_{50}$
   2. The larger the number for the TI, the safer is the drug. Drugs with lower TI numbers, such as those used to treat cancer, tend to be more toxic
   3. The more toxic drugs are usually also more hazardous for veterinary staff to handle

IV. After administration, a drug must make its way to the bloodstream (absorption) and then into the intended tissues (distribution)
A. Absorption and distribution depend on several factors in the body and the drug itself
   1. pKa (ionization tendency) of the drug
   2. pH (acidity or alkalinity) of the tissues
   3. Solubility of the drug
   4. Perfusion of the tissues
   5. Vd (volume of distribution)
   6. Other factors such as the blood-brain barrier
B. Orally administered drugs travel to the liver before reaching the systemic circulation and may be removed before they are able to affect the rest of the body
   1. This is called the first-pass effect

V. When a drug reaches its target tissues it has either a receptor-mediated or a non–receptor-mediated effect
A. Binds to a receptor site and causes the cell to react (agonist) or prevents a reaction (antagonist)
B. Interacts with ions in the body to create a chemical reaction
C. Physical presence of the drug facilitates a reaction

VI. Process of eliminating a drug from the body occurs by biotransformation (metabolism) and excretion
A. Changes in the chemical structure of drugs are caused by the liver and, to a lesser degree, other organs
   1. Resulting drug components are termed metabolites
      a. Occasionally the metabolites of a drug will be more active than the parent compound
      b. In some instances the metabolites may be toxic to the animal
B. Circulating metabolites are usually filtered into the urine through the kidneys, although they may also be excreted in the feces, sweat, or through respiration
   1. Monitoring hydration status becomes critical with drugs such as aminoglycosides, which are nephrotoxic and excreted by the kidneys
   2. Patients with decreased liver or kidney function may not be able to eliminate drugs efficiently
C. Oral drugs that are not absorbed pass through the intestine unchanged and are excreted in the feces

CLASSES OF DRUGS

I. Drugs are divided into different classes according to the effect they have on the body; drugs will often have multiple effects on different body systems

II. One drug may have multiple indications for use
   A. For example, diazepam (Valium) is used as a sedative, an appetite stimulant, and for short-term seizure control

ANTIMICROBIAL DRUGS (Table 20-1)

Antimicrobials are drugs that kill or inhibit the growth of microorganisms such as bacteria, viruses, and fungi. Antimicrobials are classified by the type of organism they fight and whether they kill *(-cidal)* the organism or only prevent its replication *(-static)*. Table 20-1 provides details about some commonly used antimicrobial drugs.

I. Antimicrobials are the most commonly prescribed drugs in veterinary medicine
   A. For an antimicrobial to be effective
      1. Organism must be susceptible to the drug selected
      2. Drug must be able to penetrate the site of infection and achieve an effective concentration for an appropriate length of time to kill or inhibit the organisms

Table 20-1 Antimicrobials

Class	Generic	Trade name(s)	Route(s)	Notes
Aminoglycosides	Amikacin	Amiglyde-V	IV	Keep animal well hydrated; possible nephrotoxic, ototoxic effects
	Gentamicin	Gentocin, Garasol	IV, IM (stings) SC (stings), PO	Keep animal well hydrated; possible nephrotoxic, ototoxic, neurotoxic effects
	Neomycin	Biosol	IV, IM, SC, PO, topical	Not absorbed well systemically; highly nephrotoxic when given parenterally
Penicillins	Amoxicillin	Amoxi-tabs, Biomox	IV, IM, SC, PO	Give with food if gastrointestinal upset occurs
	Amoxicillin w/ clavulanic acid	Clavamox	PO	An alternative for bacteria that have developed resistance to amoxicillin
	Ampicillin	Polyflex, Amoxil	IV (slow), IM, PO	Do not give orally to rabbits
	Carbenicillin	Pyopen, Geopen	IV, IM, PO, intratracheal (birds), aerosol	A penicillin of choice for exotics
	Penicillin G	Crystacillin, Flo-cillin, Dual-Pen	IV, IM, SC, PO	Route of administration depends on drug form (potassium, procaine, benzathine, etc.) Check label and do NOT give cloudy solutions intravenously unless specifically instructed
	Penicillin VK	V-Cillin-K, Pen-Vee K	PO	Best penicillin for oral administration
	Ticarcillin	Ticillin, Ticar	IV, IM, SC	Injectable penicillin often used in combination with aminoglycosides; they should not be mixed in the same syringe
Cephalosporins	Cefadroxil	Cefa-tabs	PO	First-generation cephalosporin; cephalosporins should not be used in patients with known allergy to penicillin
	Cefazolin	Anoef, Kefsol	IV (slow), IM, SC	First-generation cephalosporin
	Cefoxitin	Mefoxin	IV, IM, SC	Second-generation cephalosporin
	Cephalexin	Keflex	PO	First-generation cephalosporin
	Ceftiofur	Naxcel	IM	Third-generation cephalosporin; do not use if precipitate forms that does not dissipate with warming
Tetracyclines	Tetracycline	Panmycin	IV (slow), IM, PO	Tetracyclines may cause tooth discoloration in prenatal and neonatal animals
	Doxycycline	Vibromycin, Doxy 100	IV, PO	
	Oxytetracycline	Oxytet, Terramycin	IV, IM, PO	
Quinolones	Ciprofloxacin	Cipro	IV, IM, SC, PO	Rarely used in veterinary medicine; quinolones as a class should not be used in growing animals due to risk of damage to cartilage
	Difloxacin	Dioural	PO	Veterinary drug; approved for use in dogs, may cause gastrointestinal upset in cats
	Enrofloxacin	Baytril	IM, PO	Veterinary drug; similar to ciprofloxacin with better bioavailability in animals; avoid use in renal failure patients
	Orbifloxacin	Orbax	PO	Veterinary drug
	Marbofloxacin	Zeniquin	PO	Newest veterinary-approved fluoroquinolone

Table 20-1 Antimicrobials—cont'd

Class	Generic	Trade name(s)	Route(s)	Notes
Lincosamides/ macrolides	Clindamycin	Antirobe	IM (stings), SC, PO	Do not administer to rabbits, hamsters, guinea pigs, and horses
	Lincomycin	Lincocin	IV, IM, PO	Clindamycin is usually chosen over lincomycin because it is more bioavailable and less toxic
	Erythromycin	Erythro-100, 200	IV (slow), IM (stings), PO	Enters prostate but not central nervous system
	Tylosin	Tylan Soluable Powder	IM, PO (in food)	Powder form may be used for management of chronic colitis
Sulfonamides	Sulfadiazine/ trimethoprim	Tribrissen, Di-Trim	IV, SC, PO	Can precipitate in the kidneys of dehydrated animals; can cause keratoconjuntivitis sicca
	Sulfadimethoxine	Albon	IV, IM, SC, PO	Sulfas are coccidiostatic
Miscellaneous	Chloramphenicol	Duricol	OIV, IM, SC, PO	Penetrates central nervous system; may cause aplastic anemia in humans; do not give to food animals
	Imipenem-cilastatin	Primaxin	IV, IM	May be useful for serious infections when other antibiotics have failed; must be given parenterally; chloramphenicol may antagonize; read insert for potential adverse effects and contraindications
	Metronidazole	Flagyl	IV, PO	Antiprotozoal; may be neurotoxic and immunosuppressive at higher dosages
Antifungals	Amphotericin B	Fungizone	IV (rapid or slow bolus)	Can cause severe toxicity; should only be used to treat potentially life-threatening disease (systemic mycoses)
	Fluconazole	Diflucan	PO	Probably most useful for central nervous system infections
	Griseofulvin	Fulvicin U/F	PO	Known teratogen in cats
	Itraconazole	Sporanox	PO	Information on safety and toxicity limited
	Ketaconazole	Nizoral	PO	Much less toxic than amphotericin B; used for similar systemic fungal infections
	Nystatin	Panalog, Mycostatin	PO, topical	Used to treat gastrointestinal and skin *Candida* infections
	Miconazole	Monistat-1V	Topical	Used to treat fungal ophthalmic infections
Antivirals	Acyclovir	Zovirax	IV, PO, topical	Used for feline herpes infection and Pacheco's disease in birds
	Interferon-alpha 2A	Roferon-A	PO	For treatment of non-neoplastic FeLV infections in cats

3. Patient must be able to tolerate the treatment

B. Bacterial resistance to antibiotics is a major problem in human and veterinary medicine and can make successful treatment of a bacterial infection very difficult
   1. Resistance is created when bacteria develop the ability to survive in the presence of an antibiotic drug; they pass on this resistance to subsequent generations of bacteria
   2. When treatment with an antibiotic is insufficient to kill off a bacterial population, resistance can result

C. Technicians must educate clients about the importance of administering medications at home as directed and for the entire course prescribed—even if the animal appears to be better after a few days

II. Antimicrobials work via one of five mechanisms

A. Disruption of the development of microbial cell wall (e.g., penicillins)
   1. Interfering with the formation of the cell wall causes the cell to lyse during the growth stage
   2. Giving a bacteriostatic antibiotic (thus stopping bacterial growth) concurrently with this type of medication would prevent it from working

B. Damaging the cell membrane in static/adult populations (e.g., polymyxins)
   1. Change in permeability allows
      a. Drugs to diffuse into the bacterial cell
      b. Bacterial structures to diffuse out, collapsing the cell

C. Interference with microbial protein synthesis
   1. Aminoglycosides are bacteriocidal
      a. They make their way into the bacteria and attach to the ribosomes, rendering the bacteria unable to produce vital proteins

2. Tetracyclines, lincosamides, chloramphenicol, and macrolides use the same method but are bacteriostatic

D. Inhibition of nucleic acid production
1. Because this method interferes with DNA and/or RNA, the potential exists for mutations and birth defects to occur in patients receiving these drugs
2. Griseofulvin, ketoconazole, and metronidazole are drugs that work via this mechanism
3. Enrofloxacin (Baytril) works via this method but is selective for bacterial DNA

E. Disruption of microbial metabolic activity (e.g., sulfa drugs)
1. This usually results in bacteria being unable to divide; therefore such drugs are bacteriostatic

ANALGESIC/ANTI-INFLAMMATORY DRUGS (Table 20-2)

I. These drugs are two separate classes but are used for a similar purpose: pain control

Table 20-2 Analgesics and antiinflammatories

Class	Generic	Trade name(s)	Route(s)	Notes
NSAIDs (nonsteroidal anti-inflammatory drugs)	Acetaminophen	Tylenol	PO	Analgesia; do not use in cat; causes methemoglobinemia and liver damage
	Acetylsalicylic acid	Aspirin	PO	Analgesic, anti-inflammatory, and antipyretic; use with caution in cat; enteric coating can prevent gastric irritation
	Carprofen	Rimadyl	IV, IM, SC, PO	Labrador retriever may be more prone to severe side effects
	Neloxicam	Metacam		Used for chronic or acute musculoskeletal disorders
	Etodolac	EtoGesic, Lodine	PO	Approved for dog only
	Flunixin meglumine	Banamine	IV, IM, PO	May cause gastric ulceration, nephrotoxicity; keep patient hydrated
	Ketoprofen	Ketofen	IV, IM, SC, PO	
	Naproxen	Naprosyn	PO	Analgesic and anti-inflammatory
	Phenylbutazone	Many		Analgesic, anti-inflammatory, and antipyretic
	Piroxioam	Feldene	PO	Use in cat is as an antineoplastic
	Dimethyl sulfoxide (DMSO)		IV, topical	Teratogenic in some species; wear gloves when applying
Corticosteroids	Betamethasone	Betasone	IM	Long acting
	Dexamethasone	Azium, Dexasone	IV, IM, SC, PO	Long acting
	Methylprednisolone	Medrol, Depo-Medrol	IM, SC, PO	Intermediate acting
	Triamcinolone	Vetalog	IM, SC, PO	Intermediate acting
	Prednisone	Meticorten, Deltasone	IV, IM, SC, PO	Intermediate acting
	Hydrocortisone	Cortef	IV, IM, PO	Short acting
Glycosaminoglycans	Glucosamine	Many	PO	Often combined with chondroitin, these agents are considered nutraceuticals, not drugs
	PSGAG	Adequan	IM, IA (intra-articular)	Post injection inflammation possible when administered into the joint
Muscle relaxants	Methocarbamol	Robaxin-V	IV, PO	Skeletal muscle relaxant, may cause sedation
Opioid (narcotic) analgesics	Butorphanol	Torbutrol, Torbugesic	IV, IM, SC, PO	Partial agonist/antagonist; poorly absorbed from gastrointestinal tract; also used as an antitussive
	Buprenorphine	Buprenex	IV, IM, SC	Partial agonist; may cause respiratory depression
	Morphine	Many	IV, IM, SC, PO, rectal	May cause panting, then respiratory depression; Class II controlled substance
	Oxymorphone	Numorphan	IV, IM, SC	May cause respiratory and cardiac depression; Class II controlled substance
	Fentanyl	Duragesic	IV, transdermal	Patch gives about 3 days of analgesia; Class II controlled substance
	Pentazocine	Talwin-V	IV, IM, SC	Partial agonist/antagonist; use in cat is controversial
Local anesthetics	Lidocaine Mepivacaine Procaine Tetracaine	Many	Local infusion	These drugs are used to block nerve impulses from local or regional areas; they are available in injectable and topical forms; epinephrine is sometimes added to extend the effects

II. Examples are opioid (narcotic) analgesics, corticosteroids, and nonsteroidal anti-inflammatory drugs (NSAIDs)
  A. Opioid analgesics include morphine, meperidine, oxymorphone, butorphanol, and codeine
    1. These drugs block the pain impulse in the brain, and therefore reduce the perception of pain, but do not address the cause or source of the pain
  B. Opioids are used frequently as perianesthetic agents because of their analgesic and concurrent sedative effects
    1. A common side effect is respiratory depression, although panting may be seen initially
  C. Dexamethasone and prednisone are two commonly used corticosteroids
    1. Corticosteroids act as analgesics by reducing tissue inflammation
    2. Corticosteroid drugs can have significant effects on the endocrine and immune systems; therefore extra care must be taken with their use
  D. Phenylbutazone, aspirin, ibuprofen, etodolac, and carprofen are examples of NSAIDs
    1. NSAIDs will not produce sufficient analgesia to counteract pain associated with organs or broken bones
    2. Most NSAIDs work by blocking prostaglandin production from within the inflammatory process. They are safer but less effective than steroidal anti-inflammatories
    3. Cats lack the ability to metabolize many NSAIDs; therefore they should be used only with extreme caution on the direction of a veterinarian
  E. Narcotic agonist drugs are competitively antagonized by naloxone (Narcan) and naltrexone (Trexan)

ANESTHETIC DRUGS (Table 20-3) (See also Chapter 19)

I. General anesthetics cause the loss of all sensation
II. General anesthetics are available as injectables and inhalants
III. Overdoses of some general anesthetics are used for euthanasia, although an overdose of any general anesthetic can be fatal
  A. Pentobarbital sodium is the most common euthanizing agent
  B. By itself, pentobarbital is a C-II drug (US-DEA); controlled drug (Canada), but some euthanasia agents contain additives such as phenytoin in Beuthanasia-D or lidocaine in FP–3. These additives act as cardiac depressives and change the DEA status to C-III (U.S.)
    1. Pentobarbital sodium can cause necrosis if injected perivascularly
    2. Perivascular injection will delay or inhibit death
    3. Animals in pain may require a tranquilizer before pentobarbital sodium administration
    4. These products must not be used in food-producing animals

OTHER NERVOUS SYSTEM DRUGS (See Table 20-3)

I. There are many types of drugs having many different effects on the nervous system. They can affect both the central (brain and spinal cord) and the peripheral (autonomic) nervous systems
II. Drugs that affect the central nervous system include anesthetics, analgesics, tranquilizers and sedatives, anticonvulsants, stimulants, and psychoactives. Most of these drugs are controlled
  A. Tranquilizers and sedatives such as benzodiazepines and phenothiazine drugs reduce anxiety, produce a tranquil mental state, and cause sleepiness
  B. Anticonvulsants used to control seizures in progress are administered in the hospital and are relatively short-acting (e.g., diazepam and pentobarbital)
  C. Anticonvulsants used for long-term management of seizure-prone patients are usually given orally at home on a long-term basis (e.g., phenobarbital and potassium bromide)
  D. Doxapram is used to stimulate the respiratory center in the brain
  E. Other stimulants such as caffeine, theobromine, and amphetamines frequently cause toxicities in animals
  F. Drugs are sometimes used to treat behavioral problems in animals
    1. Many of these are human psychiatric medications that have not been approved for use in animals
    2. They may have undesirable side effects and can take a long time to work
      a. Clomipramine (Clomicalm) is a veterinary-labeled tricyclic antidepressant used to treat separation anxiety in dogs
      b. Selegiline (Anipryl) is a veterinary-labeled antidepressant used in the treatment of canine cognitive dysfunction

Table 20-3 Anesthetics and other central nervous system drugs

Class	Generic	Trade name(s)	Route(s)	Notes
Barbiturates	Pentobarbital	Nembutal	IV (slow to effect)	Used for induction of general anesthesia and to manage status epilepticus; can be used as a single agent for euthanasia; Class II controlled substance
	Pentobarbital w/phenytoin	Beuthanasia-D	IV	For euthanasia only
	Thiopental	Pentothal	IV only	May adsorb to plastic intravenous bags and lines
	Thiamylal	Bio-Tal, Surital	IV only	Reconstitution with lactated Ringer's can cause precipitation
Tranquilizers/ sedatives	Acepromazine	Atravet	IV, IM (stings), SC, PO	Do not use in conjunction with organophosphates; may cause paradoxical central nervous system stimulation, hypotension
	Diazepam	Valium	IV, IM, PO, rectal	Used as anxiolytic, muscle relaxant, appetite stimulant, and anticonvulsant
	Medetomidine	Domitor	IV, IM	Used for sedation/analgesia in young, healthy animals; adverse effects such as bradycardia can be treated by reversing the drug
	Midazolam	Versed	IV, IM	May be used in place of diazepam
	Xylazine	Rompun, Anased	IV, IM, SC	Available in 20 and 100 mg/mL; check concentration before administering; respiratory depression and vomiting are common side effects and can be treated by reversing the drug
Inhalants	Halothane	Fluothone	Inhalant	Causes increased cerebrospinal fluid pressure; rarely may cause malignant hyperthermia, hepatotoxicity
	Isoflourane	Aerrane, Forane	Inhalant	Rapid induction and recovery; noxious odor
	Sevoflurane	SevoFlo	Inhalant	Very rapid induction and recovery; no odor
Miscellaneous anesthetics	Ketamine	Ketaset, Vetalar	IV, IM	Dissociative anesthetic; most reflexes and muscle tone are maintained; no somatic analgesia
	Propofol	Rapinovet, PropoFlo	IV only	Rapid induction and recovery; drug is carried in an egg lecithin/soy base, which supports bacterial growth
	Fentanyl/ Droperido	Innovar-Vet	IV (slow), IM/SC (stings)	Fentanyl is an opiate; droperidol is a neuroleptic; used as an analgesic/tranquilizer in dogs
	Tiletamine/ zolazepam	Telazol	IV, IM	Tiletamine is a dissociative; zolazepam is a tranquilizer; most reflexes are retained
Anticonvulsants	Phenobarbital	Luminal	IV (slow), IM, PO	Usual first drug of choice for idiopathic epilepsy; may be used for status seizure
	Bromides	(Potassium, sodium)	PO	Used as an adjunct in management of idiopathic epilepsy
	Diazepam	Diazepam	IV, rectal	Used to control seizures in progress
	Pentobarbital	Nembutal	IV	Used in status epilepticus

III. Drugs that affect the autonomic nervous system can be classified in a highly simplified way by the system they affect

A. Cholinergics produce parasympathetic effects; anticholinergics block them

1. These drugs work by stimulating or blocking different receptors and/or stimulating or blocking various neurotransmitters

a. Examples of cholinergic agents include

(1) Pilocarpine, which reduces intraocular pressure

(2) Metoclopramide, which stimulates the gastrointestinal system

(3) Urecholine, which stimulates the urinary systems

IV. Adverse side effects of cholinergics are related to overstimulation of the parasympathetic nervous system
   A. Anticholinergics have the opposite effects including
      1. Slowing gastrointestinal motility (aminopentamide)
      2. Drying secretions, dilating the pupil, and speeding the heart (atropine sulfate, glycopyrrolate)
         a. Adverse side effects are dose related
            (1) For example, care must be taken not to confuse the large animal concentration with the small animal concentration of atropine sulfate
   B. Adrenergics produce sympathetic effects; adrenergic blockers inhibit them
      1. Adrenergic agents have many diverse effects according to the receptors stimulated
         a. Some of the most common include
            (1) Epinephrine stimulates the heart to beat
            (2) Dopamine is used to treat hypotension/shock
            (3) Phenylpropanolamine is used for urinary incontinence
            (4) Terbutaline and albuterol are used for bronchodilation
            (5) Xylazine and medetomidine are analgesic and sedative agents
      2. Similarly, adrenergic blockers are a diverse group. Some of the more common α-blockers include
         a. Phenoxybenzamine, for vasodilation in the urinary tract
         b. Acepromazine and droperidol, which are tranquilizers
         c. Yohimbine, the reversal agent for xylazine, and atipamezole (Antisedan), the reversal agent for medetomidine
      3. Of the β-blockers, propranolol used for cardiac arrhythmias and cardiomyopathy, and timolol, used to treat glaucoma, are most commonly used in veterinary practice

CARDIOVASCULAR DRUGS (Table 20-4)

Cardiovascular drugs affect the heart. They include antiarrhythmics, diuretics, positive inotropic drugs, catecholamines, and vasodilators. The cardiovascular system is regulated by the autonomic nervous system, and many of the drugs that affect it work by stimulating or blocking nervous impulses.

I. Antiarrhythmics
   A. When arrhythmias occur in the heart, antiarrhythmics restore normal electrical activity
   B. Drugs that work by controlling Na^+ flow include lidocaine and procainamide
   C. Drugs like propranolol, a negative inotrope, work by blocking β-receptors
   D. Verapamil and diltiazem are calcium channel blocker antiarrhythmics

II. Diuretics
   A. Furosemide and mannitol are examples of diuretics
   B. Diuretics create an osmotic force in the renal tubules, thus drawing in water and increasing urine output
      1. Removing water decreases cardiac workload
      2. Use cautiously in hypovolemic or hypotensive animals

III. Positive inotropes and catecholamines
   A. These drugs increase the strength of contraction of the heart
      1. Positive inotropes such as digoxin are used for long-term maintenance of contractility by increasing the amount of calcium available in the heart
      2. Catecholamines such as epinephrine and dobutamine are used for management of short-term increased contractility; they act by mimicking the sympathetic nervous system (adrenergics)

IV. Vasodilators
   A. Nitroglycerin, hydralazine, and enalapril are vasodilators
   B. Vasodilators cause an expansion in the diameter of blood vessel
      1. This increase in diameter allows blood to flow more easily, which in turn reduces the workload of the heart

V. Other cardiac drugs
   A. Aspirin helps to reduce the formation of blood clots
   B. Bronchodilators enable the animal to increase oxygen intake
   C. Sedatives can calm anxious patients, especially those having trouble breathing
   D. Oxygen is almost always an indicated treatment for patients with cardiac disease, but as with all drugs, it can be toxic in excess

RESPIRATORY DRUGS (Table 20-5)

I. Antitussives such as butorphanol and hydrocodone are mild narcotics that suppress the cough reflex

Table 20-4 Cardiovascular drugs

Class	Generic	Trade name(s)	Route(s)	Notes
Inotropic	Digoxin	Lanoxin, Cardoxin	IV, PO	Toxic and therapeutic doses may overlap Dobermans tend to be sensitive to digoxin
	Debutamine	Dobutrex	IV infusion	Use diluted solutions within 24 hours
Adrenergics	Epinephrine	Adrenalin	IV, IM, SC IT (intratracheal) IC (intracardiac) Inhalation	Available in several sizes for various uses: 1:100 (1% or 10 mg/mL) topical, inhalation 1:1000 (0.1% or 1 mg/mL) IV, IM, SC, IT 1:10,000 (0.01% or 0.1 mg/mL) IV, IC
	Isoproterenol	Isuprel	IV (infusion), rectal, sublingual	Do not use with epinephrine
	Dopamine	Intropin	IV (infusion)	Effects are dose dependent
Anticholinergics	Atropine	Many	IV, IM, SC	Used for cardiac support
	Glycopyrrolate	Robinul-V	IV, IM, SC	Used for cardiac support; not suitable for emergency use
β-Blockers	Atenolol	Tenormin	PO	Sympathomimetic drug effects
	Propranolol	Inderal	IV (slow), PO	can be blocked by β-blocker antiarrhythmics
Calcium channel blockers	Amlodipine	Norvase	PO	Use cautiously in animals with heart failure
	Diltiazem	Cardizem	PO	Toxicity may be treated with calcium infusion
	Verapamil	Isoptin	IV	High first-pass effect; watch for toxicity in animals with hepatic disease
Angiotensin-converting enzyme (ACE) inhibitors	Benazapril	Lotensin	PO	For adjunctive treatment of heart failure
	Captopril	Capoten	PO	Use cautiously in animals with renal disease
	Enalapril	Enacard, Vasotec	IV, PO	Give on an empty stomach
Vasodilators	Hydralazine	Apresolene	IM, PO	Use cautiously in patients with severe renal disease
	Nitroglycerin	Nitro-bid, Nitrol	topical	Wear gloves when applying ointment
	Nitroprusside	Nitropress	IV infusion	Adverse effects are due to drug's hypotensive effects
Antiarrhythmics	Lidocaine	Xylocaine	IV	Do not use lidocaine with epinephrine preparations for intravenous solutions
	Procainimide	Pronestyl, Procan	IV, IM, PO	Use with caution with other antiarrythmics
	Quinidine	Quinidex	IV, IM, PO	Use with caution with other antiarrhythmics
Diuretics	Furosemide	Lasix, Disal, Diuride, Salix	IV, IM, PO	Veterinary preparations are normally slightly yellow; if human preparations turn yellow, do not use

A. These drugs are only indicated for patients with a hacking, unproductive cough; dogs with infectious tracheobronchitis (kennel cough) may be treated with cough suppressants

B. Antitussives may be contraindicated with productive coughs due to the risk of accumulation of mucus and debris in the airways

II. Expectorants increase the fluidity of respiratory mucus, making it easier to expel; mucolytics break up mucus, decreasing its viscosity

A. Guaifenesin is a veterinary-specific expectorant

Table 20-5 Respiratory drugs

Class	Generic	Trade name(s)	Route(s)	Notes
Bronchodilators	Albuterol	Ventolin, Proventil	PO, inhalation	Most adverse effects are dose related and generally transient
	Terbutaline	Brethine	SC, PO	
	Aminophylline	Many	IV, IM (painful), PO	Do not inject air into multidose vials; CO_2 causes drug to precipitate
	Theophylline	Theo-dur, Slo-bid	IV, IM, PO	Available in sustained-release oral dose form
Antihistamines	Chlorpheniramine	Many	PO	Do not allow time-released capsules to dissolve before oral administration
	Cyproheptadine	Periactin	PO	Also used for appetite stimulation in cat
	Diphenhydramine	Benadryl	IV, IM, PO	Intravenous form used to counteract anaphylactic reactions
	Hydroxyzine	Atarax	PO	All antihistamines may cause sedation
	Clemastine	Tavist	PO	Do not use the over-the-counter product Tavist-D
Antitussives	Butorphanol	Torbutrol, Torbugesic	IV, IM, SC, PO	Narcotic cough suppressant
	Hycodone	Hycodan, Tussigon	PO	Narcotic cough suppressant
	Dextromethorphan		PO	Non-narcotic cough suppressant; available over-the-counter
Decongestants	Phenylpropana- lamine	Propagest, Pro-in	PO	Most common use in veterinary medicine is to treat urinary incontinence
Mucolytics	Acetyloysteine	Mucomyst	IV, PO, inhalation	Also antidote for acetaminophen toxicity
Stimulants	Doxapram	Dopram	IV, SC	

1. Human OTC expectorants are of little benefit to animal patients

B. Acetylcysteine is a mucolytic that is often administered via nebulization

C. Humidification of inspired air can also increase mucus fluidity

III. Bronchodilators: expand the bronchioles in the lungs, making it easier to breathe

A. Terbutaline, albuterol, and metaproterenol stimulate β_2-receptors in the lung, which in turn cause bronchodilation

B. Theophylline and aminophylline cause relaxation of smooth muscles in the lungs and, in turn, bronchodilation

IV. Other drugs used to treat respiratory problems include antihistamines, corticosteroids, diuretics, and oxygen

A. Antihistamines: also cause bronchodilation if given prophylactically by preventing histamine from affecting the respiratory tract

B. Corticosteroids are given when inflammation of the airways is severe

C. Diuretics help to remove fluid from the lungs

D. Oxygen administration is indicated whenever perfusion is compromised

GASTROINTESTINAL DRUGS (Table 20-6)

I. Emetics cause vomiting

A. Used when noncaustic poisons are eaten or as preanesthetic to prevent aspiration

B. Emetics are locally acting (cause irritation to the GI tract), such as syrup of ipecac and hydrogen peroxide, or centrally acting (stimulate vomiting center in central nervous system) such as apomorphine

II. Antiemetics prevent or decrease vomiting; the choice of antiemetic depends on the cause of the vomiting

A. Chlorpromazine, diphenhydramine, and dimenhydrinate may be used when vomiting is related to motion sickness or vestibular disturbance

B. Metoclopramide causes increased gastric motility

C. Aminopentamide is an antispasmodic

III. Antidiarrheals are used to control frequent loose stools

A. Diarrhea has various causes and treatment depending on the cause

B. These drugs work by modifying intestinal motility; adsorbing enterotoxins, and preventing intestinal hypersecretions

Table 20-6 Gastrointestinal drugs

Class	Generic	Trade name(s)	Route(s)	Notes
Antiemetics	Chlorpromazine	Thorazine	IV, IM, PO, rectal	Protect from light; may discolor urine to a pink or red-brown
	Meclizine	Antivert	PO	Primarily used for motion sickness
	Metoclopramide	Reglan	IV (slow), IM, SC, PO	Promotility agent; inhibits gastroesophageal reflux
	Ondansetron	Zofran	IV, PO	Indicated for refractory vomiting, chemotherapy sickness, and other hard-to-treat nausea
Antiulcer	Antacids	Amphogel, Maalox, Basalgel, Tums	PO	Neutralize acid; can affect absorption rates of other oral medications
	Cimetidine	Tagamet	IV, IM (stings), SC, PO	Oral form available over-the-counter; do not refrigerate injectable form
	Famotidine	Pepcid	IV, IM, SC, PO	Oral form available over-the-counter
	Ranitidine	Zantac	IV (slow), IM (stings), SC, PO	Reduces gastric acid output
	Sucralfate	Carafale	PO	Forms a protective barrier at gastric ulcer site; give 30 minutes before other antacids
	Misoproctol	Cylotec	PO	May cause gastrointestinal side effects such as diarrhea
	Omeprazole	Prilosec	PO	A proton-pump inhibitor, may affect absorption rates of drugs requiring a low stomach pH
Appetite stimulants	Cyproheptadine	Periactin	PO	Appetite stimulation in cat; may take more than one dose to be effective
	Diazepam	Valium	IV	Appetite stimulation in cats; effective immediately after injection; dose is a fraction of that used for sedation
Antispasmodics	Aminopentamide	Centrine	IM, SC, PO	Hypomotility drug; if urine retention noted as a side effect, discontinue
Stimulants	Metoclopramide	Reglan	IV (slow), IM, SC, PO	Do not use if gastrointestinal obstruction is suspected
	Cisapride	Propulsid	PO	Has been removed from U.S. market; used in managment of feline chronic constipation
Laxatives	Magnesium salts	Milk of Magnesia	PO	Hyperosmotic; holds water in gastrointestinal tract and softens stool
	Lactulose	Enulose	PO	Hyperosmotic; also used to reduce blood ammonia levels in hepatic disease
	Docuaste	Colace, DSS	PO, enema	Stool softener; watch hydration status
Antidiarrheals	Diphenoxylate/ atropine	Lomotil	PO	Opiates reduce gut motility; a small amount of atropine reduces other narcotic effects
	Kaolin/pectin	Kaopectate, K-P-Sol	PO	
	Bismuth subsalicylate	Pepto-Bismol	PO	May discolor the stool to black
Emetics	Apomorphine		IV, IM, SC, topically in conjunctiva	If vomiting does not occur with initial dose, subsequent doses are not likely to be effective and may induce toxicity; wear gloves when handling
	Syrup of Ipecac	Many	PO	Do not confuse with extract of Ipecac, which is much stronger; wait for effect of emetics to subside before administering other oral medication such as activated charcoal
Miscellaneous	Ursodiol	Actigall	PO	Used to increase the flow of bile
	Activated charcoal	Toxiban, Liquichar	PO	Adsorbant used to prevent absorption of toxic elements in the gastrointestinal tract

1. Mild narcotics such as loperamide and diphenoxylate are often very effective antidiarrheals
2. Antispasmodics such as aminopentamide are sometimes indicated
3. Protectants and adsorbents such as bismuth, kaolin, pectin, and activated charcoal are generally benign and are sometimes recommended for home use

IV. Laxatives are used to relieve constipation and to clear the lower intestinal tract
   A. Hyperosmotics such as lactulose and magnesium hydroxide draw water to the bowel, where it softens the stool
      1. Fleet enemas should NOT be used in cats
   B. Bulk-producing agents (fiber) help to increase the water content of the stool and stimulate peristalsis in the GI tract
   C. Lubricants such as mineral oil and petroleum make the passage of stool easier
   D. Stool softeners (docusate) allow water to penetrate gastrointestinal contents

V. Antacids increase gastric pH, reducing irritation
   A. Systemic antacids block gastric acid production by one of several means
      1. H-Blockers such as cimetidine, ranitidine, and famotidine prevent the production of hydrochloric acid
      2. Omeprazole is a proton pump inhibitor that prevents hydrogen ions from being pumped into the stomach
      3. Misoprostol inhibits the release of hydrogen ions and stimulates production of bicarbonate and mucus in the stomach

VI. Antiulcer medications are used to treat defects in the stomach lining
   A. Nonsystemic antacids directly neutralize acid in the stomach; usually salts of aluminum, calcium, or magnesium (Maalox, Amphogel, Mylanta, etc.)
   B. Sucralfate is a protectant that binds to the surface of gastric ulcers

ANTIPARASITIC DRUGS (Table 20-7)

I. Antiparasitics kill or inactivate internal and/or external parasites
   A. They may be drugs or insecticides

II. Rotating antiparasitic use can help prevent parasite resistance

HORMONES AND ENDOCRINE DRUGS (Table 20-8)

I. Most reproductive drugs are hormones; these include the estrogens, progestins, prostaglandins, and oxytocin
   A. Estrogens
      1. Commonly used in mismating injections
      2. Interfere with ova by not letting them reach the uterus
      3. Aplastic anemia is one of many rare but serious side effects
   B. Progestins
      1. Used for estrous cycle regulation
         a. If a mare is in transitional anestrus, progestins can return the animal to proestrus
         b. If an animal is in proestrus, progestins can prevent estrus
      2. Liquid progestins can be absorbed through the skin; technicians should use caution and wear gloves when preparing and administering
   C. Prostaglandins
      1. Lyse the corpus luteum
         a. Can initiate a new estrous cycle for animals in diestrus
         b. May cause abortion in pregnant animals and humans
      2. Prostaglandins are easily absorbed through skin; use caution and wear protective apparel
         a. See MSDS or package insert for handling precautions
   D. Oxytocin
      1. Causes uterine contraction and milk letdown
      2. Contraindicated if cervix is not dilated

II. Examples of commonly used endocrine drugs are insulin and thyroid supplements
   A. Insulin
      1. Insulin is measured as international units (IU) per milliliter
      2. Only insulin syringes should be used to measure insulin
      3. Each mark on an insulin syringe is equal to 1 IU
      4. Insulin is available in U-100 and U-40 concentrations
         a. Each concentration has a syringe-type associated with it that must be used to measure that particular concentration. If U-100 insulin is measured in a U-40 syringe the animal will be overdosed by a factor of 2.5
      5. Insulin removes glucose from circulation and stores it in tissues
      6. Insulin is available in three forms
         a. Regular insulin (short acting) is used when a rapid drop in blood sugar is needed
         b. NPH insulin (intermediate acting) is used to control diabetes mellitus on a daily basis

Table 20-7 Antiparasitics

Generic	Trade name(s)*	Route(s)	Efficacy	Notes
Ivermectin	Ivomec, Heartgard+, Iverheart +	IM, SC, PO	Effective against most internal parasites except cestodes and liver flukes; used as a heartworm preventative and microfilariocide	Collies and similar breeds may be sensitive to ivermectin; use with caution and observe for adverse reactions
Selamectin	Revolution	Topical	Dog: adult and developing fleas, heartworms, ear mites, sarcoptic mange Cat: also controls hookworm and roundworms	Safe for Ivermectin-sensitive collies
Moxidactin	Proheart 6	SC	Heartworm preventive	
Milbemycin	Interceptor, sentinel	PO	Heartworm preventive also effective against hookworms, roundworms, and whipworms	May cause shock-like reaction in dogs with large numbers of microfilaria
Lefenuron	Program, Sentinel	SC, PO	Interrupts flea lifecycle	Inhibits chitin production; does not kill adult fleas
Nitenpyram	Capstar	PO	Adult fleas	Kills 98% of adult fleas on pet within 6 hours of administration and for about 24 hours
Fipronyl	Frontline	Topical	Adult fleas and ticks	Transient irritation may occur at site of spot-on administration
Imidacloprid	Advantage	Topical	Adult fleas	May be used weekly for severe infestations
Pyrethrins (permethrin)	Many insect sprays and over-the-counter flea/tick spot-ons	Topical	Insects	Neurotoxin insecticide; many permethrin toxicity cases in cat are due to inappropriate application
Organophosphates	Many (home and yard, area, and pet products)	PO, topical	Many internal and external parasites	Use of or exposure to more than one organophosphate at a time greatly increases the possibility of toxicity; signs of toxicity include salivation, lacrimation, urination, defecation, dyspnea, and emesis
Amitraz	Mitaban	Topical	Demodex mites	Avoid contact with skin; avoid breathing fumes; can be toxic to cat and rabbit
Benzimidazole (mebendazole, fenbendazole, albendazole, etc.)	Panacur, Telmin, Valbazen	PO	Rounds, hookworms, tapes (except *D. caninum*), some lungworms, large and small strongyles	
Epsiprantel	Cestex	PO	Tapeworms	
Metronidazolo	Flagyl	IV, PO	Antiprotozoal	See Antimicrobials
Piperazine	Pipa-tabs (OTC)	PO	Roundworms	
Praziquantel	Droncit, Drontal+	IM/SC (stings) PO	Tapeworms	
Pyrantel	Nemex, Strongid, Heartgard+, Iverheart+	PO	Roundworms, hookworms	Piperuzine antagonizes the effects of pyrantel
Melarsomine	Immiticide	IM only (stings)	Heartworm adulticide	Swelling at injection site common; posttreatment thromboembolism is possible with adulticide therapy; minimize activity after treatment to reduce this risk

*Of products containing this ingredient. Many antiparasities are combination formulas that may contain two or more drugs.

Table 20-8 Hormones and other endocrine drugs

Class	Generic	Trade name(s)	Route(s)	Notes
Estrogens	Estradiol	ECP	IM	Used to prevent pregnancy after mismating in dog and cat; toxic to bone marrow; contraindicated in pregnancy
	Diethylstilbestrol	DES	PO	Used to treat estrogen-responsive urinary incontinence and other conditions in dog and cat; toxic to bone marrow; contraindicated in pregnancy
Progestins	Megestrol	Ovaban, Megace	PO	For false pregnancy, control of estrus cycle; contraindicated in pregnancy; can induce hypoadrenocorticism in cat
	Medroxyprogesterone	Depo-Provera	IM, SC, PO	Used in treatment of some behavioral and dermatologic conditions
Androgens	Testosterone	Danocrine	IM, SC	Testosterone products are now Class III controlled substances with limited use in veterinary medicine
	Mibolerone	Cheque Drops	PO	Prevention of estrus in adult dog; not recommended for cats
Prostaglandins	Dinoprost	Lutalyse	SC	Causes uterine contents to be expelled; pregnant women and asthmatics should handle only with extreme caution
	Fluprostenol	Equimate	SC	For large animal use
	Eleprostenol	Estrumate	SC	For large animal use
Pituitary hormones	Desmopressin	DDAVP	SC, intranasal	An antidiuretic hormone used in control of diabetes insipidis
	Oxytocin	Pitocin	IV, IM, SC	Induction/enhancement of uterine contractions at parturition
Steroids	Corticotropin	Cortrosyn	IV, IM	Used in the ACTH stimulation test
	Fludrocortisone	Florinef	PO	For treatment of hypoadrenocorticism
	Desoxycorticosterone (DQCP)	Percorten-V	IM	For treatment of hypoadrenocorticism
Steroid inhibitors	Mitotane	Lysodren	PO	For treatment of pituitary-dependent hyperadrenocorticism
	Selegiline (l-depranyl)	Anipryl, Eldepryl	PO	For treatment of hyperndrenocorticism; also used in the treatment of canine cognitive dysfunction
Antidiabetics	Insulin	Many	SC	Store in refrigerator; mix gently—do not shake before using; clients should be given thorough instructions on the use of insulin
	Glipizide	Glucotrol	PO	Oral hypoglycemic agent
Drugs affecting thyroid hormone	Levothyroxine	Soloxine, Thyrozine	PO	T_4 thyroid hormone supplement
	Liothyronine	Cytobin	PO	T_3 hormone supplement; may be useful in hypothyroid cases that do not respond to T_4
	Methimazole	Tapazole	PO	Used in the medical managment of hyperthyroidism

c. Protamine zinc insulin (long-acting) is used in animals, usually cats, that need a slower release of insulin to carry them through 24 hours

B. Thyroid supplements
1. The pituitary gland secretes thyroid stimulating hormone (TSH), which tells the thyroid gland to produce and secrete the hormones triiodothyronine (T_3) and thyroxine (T_4)
2. These hormones regulate the metabolic rate for the rest of the body
3. Two common conditions associated with the thyroid gland are hypothyroidism (usually seen in dogs) and hyperthyroidism (usually seen in cats)
4. Hypothyroidism occurs when thyroid function is decreased
a. This can happen when the thyroid gland is diseased (primary hypothyroidism) or when the pituitary gland is diseased (secondary hypothyroidism)
b. Hypothyroidism slows metabolic processes
c. Thyroid supplementation is the treatment of choice for hypothyroidism
d. Synthetic T_3, synthetic T_4, and thyroid extract are the supplementation choices available
(1) Thyroid extract is highly variable in its effectiveness
(2) Oversupplementation is common with T_3 administration
(3) T_4supplements are usually indicated in animals
5. Hyperthyroidism occurs when thyroid function is increased, thus speeding up metabolic processes
a. Thyroidectomy is usually indicated for hyperthyroid treatment
b. Two other courses of treatment are also available
(1) Methimazol (Tapazole), which interferes with the production of T_3 and T_4
(2) Introduction of radioactive iodine, which is taken up by the thyroid gland and destroys any tumor cells (and most of the normal thyroid cells) that are present

IMMUNOLOGIC DRUGS (Table 20-9)

I. The sheer number of vaccines available to induce active immunity limits their discussion in this chapter to general characteristics
A. Vaccines are used to prevent disease or to reduce the virulence of diseases that animals may contract
1. Vaccines cannot cure a disease process that is present before vaccination
B. Vaccines stimulate an animal's immune system by introducing an antigen derived from pathogenic agents and encouraging an anamnestic response
1. Vaccines are described as live, modified live, or killed
2. Killed vaccines are safest but tend to be less effective than the other forms
3. Modified live and live vaccines tend to be more effective, but are also more likely to induce disease and may be dangerous to pregnant animals
C. Vaccines are available in many forms, including injections, intranasal solutions, powdered feed additives, aerosol sprays, and water additives
D. Vaccine efficacy depends on several factors, including dose given, route of administration, age of animal, storage conditions, health/ immune status of animal, and breed/species of animal
E. It is not known exactly when passive immunity via maternal antibodies ceases to protect neonates; therefore multiple doses of vaccine are required at regular intervals to optimize protection for young animals
F. Most vaccines are not effective immediately after administration
1. Some take 2 weeks or more to reach maximum efficacy
G. Warming vaccines just before use reduces pain of administration

II. Vaccines that produce passive immunity by providing the animal with a short-term supply of ready-made antibodies come in two basic forms
A. Antitoxins contain antibodies to specific toxins (e.g., *Clostridium, Tetanus*)
B. Antiserums contain antibodies to specific microorganisms (e.g., *Escherichia coli, Salmonella*)

III. Drugs such as Acemannan (derived from aloe vera), Staphage Lysate, and Immunoregulin may be helpful in stimulating the immune system in certain conditions

IV. Immunosuppressants are used to treat diseases in which the animal's immune system is responding inappropriately
A. Drugs such as azathioprine, cyclosporine, cyclophosphamide, and corticosteroids are used for various immunosuppressive effects

Table 20-9 Chemotherapeutic and immunological agents

Class	Generic	Trade name(s)	Route(s)	Toxicity
Alkylating agents	Carboplatin	Paraplatin	IV	Bone marrow, gastrointestinal
	Cisplatin	Platinol	IV	Bone marrow, gastrointestinal; do not use in cats
	Chlorambucil	Leukeran	PO	Bone marrow, gastrointestinal
	Cyclophosphamide	Cytoxan	IV, PO	Bone marrow, gastrointestinal, hemorrhagic cystitis
Antimetabolites	Cytarbarine	Cytosar-U	IV, SC	Bone marrow, gastrointestinal
	Methotrexate		IV, PO	Bone marrow, gastrointestinal, renal
	5-Fluorouracil		IV	Bone marrow, gastrointestinal, central nervous system; do not use in cats
Antibiotics	Doxorubicin	Adriamycin	IV	Bone marrow, gastrointestinal, cardiac, urticaria, alopecia, vesicant
Mitotic inhibitors	Vincristine	Oncovin	IV	Gastrointestinal, peripheral nervous system, vesicant; skin contact causes irritation
	Vinblastine	Velban	IV	Bone marrow, gastrointestinal, alopecia; vesicant; skin contact causes irritation
Miscellaneous chemotherapeutics	Asparaginase	Elspar	IV, SC	Anaphylaxis, coagulation disorder
	Hydroxyurea	Hydrea	PO	Bone marrow, gastrointestinal, alopecia, dysuria
	Piroxicam	Feldene	PO	Gastrointestinal ulceration
Immunosuppressants	Azathioprine	Imuran	PO	Bone marrow, immunosuppression
	Cyclophosphamide	See above		
	Cyclosporine	Sandimmune	Topical	No significant systemic side effects
	Corticosteroids	See Table 20-2		
	Metronidazole	See Table 20-1		
Immunostimulants	*Acemannan*	Staphage Lysate		*None*
	Staphylococcus phage lysate			Lethargy, fever, chills, injection site irritation
	Propionibacterium acnes	Immunoregulin	IV	Lethargy, fever, chills
	Canine lymphoma monoclonal antibody	CL/Mab 321	IV infusion	Reactions are usually result of infusing drug too rapidly

TOPICAL DRUGS

I. Topical drugs are applied to the skin surface, including mucous membranes, and may be administered otically, ophthalmically, intranasally, sublingually, and vaginally
   A. Generally, topical drugs are not absorbed well systemically
   B. Because veterinary patients tend to lick their wounds, read package instructions carefully
      1. Extra caution is warranted when using human products because they are more likely to be toxic if consumed
   C. Wear proper protective clothing when applying topical drugs that are meant to be absorbed systemically (e.g., nitroglycerin and pour-on preparations)

II. Ophthalmic agents are usually in drop or ointment form and may require multiple applications to be effective. Read the package inserts and advise clients accordingly
   A. Mydriatics such as atropine are used to dilate the pupil
      1. Tropicamide is a rapid-acting mydriatic used in the veterinary hospital to prepare a patient for ocular fundus examination
   B. Miotics such as pilocarpine cause pupillary constriction
   C. Several drugs are used to reduce intraocular pressure and work by either reducing aqueous humor production or having a diuretic effect on the eye
   D. Proparicaine and tetracaine are ophthalmic anesthetics
   E. Cyclosporine stimulates increased tear production
   F. There are numerous ophthalmic anti-infective agents and anti-inflammatory agents

ANTIDOTES AND REVERSAL AGENTS (Table 20-10)

Table 20-10 Antidotes and reversal agents

Generic	Trade name(s)	Uses/indications
Acetylcysteine	Mucomyst	Acetaminophen toxicity
Atipamezole	Antisedan	Reversal of medetomidine (Domitor)
Atropine	Many	Organophosphate toxicity
Calcium EDTA	Calcium Disodium Versenate	Lead poisoning
Dimercaprol	BAL in oil	Arsenic, lead, mercury, gold toxicity
Ethanol	Many	Ethylene glycol toxicity
Flumozenil	Romazicon	Reversal of benzodiazepines (Valium)
Fomepizole (4-MP)	Antizol-Vet	Ethylene glycol toxicity
Methylene blue		Acetaminophen toxicity
Naloxone	Narcan	Opiod agonist reversal
Neostigmine	Stiglyn	Neuromuscular-blocking agent toxicity (pancuronium, succinylcholine)
Penicillamine	Cuprimine	Lead, copper toxicity
Pralidoxime (2-PAM)	Protopam	Organophosphate toxicity
Yohimbine	Yobine	Reversal of xylazine (Rompun)

1. Preparations containing steroids should NOT be used if a corneal ulcer could be present

III. Otic preparations are most often either anti-infective (antibacterial, antifungal, antiparasitic), anti-inflammatory, or a combination
   A. Many of these drugs should NOT be used in the presence of a ruptured eardrum, so an examination is necessary before they can be dispensed
   B. Many are also ineffective in the presence of debris, so the ear canals must be cleaned before medications are used

IV. Drugs used on the skin come in several forms
   A. Shampoos, conditioners, and sprays
   B. Wound-healing agents such as cleansers, protectants, and healing stimulators

CHEMOTHERAPEUTIC DRUGS (See Table 20-9)

I. Antineoplastic agents kill cells. They do not discriminate between "good" cells and "bad" cells or between animal cells and human cells. Therefore it is of utmost importance to wear protective clothing when administering or preparing these agents.
   A. Consult the MSDS, package insert, and hospital procedures manual for information about the safe handling of chemotherapeutic drugs
   B. These drugs target rapidly dividing cells such as tumor cells, bone marrow cells, gastrointestinal cells, and reproductive tract cells
      1. They can cause permanent alterations to DNA
   C. Doses are administered according to body surface (measured in meters squared, not body weight)
   D. There are five basic types of antineoplastic drugs: alkylating agents, antimetabolites, plant alkaloids, antibiotics, and hormonal agents
      1. Chemotherapy is often a scheduled combination or alternation of two or more of these agents, depending on the cancer type and stage
      2. This complicated treatment system is often best left to cancer specialists

II. Hemantics are substances that promote an increase in the oxygen-carrying capacity of the blood
   A. Iron, copper, and B vitamins support the formation of hemoglobin
   B. Erythropoietin is a growth hormone produced by the kidneys that stimulates red blood cell production
      1. A synthetic form is available for injection
   C. Androgens (anabolic steroids), although rarely used because of the problems associated with them, may be beneficial in certain chronic anemias
   D. Blood substitutes such as Oxyglobin can increase oxygen-carrying capacity temporarily while the body grows new red blood cells

III. Anticoagulants such as heparin and coumarin derivatives are sometimes used to treat thrombotic disease in vivo, but anticoagulants in general are more commonly used to preserve blood samples in vitro

IV. Thrombolytics such as streptokinase have largely proved minimally effective and cost-prohibitive in the treatment of thromboembolic disease in animals

SUMMARY

Pharmacology is an inexact science. Any given drug may affect different animal species, or even individual animals within one species, unpredictably. Remember to treat each patient as an individual and pay attention to any abnormal behavior displayed by an animal being treated with any pharmaceutical. Used correctly, drugs are a great benefit to veterinary medicine; used incorrectly they can be equally detrimental.

ACKNOWLEDGMENT

The editors and author recognize and appreciate the original work of Cathy Painter, on which this chapter is based.

Glossary

absorption Movement of drug from the site of administration to the bloodstream

adrenergic Agent that acts like adrenaline (epinephrine)

adverse effect Any effect a drug causes other than the intended effect; may be mild to severe or fatal

agonist Drug that binds to a specific receptor site and causes the cell to react

alkylating agent Compounds that combine readily with other molecules and are used in chemotherapy of cancer

α-blockers Agents that inhibit the activities of α-receptors in the sympathetic nervous system

analgesics Pain relievers

antagonist Drug that binds to a specific receptor site and prevents a cell reaction

antiarrhythmic Agent that prevents or stops cardiac arrhythmias

anticholinergics Drugs that block stimulation of the parasympathetic nervous system; also called parasympatholytics

antiemetic Agent that relieves vomiting

antimetabolite Substance that interferes with the utilization of an essential metabolite

antimicrobial Suppression of microorganism either by killing or stopping the multiplication or growth

antineoplastic Agent that inhibits the maturing and growth of tumor cells

antispasmotic Preventing or relieving spasms

antitussive Cough suppressants

bacteriocidal Kills bacteria

bacteriostatic Prevents the growth or reproduction of bacteria

β-blockers A drug that blocks the action of adrenaline; effects include: increased heart rate and contractions, vasodilation of the arterioles that supply the skeletal muscles, and relaxation of the bronchial muscles

biotransformation See Metabolism

bronchodilator Agent that causes dilation of the bronchi

catecholamine Chemical released by the body to respond to stress

cholinergics Drugs that stimulate the parasympathetic nervous system; also called parasympathomimetics

contraindications Situations in which a drug should NOT be used

DEA, Drug Enforcement Administration (U.S.) Controls drugs that have the potential for abuse

diffusion Process of spreading, especially from areas of greater concentration to areas of lesser concentration

distribution Movement of drug from the bloodstream into tissues

diuretic Drug that promotes water loss via increased urine formation

drug Any substance used in the diagnosis, treatment, or prevention of disease or other pathological condition

ED_{50} Dose of a drug that is effective in 50% of the animals to which it is administered in a trial

efficacy Ability of a drug to create its intended effects

emetic Substance that promotes vomiting

excretion Elimination of circulating drug metabolites from the body, usually in urine, but also in feces, sweat, or breath

expectorant Agent that promotes coughing or swallowing material from the trachea, bronchi, or lungs

extra-label Use of a drug for any other than its indicated uses

first-pass effect Orally administered drugs travel to the liver before reaching the systemic circulation and may be removed before getting into the general circulation

generic Nonproprietary drug name usually derived from its chemical structure

helmintic Pertaining to a parasitic worm

indication An approved use of a drug

ingesta Stomach contents

inotropic Affecting the force of the cardiac contraction

LD_{50} Dose of a drug that is lethal to 50% of the animals to which it is administered in a trial

metabolism Changes in the chemical structure of a drug caused by the liver and, to a lesser degree, other organs from the form in which it was administered to one that can be eliminated from the body

miotic Drug that contracts the pupil

mucolytic Destroying or dissolving mucus

mydriatic Drug that dilates the pupil

OTC (over-the-counter) Drugs that do not require a prescription for purchase

overdose Condition of having too much drug in the body, due to incorrect administration or drug accumulation, which leads to toxicity

parasympathetic Part of the nervous system concerned with maintaining homeostasis

perfusion Passage of blood through the vessels of a tissue

perianesthetic Period of time before, during, and after an anesthetic episode

pH Degree of acidity or alkalinity

pharmacokinetics Study of drug actions and affects on the body

pKa Specific pH at which a drug is equally composed of ionized and nonionized molecules

poison Substance that may cause structural damage or functional disturbance within the body

precautions On a drug label or package insert, usually mild side effects or rare adverse reactions

proprietary Drug name assigned and owned by a particular manufacturer
psychoactive Affecting the mind
resistance Ability of an organism to adapt and survive in an environment containing an antimicrobial to which it was previously susceptible
solubility Ability of a solid to dissolve in a liquid
susceptibility Vulnerability of an organism to an antimicrobial
suspension Solid particles suspended in, but not dissolved in a liquid
TI (therapeutic index) Relationship between ability of a drug to achieve its desired effect compared with its tendency to produce toxic effects
therapeutic range Ideal range of drug concentration in the body, where it is effective but not toxic
thrombolytic Agent that dissolves a blood clot
thyroidectomy Removal of the thyroid gland
vasodilator Causing dilation of blood vessels
Vd (volume of distribution) Body space in which a drug will be distributed; a calculated number representing the amount of drug/amount of body space
withdrawal time Time after administration of a drug to a food-producing animal during which the products of that animal cannot be sold for human consumption

Review Questions

1 Insulin is dosed in what unit of measurement?
   a. mL
   b. tsp
   c. IU
   d. g

2 In what class of drugs are nephrotoxicity, neurotoxicity, and ototoxicity problems?
   a. Barbiturates
   b. Aminoglycosides
   c. Phenothiazine tranquilizers
   d. Dissociative anesthetics

3 With what group of animals is withdrawal time especially important?
   a. Food animals
   b. Exotics
   c. Equids
   d. Pets

4 What is the primary organ involved in excretion of drugs?
   a. Liver
   b. Intestine
   c. Kidney
   d. Spleen

5 A cow is accidentally dosed with an equine dose of xylazine. What drug should be immediately administered?
   a. None: the cow cannot survive that amount of xylazine
   b. Epinephrine followed by naloxone
   c. Yohimbine
   d. Do nothing

6 The therapeutic index is
   a. The comparison between the ability of a drug to reach the desired effect and its tendency to produce toxic effects
   b. The dose of a drug that produces the lethal dose in 50% of the animals tested
   c. The comparison between the ability of a drug to reach a toxic effect and a lethal effect
   d. The dose of a drug that produces the effective dose in 50% of the animals tested

7 The "first-pass effect" is
   a. Blood-brain barrier
   b. Metabolization of drugs containing proteins
   c. Reduction of drugs reaching the systemic circulation by the liver
   d. Ionization of drugs

8 Which drug requires protective clothing when handled?
   a. Xylazine
   b. Torbugesic
   c. Prostaglandin
   d. Lidocaine

9 Vaccines may fail because
   a. Animal is too young for the vaccine to be effective
   b. Vaccine was improperly stored
   c. Animal was febrile at the time of administration
   d. All of the above

10 A dog is seen eating battery acid
   a. Emesis should be induced as soon as possible
   b. Emesis should not be induced
   c. The veterinarian may prescribe a laxative to relieve the dog of the gastrointestinal upset
   d. The veterinarian may prescribe an antacid such as Magnalax or Maalox

REFERENCES

1. Taylor EJ, editor: *Dorland's illustrated medical dictionary,* ed 27, Philadelphia, 1988, WB Saunders.
2. O'Toole M, editor: *Miller-Keane encyclopedia and dictionary of medicine, nursing, and allied health,* ed 5, Philadelphia, 1992, WB Saunders.
3. Wanamaker B, Pettes CL: *Applied pharmacology for the veterinary technician,* ed 2, Philadelphia, 2000, WB Saunders.

BIBLIOGRAPHY

Allen DG et al: *Handbook of veterinary drugs,* ed 2, Philadelphia, 1998, Lippincott-Raven.
Bill R: *Pharmacology for veterinary technicians,* ed 2, St Louis, 1997, Mosby.
Fraser CM, editor: *The Merck veterinary manual,* ed 7, Rahway, NJ, 1991, Merck & Co, Inc.
McCurnin DM, Bassert JM: *Clinical textbook for veterinary technicians,* ed 5, Philadelphia, 2002, WB Saunders.
Muir W, Hubbell J et al: *Handbook of veterinary anesthesia,* ed 3, St Louis, 2002, Mosby.
O'Toole M, editor: *Miller-Keane encyclopedia and dictionary of medicine, nursing, and allied health,* ed 5, Philadelphia, 1992, WB Saunders.

Plumb D: *Veterinary drug handbook,* ed 3, Ames, 1995, Iowa State University Press.

Pratt PW: *Principles and practice of veterinary technology,* St Louis, 1998, Mosby.

Rawlings CA, McCall JW: Melarsomine: a new heartworm adulticide, *Compendium,* April:373, 1996.

Taylor EJ, editor: *Dorland's illustrated medical dictionary,* ed 27, Philadelphia, 1988, WB Saunders.

Wanamaker B, Pettes CL: *Applied pharmacology for the veterinary technician,* ed 2, Philadelphia, 2000, WB Saunders.

CHAPTER 21

Pharmaceutical Calculations

Monica M. Tighe

OUTLINE

LEARNING OUTCOMES

After reading this chapter you should be able to:

1. Describe the rules for writing metric, dates, and symbols.
2. Perform conversion of numbers to various metric units.
3. Calculate dosages.
4. Calculate dilutions.
5. Calculate concentrations of solutions.
6. Describe parts per million and calculate a parts per million dose.
7. Calculate drip rates.
8. Define the technician's role in dispensing medication.
9. Define the information that must be included on a prescription label.

This chapter contains basic information on the metric system, including the conversion of metric units. Formulas for calculating dosages, preparing solutions and dilutions, and estimating drip rates are also included with examples. This chapter also includes a brief section on prescription labels, an abbreviations list, and an equivalent chart. Check appendixes for further information.

METRIC SYSTEM

The metric systeme can also be referred to as the SI system, or Système International d'Unités.

Metric Conversions

I. Abbreviations of commonly used units are shown in Table 21-1. The prefix and a base unit are also shown

II. Metric unit conversion methods
   A. Step method
      1. Move the decimal place to the right if converting to a smaller unit and to the left if converting to a larger unit
      2. Example: to convert 500 milligram (mg) to gram (g)
         a. As shown in Table 21-2, 1 mg × 1/1000 of a gram
         b. Therefore the decimal must move 3 decimal places
         c. Also, 1 g is larger than 1 mg—therefore the decimal place must move to the left
         d. The answer is 0.5 g
   B. Proportion equation
      1. Example: to convert 500 mg to g
         a. According to the chart, 1 g = 1000 mg
         b. Therefore x g/500 mg = 1 g/1000 mg
         c. (x = unknown number)

$$\frac{x\text{g}}{500\text{ mg}} = \frac{1\text{g}}{1000\text{ mg}}$$

$$1000\text{ mg} \times x\text{g} = 500\text{ mg} \times 1\text{g}$$

$$x = 500\text{ mg} \times 1\text{g} \div 1000\text{ mg}$$

$$x = 0.5\text{ g}$$

Metric Date

I. A metric date is written in the following format: year/month/day/time (24-hour clock)

Table 21-1 Prefix, abbreviation, and a base unit for metric units

Prefix	Symbol	Value
giga	G	base unit × 10^9 Largest unit
mega	M	base unit × 10^6
kilo	k	base unit × 10^3
hecto	h	base unit × 10^2
deca	da	base unit × 10
Base unit		
gram	g	
meter	m	1
liter	L	
deci	d	base unit × 10^{-1}
centi	c	base unit × 10^{-2}
milli	m	base unit × 10^{-3}
micro	µ	base unit × 10^{-6}
nano	n	base unit × 10^{-9}
pico	p	base unit × 10^{-12} Smallest unit

Table 21-2 Common medical units and conversions

Unit	Value
liter (L) to milliliter (mL)	1 L = 1000 mL
gram (g) to milligram (mg)	1 g = 1000 mg
milliliter (mL) to microliter (uL)	1 mL = 1000 µL
meter (m) to centimeter (cm)	1 m = 100 cm
kilometer (km) to meter (m)	1 km = 1000 m
microgram (ug) to milligram	1 µg = 0.001 mg

A. Example: January 24, 2003, 5:50 PM, is written 2003/01/24 17:50

II. There may be a slash, dot, or space between the numbers

III. In the United States the date is commonly written month/day/year
   A. Example: 01/24/03

Metric Time

I. Measured in hours, minutes, and seconds using a 24-hour clock
   A. The 24-hour clock expresses the time in four digits beginning at midnight with 00:00 or 24:00
      1. The first two digits express the number of hours since midnight, and the second two digits express the number of minutes in that hour
   B. Example: The time at 2:53 PM is written 14:53
      1. There is no need to write AM or PM because it is expressed in the value of time

Metric Temperature

I. Celsius or C (Capital C)
   A. Freezing point = 0° C at 1 atmospheric pressure
   B. Boiling point = 100° C at 1 atmospheric pressure

II. Fahrenheit or F
   A. Freezing point = 32° F at 1 atmospheric pressure
   B. Boiling point = 212° F at 1 atmospheric pressure

III. To convert from ° C to ° F use the formula
   A. ° F = ° C × 9/5 + 32

IV. To convert from ° F to ° C use the formula
   A. ° C = ° F – 32 × 5/9

Metric Mass

I. Gram (g) is the standard unit

II. Nonmetric unit is the pound (lb)

III. 1 kg = 2.204 lb

IV. To convert lb to kg
   A. kg = lb ÷ 2.204

V. To convert kg to lb
   A. lb = kg × 2.204

VI. One ton = 1000 kg or 2204 lb

DOSAGE CALCULATIONS

I. Definitions
   A. Dose is the amount of medication measured (i.e., mg, mL, units, etc.)
   B. Dosage is the amount of medication based on units per weight of animal (i.e., 50 mg/kg, mL/kg, or tablets/kg)
   C. The concentration of a drug is calculated by the manufacturer (i.e., mg/mL, mg/tablet)

II. To calculate the dose in milligrams (mg) use the following formula
   A. Dose (mg) = weight (kg) × dosage (mg/kg)
   B. Example: What is the dose if a patient weighs 30 kg and the dosage is 10 mg/kg?
   C. Dose (mg) = 30 kg × 10 mg/kg
   D. Therefore dose = 300 mg

III. To calculate the dose in mL use the formula
   A. Dose (mL) = dose (mg) ÷ concentration (mg/mL)
   B. Example: What is the dose in milliliters (mL) of a drug if the dose is 300 mg and the concentration of the drug is 50 mg/mL?
   C. Dose (mL) = dose (mg) ÷ concentration (mg/mL)
   D. Therefore dose = 300 mg ÷ 50 mg/mL = 6 mL

IV. To calculate the dose in tablets use the formula:
   A. Dose (tablets) = dose (mg) ÷ concentration (mg/tablet)
   B. Example: What is the dose (in tablets) of a drug if the required dose is 100 mg and the concentration of the drug is 50 mg/tablet?
   C. Dose (tablets) = dose (mg) ÷ concentration (mg/tablet)

D. Dose = 100 mg ÷ 50 mg/tablet = 2 tablets

V. Because drugs are manufactured in various concentrations, the milligram dose of a drug should always be recorded on the patient file (rather than the administered dose or mL/tablets)
   A. Example: 1 mL of acepromazine maleate is administered to a patient. If the concentration of acepromazine maleate is 10 mg/mL, the patient will receive 10 mg of the drug. However, if the concentration of acepromazine maleate was 25 mg/mL, and the patient was administered 1 mL, the patient would have received 25 mg, or 2.5 times the prescribed amount

DILUTIONS/SOLUTIONS

I. Definitions
   A. Solution: mixture of substances made by dissolving solids in liquid or liquids in liquids
   B. Solvent: solution capable of dissolving other substances
   C. Solute: substance that is dissolved in a liquid
   D. Dilution: reduction of a concentration of a substance
   E. Diluent: agent that dilutes

II. When working with solutions/dilutions, the concentration of the substance is the amount of solute dissolved in the solvent

III. Concentrations may be expressed as
   A. Volume per volume (or v/v) for liquids: percent volume in volume expresses the number of milliliters of solute in 100 mL of solution
   B. Weight per volume (or w/v): percent weight in volume expresses the number of grams (weight) of solute in 100 mL of solution (volume)
   C. Weight per weight (or w/w) for solids: percent weight in weight expresses the number of grams of a solute in 100 g of solution

IV. Calculating the percent strength of a solution (w/v)
   A. Use the formula: concentration (g/mL) = mass (g) ÷ volume (mL)
   B. Example: What is the strength of a solution if 20 g of powder is dissolved in 500 mL of liquid?
      1. Concentration (g/mL) = mass (g) ÷ volume (mL)
      2. Concentration = 20 g ÷ 500 mL = 0.04
      3. To find percent multiply the concentration by 100 (0.04 × 100 = 4%)
   C. Any of the quantities can be substituted in the equation (i.e., mass or volume or percent)
      1. Variations in the formula include
         a. Mass (g) = volume (mL) × concentration (g/mL)
         b. Volume (mL) = mass (g) ÷ concentration (g/mL)
   D. Percent (w/v) means that there are a number of grams of solute in 100 mL of solution
      1. Example: A 5% (w/v) solution means that there are 5 g of solute in 100 mL of solution
      2. A pure solution is assumed to be 100% or 100 g of solution in 100 mL of solution
   E. Concentration of a solution can also be expressed as a ratio
      1. 1:100 = 1 g/100 mL = 1% = 10 mg/mL

V. Calculating the strength of diluted solutions (v/v)
   A. If a pure solution is diluted, the result is a stock solution
   B. A weaker solution can be made by diluting it with solvent; however, a stronger solution requires the preparation of a new solution or the addition of pure solution
   C. Use the formula

Concentration of desired solution × volume of desired solution = concentration of stock × volume of stock

   D. Example: Prepare 2 L of a 25% solution given a 50% solution and sterile saline
      1. Substitute all known quantities and solve for the unknown *(x)*
         a. Concentration of desired solution is 25%
         b. Volume of the desired solution is 2000 mL or 2 L
         c. Concentration of the stock solution is 50%
         d. Volume of stock solution needed to prepare the solution is the unknown *(x)*

Concentration of desired solution × volume of desired solution = concentration of stock × volume of stock

$$25\% \times 2000 \text{ mL} = 50\% \times x$$
$$25 \times 2000 = 50x$$
$$50{,}000 = 50x$$
$$50{,}000 \div 50 = x$$
$$1000 \text{ mL of the } 50\% \text{ solution} = x$$

         e. To calculate amount of sterile saline or diluent to add to the 1000 mL of 50% solution to make 2000 mL of 25% solution
            (1) Use the formula: Diluent = volume of desired solution − volume of stock solution 2000 mL − 1000 mL = 1000 mL
            (2) Thus 1000 mL of 50% solution is added to 1000 mL of diluent to prepare 2000 mL of 25% solution

PARTS PER MILLION (PPM)

I. Parts per million (ppm) is defined as the number of parts of solute contained in 1 million parts of solution. One part per million is 1 g solute in 1,000,000 mL or 1 part/10^6

A. Example: What is the ppm for a 0.6% solution?

B. Knowing that a 0.6% solution = 0.6 g/100 mL = x/1,000,000
   1. 0.6 g × 1000000 = 100 mL × x
   2. x = 0.6 × 1,000,000 ÷ 100
   3. x = 6000 ppm

DRIP RATES

I. Use this formula

$$\text{Drip rate} = \frac{\text{Volume of solution (mL)} \times \text{drops/mL}}{\text{time (seconds)}}$$

A. Volume of solution (mL) is the amount of solution to be administered

B. Drops/mL is the calibrated amount of an administration set determined by the company that produces it
   1. The drop/mL value is usually written on the administration set package

C. Time (seconds) is the amount of time that the fluids are to be administered
   1. Time could be expressed as seconds, minutes, or hours; however, the drip rate is usually expressed as drops/min
   2. To calculate how many minutes there are in a value expressed in seconds, divide the seconds by 60

D. Drip rate (drops/min) is the amount of drops that are administered per 1 minute

E. Example: What is the drip rate if the volume of the solution is 1 L, the drops/mL = 20, and the time is 4 hours?

$$\text{Drip rate} = \frac{1000 \text{ mL} \times 20 \text{ drops/mL}}{4 \text{ hours} \times 60 \text{ minutes}}$$

(There are 60 minutes in 1 hour)

$$= \frac{20{,}000 \text{ drops}}{240 \text{ minutes}}$$

$$= 83.33 \text{ drops/min}$$

II. Variations on the formula include

A. Time = (volume × drops/mL) ÷ drip rate
   1. Example: How long will it take for 2 L of normal saline to be administered to a patient if the drops/mL is equal to 20 and the drip rate is 60 drops/min
   2. Time = 2 L × 20 drops/mL ÷ 60 drops/min
   3. Before continuing, 2 L must be converted to 2000 mL
   4. Therefore time = 2000 mL × 20 drops/mL ÷ 60 drops/min
   5. Time = 40,000 drops ÷ 60 drops/min
   6. Final answer is time = 666.666 minutes = 11.11 hours = 11 hours 6.6 minutes

B. Volume = (drip rate × time) ÷ drops/mL
   1. Example: How much normal saline can be administered if the drip rate is 60 drops/min, the veterinarian would like the patient to receive the fluids in 4 hours, and the drops/mL is equal to 20?
   2. First convert the time of 4 hours to 240 minutes
   3. Volume = 60 drops/min × 240 minutes ÷ 20 drops/mL
   4. Volume = 14,400 drops ÷ 20 drops/mL
   5. Volume = 720 mL = 0.720 L

PRESCRIPTIONS

Guidelines

I. The American Veterinary Medical Association (AVMA) has approved the following guidelines

A. "A prescription drug can only be dispensed by or upon the lawful written order of a licensed veterinarian within the course of his or her professional practice where a valid veterinarian-client-patient relationship (VCPR) exists
   1. A VCPR exists when the following conditions have been met
      a. The veterinarian has assumed the responsibility for making clinical judgments regarding the health of the patient and the need for medical treatment, and the client has agreed to follow the veterinarian's instructions
      b. The veterinarian has sufficient knowledge of the animal to initiate at least a general or preliminary diagnosis of the medical condition of the animal
      c. The veterinarian is readily available for follow-up evaluation or has arranged for emergency coverage in the event of adverse reactions of failure of the treatment regimen

B. All veterinary prescription drugs must be properly labeled when dispensed" (McCurnin and Bassert, 2002, p 551)

Veterinary Technician's Role in Dispensing Medications

I. The technician should not issue or refill medications without the veterinarian's approval

A. If medication is dispensed by a technician, this is in violation of federal law

II. The ultimate responsibility for any medication dispensed lies with the prescribing veterinarian

Table 21-3 Abbreviations commonly used in veterinary medicine

Abbreviations	Definition
ad lib.	Freely; as much as is wanted
$\overline{aa}$	Of each
a.c.	Before meals
aqua	Water
aqua dist.	Distilled water
at diet.	As directed
b.i.d.	Twice daily
caps	Capsules
chart.	Powder
$\bar{c}$	With
cc	Cubic centimeter
d.t.d.	Give such doses
D_5W	5% Dextrose in water
gtt	A drop; drops
h	Hour
h.s.	Hour of sleep; at bedtime
IM	Intramuscular
IV	Intravenous
K	Potassium
M	Mix
non. rep. or N.R.	Do not repeat
No.	Number
o.h.	Every hour
O.D.	Right eye
O.S.	Left eye
os	Mouth
per os	Oral
pil.	Pill
p	After
p.c.	After meals
p.o.	By mouth
p.r.n.	According to circumstances; occasionally
q.2h	Every 2 hours
q.s.	A sufficient amount
q.i.d.	Four times a day
Q.R.	Quantity required
R_x	Dispense
SC	Subcutaneous
sq	Subcutaneous
ss	One-half
s.i.d.	Once daily
sig.	Write on label
s	Without
S_x	Surgery
stat	Immediately
T_x	Treatment
tab	Tablet
t.i.d.	Three times a day
Tr.	Tincture
Ung.	Ointment

Sometimes these abbreviations are written without periods: for example, bid or po.

A. Technicians may prepare labels, count tablets or pour medication, attach labels, and price the dispensed medication

Prescription Labels

I. Even though most prescription labels are now generated by a computer, the label should be checked for accuracy before dispensing the drug

II. The label should contain the following information
   A. Name, address, and telephone number of clinic
   B. Prescribing veterinarian's name
   C. Name of patient and client's last name (the species in some provinces/states)
   D. Name of drug
   E. Concentration of drug and amount of drug dispensed
   F. Date
   G. The drug identification number (DIN) (check provincial/state regulations to determine if required)
   H. Refills should be noted
   I. Specific instructions (Sig)
      1. No abbreviations should be used (Table 21-3)
         a. Example: b.i.d. should be written two times a day or every 12 hours
      2. If the medication is for the left or right eye, it should be noted on the label
      3. If the drug should be administered with food or without food, it should also be noted
      4. The instructions should be clearly typed
   J. The vial may also need additional labels such as
      1. *For veterinary use only*
      2. *Keep refrigerated*
      3. *Keep out of reach of children*
      4. *Withdrawal time*
      5. *Shake well*
      6. *Do not use after* [date]
      7. *Poison*
      8. *External use only*
   K. A childproof container may be necessary in some states/provinces due to state/provincial laws
      1. The vial may also need to be amber in color to prevent the breakdown of some drugs due to ultraviolet light

III. Also see Appendixes A and B for further information

Review Questions

1 How much sterile water is needed to make a 4% solution using 1 g of drug?
a. 25 mL
b. 400 mL
c. 100 mL
d. 50 mL

2 Convert 6 µm to m
a. 0.006 m
b. 0.000006 m
c. 6000 m
d. 600 m

3 Given a 45% solution and sterile diluent, how would you prepare 3 L of 15% solution?
a. Take 200 mL of 45% and add 2000 mL of sterile diluent
b. Take 1000 mL of sterile diluent and add 2 L of 45% solution
c. Take 1000 mL of 45% solution and add 2 L of sterile diluent
d. Take 2 L of water and add 4.5 L of 45% solution

4 A previous client calls to report that their new pet needs some antibiotics. They will be by in 1 hour to pick up the prescription. What should the technician do?
a. Explain to the client that a veterinarian must examine the animal first before any medication can be dispensed
b. Explain to the client that a technician cannot dispense medication and suggest that the client speaks with the veterinarian
c. Explain to the client that antibiotics require a prescription to be dispensed
d. All of the above

5 Given the following information: 1987 mL of saline at 15 drops/mL over an 8-hour period, the approximate drip rate should be
a. 10.3/10 sec
b. 1.05/10 sec
c. 20/10 sec
d. 1.92/sec

6 Given a pure solution, how would you make 500 mL of 50% solution?
a. Add 500 mL of 100% solution to 500 mL of water
b. Add 100 mL of sterile water to 400 mL of pure solution
c. Add 5000 mL of sterile water to 500 mL of 50% solution
d. Take 250 mL of pure solution and add 250 mL of sterile water

7 What is the concentration (mg/mL) and percentage of the following solution (w/v): 5 g added to 200 mL of sterile water
a. 25 mg/mL, 2.5%
b. 250 mg/mL, 2.5%
c. 50 mg/mL, 5%
d. 4 mg/mL, 40%

8 What is the percent of the final solution (v/v) if 30 mL of solution is added to 70 mL of water?
a. 30%
b. 100%
c. 10%
d. 3%

9 A dog weighs 20 kg, the dose rate is 5 mg/kg, and the tablet size is 50 mg. The prescription reads "100 mg bid for 10 days a.c." How many tablets are needed for 1 dose and for a 24-hour period?
a. 2 tablets, 8 tablets
b. 1 tablet, 2 tablets
c. 2 tablets, 4 tablets
d. 4 tablets, 8 tablets

10 How would you prepare 1.5 L of a 1:200 (w/v) solution given a 12% solution and sterile water?
a. Take 625 mL of the 12% solution and add 875 mL of sterile water
b. Take 1437.5 mL of the 12% solution and add 62.5 mL of sterile water
c. Take 62.5 mL of the 12% solution and add 1 437.5 mL of sterile water
d. Take 875 mL of 12% solution and add 635 mL of sterile water

BIBLIOGRAPHY

Bill RL: *Medical mathematics and dosage calculations,* Ames, 2000, Iowa State University Press.

Bill RL: *Pharmacology for veterinary technicians,* St Louis, 1997, Mosby.

McConnell VC, Ritchie BW: *Calculations for the veterinary professional,* Ames, 2000, Iowa State University Press.

McCurnin DM, Bassert JM: *Clinical textbook for veterinary technicians,* ed 5, Philadelphia, 2002, WB Saunders.

Petrie A, Watson P: *Statistics for veterinary and animal science,* Oxford, 1999, Blackwell Science.

Pratt PW: *Principles and practice of veterinary technology,* St Louis, 1998, Mosby.

Stoklosa MJ, Ansel HC: *Pharmaceutical calculations,* ed 8, Philadelphia, 1986, Lea & Febiger.

PART V

Medical and Surgical Nursing

CHAPTER 22

Surgical Preparation and Instrument Care

Melanie K. Gramling

OUTLINE

LEARNING OUTCOMES

After reading this chapter you should be able to:

1. Recognize common surgical instruments and define their intended use.
2. Identify types of surgical needles.
3. Identify suture material.
4. Understand the sizing of suture material.
5. Describe proper instrument care.
6. Describe pack preparation for sterilization.
7. Understand the principles of sterilization monitors.
8. Describe aseptic technique while performing a patient surgical preparation and patient positioning.
9. Describe how to maintain asepsis in a surgical suite.
10. Describe correct surgical scrubbing and conduct in the operating room.
11. List possible duties of a sterile surgical assistant.

This chapter contains basic information on identification of instruments, instrument care, and sterile technique. The chapter also includes a summary of aseptic patient preparation, pack preparation, and preparation of the surgical suite.

Acting as sterile assistant to a surgeon or as a circulating nurse during surgery is an important aspect of the veterinary technician's role in a veterinary hospital. These concepts are not only learned and memorized but by experience become second nature.

SURGICAL INSTRUMENTS

The veterinary technician should be familiar with basic surgical instruments and their intended use (Figure 22-1). The following are some common instruments used in veterinary surgery.

Scissors

I. Operating scissors are for the general purpose of cutting suture and drape material and are classified in three ways
   A. Type of point (e.g., blunt/blunt, sharp/blunt, or sharp/sharp)
   B. Shape of the blade (e.g., straight or curved)
   C. Cutting edge (e.g., plain or serrated)

II. Mayo scissors work well for cutting and dissecting dense tissue (Figure 22-2)

III. Metzenbaum scissors have fine tips and long handles for cutting and dissecting more delicate tissue

IV. Iris scissors are small, sharp, delicate scissors commonly used for intraocular surgery

V. Wire-cutting scissors have short, thick jaws with serrated edges for cutting wire suture material

VI. Littauer and Spencer suture removal scissors are used to cut and remove sutures postoperatively
   A. Blunt tips with one blade terminating into a thin curved hook

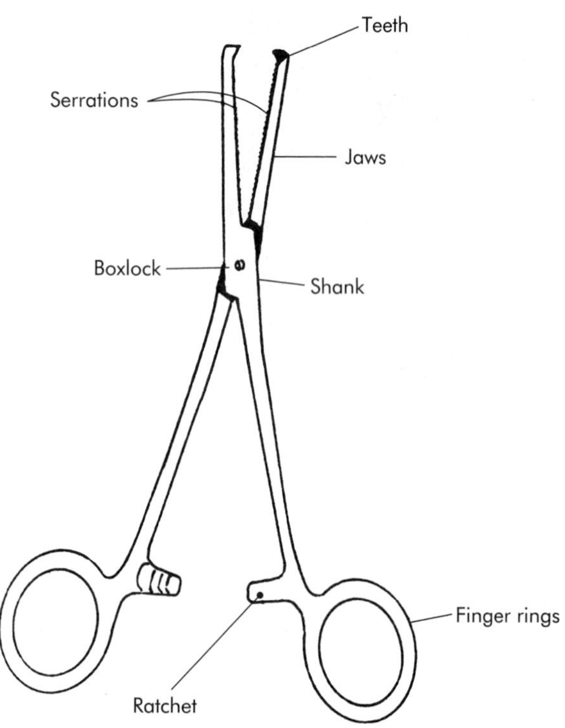

Figure 22-1 Parts of surgical instruments. (Courtesy The Ohio State University. In Tracy DL: *Small animal surgical nursing,* ed 3, St Louis, 2000, Mosby.)

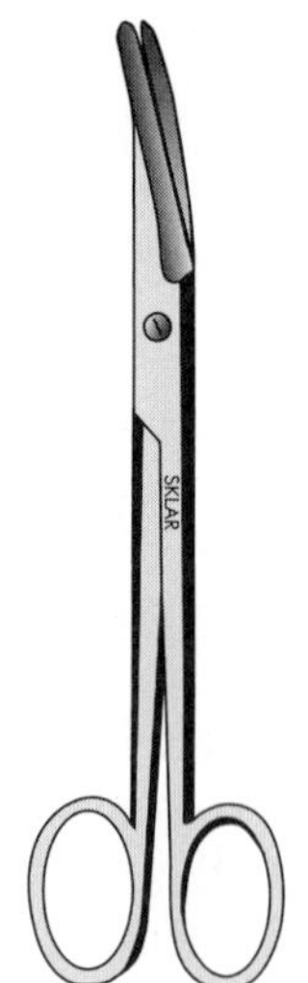

Figure 22-2 Mayo dissecting scissors.

B. Spencer scissors are smaller than Littauer scissors

VII. Lister bandage scissors are used to cut under a bandage without puncturing the patient's skin (Figure 22-3)
   A. One blade has a flat, thick edge and a blunt tip
   B. Available in various sizes

Forceps

I. Thumb forceps are hand held in a pencil grip to hold tissue
   A. Adson tissue forceps provide good tissue grip with minimal damage to tissue due to tiny "rat tooth" tips
   B. Brown-Adson tissue forceps have multiple fine intermeshing teeth on edges of the tips (Figure 22-4). The sides of the blades are wider for ease of handling
   C. Dressing forceps have serrations but no teeth on the jaws; they are useful for handling dressing material
   D. Russian tissue forceps have rounded tips and are used for holding hollow viscera

II. Self-retaining forceps use a ratchet-locking device to grasp and retract tissue
   A. Allis tissue forceps have intermeshing teeth that ensure a secure grip
   B. Babcock tissue forceps are similar to the Allis forceps but have no gripping teeth
   C. Doyen intestinal forceps are useful for holding bowel
   D. Ferguson angiotribe forceps assist in holding large bundles of tissue
   E. Sponge forceps have a hole in the center of its circular tips and hold gauze to provide hemostasis during surgery or when performing patient preparation
   F. Backhaus towel clamps are considered forceps and are used to secure drapes to the patient's skin (Figure 22-5)

III. Hemostatic forceps can be straight or curved and are used for ligating vessels and tissues
   A. Halsted mosquito forceps control capillary bleeders (Figure 22-6)
      1. Length: up to 10 cm (4 inches)
      2. Transverse serrations cover the entire jaw length
   B. Kelly and Crile forceps are used to grasp intermediate-size vessels
      1. Standard length: 12.5 cm (4.5 in)
      2. Kelly forceps have distal transverse grooves
      3. Crile forceps have complete transverse grooves
   C. Rochester-Pean and Rochester-Carmalt forceps are commonly used in stump and pedicle ligation (Figure 22-7)
      1. Larger forceps 20 cm (9 inches)
      2. Carmalts have longitudinal grooves and distal transverse grooves
      3. Peans have transverse grooves
   D. Rochester-Oshner forceps are similar to Rochester-Pean but in addition have 1:2 teeth at the tips

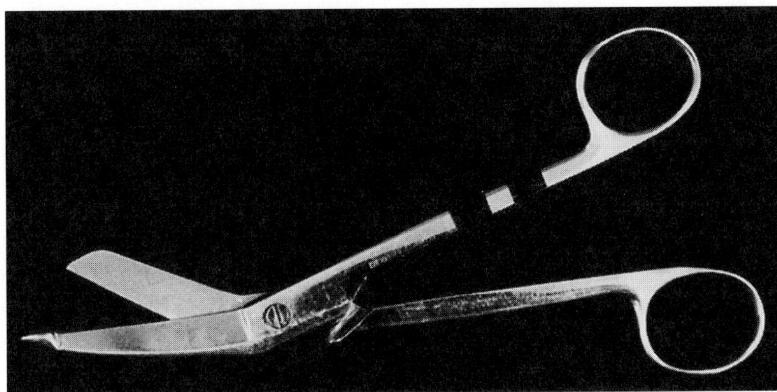

Figure 22-3 Lister bandage scissors. (In Tracy DL: *Small animal surgical nursing,* ed 3, St Louis, 2000, Mosby.)

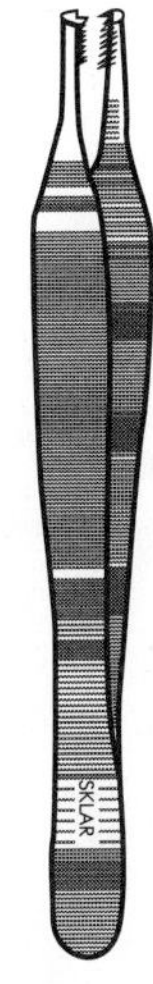

Figure 22-4 Brown-Adson tissue forceps.

1. 1:2 means one tooth and two teeth at the tip of the instrument

Needle Holders

I. Type of forceps used to hold curved needles and aid in tying sutures

II. Surgical preference determines the type of needle holder used

III. Mayo-Hegar (Figure 22-8) and Olsen-Hegar are commonly used in veterinary surgery
   - A. Olsen-Hegar combine a needle holder with scissors to cut suture without using a separate scissor
   - B. Mayo-Hegar can be used only as a needle holder (no scissors)
   - C. Crisscross grooves assist in grasping the needle

IV. Mathieu needle holders do not have rings for the fingers and spring open and closed by finger pressure

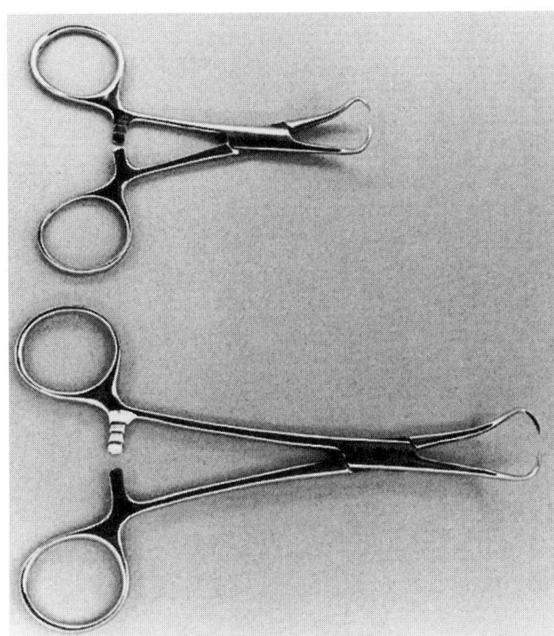

Figure 22-5 Backhaus towel clips. (In Tracy DL: *Small animal surgical nursing,* ed 3, St Louis, 2000, Mosby.)

Retractors

I. Senn retractors are double ended and useful for skin and superficial muscle retraction

II. Meyerding, Hohmann, and U.S. Army retractors are hand held for larger muscle masses (Figure 22-9)

III. Malleable retractors are made of a soft metal that can be bent to accommodate hard-to-retract areas

IV. Self-retaining retractors have a locking mechanism
   - A. Gelpi retractors have a single tip that extends outward to retract muscles
   - B. Weitlanders are similar but have multiple prongs at the tips
   - C. Balfour retractors are useful in abdominal surgery; several sizes are available

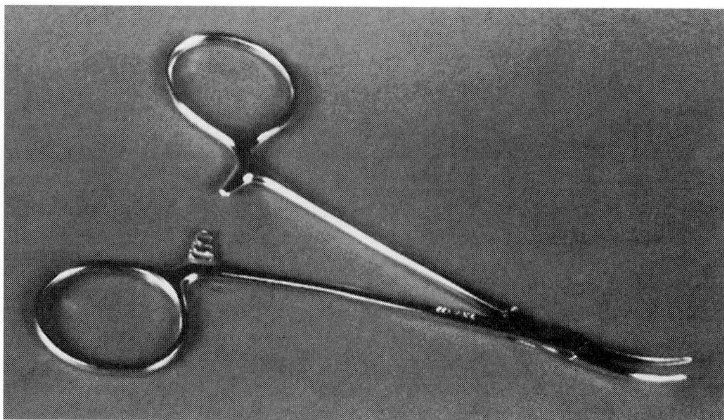

Figure 22-6 Halsted mosquito forceps, curved. (Courtesy The Ohio State University. In Tracy DL: *Small animal surgical nursing,* ed 3, St Louis, 2000, Mosby.)

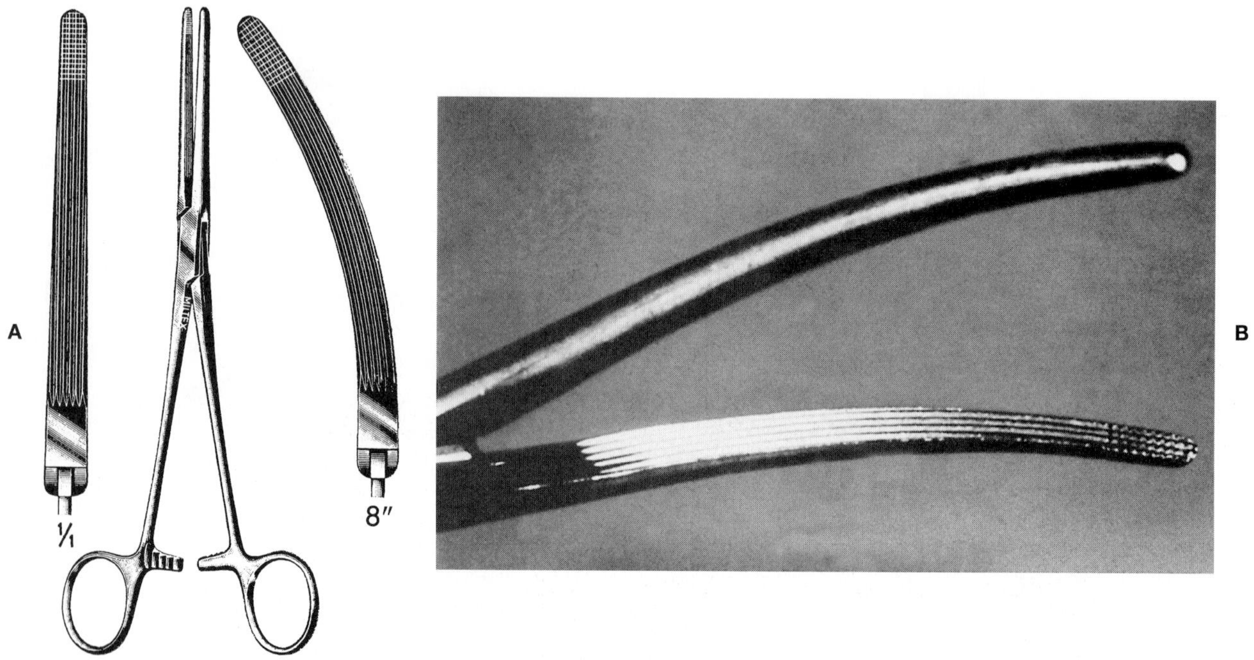

Figure 22-7 **A,** Rochester-Carmalt forceps. **B,** Rochester-Carmalt forceps have longitudinal serrations and cross-hatched pattern at tips of each jaw. (Courtesy Miltex and The Ohio State University. In Tracy DL: *Small animal surgical nursing,* ed 3, St Louis, 2000, Mosby.)

D. Finochetto retractors are for thoracic surgery

V. Ovariohysterectomy hook or spay hook is a type of retractor (Figure 22-10)
   A. Snook has a broad, flat handle and a flat, curved tip
   B. Covault has an octagonal handle and a buttoned tip

Common Orthopedic Instruments

I. Kern and Richards forceps have strong gripping teeth; some have a ratchet to manipulate bone fractures to reduction

II. Verbrugge and reduction forceps can hold bone fragments in reduction while inserting fixators such as screws

III. Wire twisters look like larger needle holders

IV. Jacobs chucks are used to advance pin placement

V. Rongeurs, such as the Lempert, are used to break up and remove bone

VI. Bone-cutting forceps, such as the Liston, are used to cut bone

VII. Ostotomes and mallets are also used to cut bone

VIII. Bone curettes have a sharp edge to remove bone

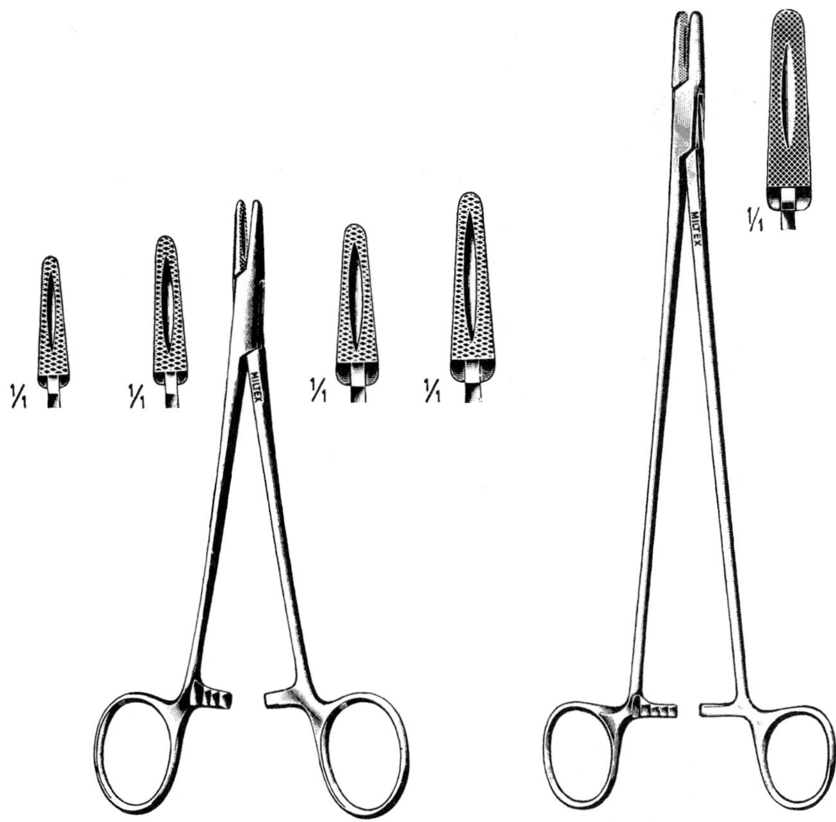

Figure 22-8 Mayo-Hegar needle holder. (Courtesy Miltex. In Tracy DL: *Small animal surgical nursing,* ed 3, St Louis, 2000, Mosby.)

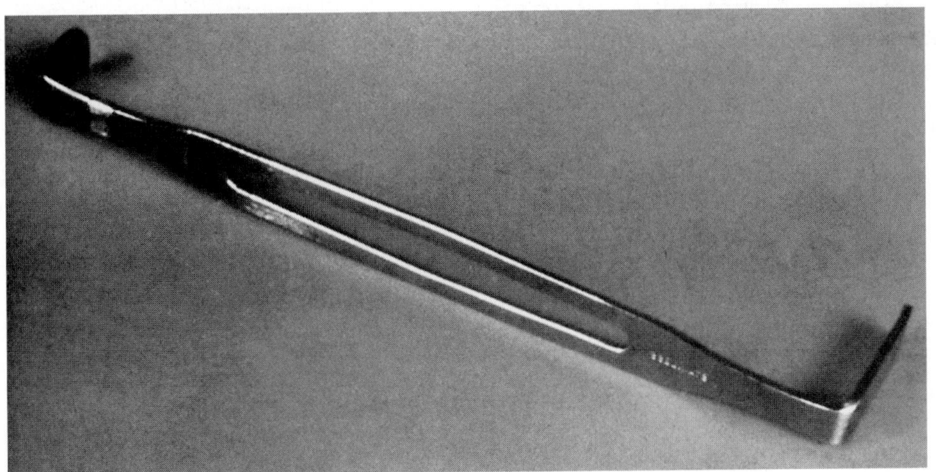

Figure 22-9 U.S. Army retractor. (Courtesy The Ohio State University. In Tracy DL: *Small animal surgical nursing,* ed 3, St Louis, 2000, Mosby.)

IX. Bone rasps are used to smooth bone

X. Periosteal elevators, such as the Freer and Langbeck, are used to remove muscle from bone by releasing the periosteum

Miscellaneous Instruments

I. Suction tip chosen depends on its intended use

A. Poole tips work well to remove abdominal fluid without being plugged by omentum

B. Frazier-Ferguson tips allow variable suction strength for removing blood

C. Yankauer tips are best for removing fluid but not blood

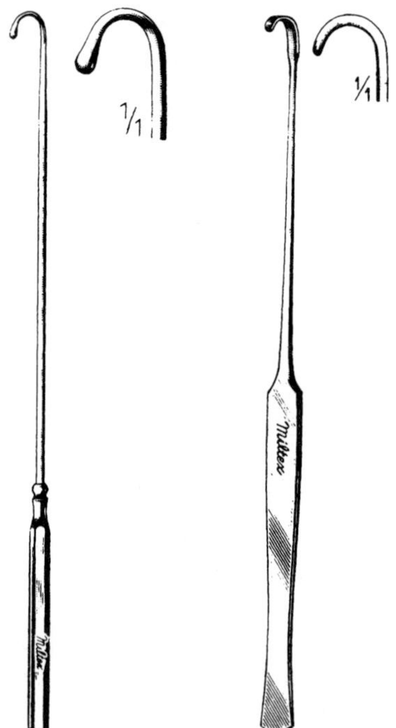

Figure 22-10 Spay hook. (Courtesy Miltex. In Tracy DL: *Small animal surgical nursing,* ed 3, St Louis, 2000, Mosby.)

II. Bard-Parker scalpel handle is used with a detachable blade
   A. Use a needle holder to attach and remove the blade
   B. A no. 3 handle and a no. 10, 11, 12, or 15 blade are most commonly used in small animal surgery
   C. A no. 4 handle and a no. 20 blade can also be used
III. Groove directors are sometimes used to assist in making an incision

Needles and Suture Material

I. Surgical needles are available in several sizes and forms
   A. Can be straight, curved, half curved, or half circle
      1. Curved needles are most commonly used
      2. Curved needles are described by their circle size (i.e., ¼, ⅜, ½, ⅝ circle)
      3. One-half curved needles are straight except for a curved tip
   B. Needle points are cutting or tapered (noncutting)
      1. Type of cutting points can be reverse, triangular, or side cutting for skin, cartilage, or tendons
      2. Taper point needles are round or oval with reverse cutting points for tissues that may tear easily
   C. Needles can be eyeless (swaged) or with an eye (round, square)
      1. Needles "swaged on" to the suture are less traumatic because needle size is relative to suture size
      2. A separate needle and suture can cause tissue damage if used improperly
         a. Needle and suture should be close to the same size
         b. Thread suture through curved needles from the inside without tension
II. Commonly used absorbable suture material
   A. Surgical gut is the most common nonsynthetic material
   B. Examples of synthetic suture material
      1. Polyglycolic acid (Dexon, Davis-Geck): synthetic polyester from hydroxyacetic acid
      2. Polygalactin acid (Vicryl, Eithicon): copolymer of lactic and glycolic acids
      3. Polydioxanone (P.D.S., Ethicon) and polyglyconate (Maxon, Davis-Geck): synthetic polyester
III. Nonabsorbable suture material can also be natural or synthetic
   A. Examples of natural fibers for suture material
      1. Silk is considered nonabsorbable even though its tensile strength is usually lost after 6 months
      2. Cottons and linens have been used for suture material
      3. Stainless steel is used in veterinary surgery but can be difficult to work with due to decreased flexibility
   B. Examples of synthetic nonabsorbable suture material
      1. Polypropylene (Prolene, Ethicon): synthetic plastic
      2. Polyamide/nylon (Ethilon, Ethicon): polymerized plastic
      3. Polymerized caprolactrum (Vetafil, B. Braun, Melsungen AG): coated synthetic fiber commonly used for skin closure
IV. USP (Pharmacopeia) sizing is generally used when asking for suture material
   A. Example: 4-0 (pronounced "4 ought"), 3-0, 2-0, 0, 1, 2 . . .
   B. As the number increases to the right after 0, the diameter of the suture becomes thicker; thus the size increases (i.e., size 3 suture is larger than size 2 suture)
   C. As the number increases to the left of 0, the diameter of the suture is thinner; thus the size decreases (i.e., size 2-0 is larger than size 3-0)
   D. Wire suture is also sized by gauge

1. Size varies from 18 to 40 gauge
2. The lower the gauge number, the thicker the diameter of the wire suture

V. Suture material and needle size used are based on many factors determined by the surgeon

INSTRUMENT CARE AND PACK PREPARATION

Stainless steel instruments are in general expensive and of high quality. If maintained well, stainless steel instruments will last a lifetime.

Instrument Care

I. Instruments should be kept moist or washed immediately after use to prevent residue from drying, which can cause staining, pitting, and corrosion

II. Clean instruments in distilled water and approved cleaning agents
  A. Tap water should be avoided because it can leave mineral deposits on the instruments during the sterilization process
  B. Cleaning agents should have a neutral pH (between 9.2 and 11) to prevent spotting and corrosion
  C. Instrument-cleaning brushes are helpful in removing debris from boxlocks, ratchets, and teeth

III. Use an ultrasonic cleaner to clean instruments because it is 16 times more effective than manual cleaning
  A. Instruments should be placed in cleaner with boxlocks and ratchets open
  B. Do not overpack the cleaner with too many instruments
  C. To prevent electrolytic corrosion, do not mix different metals in the same cycle
  D. Run the cycle for approximately 10 minutes

IV. Place instruments in a surgical milk solution
  A. The surgical milk solution is an excellent lubricant and rust inhibitor
  B. In general, surgical milk must be used on all instruments cleaned by ultrasound because all traces of lubricants are lost in cleaning
  C. After immersion in instrument milk, the instruments should be put on a clean paper or cloth towel to drain

V. Additional use of a surgical lubricant on the instrument's moving parts can help to ensure a better working condition

VI. Instruments should be examined before being packed for resterilization
  A. Check that all surfaces are clean and free of foreign material
  B. Make certain that boxlocks work smoothly and are not loose
  C. Instrument tips should close tightly and evenly, especially on all forceps and needle holders
  D. Scissors should be sharp along the entire edge of the blade

Preparing Instrument Packs and Linens

I. Reusable linens, such as gowns, drapes, and skin towels, should be laundered in a separate washer and dryer with minimal detergent
  A. An extra rinse cycle should be used to ensure that no detergent residue is left
  B. Leftover detergent residue can transfer via steam to surgical instruments during the sterilization process

II. The packing of instruments and linens should be consistent and allow the greatest amount of steam sterilization
  A. Use of pans or trays with perforations to hold instruments can allow better steam penetration and drying
  B. Leave boxlocks and ratchets in the open position or locked no more than one click
  C. Place heavier instruments on the bottom of the packs and place items that are used first, such as towel clamps, on top
  D. Fold linens by the accordion style method (fan fold)
    1. Surgical gowns should be laundered and untorn
      a. Wrap inside out with all ties folded inside neatly and sleeves on top of the gown
      b. Gown pack can also include a towel for drying hands after a surgical scrub
    2. Laporatomy sheets, drapes, and skin towels should be laundered and lint free
      a. Wrap using the accordian pleat method and then fold into three sections
      b. Some surgeons prefer to have one corner of the drape folded over for easier grasping of the drape
  E. Packs must fit the size of the autoclave and allow ample room for steam movement and penetration
    1. Size should not exceed 30 × 30 × 50 cm
    2. Weight should not exceed 5.5 kg
    3. Density should not exceed 115.3 kg/m^3
    4. Space between packs should be 2.5 to 7.5 cm

III. The wrapping of instrument packs and linens should be consistent for proper sterile handling technique when opened
  A. Place a minimum of two appropriate-sized wrapping materials in front of you in a diamond shape

B. Place the instrument pack or linen in the center of the first or inner wrapper
C. Begin with the corner nearest you and fold over the top of the pack
D. Take a small part of that corner and fold it back toward you to leave a tab
E. Do the same with one of the side corners, then the opposite side
F. The side farthest from you should always be folded over last
G. Tuck this last corner inside the two sides, leaving a tab that can be pulled to open
H. Repeat the same folding technique with the second or outer wrapper

IV. Indicator tape should be used on the outside of every pack and linen
A. Tape keeps the packs sealed tighter and prevents corners from unfolding
B. Useful for labeling information
1. Contents of item (i.e., large gowns, general packs, etc.)
2. Date item was sterilized and anticipated expiration date
3. Initials of the technician who prepared and sterilized the pack

V. Sterilization pouches made of paper and/or plastic are useful for sterilizing individual item
A. Pouches can be sealed by heat or by rolling the ends three times and securing with indicator tape
B. Sterilize in an upright position to allow the best steam sterilization and drying

VI. Types of sterilization monitors

More than one sterilization monitor should be used to ensure optimum sterility of the pack.

A. Indicator tape indicates only that an item has been exposed to steam or ethylene oxide
1. Lines on the tape will change color
2. Color change does not indicate that temperature has been met and maintained for a certain period of time
3. Indicator tape on the outside of the pack means only the outside of the pack has been exposed to steam
B. Chemical indicator strips change color when exposed to steam or ethylene oxide for a certain period of time
1. Place in the center in the least accessible place for steam: between folds of drapes or gown. Do not place the indicator directly on instruments
2. Must remember to check the strip as soon as pack is open
C. Bowie Dick test is a prepurchased dense pack with indicator tape in the center
1. Place test in the most inaccessible location in the autoclave
2. Verifies steam penetration
D. Biological indicators are excellent monitors of sterility
1. Tests for the most heat-resistant bacteria
2. However, it does not give an immediate answer
E. Visual monitoring of sterilization should always occur to ensure that adequate time, temperature, and pressure have been achieved

VII. Length of time a steamed autoclaved item remains sterile can be extended by the type of wrapping material and where they are stored
A. Textile wrapping material can be bulky to use and must be laundered and in good repair
1. Cotton muslin should be double layered, and two wraps should be used for pack preparation
2. Higher thread count cottons can use two single-layered wraps
3. If kept in open shelving, the items can remain sterile for 3 weeks
B. Disposable paper wraps can be crepe, or non-crepe material that can be cut to the desired size
1. Crepe paper is easier to work with and more durable
2. Crepe paper is more expensive
3. Single-wrapped two-way crepe paper can remain sterile for 3 weeks with open shelving
C. You can double the sterilization shelf life by keeping items in a clean, closed cabinet
D. For infrequently used items, wrap and store in sterilization pouches to extend the shelf-life to 1 year in a closed cabinet
E. Ethylene oxide sterilization can also prolong the shelf-life of sterile items

PATIENT PREPARATION

The goal of patient preparation is to achieve asepsis or a preparation site free of germs that could cause disease or decay.

I. Patient preparation should be performed outside of the operating room

II. Before clipping, the bladder may need to be emptied, either by walking the patient outside or manually expressing the bladder
A. Caution may be warranted when expressing a patient's bladder, and the surgeon should be consulted before performing the procedure
B. An empty bladder can increase the space in the abdominal cavity and prevents the animal from eliminating on the surgery table while under anesthesia

III. Surgical hair removal should be completed with electric clippers and a no. 40 blade
   A. Blades should be clean and well lubricated and have no missing teeth that may tear the skin
   B. Coolants prevent clipper blades from overheating
IV. Start clipping at the proposed incision and work laterally against the direction of hair growth
   A. Thick-coated animals sometimes require clipping with the direction of hair first, perhaps using a no. 10 blade initially
   B. Try not to allow clipped areas to touch unclipped areas
   C. In general, clip more hair rather than too little hair
   D. By consulting the surgeon and the patient file, determine the proper site and the size of the site before clipping
V. Technicians should be familiar with common general surgical clips and animal placements for surgery
   A. Most laparotomies such as the ovariohysterectomy and splenectomy have a standard preparation site
      1. Animals are placed in dorsal recumbency
      2. Hair is removed cranially to the xiphoid process and caudally to the pubis
      3. Hair is removed laterally
         a. For cats, approximately one clipper blade width past the nipple line
         b. For large dogs, at least 4 inches (10 cm) of hair either side of the midline should be removed
   B. Canine castrations require hair removal from the scrotum and prepuce extending into the inguinal area
      1. Some surgeons prefer that the tip of the prepuce remain unshaven to reduce irritation
   C. Feline castrations require less hair removal and can be done by plucking the hair from the testes and around the scrotum
   D. Puppy dewclaw removal and tail docking, as well as feline declawing, do not require hair removal before surgical scrub
   E. For perineal urethrostomies, rectal fistulas, and anal sac surgeries, the animal is in ventral recumbency with its hindlegs hanging down over the edge of the table. The tail is tied or clipped to the top or side of the body
      1. Some surgical tables can be tilted upward for the surgeon's comfort
      2. Hair removal should be outward from the rectum and extended up the base of the tail and down both legs
   F. Orthopedic surgeries require a larger surgical area prepared to enable the surgeon to manipulate the limb (e.g., lateral and medial hindlimb for a femoral intramedullary pinning)
VI. After clipping, a dust buster or central vacuum is useful to remove all loose hair from the surgery site and the surrounding area of the preparation table
VII. If performing a limb surgery, the unclipped area of hair on the foot should be wrapped
   A. Plastic wrap or examination gloves secured with tape work well
   B. Wrapping after the hair is clipped prevents loose hair from sticking to the tape
      1. Hanging leg preparation can be used or shoulder and hip surgeries
         a. Operated limb is suspended by tape/rope for the surgical scrub
         b. After prep is finished, paw is wrapped with a sterile towel for easy handling by the surgeon
VIII. Recommended scrub solutions are chlorhexidine or povidone-iodophor products
IX. Surgical Scrub Procedure with sterile gloves, gauze, sponge forceps, and scrub bowl
   A. Begin at the incision and work outward in a circular motion
   B. Never return to the incision area without getting a new gauze square
   C. Produce a good lather but do not scrub too hard
   D. Scrubbing process should be completed a minimum of three times
      1. Gauze squares should appear clean after the final scrub
      2. Ask yourself if the skin is aseptic for surgery before continuing to the next step
   E. A procedure of alternating each scrub with sterile saline is helpful
   F. Final preparation should be completed in a manner such that the area of the incision is the most aseptic
      1. Apply chlorhexadine or povidone-iodine as an antiseptic
      2. There are at least three methods to accomplish the final aseptic application
         a. Method 1: using a nonsterile gauze square with antiseptic, make the first stroke medially down the incision line. Each subsequent stroke of antiseptic is to the right or left of the incision site, ending at the outermost border
         b. Method 2: begin similar to method 1, complete one side, and use a new sponge soaked with antiseptic to complete the opposite side in the same manner

(1) The objective is that no stroke of antiseptic is repeated, thereby maintaining asepsis

c. Method 3: at many practices, antiseptic spray is used as the final prep in the operating room

X. Once surgical preparation is completed, carefully move the patient (by gurney if available) into the operating room, trying not to contaminate the surgical scrub

XI. The patient should be tied to the table in the appropriate position

A. The knot should be a half hitch on the limb to facilitate easy release in case of an emergency

1. Apply ties with two contact points per limb to reduce pressure problems
2. Do not secure too tightly; this may cause muscle problems

XII. Once patient is positioned and necessary monitoring equipment is in place, a final surgical preparation is performed

A. Reapply antiseptic using one of the methods given

B. Repeat entire preparation if contamination occurs

DRAPING

After the animal is secured on the table and the final skin preparation is complete, the patient is ready to be draped.

I. Drapes maintain a sterile field

II. Draping is performed by a gowned and gloved surgical assistant or team member

III. Draping begins with the placement of field drapes (also called quarter drapes)

A. Field drapes are placed on the unprepared portion of the animal

B. These drapes are placed one at a time at the very periphery of the prepared area

C. After the drapes are in place, they should not be readjusted toward the incision site

1. Readjustment carries contaminants onto the prepared skin

D. Towel clamps are placed to secure the four-corners of the drapes

1. Towel clamps secure the drapes to the skin and surround the incision site

E. Finally, a large drape or laparotomy sheet is placed over the animal with the center or fenestration over the surgical site

1. Final drape provides a continuous sterile field

SURGEON AND STERILE ASSISTANT SURGICAL SCRUB

I. Purpose: remove dirt, grease, and decrease bacterial flora from the hands and arms

II. Before scrubbing, set out sterile scrub brush and any packs and surgical equipment that may be needed. Put on cap and mask, remove jewelry, and ensure nails are fingertip length and that fingernails are free of nail polish

A. There are many variations of a surgical scrub. All variations are based on timed or stroke methods of scrubbing the surface of the hands and arms. For the purposes of this text, a stroke method will be used as an example

1. Turn on water, checking for comfortable water temperature; thoroughly wash both hands and arms; clean nails
2. Begin with a sterile scrub brush or prepackaged soap/brushes; wet the brush and/or apply antiseptic soap to it
3. Begin with one hand, scrubbing fingertips, using 12 strokes. Proceed in a methodical fashion from the baby finger to the thumb, scrubbing each plane of each finger 12 times
4. Progress to the palm and then the back of the hand and lateral hand
5. Move to wrist area, scrubbing all four planes
6. Scrub the remaining portion of the arm, ending 2 inches (5 cm) proximal to the elbow
7. Rinse the brush, apply more antiseptic to the brush, and begin the same procedure on the opposite hand and arm
8. After right and left arms have been scrubbed, rinse hands and arms from the fingertips to the elbows, continuing to hold hands upward
9. Drying of hands and arms: hold sterile towel away from the body. Using one side of the sterile towel, dry one hand first, followed by the arm. Use the other side of the towel for the opposite hand and arm

III. Gowning and gloving should be completed immediately after drying hands

A. Gowning

1. Hold gown by inside shoulder seams; carefully pick the gown up and away from the counter
2. The gown will unfold open
3. Slide one arm into the sleeve and then the opposite arm into the remaining sleeve
4. Allow unsterile personnel to tie the gown

B. Gloves should fit snugly but not so tightly as to cut off circulation of the hands

C. There are two standard methods of gloving: open and closed

1. Open gloving

a. With left hand, grasp inside cuff of the right glove; pull glove over the right hand and cuff of the gown

b. The left glove can now be handled with the gloved right hand by placing the fingertips on the inside of the folded back cuff of the glove and pulling it on the left hand and over the cuff of the gown
2. Closed gloving (minimizes contamination)
   a. With fingertips of the right hand covered by the cuff of the gown, pick up the glove and place it on the covered left hand with fingertips of the glove facing the shoulder
   b. The thumb of the glove is on top of the left thumb
   c. Pull the glove over the cuff and push the hand into it while pushing out of the gown cuff
   d. The same procedure is used for the right hand glove
   e. After both gloves are in place, the gloves can be repositioned for comfort
3. After gloving is completed the hands should be held above the waist and in front of the body

OPERATING ROOM CONDUCT

All operating rooms have the same strict rules that must be followed. Knowing and understanding aseptic technique will help any technician adapt to any operating room.

I. Aseptic conditions must be applied to the surgical suite and the patient
   A. Patients and surgery staff prep in another room
   B. Only surgery-related equipment belongs in the operating room
   C. Always clean from ceiling to floor. Every item in the operating room must be removed and cleaned regularly with disinfectants
   D. Clean daily before surgeries begin and between cases
II. Proper surgical attire is a must
   A. Scrubs are specially designed for operating rooms
      1. Street clothes should never be worn
      2. Smocks should be worn over scrubs while clipping hair and when outside the surgical area
   B. Surgical head attire should be a bouffant cap or a hooded cap
      1. No hair should be exposed
      2. Hooded caps cover both the head and neck and are useful for those with facial hair
   C. Surgical masks are either molded or flat
      1. Molded masks have a metal nose band to assist with fit but provide less facial coverage and can allow air to escape
      2. Flat-style masks have pleats and a metal nose band to provide a more custom fit and decrease the chance of allowing air to escape
   D. Foot covers or surgery shoes must be worn
III. Talking in the operating room should be minimal
   A. Talking can distract a surgeon's concentration
   B. Saliva weakens the filtration of the surgical mask
IV. Movement within the operating room should be limited because the increased air movement can increase the risk of contamination
   A. Prepare any equipment that may be used before the surgery begins
   B. An organized surgery suite layout will prevent movement in the room to retrieve needed equipment and material
   C. The surgery suite should be located in an isolated area of the hospital with decreased traffic volume
V. An imaginary line should be drawn around the sterile field of the surgeon, operating table, and instrument tray
   A. When passing sterile equipment, do not cross that line but stand near it
   B. Stand to the right or to the left, so the surgeon does not have to turn his or her back to the patient
   C. Hold a sterilized packaged item away from your body when opening
   D. When opening items wrapped as described earlier
      1. Open the side farthest away from you using the tab
      2. Proceed to do one side and then the other without allowing your arms to pass over the top of the item
      3. Then pull the last tab (one closest to your body) toward you, exposing the item or second sterile wrap
      4. Only outer pack wrappers should be opened by unsterile personnel before surgery: keeping the inner wrap closed ensures sterility of the contents
   E. How to open items in sterilization pouches
      1. Determine which end is marked to be opened
      2. Hold both hands in fists with thumbs on top of your index finger
      3. Grab each side of the pouch, holding it between your thumb and index finger
      4. Separate the seal by rolling your fists outward
      5. Lower part of your fist can apply pressure to the item in the pouch to prevent it from sliding out

F. Always allow the surgeon to approach you to retrieve a sterile item or place the item in a sterile manner on the pack

VI. Surgical gowns should be considered sterile only on the front side above the waist to the shoulder and down the arms
   A. Keep hands clasped in front, close to the body, and above the waist or above the surgery table
   B. If trading places, pass back to back with hands folded; never turn your back toward the patient

VII. A sterile surgical assistant can perform the following functions
   A. Receive sterile equipment
      1. Lift items up and out
      2. Do not reach over a patient or sterile field
   B. Keep the surgical table organized and instruments clean
   C. Anticipate and pass needed equipment and instruments
      1. Hand in the correct position for immediate use
      2. Tap the surgeon's palm with the instrument to ensure proper contact
   D. Maintain hemostasis for the surgeon
      1. Place suction tip near tissue, not directly on the tissue
      2. Dab area with gauze square; do not wipe
      3. Keep an accurate count of the gauze squares used and discarded
   E. Provide retraction of muscles and tissues with minimal trauma and good surgical exposure
   F. Cut suture material after suture placement

VIII. If a sterile item touches an unsterile item, it immediately becomes unsterile and is discarded
   A. Any item that is dropped, punctured, or wet is unsterile
   B. The patient's skin is aseptic, not sterile; avoid contact
   C. *If in doubt, it is not sterile*

Glossary

asepsis In surgery, refers to the destruction of organisms before they enter the body

fenestration To perforate or make an opening into

fistulas Any abnormal passage within body tissue; generally a passage leading from two internal organs or an internal organ to the body surface

intramedullary Within the marrow cavity of a bone

laparotomies An incision into the abdominal wall; exploratory laparotomy often used to physically examine the abdominal organs (also referred to as celiotomy)

ligating Application of a ligature or material such as wire or suture material to tie off blood vessels to prevent bleeding or constrict tissue

ovariohysterectomy Surgical excision of the ovaries and uterus; commonly called a "spay"

pedicle Stem or stemlike structure

perineal Situated on the perineum

perineum External region between the vulva and the anus in the female or between the scrotum and anus in the male

ratchet Step-locking device on surgical instruments. The ratchet consists of a notched bar on each handle of an instrument; the notches are facing and overriding when the handles are closed and locked

reduction Correction of a hernia, luxation, or fracture

serrations Having a sawlike edge or border

splenectomy Excision of the spleen

swaged-on Type of suture material that is fused to the end of the needle

transverse Extending from side to side or at right angles to the long axis

urethrostomies Creation of a permanent hole for the urethra in the perineum

viscera Internal organs enclosed within a cavity

Review Questions

1 Type of scissors with long handles used for cutting delicate tissue are
a. Littauer
b. Metzenbaum
c. Mayo
d. Lister

2 Forceps that are 20 cm (9 inches) with longitudinal grooves are
a. Rochester-Pean
b. Rochester-Carmalt
c. Kelly
d. Crile

3 A needle holder combined with a scissor is called
a. Mathieu
b. Rochester-Pean
c. Mayo-Hegar
d. Olsen-Hegar

4 Self-retaining tissue forceps with multiple fine intermeshing teeth at the tips are called
a. Allis
b. Babcock
c. Adson
d. Brown-Adson

5 Which of the following is *not* a type of needlepoint?
a. Reverse cutting
b. Taper
c. Side cutting
d. Swaged

6 An example of a nonsynthetic absorbable suture material is
a. Surgical gut
b. P.D.S.

c. Silk
d. Nylon

7 What is the scientific name for Vetafil?
a. Polyglycolic acid
b. Polypropylene
c. Caprolactrum
d. Polydioxanone

8 What type of detergent should be used to clean instruments?
a. Slightly acid pH
b. Neutral pH
c. Slightly alkaline pH
d. Does not matter

9 The minimum number of surgical scrubs on a surgical site that should be completed is
a. One
b. Two
c. Three
d. Four

10 Which of the following is a recommended antiseptic for patient preparation?
a. Chlorhexidine
b. Hydrogen peroxide
c. Roccal
d. Dish detergent

BIBLIOGRAPHY

Berg J: Sterilization. In Slatter DJ, editor: *Textbook of small animal surgery,* ed 2, vol 1, Philadelphia, 1993, WB Saunders.

Boothe HW: Suture material, tissue adhesives, staplers and ligating clips. In Slatter DJ, editor: *Textbook of small animal surgery,* ed 2, vol 1, Philadelphia, 1993, WB Saunders.

Egger EL: Surgical assistance and suture material. In McCurnin DM, Bassert JM, editors: *Clinical textbook for veterinary technicians,* ed 5, Philadelphia, 2001, WB Saunders.

Fahie MA: Thoracic and abdominal surgery: the technician's role, *Vet Tech* 18:565, 1997.

Fitch R, Davidson JR, Burba DJ: Surgical instruments and aseptic technique. In McCurin DM, Bassert JM, editors: *Clinical textbook for veterinary technicians,* ed 5, Philadelphia, 2001, WB Saunders.

Fries CL: Assessment and preparation of the surgical patient. In Slatter DJ, editor: *Textbook of small animal surgery,* ed 2, vol 1, Philadelphia, 1993, WB Saunders.

Hobson HP: Surgical facilities and equipment. In Slatter DJ, editor: *Textbook of small animal surgery,* ed 2, vol 1, Philadelphia, 1993, WB Saunders.

Khachatoorian L, Brady M: Aseptic surgical technique, *Vet Tech* 18:115, 1997.

Knecht CD et al: Operating room conduct. In Pederson D, editor: *Fundamental techniques in veterinary surgery,* ed 3, Philadelphia, 1987, WB Saunders.

Knecht CD et al: Selected small animal surgical procedures. In Pederson D, editor: *Fundamental techniques in veterinary surgery,* ed 3, Philadelphia, 1987, WB Saunders.

Knecht CD et al: Surgical instrumentation. In Pederson D, editor: *Fundamental techniques in veterinary surgery,* ed 3, Philadelphia, 1987, WB Saunders.

Knecht CD et al: Suture material. In Pederson D, editor: *Fundamental techniques in veterinary surgery,* ed 3, Philadelphia, 1987, WB Saunders.

McCurnin DM, Jones RL: Principle of surgical asepsis. In Slatter DJ, editor: *Textbook of small animal surgery,* ed 2, vol 1, Philadelphia, 1993, WB Saunders.

Miltex Instrument Co Inc: *Miltex surgical instruments,* Lake Success, NY, 1986, The Company.

Nieves MA, Merkley DF, Wagner SD: Surgical instruments. In Slatter DJ, editor: *Textbook of small animal surgery,* ed 2, vol 1, Philadelphia, 1993, WB Saunders.

Oakes AB, Oakes MG, Seim HB III: Small animal surgical nursing and dentistry. In McCurnin DM, Bassert JM, editors: *Clinical textbook for veterinary technicians,* ed 5, Philadelphia, 2001, WB Saunders.

Schultz R: The ten commandments of surgical instrument care, *Vet Tech* 19:696, 1998.

Tracy DL: *Small animal surgical nursing,* ed 3, St Louis, 2000, Mosby.

Wagner SD: Preparation of the surgical team. In Slatter DJ, editor: *Textbook of small animal surgery,* ed 2, vol 1, Philadelphia, 1993, WB Saunders.

CHAPTER 23

Small Animal Nursing

Monica M. Tighe

OUTLINE

LEARNING OUTCOMES

After reading this chapter you should be able to:

1. Explain how to perform a basic physical examination.
2. Define the importance of fluid therapy and why and how patient requirements may change.
3. Explain and identify the signs and degrees of dehydration.
4. Describe the various routes of fluid administration and why a specific route may be used.
5. Describe various routes of drug administration.
6. Define contraindications of certain routes of drug administration.
7. Describe venipuncture procedure in the canine or feline patient.
8. Describe the collection and transfusion of blood in the canine and the feline patient.
9. Define electrocardiography.
10. Describe the equipment needed and procedure for producing an electrocardiogram.
11. Describe various abnormal electrocardiographic tracings and their etiology.
12. Describe the precautions and procedure for inserting an orogastric tube.
13. Describe the indications, equipment, procedure, and precautions involved in male dog catheterization.
14. Describe the indications, equipment, procedure, and precautions involved in female dog catheterization.
15. Describe the indications, equipment, procedure, and precautions involved in performing a cystocentesis.
16. Describe the indications, procedure, and precautions involved in performing manual compression of the urinary bladder.
17. Describe the indications, equipment, procedure, and precautions involved in anal sac expression.
18. Describe the indications, equipment, procedure, and precautions involved in enema administration.
19. Define the difference between a contaminated and an infected wound.
20. Differentiate and describe the four phases of wound healing.
21. Describe the different types of wound healing.
22. Define the treatment protocol for wound management.
23. Describe various types of bandages.
24. Define the indications and complications in bandaging various areas in small animals.
25. Define the classification method of tumors.
26. Describe the possible therapies that are available for cancer treatment.

As a paraprofessional, the veterinary technician works with the veterinarian and performs many diagnostic and technical procedures to aid the veterinary patient. Veterinary technicians are very versatile and perform numerous technical skills. This chapter outlines many basic clinical techniques.

PHYSICAL EXAMINATION

Introduction

I. Under the supervision of a veterinarian, veterinary technicians may conduct physical examinations
   A. To provide information to assess a patient's anesthetic risk and prepare an anesthetic plan
   B. To obtain a status or progress report for monitoring an animal's recovery
   C. To verify medical record entries
   D. To evaluate abnormalities or conditions that should be brought to the attention of the veterinarian
II. A physical examination is the first step in assessing a patient and may indicate possible health problems
III. All body systems should be checked
IV. A consistent routine should be followed to ensure that each area is thoroughly examined
   A. Example: evaluating from the nose to tail, or system by system

General Appearance

I. Note the animal's general appearance, gait and behavior, temperament, and attitude
II. The environment of the animal should be noted
   A. Vomiting/diarrhea, urination, defecation in the cage
III. An accurate weight should be recorded, as well as temperature, pulse, and respiratory rate

Examination by System

The detection of physical problems is usually due to observing the animal and palpating, smelling, and listening. The description of what is detected is also important. Size, color, rate, and appearance should also be included in the record. For the following systems, various clinical signs should be noted on the patient's file.

I. Skin and coat
   A. Examine the skin and coat
      1. Shiny or dull
      2. Skin turgor
         a. Normal skin pliability depends on hydration of the tissues
         b. To assess turgor: tent the skin at the thoracolumbar junction
         c. Avoid cervical area due to the extra skin in this area
         d. If the skin returns rapidly to normal position, it is normal

e. If the skin remains tented or returns slowly to normal resting position, it is a sign of dehydration
f. Mild, moderate, and severe dehydration are graded at 6% to 8%, 10% to 12%, and 12% to 15%, respectively
3. Alopecia or dryness
4. Lesions or obvious parasites such as fleas, lice, mites, or ticks
B. Palpate the entire animal; note any lumps, swelling, or painful reactions to palpation
II. Eyes, ears, and nares
A. Examine the eyes and note the following
1. Reflexes and response to visual stimuli
2. Discharge from the eyes
a. Clear or purulent
3. Corneal changes
4. Color of conjunctiva
B. Manipulate the ear and note the following
1. Response to auditory stimuli
2. Debris in the ear canal or unusual or excessive odor
3. If the animal is shaking or tilting its head to one side
C. Nares
1. Discharge: color and consistency
2. Sneezing and patency
III. Gastrointestinal
A. Examine mouth, teeth, and gums
1. Signs of periodontal disease and halitosis
2. Fractured, missing, or discolored teeth
3. Verify age in young animals
4. Check tonsils for enlargement
5. Excessive salivation or difficulty swallowing
6. Signs of malocclusion
B. Note color of mucous membrane
1. Mucous membranes should be a pale pink color
a. Abnormal colors are blue-purple (cyanotic), yellow (jaundice), pale, bright red, or muddy brown
C. Capillary refill time (CRT)
1. Press on gums and note when the color returns
2. If color returns in less than 1 second, CRT is normal
3. If color returns in greater than 1 second, CRT is increased and abnormal
D. Palpate the abdomen gently
1. Check symmetry from side to side
2. Distention
3. Signs of discomfort during palpation
4. Assess the bladder size
5. Lymph node abnormalities
E. Examine the anal area for any abnormalities
1. Color
2. Anal gland abscesses, discharge, or inflammation
IV. Respiratory
A. Auscultate the chest
1. Using a stethoscope, auscultate the thorax dorsally and laterally
2. Listen for abnormal sounds such as crackles, wheezes, stridor, and rales
3. Be aware of referral sounds from the upper airway
a. Listen to the trachea to rule out this source
4. Be aware of a decrease or lack of breath sounds
B. Note pattern, rate, depth, and effort of breathing
1. Hyperventilation or hypoventilation
2. Panting or shallow breathing
3. Open mouth breathing or panting in cats is especially abnormal
4. Watch for dyspnea
V. Musculoskeletal
A. Observe the animal's gait
1. Lameness, dysplasia, or pain
B. Note obvious signs of joint swelling or displacement of joints
C. Flex the limbs
1. Painful reactions
2. Range of motion
VI. Cardiovascular
A. Palpate femoral and dorsal pedal pulses
1. Strength and rate of pulses
B. Auscultate the heart and check pulses at the same time
1. Note irregularities between pulse rate and heart rate, which can indicate pulse deficits
VII. Reproductive and urinary
A. Examine external genitalia
1. Redness or irritation
2. Abnormal discharge, growths
3. Symmetry of testicles
VIII. Lymphatic
A. Lymph nodes may or may not be palpable
1. Lymph nodes should not be painful when palpated
2. Note any signs of enlargement
B. Major lymph nodes and locations
1. Submandibular: located cranial to the angle of the mandible
2. Prescapular: cranial to the shoulder joint
3. Axillary: where the forelimb meets the body

4. Popliteal: dorsal stifle
5. Inguinal: in the inguinal area near the femoral artery and vein, where the hind limb meets the body

IX. Neurological
   A. Bright and alert
   B. Check pupil size
      1. Response to light
      2. Pupils are of equal size
      3. Nystagmus
   C. Look for signs of ataxia or weakness
   D. Check tail response and/or if there is anal tone
   E. Response in all four limbs to painful stimuli
   F. Levels of consciousness
   G. Knuckling when walking

DRUG ADMINISTRATION

Introduction

I. Drugs are administered in several ways
II. The route depends on type of medication and health status of the animal
III. Most common routes: oral, parenteral, and topical
IV. Whichever method is used, it is important to verify correct drug, patient, dosage, time, and route

Oral Route

I. It is important to note that oral medications are contraindicated in the following situations
   A. If patient is vomiting
   B. There are injuries to the oral cavity or esophagus
   C. Patient has decreased swallowing reflex
   D. Any disease process is present that prohibits oral intake, such as pancreatitis
II. Medication can be a liquid, semisolid, tablet, or capsule
III. Liquid is administered via syringe in the cheek pouch
IV. Tablets or capsules are administered by
   A. Holding the patient's mouth open with one hand
   B. Placing the pill at the base of the tongue with the opposite hand
   C. Closing the mouth
   D. Observing the animal swallowing

Parenteral Route

I. Includes all medications that are injected
II. These drugs are not absorbed through the gastrointestinal tract
III. Commonly includes three routes
   A. Subcutaneous (SQ or SC)
   B. Intramuscular (IM)
   C. Intravenous (IV)
IV. Occasionally, drugs may also be administered
   A. Intradermally (ID)
   B. Intraperitoneally (IP)
   C. Intracardiac (IC)
   D. Intratracheal (IT) (this route is used for emergency drug administration)
   E. Intramedullary or intraosseous (IO)
   F. Intranasal (IN)
   G. Intra-arterial (IA)
V. Subcutaneous injections
   A. Solutions are injected under the skin using a 22- to 25-gauge needle
      1. Vaccines are most commonly administered via this route
         a. Due to possibility of vaccine-induced tumors, the intrascapular region in cats should be avoided
   B. Usually where excess skin is available
      1. Dorsally from the neck to the hips
   C. Bulk fluids may also be administered subcutaneously
      1. From 50 to 100 mL of isotonic body temperature fluids may be administered per site
      2. The preferred sites are dorsal left and right thoracic region and dorsal left and right lumbar region
VI. Intramuscular injections
   A. Injections into the lumbar muscles or biceps femoris using a 22- to 25-gauge needle
   B. Small volumes of up to approximately 2 mL are recommended
   C. Multiple sites may be necessary
VII. Intravenous injections
   A. Via a needle or catheter inserted into a blood vessel
   B. Most common sites: cephalic, femoral, saphenous, and jugular
   C. Alcohol is applied to the site before venipuncture to disinfect and part the fur
   D. A restrainer or a tourniquet is used to apply proximal pressure to vein
   E. By drawing blood into the syringe before injecting, correct placement may be ensured before administering medication
      1. Best to enter at a distal point on the limb
   F. Fastest route of absorption, and large volumes can be rapidly administered
   G. Fewer problems if solutions are caustic, irritating, or hypertonic
   H. IV catheters can also be inserted for long-term administration of medications or fluids
VIII. Intraosseous route
   A. Needles are placed directly into the bone cavity for administration of fluids, drugs, or blood products

B. This method is most commonly used for neonatal and smaller animals and animals with circulatory problems
C. Sites of administration
   1. Femur, humerus, tibia, and sometimes the ilial wing or ischium
D. A 15- to 18-gauge bone marrow needle is commonly used
   1. In small neonatal animals, an 18- to 22-gauge hypodermic needle may also be used
E. Sterile technique must be used to prepare the skin for needle placement

Topical Route

I. Medications applied directly to the skin
II. Can be applied directly on top of lesions
III. The area must be clipped and clean before applying medication
IV. Directions must be followed carefully
   A. Absorption rate is variable and depends on the amount applied and how quickly it is absorbed
V. Wearing gloves as a precautionary measure is sometimes advisable for certain medications

FLUID THERAPY

Introduction

I. Fluid therapy is one of the most common procedures performed in veterinary medicine
II. It is used as supportive therapy in sick and injured patients

Normal Fluid Balance

I. The body is made up of approximately 60% water
II. This is divided into intracellular and extracellular fluids
III. The body maintains fluid balance on a constant basis
IV. Fluids are gained via
   A. Oral intake
   B. Metabolism in the body
V. Fluids are lost by
   A. Respiration
   B. Excretion
   C. Minor routes such as sweating and milk production

Abnormal Fluid Losses

I. Vomiting and diarrhea
II. Increased respiration (panting) in dogs
III. Disease with accompanying polyuria
IV. Any chronic or acute injury or disease that causes fluid loss
V. Any disease state or injury that prevents or decreases the oral intake of fluids

Signs of Dehydration

I. Indicators of dehydration can be found during physical examination
   A. Evaluating weight
   B. Skin turgor
   C. Moistness of mucous membranes
   D. Heart rate
   E. CRT

Estimating Degree of Dehydration

I. 5% Dehydration
   A. Not detectable
II. 5% To 6% dehydration
   A. Slight loss in skin turgor
III. 8% Dehydration
   A. Definite increase in skin turgor
   B. Slight increase in CRT
   C. Possibly dry mucous membranes
IV. 10% To 12% dehydration
   A. Skin turgor remains
   B. Sunken eyes
   C. Increased CRT
   D. Dry mucous membranes
   E. Increased heart and respiratory rates
   F. Cold extremities
   G. Possible signs of shock
      1. Signs include rapid thready pulse, tachycardia, and tachypnea
V. 12% To 15% dehydration
   A. Shock and its clinical signs
   B. Very depressed patient
   C. Imminent death
VI. Other indicators of dehydration
   A. Packed cell volume (PCV) and total plasma protein (TPP)
      1. PCV and TPP increase with all types of fluid loss, except in cases of severe hemorrhaging, when both will decrease
   B. Urine specific gravity
      1. Can be greatly increased (1.045)
   C. Decreased urine production
      1. Normal production is 1 to 2 mL/kg/hr

Calculation of Fluid Replacement Volume

I. Emergency fluid therapy
   A. For hypovolemic, shocky, or severely dehydrated patients, fluids should be administered at 60 to 90 mL/kg/hr
II. Replacement fluids
   A. Replacement fluids can be given over a 12- to 24-hour period
   B. Daily fluid requirement = replacement + maintenance + ongoing losses
      1. Replacement requirement = % dehydration × body weight (kg) × 10

a. Examples of replacement fluids include Normosol R or lactated Ringer's solution (LRS)
2. Maintenance requirement = 40 to 60 mL/kg/day
3. Ongoing losses can be estimated by the daily volume of excretion of urine, diarrhea, vomit, or fluid drainage from a wound over a 24-hour period

III. Maintenance fluids at the rate of 40 to 60 mL/kg/day
A. Examples of maintenance solutions include Normosol M or normal saline with KCl
B. When the patient only needs to be on maintenance fluids, saline with KCl should be used
1. Replacement fluids do not have the required amount of KCl

Contraindications for Fluid Therapy

I. Patients may have existing conditions that may contraindicate the rapid replacement of fluid
II. Conditions that carry a risk of pulmonary edema from fluid shifting into the lungs necessitate the need for caution and frequent monitoring
III. Some conditions that are contraindicated for rapid fluid therapy are
A. Pulmonary contusions
B. Existing pulmonary edema
C. Brain injury
D. Congestive heart failure
IV. Signs of overhydration
A. Restlessness
B. Increased respiratory rate
C. Increased lung sounds (crackles and wheezes)
D. Increased blood pressure
E. Chemosis (edema of ocular conjunctiva)
F. Pitting edema
V. Subsequent weights should be taken, and urine production and specific gravity should be monitored regularly
VI. Fluid rates should be adjusted according to patient response and veterinarian orders

Routes of Fluid Administration

I. Oral
A. Contraindicated if animal is vomiting and/or has a disease such as pancreatitis
B. Can be given by syringe
C. Can be given by feeding tube
1. Nasoesophageal or gastric tube directly into the stomach or intestinal tract
II. Subcutaneous
A. Useful for mild dehydration
B. Fluids must be isotonic; therefore cannot contain dextrose
C. Contraindicated with patients in shock or with more severe cases of dehydration
1. In these cases, peripheral circulation is very poor and very little absorption will take place
D. Absorption can take up to 6 to 8 hours
E. Approximate guidelines: body temperature fluids in the amount of 50 to 150 mL at each site
F. Administration can be by large-gauge needle and syringe or needle attached to an administration set and IV bag
G. Can be administered anywhere there is excess skin
1. Dorsally, between the scapulas
2. Dorsal flank area
III. Intravenous
A. Preferred method for correction of moderate to severe dehydration and patients in shock
B. Commonly administered via catheter through cephalic, saphenous, or jugular veins
IV. Intramedullary
A. Useful in small or young patients where quick venous access is not possible
B. Fluids administered directly into the bone marrow cavity, for rapid absorption
C. Injected through the head of the femur or humerus
D. Strict aseptic technique must be used and local anesthetic may be needed because this procedure can be painful

Types of Fluid

I. Crystalloids
A. Isotonic electrolyte solutions
B. Most commonly used
C. Examples
1. LRS
2. 0.9% Saline or normal saline, also called physiological saline
II. Colloids
A. Solutions containing protein or starch molecules
B. Stay in vascular space and expand volume
C. Useful in patients with cerebral or pulmonary edema, and hypoproteinemia
D. Examples
1. Plasma
2. Pentastarch

VENIPUNCTURE

I. Purposes
A. For clinical pathology tests such as complete blood cell count (CBC) or serum chemistry tests
B. To administer medications or fluids

II. Equipment and supplies
  A. Cotton balls soaked with 70% alcohol (isopropyl)
  B. 3- Or 12-mL syringe or Vacutainer holder
  C. 20 To 22 gauge
  D. Blood collection tubes, with or without anticoagulant (EDTA)
    1. Blood collection tube selection will depend on which laboratory tests are requested by the veterinarian

III. Restraint and handling
  A. Jugular vein
    1. Animal should be in sternal recumbency on table
    2. The restrainer should grasp the animal's front legs with one hand and the animal's head with the other hand, extending the neck to expose the jugular vein
      a. It may be easier to facilitate venipuncture if the patient is positioned hanging over the edge of the table with legs below the table surface
    3. Cephalic vein
      a. The animal should be in sternal recumbency on an examination table
      b. The restrainer should extend the animal's front leg by placing the fingers of one hand behind the animal's elbow
      c. To compress the vein
        (1) Use a tourniquet tightened cranial to elbow; or
        (2) The restrainer can use their thumb or first two fingers to roll and compress or "hold off the vein"
  B. Lateral saphenous vein
    1. The animal should be in lateral recumbency
    2. The restrainer can extend the stifle and compress the vein by grasping the animal's distal thigh or proximal tibia
  C. Femoral vein (feline patients)
    1. Place animal in lateral recumbency
      a. For cats, they may prefer sitting on a table with hind leg extended
    2. The restrainer can place one hand on the medial side of the upper thigh to compress the vein

IV. Procedure
  A. Prepare venipuncture site
    1. Clip the site with a no. 40 blade
    2. Check that the needle, syringe, and Vacutainer sizes are appropriate for collection
      a. Also check for needle burs and sterility
      b. Bevel of needle should be toward the venipuncturist
        (1) This is so the needle facilitates the incoming blood and is not occluded by the vein
    3. Swab the area with alcohol
    4. Have restrainer hold off vein
    5. Insert the needle bevel up approximately three fourths of the its length into the vein
      a. It is preferred to bury the needle in most medium to large dogs' veins so that if there is movement or a change in the position of the animal, the needle will remain in the vein
      b. For smaller animals, approximately half of the needle should be inserted
    6. Pull back on the plunger and check for a small amount of blood in the hub of the needle
    7. Using a gentle force, continue to pull back on the plunger of the syringe until the syringe is full or the required amount of blood is collected
      a. The restrainer should continue to hold off until the required amount of blood is collected or until the venipuncturist directs them to remove the compression
    8. After the blood is collected, the restrainer should be directed to stop the compression of the vein and the venipuncturist can then remove the needle
      a. It is best to have the restrainer at this point apply light pressure over the venipuncture site for hemostasis
    9. The blood is then placed in a Vacutainer using sterile technique
      a. The top can be removed from the Vacutainer and the blood can be gently squirted into the Vacutainer
      b. The Vacutainer can be punctured using the needle and the blood can be injected into the Vacutainer (the Vacutainer should have a vacuum and therefore the blood will automatically be suctioned into the Vacutainer)
      c. If the venipuncturist used a Vacutainer, it should be completely filled for the sample to be viable
    10. At this time the Vacutainer should be gently rocked for all of the blood to be mixed with EDTA (lavender top Vacutainer) or left in a rack for the blood to clot (red top Vacutainer)
    11. The Vacutainer should be labeled with the name of the patient, date, and the initials of the venipuncturist

V. Administration of drugs

A. The procedure for the administration of drugs is the same as for a collection except that after the venipuncturist is positive that the needle is in the lumen of the vein (blood in hub of needle), the restrainer must remove the compression of the vein to facilitate the induction of the drug

BLOOD COLLECTION AND TRANSFUSION

Canine Blood Collection

I. Dogs have two identified canine blood groups
  A. They are A– or A+
    1. A– is the universal donor
II. Canine donor requirements
  A. Any breed or sex may be used
  B. A dog with a good temperament and easily accessible veins is a prime candidate
  C. Blood typing should be performed on each donor
    1. Blood typing can be performed by using a commercially prepared blood typing card
  D. Ideally donors should be neutered and weigh more than 25 kg (55 lb)
  E. Donors can be between 1 and 7 years old
  F. Donors should be tested every 6 months for parasites, including
    1. Heartworms (and maintained on a preventive medication)
    2. Intestinal parasites
  G. Donors should be fully vaccinated
  H. Donors must be in excellent health with yearly normal blood chemistry, CBC, and urinalysis
  I. Donors must be free of the following infectious diseases
    1. Blood parasites: *Babesia canis, Hemobartonella canis*
    2. Rickettsial diseases: *Ehrlichia canis, Ehrlichia platus, Borrelia burgdorferi,* and *Rickettsia rickettsii*
  J. Donors should be fasted before donation to decrease lipemic samples of blood
III. Supplies
  A. Sedation depends on each individual animal
    1. Do not use acepromazine maleate because it causes hypotension
    2. The sedation of choice regularly used is oxymorphone given approximately 15 to 20 minutes before blood collection
  B. A blood collection bag with anticoagulant added is required
    1. The most common anticoagulants are
      a. CPDA-1 (citrate, phosphate, dextrose, adenine) (storage life of 21 days)
      b. ADSOL (dextrose, sodium chloride, mannitol, adenine); will preserve the blood product for a longer period of time
      c. ACD Evacuated Blood Collection Bottle (storage life of 14 days)
  C. Clippers and surgical scrub solutions for preparation of the veins
  D. All supplies for IV fluid administration should also be available
  E. Scale to measure the blood
    1. The total weight of the blood (470 g) plus the weight of the collection bag and anticoagulant (117 g) should be 587 g
IV. Procedure
  A. Sedate animal
  B. Place animal in lateral recumbency with neck extended
  C. Clip a wide area around the jugular vein to be used for collection
  D. Clip and prep the cephalic vein for an IV catheter for fluid replacement after blood collection
  E. Place cephalic catheter
  F. Prepare jugular vein for blood collection
  G. Restrainer should be prepared to hold off the jugular vein in preparation for the blood collection
  H. Insert 16-gauge needle attached to the blood collection bag into the jugular vein in a cranial direction
    1. Blood bags are manufactured with the needle and tubing attached
  I. As blood enters the collection bag, move the bag slightly to mix the anticoagulant with the blood
  J. 450 mL of blood constitutes one entire blood collection
  K. Use the scale to measure the volume of blood in the collection bag so that it is not overfilled or underfilled
    1. Overfilling or underfilling the blood collection bag results in an improper ratio of anticoagulant to blood volume
  L. After completion of blood collection, apply pressure to the jugular vein for 2 minutes to minimize hematoma formation
  M. The amount of blood collected from a canine donor should not exceed 10 to 20 mL/kg
    1. A dog can donate blood approximately every 3 weeks if necessary; however, in general most facilities bleed a donor no more than once per month
  N. Replace blood volume loss from the patient with three times the volume of replacement IV fluids
  O. Clearly label the collection bag with the donor's name, date of collection, date of

expiry, and the donor's PCV, TP (total protein), and blood type

P. The donor should be observed for 1 hour after donation; mucous membrane color, pulse, and CRT should be monitored

Feline Blood Collection

I. Feline donors are not routinely typed before blood collection
   A. The AB system of blood typing is used for cats
      1. There are three recognized blood types: A, B, and AB
         a. The most common blood type is A
         b. Nearly all domestic shorthair and longhair cats have type A
         c. Many purebred cats have type B blood
II. Donor requirements
   A. Less than 8 years of age
   B. A lean body weight of no less than 4.5 kg (10 lb)
   C. Donor must be neutered
   D. A good-natured indoor cat makes donation smoother and less stressful
   E. The donor should be fully vaccinated
   F. Excellent health must be maintained by monitoring serum biochemistry, CBC, urinalysis, and fecal tests on a yearly basis
   G. All donors must be negative for feline leukemia, feline infectious peritonitis, feline immunodeficiency virus, and *Hemobartonella felis*
   H. A donor may provide 60 mL of blood no more than once a month
III. Supplies
   A. Sedation
   B. Clippers and surgical scrub solutions
   C. Appropriate size catheter and butterfly (19 gauge)
   D. Anticoagulant
   E. IV fluids
IV. Procedure
   A. The area is aseptically prepared and a catheter is placed in the cephalic vein for fluid therapy
   B. Animal is sedated "to effect"
   C. Monitor vital signs: pulse, respiration, and blood pressure throughout the procedure
   D. Administration of replacement fluids can begin approximately halfway through the donation
   E. Clip jugular vein and aseptically prepare the area
   F. Place cat in lateral recumbency with neck extended, or place cat in sternal recumbency with neck extended and legs over the edge of the table
   G. Insert 19-gauge butterfly into the jugular vein
   H. Connect the butterfly to a 60-mL syringe containing 8.5 mL of anticoagulant
   I. Always try to minimize movement of the needle in the jugular vein
   J. Mix anticoagulant and blood often throughout the donation
   K. Blood collection from cats is a slow process; patience is a must
   L. Collection is complete when the syringe reaches a volume of 60 mL
   M. Remove butterfly and apply pressure to the vein to minimize hematoma formation
   N. Replace fluid volume lost by donation with approximately three times the amount of fluids (180 mL)
   O. Clearly label the syringe with the donor's name, PCV, TP, volume, and date of collection

Administration and Reactions

I. Patient history should be checked for previous transfusions
   A. Before the transfusion all vital signs are observed and recorded
II. All blood products should be administered at room temperature using an in-line filter to remove debris and clots
III. Flush IV lines with only sodium chloride during transfusions of blood products
   A. Flushing IV lines with any other fluid or solution may cause red blood cells to clump, swell, or cause subsequent hemolysis
IV. For platelet administration, administration sets should not contain Latex because platelets will adhere to it
V. Initial administration should be slow (0.25 mL/kg) for the first 15 to 20 minutes
VI. If there are no signs of a transfusion reaction, the transfusion can be continued at the rate of 5 to 10 mL/kg/hr to a maximum of 22 mL/kg/dog
VII. Transfusion reactions can be either immunological or nonimmunological
   A. Immunological
      1. Acute immunological transfusion reaction signs include hypotension, vomiting, salivation, muscle tremors, and tachycardia
      2. At 7 to 10 days posttransfusion, the recipient's body will destroy red blood cells
      3. Delayed hemolytic reactions sometimes follow multiple transfusions
         a. A key indicator of delayed reaction is if the PCV drops unexpectedly 2 to 21 days posttransfusion

•

b. Reactions may also be due to blood element incompatibilities

B. Nonimmunological signs are due to vascular overload

1. Signs include respiratory disease and vomiting

VIII. For further information see Chapter 19

Shelf-Life

I. Packed red blood cells

A. Blood should be stored at 1° to 6° C (33° to 36° F)

B. Can last up to 42 days in preservative when refrigerated

II. Packed red cells without preservative

A. 21 Days refrigerated (reconstitute with 120 mL saline)

B. Cannot be frozen

III. Fresh or frozen plasma

IV. Platelets

A. Stored at room temperature for 5 days

Indications for Use of Blood Component Therapy

I. Fresh whole blood (should be transfused within 4 to 6 hours)

A. Used for hemorrhagic shock, anemia, excessive surgical hemorrhage, bleeding disorders (due to thrombocytopenia or clotting factor deficiencies), non–immune-mediated hemolytic anemia, and in some circumstances immune-mediated hemolytic anemia

II. Packed red blood cells

A. Fluid balance and osmotic pressure are maintained with crystalloid given with packed cells

B. Used for hemolytic anemias and nonregenerative anemias

C. The preservative ADSOL will maintain cells without having to reconstitute them

1. Approximately 200 mL packed red blood cells in 100 mL of ADSOL

2. Always add ADSOL to the packed red blood cells

a. If packed red blood cells are added to the ADSOL, the cells may be damaged in the process

III. Plasma

A. Used for volume expansion (shock and burn patients), hypoproteinemia, pancreatitis, and sepsis

IV. Platelet concentrated or platelet-rich plasma

A. Mainly used for thrombocytopenia cases

B. One year in 220° C freezer (25° F)

V. Oxyglobin can be substituted as outlined in Chapter 19

ELECTROCARDIOGRAPHY

Definition

I. Recording of the electrical activity on the surface of the body generated by the heart

II. Electrocardiograph: a machine that makes a recording of the bioelectrical signals on the surface of the body that arise from within the heart

A. Electrocardiogram (ECG or EKG): a recording on heat-sensitive paper or on a monitor

III. The ECG represents amplitude (amount of electrical activity) and duration (length of time) of electrical activity

IV. Each contraction of the heart is preceded by an electrical wave front that stimulates the heart muscle to contract (systole) and then relax (diastole) in preparation for the next heartbeat

A. Depolarization: contraction of the myocardium

B. Repolarization: relaxation of cells after depolarization

V. The continuous wave of electricity through the heart is organized, rhythmic, and repetitive

A. The sinoatrial node, or pacemaker of the heart, is the point of origin of electrical activity

B. The cells of the heart are linked closely together; therefore the depolarization spreads quickly from the sinoatrial node to the atria in a caudal direction toward the ventricles, finally reaching the atrioventricular (AV) node

C. Electrical activity moves slowly from the AV node and into the proximal portions of the ventricular conduction system known as the bundle of His

D. From the bundle of His, the depolarization moves to the interventricular septum, which is depolarized in a left-to-right direction

E. The current then moves along the left and right bundle branches to the apex of the heart, where the Purkinje fibers direct the wave of depolarization through the ventricles in a cranial direction

VI. The parts of an ECG tracing are associated with the waves of electrical activity that spread through the heart. The parts are labeled P, QRS, and T (Figure 23-1)

A. P wave: ECG representation of the depolarization of right and left atria

B. PR interval: ECG representation of the beginning of atrial depolarization into ventricular depolarization

1. This interval is mainly a result of slow conduction through the atrioventricular node

2. This interval is only the measurement of time

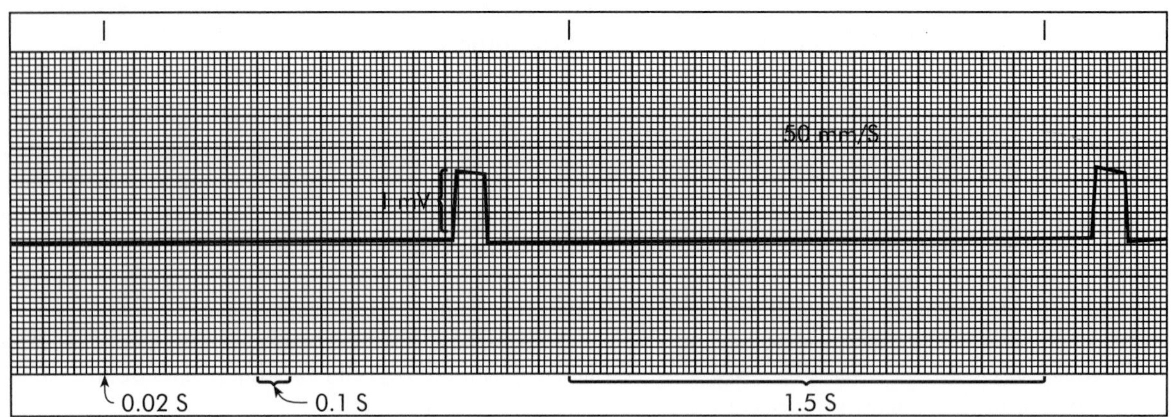

Figure 23-1 Time intervals at 50 mm/sec and 1 mV standard. (Courtesy of Loncke D, Rivait P, Tighe M: *Clinical procedures handbook*, Windsor, Ontario, 2001, St Clair College of Applied Arts and Technology, Veterinary Technician Program.)

C. QRS complex: ECG expression of ventricular depolarization
D. T wave: ECG expression of repolarization of the ventricular myocardium
E. Atrial repolarization is not seen on an ECG because it is hidden by ventricular depolarization or the QRS complex

Supplies

I. Protective padding, blanket, or mat for steel tables (stainless steel conducts electricity)
II. Alcohol or conducting gel or paste for increased skin contact
  A. Note: alcohol should not be used in an emergency situation if defibrillation is a possibility
III. ECG machines that are manufactured for human use may need to be modified
  A. Change the snap end to an alligator clip
    1. Alligator clips should be filed or bent slightly to prevent pinching and bruising
  B. For continuous monitoring, pads or wire may be used
    1. Clip fur so that pad may be applied directly to the skin
    2. For surgical wire placement, which is less painful
      a. Swab area and wire with alcohol
      b. Use a 20-gauge needle to enter and exit the skin subcutaneously
      c. The wire is then passed through the eye of the needle
      d. The needle is removed leaving the wire through the skin
      e. The ends of the wire should be twisted together and taped to prevent injury and ease retrieval in long-haired animals

Procedure

I. Ideally the animal should be in right lateral recumbency during the recording of an ECG
  A. For large animals, standing position is acceptable and should be noted on the recording
  B. Cats sometimes prefer crouching on the table
II. Using manual restraint, the animal should be placed on a mat or blanket with limbs separated by paper towels or a blanket to reduce contact
III. Using alcohol or electrode gel to increase contact at the site, attach the five electrodes by alligator clips to the skin at the following locations (if using surgical wire method, attach electrodes to wire)
  A. Proximal left and right olecranons
  B. Proximal left and right stifles
  C. Chest lead: dorsal thorax near the seventh thoracic vertebra
    1. The chest lead is not universally used; however, it may provide additional data to diagnose right and left cardiac enlargement
IV. A three-lead ECG can be used
  A. The leads are labeled RA (right arm), LA (left arm), and LL (left leg)
V. Ideally, the animal should be drug free and without stress; however, sedation can be provided to a fractious animal
  A. If sedation is needed to perform the ECG, the drug and dosage (in mg) should be recorded on the ECG because the tracing could change
VI. Monitor the patient's color and respiration throughout the procedure because many patients have already compromised cardiac output and may have problems when in lateral recumbency or stressed
VII. ECG machine calibration and recording
  A. A mV "standard" should be recorded at the speed of 25 mm/sec on the strip before the ECG

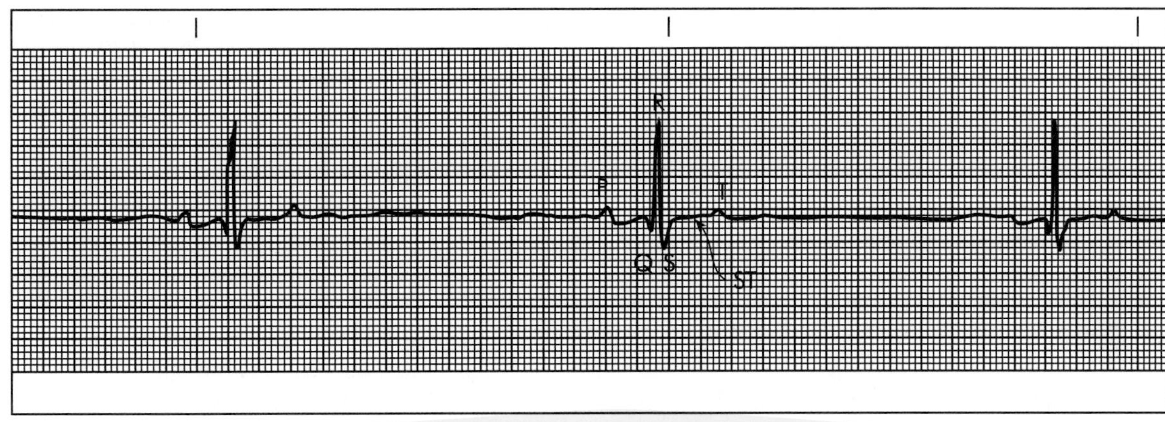

Figure 23-2 Normal lead II complex. (Courtesy of Loncke D, Rivait P, Tighe M: *Clinical procedures handbook*, Windsor, Ontario, 2001, St Clair College of Applied Arts and Technology, Veterinary Technician Program.)

1. The mV "standard" is the measurement of the sensitivity of the machine (Figure 23-2)

B. The paper speed should also be recorded
  1. The paper speed should be changed to 50 mm/sec for tracings
  2. A rhythm strip is run at 25 mm/sec

C. A complete ECG consists of about 30 cm (12 inches) of each lead
  1. In general six leads are recorded: I, II, III, aVR, aVL, and aVF
  2. A rhythm strip consisting of 30 cm or 12 inches of lead II at 25 mm/sec

D. After completing all lead tracings, the following information should be recorded on the tracing
  1. Date of ECG
  2. Patient name, client name, and species
  3. Other relevant information
    a. Recumbency
    b. Drugs used in mg

E. The tracing may then be "mounted" for filing purposes

Normal Electrocardiographic Interpretation

I. A normal heartbeat should include a P, Q, R, S, and T segment
  A. There is a P wave for every QRS complex
  B. The PR interval is relatively constant
  C. The P wave has a positive deflection (above the baseline) in lead II
  D. The T segment can have a positive or a negative deflection

II. A sinus rhythm is the normal cardiac rhythm in domestic animals

III. After completion of an ECG, the veterinarian/technician can measure the complexes and compare the measurement with normal values for each species

IV. The veterinarian/technician can also calculate the heart rate by counting the complexes in a 3-second period
  A. Most ECG paper has specific markings for duration of time on the top of the grid

Abnormal Rhythms

I. Sinus arrhythmia
  A. An irregular ventricular rhythm, which is sinoatrial in origin
  B. On the ECG, the QRS-to-QRS interval varies and there is a P wave for every QRS complex
  C. Most cases of sinus arrhythmia are phasic and associated with respiration
    1. The rate increases with inspiration and decreases with expiration
    2. The sinus arrhythmia of respiratory origin occurs due to the influence of vagal tone
    3. Individuals with respiratory disease tend to have augmented sinus arrhythmia
  D. Most sinus arrhythmias are associated with slow rates
  E. Sinus arrhythmia is normal in the dog

II. Sinus bradycardia
  A. Ventricular rate is decreased
    1. If a dog less than 20 kg (45 lb) has a heart rate of less than 70 beats per minute or if a dog greater than 20 kg (45 lb) has a heart rate of less than 60 beats per minute
    2. Cat: approximately 100 beats per minute or less
  B. Profound bradycardia will cause weakness, hypotension, and syncope
  C. Etiology of sinus bradycardia
    1. Enhanced parasympathetic tone due to
      a. Increased inspiratory effort as a result of respiratory disease
      b. Gastric irritation

c. Increased cerebrospinal fluid pressure, hypothyroidism, hypothermia, hyperkalemia, hypoglycemia, and drug therapy

III. Sinus tachycardia
   A. Sinus rhythm with an increased ventricular rate
   B. A heart rate of 180 beats per minute or greater in dogs that are less than 20 kg (45 lb)
   C. A heart rate of 160 beats per minute or greater in dogs that are more than 20 kg (45 lb)
   D. Puppies with heart rate greater than 220 beats per minute
   E. Cats with heart rate greater than 240 beats per minute
   F. Etiology of sinus tachycardia
      1. Pain
      2. Fever
      3. Anemia
      4. Reduced cardiac output
      5. Hyperthyroidism
      6. Excitement

IV. Atrial flutter
   A. Atrial flutter appears as a regular, saw tooth formation between the QRS complexes
   B. Occurs as the ventricular rate differs from the atrial rate
   C. Is the precursor to atrial fibrillation

V. Atrial fibrillation
   A. No P waves are evident, and the baseline is irregular due to many erratic impulses passing through the atrial myocardium
   B. The ventricular depolarization rate is also irregular and rapid

VI. Premature ventricular contractions or complexes (PVCs)
   A. Premature beats
   B. The ventricle discharges before the arrival of the next anticipated impulse from the sinoatrial node
   C. PVCs can occur at any rate but pose a greater danger when occurring with a sustained heart rate that is tachycardic
   D. The P wave is often not seen on the ECG tracing
   E. A wide distorted QRS complex is also evident
   F. The beat preceding the PVC and the beat following the PVC are equal to the time of two normal beats
   G. Etiology of premature ventricular contraction
      1. Associated with the following
         a. Ventricular concentric hypertrophy or eccentric hypertrophy
         b. Hypoxemic states such as anemia, gastric dilation/volvulus, and heart failure
         c. Acidosis
         d. Drugs such as digitalis, barbiturates, and antiarrhythmic agents
         e. Hypokalemia
   H. Possible consequences of PVCs
      1. May initiate repetitive ventricular firing in the form of ventricular tachycardia or fibrillation
      2. Cardiac output may fall if sufficient premature beats are present
      3. Treatment of PVCs should occur if the patient shows signs due to dysrhythmia

VII. Atrial premature contraction
   A. The PR interval may be short, normal, or long, depending on the area of origin of the premature beat
      1. The origin could include the sinoatrial node or ectopic locations in the atria
   B. The atrial premature contraction may or may not be conducted to the ventricles
      1. If the beat is not conducted to the ventricles and reaches the AV node before repolarization, premature P waves without QRS complexes will appear on the ECG
      2. If depolarization is conducted through the ventricles, the QRS complex will appear normal

VIII. Ventricular tachycardia
   A. A series of four or more PVCs in sequence

IX. Ventricular fibrillation
   A. The mechanical pumping of the heart is not evident on the ECG
   B. The ECG has a bizarre baseline with prominent undulations
   C. There are no recognizable P or QRS complexes
   D. Unless controlled immediately, ventricular fibrillation will result in cardiac arrest

X. First-degree AV block
   A. The PR interval is longer than normal
   B. This type of heart block is a result of a minor conduction defect

XI. Second-degree AV block
   A. Some atrial pulses are not conducted through the AV node and therefore do not cause depolarization of the ventricles
   B. There are two types
      1. Type I (Mobitz type I or Wenckebach AV block): progressive lengthening of the PR interval on successive beats and then P waves occurring without QRS complexes

a. P waves occurring without QRS complexes is called a "dropped beat"

2. Type II: a constant PR interval that is usually of normal duration with random dropped beats

XII. Third-degree AV block
- A. Also known as a complete heart block; the most severe heart block
- B. A lack of any relationship between P waves and QRS complexes; the atria beat at their own rate and the ventricles beat at their own rate

XIII. Asystole
- A. Cardiac arrest
  1. The ECG tracing will appear as a flat line

OROGASTRIC INTUBATION

Indications

I. To remove stomach contents
II. To administer food/nutrients for orphaned or neonatal animals
III. To perform gastric lavage
IV. To administer medication or radiographic contrast material (barium)

Equipment

I. Stomach tube
- A. 12 F to 18 F infant feeding tube for puppies and kittens
- B. 18 F foal stomach tube for dogs greater than 10 kg (22.2 lb)
- C. Foal stomach tube for large dogs

II. Speculum
- A. Canine speculum
- B. Roll of 2-inch (2-cm) wide adhesive tape can be used

III. Adhesive tape for marking the tube
IV. Lubricant
V. Syringe containing sterile saline
VI. Syringe or funnel for administering drugs or other materials

Procedure

I. Most animals will tolerate this procedure without tranquilization; however, light tranquilization may be required
- A. Note that the use of atropine as part of a tranquilizer will slow the motility of the intestines and should not be administered before a barium study
- B. If an animal is anesthetized during this procedure, a cuffed tight-fitting endotracheal tube should be used
  1. A tight-fitting endotracheal tube will prevent aspiration of the administered material

II. Premeasure the stomach tube
- A. The animal can be in either sternal recumbency or standing
- B. Using the tube, estimate approximately the location of the stomach (or last rib) by holding the tube next to the animal
  1. Mark the measurement on the tube at the oral end with adhesive tape

III. Lubricate the tube

IV. Insert the speculum into the mouth and have the restrainer hold the animal's jaws shut on the speculum

V. Pass the lubricated tube into the speculum and then advance to the premarked point on tube
- A. If the tube cannot be passed to the premarked point
  1. The tube is in the trachea
  2. There is an obstruction in the esophagus. There is a volvulus, which is preventing the tube from passing

VI. Check the placement of the tube before administration of fluids or other material
- A. Note: If an animal is heavily sedated, check the tube placement by more than one method
  1. Palpate the neck to check for a trachea and the stomach tube
  2. Blow into the tube and listen for gurgling either on the outside of the body or within the tube
  3. Inject 5 mL of sterile saline into the tube while holding the tube toward the ceiling; if the animal does not cough, the tube is in the esophagus
  4. Smell the end of the tube for gastric odors
- B. If there is *any* evidence that the tube is in the trachea, such as coughing, remove the tube and reinsert it

VII. Administer materials

VIII. After administration of material, administer 6 mL of water to flush the tube or kink the tube

IX. Before removing the tube, seal the end with a thumb and then remove or kink the tube
- A. This will help to prevent the leakage of the administered material and water while removing the tube
  1. The animal could aspirate the material if leakage occurs

Precautions

I. Administration of material into the respiratory tract, causing aspiration pneumonia
II. Esophageal trauma
III. Gastric irritation
IV. Gastric perforation

NASOGASTRIC INTUBATION

Definition

I. Placement of a tube through the external nares, the nasal cavity, pharynx, and esophagus and into the stomach

Indications

I. Used for liquid nutritional support and water administration for an extended period of time
   A. For anorexic animals or animals too stressed to force feed
II. To administer medication or radiographic contrast medium

Equipment

I. Nasogastric feeding tube, infant feeding tube, red rubber tube, or polyurethane tube
   A. The tube must be soft and flexible
      1. Animals less than 5 kg (12 lb) require a 5 F feeding tube
      2. Animals 5 to 15 kg (12 to 33 lb) require an 8 F feeding tube
II. Topical ophthalmic anesthetic
III. Lubricating jelly
IV. Syringe with 1 mL of sterile saline
V. Bandaging material if feeding tube is going to be used for an extended period of time
   A. Gauze squares and adhesive tape or elastic adhesive tape
VI. Injection cap
VII. Medication or liquid to administer

Procedure

I. Patient should be awake
II. Pre-measure the tube by placing it on the side of the patient with the tip at the thirteenth rib and the end of the tube at the nares
   A. Mark the tube with a permanent marker for future reference
III. Instill 4 to 5 drops of topical anesthetic into one nostril
   A. The patient may sneeze
   B. The patient's head should be pointed toward the ceiling
IV. Wait 2 to 3 minutes and apply a few more drops of topical anesthetic to the same nostril
V. Apply a small amount of lubricating jelly to the tip of the nasogastric tube
VI. Hold the head with one hand and insert the tube into the anesthetized nostril
VII. Advance the tube approximately 20 to 25 cm (10 inches)
   A. Gently rotate the tube until it is in place
VIII. Check the placement of the tube by instilling 1 mL of sterile saline into the tube
   A. If the animal coughs, the tube is in the trachea
   B. If the tube is in the trachea, remove the tube and start the procedure again
IX. If the tube is to remain in place for an extended period of time, bandage the tube in place on one side of the patient's neck
   A. Cachexic or debilitated cats will usually tolerate a tube for extended periods of time
   B. The tube can remain in place for approximately 1 week or until the animal tolerates force feeding or is eating on its own
X. The end of the tube should be covered with a cap to prevent the aspiration of air into the patient's stomach
XI. Aspirate the tube before each feeding and instill 1 mL of sterile saline into the tube to check for coughing
   A. There should be negative pressure on the tube if the tube is in the stomach
XII. Before removing the tube, seal the end with a finger or thumb to prevent leakage into the pharynx when the tube is removed
XIII. Write in the patient record the location and time that the procedure was performed and if any medication was administered

Precautions

I. Possible administration of materials into the respiratory tract, causing aspiration pneumonia
II. Esophageal trauma
III. Gastric irritation
IV. The procedure can be stressful to some patients
V. Contraindicated in patients with nasal tumors, esophageal disorders, or no gag reflex
VI. Possible epistaxis (nosebleed) when the tube is first inserted
VII. The tube can become obstructed by medications or nutritional supplements

CANINE MALE URINARY CATHETERIZATION

Indications

I. To collect a sterile sample of urine for analysis and culture
II. To measure urine output and drainage of urine from the urinary bladder
III. To relieve a urethral obstruction
IV. To administer medication or radiographic contrast medium into the bladder or perform pneumocystography

Equipment

I. Mild soap
II. Sterile polyethylene, vinyl, or rubber urethral catheter

A. These can be purchased in a variety of sizes: 3.5 F, 5 F, 8 F, and 10 F
   1. Less trauma with a smaller and more flexible catheter
B. Sterile lubricant
C. Sterile syringe(s) or sterile container to collect urine

Procedure

I. The patient may be in lateral recumbency or standing
II. Clip the area free of long hairs and cleanse the prepuce with a mild soap
III. Select an appropriate size of sterile catheter for the patient
   A. Dogs less than 12 kg: 3.5 F or 5 F catheter
   B. Dogs greater than 12 kg: 8 F
   C. Dogs greater than 35 kg: 10 F or 12 F
   D. Foley catheter, which has inflatable tip for long-term use
IV. Estimate the length of the catheter, which will be needed to enter the urinary bladder by measuring the catheter against the dog in the approximate position of the penis and bladder
V. A restrainer can lift the dog's upper leg away from the body
VI. Open the package containing the catheter in a sterile manner
VII. Advance the catheter out of its sterile sleeve and lubricate the end of the catheter with sterile lubricant; the restrainer can then hold the catheter, which is still in the sterile sleeve
VIII. With one hand, retract the dog's prepuce so that approximately 1 to 2 inches (5 cm) of glans penis is exposed
   A. The glans penis may be cleansed again at this time
IX. With the other hand, insert the lubricated catheter into the urethral orifice, advancing slowly into the bladder
   A. Slight resistance or stoppage may be felt as the catheter passes the area of the ischial arch
   B. If this does occur, direct the penis toward the cranial end of the animal and slightly lift the penis off the body
X. Attach a syringe to the end of the catheter; extract urine by pulling back on the plunger
   A. If there is no urine entering the catheter, advance the catheter further into the bladder
XI. After the sample is obtained, label the syringe or container with name, date, time, type of sample (sterile) or catheterized, and initials
XII. An acceptable alternative is to remove the entire catheter from the package while wearing sterile gloves
   A. If this method is chosen, sterile technique must be used

Precautions

I. Urinary tract infections due to a break in sterility procedure
II. Trauma to the urethra or urinary bladder by rough handling or incorrect size of the catheter

CANINE FEMALE URINARY CATHETERIZATION ■

Indications

I. The same as for the male dog

Equipment

I. The same as for male dog with the addition of a vaginal speculum, sterile gloves, small amount of viscous Xylocaine or 0.5% lidocaine jelly, and possibly a steel catheter
   A. A human bivalve nasal speculum with a halogen bulb attached may be used instead of a vaginal speculum
      1. The use of an otoscope or a modified syringe casing as a speculum is also acceptable

Procedure

I. Dog can be in sternal or lateral recumbency if anesthetized or standing if awake
II. The restrainer should hold the dog's tail out of the field of view
III. For visual technique
   A. Before performing the procedure, the area can be anesthetized with lidocaine jelly for the comfort of the patient
   B. Check the vulva and vaginal opening using a speculum
      1. Insert the closed speculum first, aiming dorsally and then cranially to avoid the clitoral fossa (blind sac at the ventral opening of the vulva)
   C. Insert lubricated sterile catheter by passing it through the speculum into the urethral orifice and advancing the catheter into the bladder
      1. The urethral tubercle leading to the urethral orifice is on the ventral surface of the vagina approximately 1 to 2 cm (0.5 to 1 inch) from the clitoral fossa
         a. Often the urethral tubercle is white or red and appears to be puckered or in the form of a cross
   D. The catheter should be directed ventrally; if the catheter is moving in a dorsal position, it is entering the cervical area of the uterus and will not pass farther than approximately 4 to 5 cm (2 inches)
   E. If no urine is entering the catheter, advance the catheter further into the bladder

F. Collect the urine in a sterile container and label accordingly
    1. The urine can be collected in a sterile container or with a sterile syringe

IV. Touch technique
   A. Prepare the area as in the visual technique
   B. Lubricate the gloved index finger of one hand and palpate the urethral tubercle
   C. Pass the sterile lubricated catheter ventrally to the gloved finger in the vagina and use a finger to guide the catheter down to the urethral tubercle and into the urethral orifice

V. A small amount of dilute povidone-iodine solution may be infused into the bladder before removing the catheter to prevent infection

Precautions

I. The same as for the male dog

CYSTOCENTESIS

Indications

I. To puncture the urinary bladder for the purpose of obtaining an uncontaminated sample of urine for analysis or culture

II. To relieve distension of the urinary bladder when an obstruction cannot be relieved by catheterization

Equipment

I. Large syringe (6 or 12 mL), 22-gauge needle, and isopropyl alcohol

Procedure

I. This procedure can be performed on an awake, tranquilized or anesthetized cat or dog

II. The animal should be in dorsal or lateral recumbency with the upper leg lifted away from the body to expose the inguinal area
   A. Cats and dogs may also be in standing position

III. Palpate the bladder in the ventral abdominal area just cranial to the pubis to assess whether there is urine in the bladder

IV. The location of the approximate puncture site can then be swabbed with isopropyl alcohol

V. Try to immobilize and hold the bladder in place with one hand; use the other hand to puncture the bladder with a sterile needle and syringe

VI. Puncture the bladder and direct the needle in a caudodorsal direction

VII. Using the syringe plunger and negative pressure, withdraw the sample of urine from the bladder
   A. Do not squeeze the bladder while performing cystocentesis
   B. If no fluid is obtained, remove the needle from the body and perform a second puncture using a different needle

VIII. Withdraw the needle and syringe quickly from the body after releasing the plunger

IX. Transfer the sample to a sterile collection container and label the container with the name of the patient, date, initials, and type of sample

X. An alternate method is the "pooling" technique, which may help to locate the ideal location for cystocentesis
   A. The animal is in dorsal recumbency
   B. A small amount of alcohol is poured on the abdomen
   C. The area where the alcohol pools on the ventral midline is the ideal location for the puncture
   D. Withdraw the sample as described earlier
      1. In male dogs, the prepuce may be moved to one side to allow room for insertion of the needle

Precautions

I. Urine leakage and peritonitis due to a ruptured bladder

II. Contamination of urine by blood due to a bladder hemorrhage

III. Contamination of the bladder with fecal material is possible due to the accidental intestinal penetration

IV. Cystocentesis is contraindicated in patients with a suspected pyometra, bladder neoplasias, and bleeding disorders

MANUAL COMPRESSION OF THE URINARY BLADDER

Indications

I. Urine collected by manual compression is unsatisfactory for urine culture but can be used to examine solute concentration, physical properties, and chemical constituents

Procedure

I. Locate the bladder
   A. Begin palpating the abdomen starting at the last rib and move caudally; or
   B. Begin palpating the abdomen slightly cranial to the rear legs
      1. Begin dorsally and move ventrally

II. After palpating and immobilizing the bladder, exert moderate, gentle, steady pressure over the bladder

III. Direct the expressed urine into a container for analysis

Precautions

I. Do not apply excessive force on the bladder, especially in cases of urethral blockage, because the bladder might rupture

ANAL SAC EXPRESSION

Definition

I. The anal sacs are located on either side of an animal's anus at approximately the 4 and 8 o'clock positions
II. The anal sacs are filled with odorous secretions and should normally be expressed when the animal defecates
III. This procedure is commonly performed on dogs, rarely on cats

Indications

I. To decrease irritation to the animal caused by distention or inflammation
II. To instill medication into diseased anal sacs
III. Removal of material from anal sacs

Procedure

I. The dog may have to be muzzled and/or securely restrained
II. There are two methods for anal sac expression
  A. External
    1. Using rolled cotton over the dog's anus, apply pressure in a medial and slightly dorsal direction of the external anus
    2. This method does not guarantee full expression of anal sacs
  B. Internal
    1. Insert a gloved, well-lubricated index finger into the anus
    2. With cotton covering the sac, gently squeeze together index finger and thumb to milk contents of the anal sac toward the medial anus
    3. After examining the contents of secretions, roll the glove over the cotton, remove from the hand, and discard
      a. Normal anal sac material should contain granular brown, malodorous material

Precautions

I. Rupture of abscessed anal sac
II. Perforation of rectum

ENEMAS

Definition

I. An enema is the infusion of fluid into the lower intestinal tract through the anus
II. Enemas are used to remove fecal material from the colon

Indications

I. To prepare for radiographs with or without contrast medium involvement
II. To irrigate the colon of a patient who has been poisoned
III. To relieve constipation

Procedure

I. Sedation or anesthesia may be needed in cases of severe blockage or fractious animals
II. An abdominal radiograph should be completed to rule out perforation or foreign body
III. Use an enema container with a rounded, soft, pliable piece of connected tubing
IV. Place the animal in sternal or lateral recumbency, preferably on a tub table
V. Put on examination gloves
VI. Place the enema preparation into the enema container
  A. Examples of enema preparations
    1. Mild soap and water
    2. Saline for irrigation
    3. Commercial enema preparation
  B. Hyperphosphate enema solutions should not be used in cats or small dogs
    1. These solutions may cause acute collapse associated with hypocalcemia
VII. Lubricate well the end of the flexible tubing
VIII. Insert the tip of the enema tubing to the colorectal junction
IX. Place the enema container above the animal to aid the solution in flowing into the animal by gravity
X. More than one enema may be required to adequately evacuate the animal's bowels
XI. Do not continue to administer enemas if there is no sign of fecal material
XII. Do not proceed with enema if there is evidence of abdominal pain that could be associated with intestinal perforation or obstruction

Precautions

I. Rupture of the colon
II. Leakage of enema fluid into peritoneal cavity through already ruptured intestinal tract
III. Hemorrhage in cases of ulcerative colitis
  A. Enemas are contraindicated in cases of ulcerative colitis because they may increase bleeding

WOUND MANAGEMENT

Wound Contamination Versus Infection

I. All wounds are contaminated; however, a contaminated wound elicits no immune response from the host body

A. A surgical wound is considered contaminated by microbes on the tissue and surrounding area

II. Infection is the term used for a wound where microorganisms are invading tissue and therefore elicit an immune response from the host body
   A. A wound is considered infected if the patient is presented for treatment more than 12 hours postinjury
      1. Signs of infection can include edema, pus, fever, neutrophilia, pain, color change, exudates, and odor

III. Contaminated wound can become infected due to the addition of foreign material in the wound, necrotic tissue, or excessive bleeding

Wound Healing

I. The four phases of wound healing are the inflammatory phase, the debridement phase, the repair phase, and the maturation phase
   A. Inflammatory phase: begins directly after the injury
      1. Vasoconstriction is followed by vasodilation to control hemorrhage and then produce a clot
      2. The blood clot will dry and form a scab, which allows healing to begin
   B. Debridement phase: begins approximately 6 hours postinjury
      1. Neutrophils and monocytes travel to the site to remove foreign material, bacteria, and necrotic tissue
      2. An exudate is formed from fluid and white blood cells
   C. Repair phase: begins 3 to 5 days postinjury and depends on the debridement stage and the removal of foreign material in the wound
      1. The debridement and inflammatory phases, or the first 3 to 5 days postinjury, can also be called the "lag phase"
         a. The lag phase is characterized by minimal wound strength
      2. At this point, fibroblasts produce collagen that after maturation will become scar tissue and strengthen the wound
      3. Granulation tissue starts to appear due to new capillaries, fibroblasts, and fibrous tissue formation
         a. Granulation tissue appears under the scab as red, fleshy material
      4. Epithelialization, or the formation of new epithelial tissue, on the wound surface becomes visible 4 to 5 days postinjury
         a. Epithelial cells at the edge of the wound divide and migrate across the granulation tissue
         b. The new tissue is only one cell thick; however, over time it thickens through the formation of more cell layers
      5. Wound contraction, reducing the size of the wound, occurs 5 to 9 days postinjury
   D. Maturation phase: the final phase, this is the longest phase
      1. During this phase, wound strength increases to its maximum level due to remodeling of the collagen fibers and fibrous tissue
         a. Cross-linking increases and improves wound strength
      2. The scar gradually disappears due to the number of capillaries in the fibrous tissue
      3. This phase may continue for many years
   E. Wound healing is a series of overlapping events; more than one phase may be occurring at one time

Types of Wound Healing

I. Primary or first-intention healing
   A. Characterized by noncomplicated healing
      1. Examples: small lacerations, minor wounds, and clean wounds
      2. In the case of fractures, using pins or plates

II. Second-intention healing
   A. Wounds that are left open and allowed to heal from the internal to external areas
      1. Examples: larger wounds, infected wounds
      2. Healing of fractures through the normal formation of a callus

III. Third-intention healing
   A. Initial second-intention healing (open wound) followed by surgical repair
      1. Examples: severely contaminated wounds, very large wounds

Wound Treatment

I. First aid
   A. Protection of the wound is important either by bandaging or by a makeshift splint

II. Wound evaluation
   A. Control of hemorrhaging should be the first priority, followed by an evaluation of the wound for possible contamination and infection
   B. The injury should then be assessed by obtaining a history and checking the location and size of the wound

III. Clipping, scrubbing, and wound lavage
   A. All wounds should be clipped before treatment
      1. A sterile lubricant can be put into any open wounds to avoid further contamination of the site by loose hair

2. Ophthalmic ointment may be applied in the eye before clipping and cleaning for protection of the cornea and globe
B. The outer edges of the wound can then be gently scrubbed using a detergent/antimicrobial surgical scrub
1. Povidine-iodine or chlorhexidine base type of agent is recommended
C. Wound lavage is most effective when performed using at least 7 pounds per square inch (psi) of pressure
1. Equipment
a. A 35- to 60-mL syringe with an 18-gauge needle attached
b. WaterPik at low pressure
c. Spray bottle
d. Lavage solutions include
(1) Isotonic saline, LRS, or plain Ringer's solution
(2) Hydrogen peroxide
(a) Can cause damage to tissues due to the foaming effect
(b) Is not antimicrobial, just sporicidal
(c) Should only be used for first-time irrigation of dirty wounds
(d) Should not be used under pressure due to foaming
(3) Chlorhexidine diacetate solution 0.05% solution
(a) Broad-spectrum antimicrobial
(b) Microbial effect is immediate with a lasting residual effect
(c) Not inactivated by organic material
(4) Povidone-iodine 1% to 2% solution
(a) Broad-spectrum antimicrobial
(b) Antimicrobial effect lasts approximately 4 to 6 hours
(c) It is inactivated by blood, exudates, and organic material
(d) The detergent form is not recommended for wounds because it causes irritation and potentiation of wound infections

IV. Debridement
A. Debridement is the removal of necrotic tissue
B. Necrotic tissue must be removed for new tissue to migrate over the wound
1. Necrotic tissue is also considered a growth medium for bacteria, so if removed the chances of infection are reduced
C. Debridement is considered complete when the wound is free of necrotic tissue
1. The wound is then considered a "clean wound"
D. Mechanical debridement includes the use of surgical instruments, dry-to-dry bandages, wet-to-dry bandages, and irrigation
E. Nonmechanical debridement is generally the addition of enzymatic agents or chemicals to the wound
1. Both mechanical and nonmechanical methods may be used to treat a wound
F. The procedure should be performed aseptically

V. Drainage
A. Drains are implanted in a wound to help relieve the buildup of air or fluid
1. The drain will reduce the possible formation of seromas, hematomas, tissue pockets, or dead space
B. Drains are usually indicated for
1. Treatment of an abscess
2. When foreign material is in a wound and cannot be removed
3. When contamination is probable
4. When necrotic tissue cannot be excised
5. Prevention of the creation of dead space and to remove fluid or air after a surgical procedure
C. Penrose drains are used most commonly
1. They are composed of soft, latex rubber
2. Fluid flows through the lumen of the drain and around the drain
3. Penrose drains should not be left in place for longer than 3 to 5 days

BANDAGING

Types of Bandages

I. Bandages are made up of three layers: primary, secondary, and tertiary
A. Primary layer is next to the wound
B. Secondary layer is present to absorb exudates and provide padding
C. Tertiary layer is the outer layer, which is used for support

II. Primary layer material
A. Adherent bandages are used to remove necrotic tissue and wound exudates when it is taken off
1. These types of bandages (usually sterile gauze) are used in the very early stages of wound healing
a. Dry-to-dry dressings are used when loose necrotic tissue is evident
(1) Dry sterile gauze is placed over the wound with an absorbent wrap holding it in place

(2) Bandage removal may be painful because dead tissue is adhered to the bandage

b. Wet-to-dry dressings are used for wounds with dried or semidry exudates

(1) The bandage is applied wet, and it absorbs the material from the wound

(2) The exudate then adheres to the bandage and is removed when the bandage is removed

(3) Saline or chlorhexidine can be used to moisten the bandage

c. Wet-to-wet dressings are used on wounds with large amounts of exudates and transudate

(1) Wet dressings tend to absorb fluid easily

(2) Wet dressings can be used to heat the wound, which will enhance capillary action and therefore increase the drainage of the wound

(3) These bandages are removed wet and therefore cause less pain on bandage removal

(4) The negative aspect of this type of bandage is that there is little wound debridement because of the decreased adhesion to necrotic tissue

B. Nonadherent primary layer

1. Used when granulation tissue is starting to form
2. Commonly used to minimize tissue injury during bandage changes
3. There are many commercial products on the market

III. Secondary layer provides extra absorbency to draw fluids away from the wound and adds padding for support

A. Generally, gauze bandaging is used, such as Kling or Sof-Kling (Johnson & Johnson)

IV. Tertiary layer holds the primary and secondary layers in place

A. Generally made up of adhesive tapes, elastic bandages, Vet Wrap (3M) and a conforming stretch gauze (Conform; Kendall)

Head and Neck

I. Reasons for bandaging

A. Postocular surgery
B. Repair of an aural hematoma
C. Ear surgery
D. To secure a jugular catheter or pharyngostomy tube

II. Precautions

A. The bandage should be frequently checked postoperatively because edema, which could be life threatening, may occur

B. Respiration and mucous membrane color must be monitored closely

1. The bandage should be loose enough to enable two fingers to fit under the bandage
2. If there are any changes in respirations, the bandage should be loosened or changed immediately

C. If the animal tries to remove the bandage, an Elizabethan collar can be used for restraint

Thorax

I. Reasons for bandaging

A. To secure chest drains
B. To protect large thoracic wounds
C. Spinal surgery

II. Precautions

A. If impairment of respiration occurs, the bandage should be removed or cut to loosen it immediately

Abdomen

I. Reasons for bandaging

A. To secure a gastrostomy tube
B. After a radical mastectomy
C. For extensive wounds or dissection of the abdominal region

II. Precautions

A. Care must be taken when applying the bandage not to incorporate the prepuce in male dogs because this can interfere with urination
B. Steps should be taken also to keep the bandage clean and dry from urine and feces

Limbs

I. Reasons for bandaging

A. Immobilization of fractures
B. Wound protection
C. Stabilization for fluid therapy

II. Most common type: Robert Jones pressure bandage

A. A Robert Jones bandage can be used to temporarily stabilize fractures before surgical repair
B. This bandage consists of several layers of rolled cotton compressed tightly with elastic gauze and elastic tape
C. The underlying layers of cotton prevent constriction of the limb

III. Precautions

A. When bandaging the upper portion of a limb, the entire limb should be incorporated in the bandage

B. This allows for even distribution of pressure along the limb and maintains venous return from the paw
C. The toes should be checked routinely for swelling, coldness, and pallor of the nail beds (where possible)
   1. If any of these changes occur, the bandage should be loosened or changed because these signs may indicate poor venous return
D. The bandage should be loose enough to allow two fingers to slip under the bandage at all times
E. To keep the bandage clean and dry when walking the animal
   1. A small bag, an examination glove, or an empty fluid bag can be taped onto the proximal end of the limb and then removed after exercising

Paw

I. Reasons for bandaging
   A. Declawing of cats
   B. Dewclaw removal in dogs
   C. Repair of lacerations
II. Precautions
   A. The accessory pad should be included when bandaging the paw
   B. A piece of cotton under the pad, as well as between the digits, helps to prevent irritation or chafing

Tail (Figure 23-3)

I. Reasons for bandaging
   A. Partial tail amputation
   B. Protection of wounds
   C. Tumor removal
   D. To wrap long-haired cats or dogs with severe diarrhea to keep the area as clean as possible
II. Precautions
   A. Sedation may be needed if bleeding persists from excessive tail wagging or from hitting the remaining portion of tail on a hard surface after amputation
      1. In cases of amputation, a hard tubular object fastened to the base of the tail protecting the sight is often helpful
         a. Objects such as an empty cardboard roll can be useful
         b. Analgesics may be required for pain

Specialized Bandaging Techniques

I. Ehmer sling to support the hind limb postreduction of hip luxation
II. Velpeau sling (Figure 23-4) to support the shoulder joint after surgery
III. Hobbles can be applied to hind limbs to prevent them from abducting excessively

Casting Materials

I. Fiberglass cast
   A. Lightweight and strong
   B. Fast-setting cast
II. Plaster of Paris
   A. Gauze roll impregnated with calcium sulfate dihydrate

Aftercare of Bandages, Slings, and Casts

I. Close monitoring is essential
   A. Note evidence of odor, edema, discharge, or skin irritation
   B. Note warmth, color, and swelling of toes
II. Prevent the animal from chewing or licking the bandage
   A. Use discipline, sedation; Elizabethan collar, T-shirt, sock, or foul-tasting substances that can be applied to the dressing

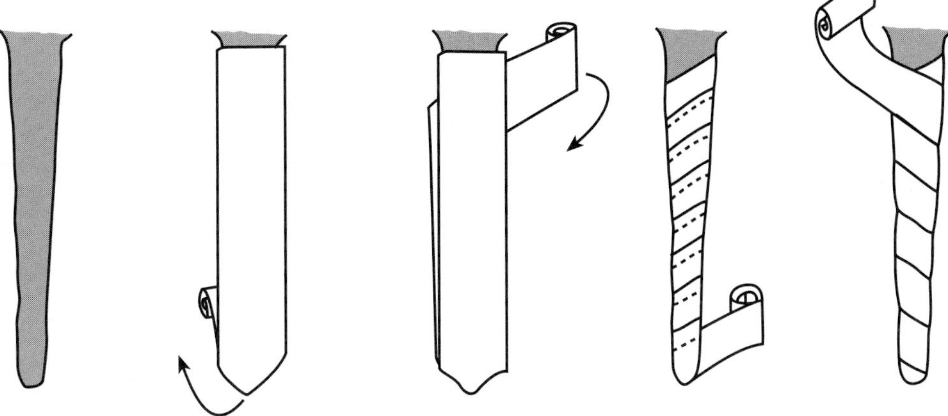

Figure 23-3 Tail bandage. (From Lane DR, Cooper B: *Veterinary nursing, formerly Jones' animal nursing,* ed 5, Woburn, Mass, 1998, Butterworth Heinemann.)

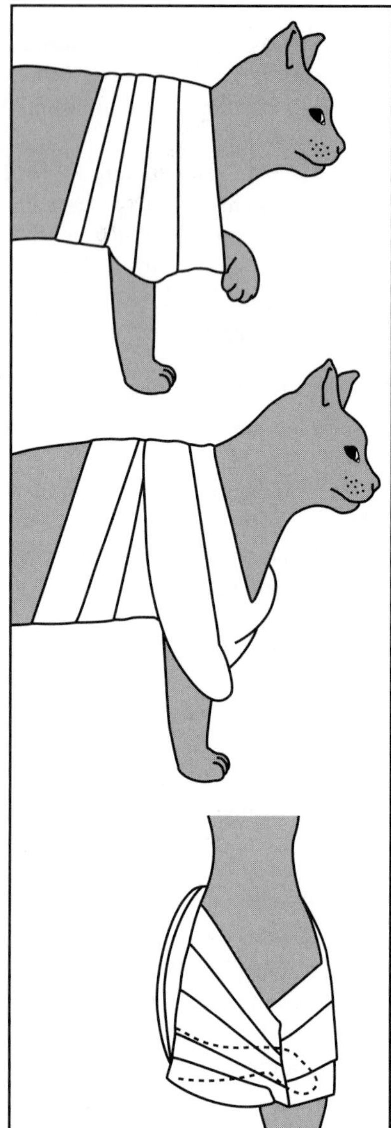

Figure 23-4 Making a Velpeau sling. (From Lane DR, Cooper B: *Veterinary nursing, formerly Jones' animal nursing,* ed 5, Woburn, Mass, 1998, Butterworth Heinemann.)

III. When outdoors, protect the bandage from dirt and moisture by covering it with a plastic bag
IV. Exercise should be limited

ONCOLOGY

The cause of tumors is not known; however, genetic factors, carcinogens, radiation, trauma, foreign material, or infectious agents may play a role in the development of some types of neoplasia.

Definition

I. Oncology is the study of cancer
II. Cancer is defined as any malignant, cellular tumor
   A. Other terms used to describe cancer include neoplasia, neoplasm, growth, tumor, and malignancy
III. Carcinogenic means a substance that produces cancer
IV. Benign or malignant
   A. A benign neoplasm is localized, does not infiltrate another area, and can be easily excised due to encapsulation
      1. The harm in the neoplasm is generally due to the space the tumor is occupying
      2. Benign in latin means "innocent"
   B. A malignant neoplasm has the ability to be metastatic and infiltrative
      1. Metastasis is the process in which cancer cells spread from the primary location to a secondary area such as lymph nodes, lungs, or other viscera
         a. The secondary location is not directly connected to the primary location
      2. Often tumors are classified as primary and secondary to denote which type of neoplasm was identified first

Classification

I. Tumors are classified as malignant or benign and by their origin
   A. Example: carcinomas are malignant and arise from epithelial tissues such as skin, mucous membranes, glandular tissue, and organs such as liver and kidneys
   B. Example: sarcomas are also malignant tumors and arise from mesenchymal tissues such as connective tissue, cartilage, or bone
II. Tumors are also classified by their tissue of origin
   A. The prefix of a name generally indicates the specific area of origin; the suffix indicates whether it is benign or malignant (Table 23-1)
   B. The suffix *-oma* generally indicates a benign tumor
      1. Example: fibroma is a benign tumor of fibrous tissue
   C. The suffix *-sarcoma* or *-carcinoma* indicates malignancy
      1. Example: chondrosarcoma is a malignant tumor of cartilage
   D. Exceptions to this rule are melanoma, insulinoma, and thymoma; all of these tumors are malignant

Diagnostics

I. Early warning signs
   A. Bleeding or discharge
   B. Difficulty eating, swallowing, loss of appetite, weight loss
   C. Dyspnea, dysuria, abnormal stool or problems defecating

Table 23-1 Examples of common neoplasias

Name	Location	Malignant or benign
Mast cell	Skin	Both
Osteosarcoma	Bone	Malignant
Hemangiosarcoma	Blood vessels	Malignant
Malignant melanoma	Arising from melanocytes of the skin, eye, or oral cavity	Pigs and cattle benign; all other species usually malignant
Squamous cell carcinoma	Conjunctiva, mouth, stomach, vulva, penis, and skin	Malignant
Lymphosarcoma	Lymph tissue	Malignant
Leukemia	Blood forming organs	Malignant
Mammary adenocarcinoma	Mammary tissue; generally glandular tissue	Malignant
Fibrosarcoma	Fibrous tissue	Malignant

D. Loss of stamina, lameness, stiffness, decreased exercise

E. Abnormal swelling, sores that do not heal, or a bad odor

II. Evaluation

A. Obtain an patient history from the owner

1. The history should include the duration of the problem, observations, clinical signs, previous medical problems, husbandry, and vaccination history

B. A complete physical examination should be performed

1. After a physical examination, which includes palpation of all lymph nodes, all masses should be checked and measured and a detailed record should be completed

C. A CBC, serum chemistry profile, urinalysis, thoracic radiograph, abdominal radiograph, and possibly abdominal ultrasound should also be included in the evaluation of the patient

D. Cytology

1. To determine the cell morphology of a tumor, cytology may be performed

a. The most common method to collect samples is a fine needle aspiration biopsy

(1) The neoplasm is cleansed with alcohol

(2) A 22-gauge needle attached to a 6-mL syringe is inserted into the center of the neoplasm

(3) Using suction, a sample of the tumor is obtained

(4) The sample is then squirted onto a slide, air dried, and fixed with Wright's stain, new methylene blue, or a Diff-Quick type stain

(5) If the sample is to be shipped in a commercial laboratory pack, the slides are packed in a plastic container to protect them

(6) The history of the patient and size, location, and duration of the neoplasm should be included with the slides

E. Histopathology is the definitive method of diagnosis

1. Entire masses or large sections of a tumor may be submitted for testing

2. Biopsy techniques include

a. Needle core biopsy: a small incision is made in the mass, and the specialized needle is inserted to obtain a small sample

(1) The TruCut biopsy needle is commonly used for this procedure

b. Incisional biopsy: removal of a small wedge of tissue

c. Excisional biopsy: removal of the entire tumor and margins of surrounding tissue are included to check for cancer cells

Therapy

I. Surgery: removal of the entire tumor

A. Surgery is most commonly used to treat localized neoplastic disease

B. If a tumor is malignant, the surgeon should remove approximately 2 to 3 cm (1 to 2 inches) of normal tissue along the margin of the tumor if possible

C. Surgery could alter organ function, change the appearance of the patient, and cause hemorrhaging

II. Cryosurgery: use of liquid nitrogen, or N_2O, (cold) to freeze cancerous tissue

A. This method is generally used for small lesions on the external epithelium

III. Chemotherapy: the treatment of cancer with cytotoxic agents

A. Generally used for systemic or metastatic cancer and is not usually a cure

1. Often chemotherapy is used to produce remission in the patient; this method does not always eradicate cancer cells

B. Can be used after surgical excision of a malignant tumor to prevent further metastasis
C. Also used for tumors that cannot be surgically removed and to improve the quality of the patient's life
D. Can be used in conjunction with other methods such as surgery, radiation, or hyperthermia
E. Chemotherapy is often used to decrease the size of a neoplasm, to decrease the patient's pain
F. Technique
  1. A combination of chemotherapeutic drugs is used most often
    a. Ideally the combined drugs should have different toxicities, work through different mechanisms, and have different efficacies
  2. Examples of chemotherapeutic drugs
    a. Hormones, antineoplastic antibiotics, antimetabolites, alkylating agents, plant alkaloids
G. Complications
  1. Most cytotoxic agents kill neoplastic cells and rapidly divide noncancerous cells
    a. Examples: bone marrow cells, intestinal cells
  2. There are many side effects from chemotherapeutic agents
    a. The most common are alopecia, cardiotoxicity, vomiting, diarrhea, pancreatitis, hepatosis, neutropenia, thrombocytopenia, anemia, neurotoxicity, and renal toxicity
  3. Side effects also apply to technical staff who administer the drugs
    a. Protective equipment should be used for safety
      (1) Disposable latex gloves, long-sleeved coat or surgical gown with tight-fitting cuffs, and safety eyewear are necessities
    b. Biomedical waste should be placed in a sealable plastic bag and held for biomedical waste pickup
      (1) Biomedical waste includes syringes, IV administration sets, gauze, and gloves
      (2) Cytotoxic waste includes urine, feces, vomitus, and other body fluids
        (a) Waste from animals that have received cytotoxic drugs within the previous 48-hour period is the most harmful
        (b) Patient waste may be disposed of through the sewage system

IV. Radiotherapy: the use of ionizing radiation
A. The cell is killed by the disruption of its DNA
B. Radiation can be used in conjunction with another therapy method such as surgery or chemotherapy
C. Radiation may be used to treat localized or regional neoplasias or as a palliative therapy in patients with terminal disease
D. Radiation is administered in frequent small doses to minimize the toxic effects and maximize the therapeutic effects

V. Hyperthermia: using a cautery unit to burn small epithelial tumors
A. This method causes necrosis and vascular thrombosis of the area
B. Hyperthermia is sometimes used with chemotherapy or radiation therapy

ACKNOWLEDGMENT

The editors recognize and appreciate the original contributions of Julie Ball-Karn and Kathy Taylor, on which this chapter is based.

Glossary

abducting To draw away from the median plane
alkylating Compound that is used as a chemotherapeutic agent
alopecia Absence of hair from skin in areas in which it is normally present
anaphylaxis Manifestation of immediate hypersensitivity in which exposure of a sensitized individual to a specific antigen or protein results in life-threatening respiratory distress, usually followed by vascular collapse and shock
antimetabolite Substance that interferes with the utilization of an essential metabolite
antineoplastic Drug that inhibits the proliferation and maturation of malignant cells
anuria Complete suppression of urinary secretion from the kidneys
aseptic In a sterile manner
aspirate To apply suction and withdraw fluid
ataxia Lack of muscle coordination
auscultate To listen to thoracic and abdominal sounds
capillary refill time (CRT) After applying pressure to the gum line to blanch them, it is the time it takes for color to return to the area, normally 1 to 2 seconds
cautery unit Used in surgery to burn tissue with an electrical current
chondrosarcoma Malignant tumor of cartilage cells or their precursors
colloid An intravenous solution containing starch or protein molecules
conjunctiva Delicate membrane lining the eyelids and surrounding the eyeball
crackles A sharp sound heard on auscultation; usually a sign of emphysema
crystalloid Isotonic electrolyte solution
cytotoxic Toxic to cells

debridement Removal of necrotic or devitalized tissue
depolarization Process of neutralizing polarity. Depolarization phase of the cardiac cycle means the resting phase
distention Abnormal swelling or size
dressing Bandage; material that covers a wound
dry-to-dry bandage Primary layer of an adherent bandage that is used on open wounds to remove necrotic tissue
edema Abnormally large amounts of fluid in the intercellular tissue spaces of the body
Elizabethan collar Special collar used in small animals to prevent self-mutilation
epithelialization Growth of epithelium to heal a wound
extracellular Outside a cell or cells
exudate Fluid containing protein and cells that is excreted from the body on tissue surfaces
F (French) Unit; used to describe the circumference of a tube. Each gauge unit is about 0.33 mm diameter
fibroblasts Immature fiber-producing cell of connective tissue
fibroma Tumor of fibrous tissue, usually benign
gait Manner or style of walking
granulation Formation of small masses of tissue that are formed during the healing process of wounds
hemangiosarcoma Malignant tumor of the blood vessels
hemorrhagic shock Hypovolemic shock resulting from hemorrhage
hepatosis Disorder of the liver
hypoproteinemia Abnormal decrease in the amount of protein in the blood, sometimes resulting in edema and fluid accumulation in serous cavities
hypotensive Abnormally low blood pressure
hypovolemic Abnormally decreased volume of circulating fluid (plasma) in the body
hypovolemic shock Shock resulting from insufficient blood volume for the maintenance of adequate cardiac output, blood pressure, and tissue perfusion
intracellular Situated or occurring within a cell or cells
intradermal In the dermis layer of the skin
intramedullary Within the marrow cavity of the bone
intraperitoneal Within the peritoneal cavity
isotonic A solution that has equal tonicity as another solution with which it is compared
lavage Irrigation or washing of an organ or wound
malocclusion Absence of proper alignment of teeth when the jaws are closed
malodorous Bad odor
mesenchymal Embryonic connective tissue such as muscle
metastatic Disease that is transferred from one organ to an unrelated organ
Mobitz type 1 block Variation of second-degree heart block
myocardium Middle and thickest layer of the heart wall, composed of cardiac muscle
nystagmus Involuntary rapid horizontal or vertical movement of the eyeball
oncology Study of cancer
oncotic pressure Osmotic pressure due to presence of colloids in a solution; it is the force that tends to counterbalance the capillary blood pressure
orogastric Pertaining to the mouth and stomach
osteosarcoma Malignant tumor of bone cells
palliative Affording relief
palpation Using the fingers with light pressure on the surface of the body to determine consistency of the parts beneath
pancreatitis Inflammation of the pancreas
parenteral Not through the gastrointestinal tract but via another route, such as intravenous
peripheral Outward structure or surface as in the limbs of the body
polyuria Production of a large volume of urine over a specific period of time
premature ventricular contraction (PVC) Premature beats where the QRS complex usually has wide and bizarre complexes
pruritus Itching
purulent Containing or forming pus
pyrexic Abnormal elevation of body temperature
rales Abnormal respiratory sound heard on auscultation. Rales are classified by their point of origin and whether the sound is dry or moist with fluid involvement
repolarization After depolarization, the cells reestablishment of polarity
sarcoma Type of tumor that is highly malignant
sinus arrhythmia Variation in the heart rate that is normal in the dog
stridor Harsh, shrill respiratory sound usually heard on inspiration that is due to a laryngeal obstruction
tachycardia Increased heart rate
turgor Normal consistency of tissue or how quickly it returns to normal after being slightly pulled
urticaria Vascular reaction, usually transient, involving the upper dermis and representing localized edema caused by dilatation and increased permeability of the capillaries and marked by the development of wheals
volvulus Torsion or twisting of a loop of intestine causing obstruction
Wenchenbach AV block Repetitive sequence seen in a partial heart block. The PR interval becomes progressively longer until ventricular response occurs
wet-to-dry bandage Wet dressing that is used on wounds to extract exudates
wheeze Whistling respiratory sound

Review Questions

1 What is a pulse deficit?
a. Increased heart rate
b. Pulse rate and heart rate are the same
c. Pulse rate lower than heart rate
d. Weak pulses

2 Where are the popliteal lymph nodes located?
a. Cranial to the scapula
b. On the sternum
c. Behind the stifle
d. Just below the hock

3 Referred sounds are generally
a. From the diaphragm
b. From the trachea
c. From the lung lobes
d. Digestion noises

4 Oral medications would be contraindicated when
a. Fractured ribs are evident
b. Pancreatitis is diagnosed
c. Blood loss is chronic
d. The treatment is chronic

5 A parenteral drug is administered
a. Topically
b. Orally
c. Not via the gastrointestinal tract
d. Intramuscularly only

6 What is a sign of overhydration?
a. Decreased respiratory rate
b. Decreased capillary refill time
c. Increased respiratory rate
d. Increased salivation

7 Which fluid would be considered a colloid?
a. Ringer's lactate
b. 5% Dextrose
c. Plasma
d. Saline

8 Subcutaneous fluids are contraindicated when
a. There is evidence of mild dehydration
b. The patient needs dextrose
c. The patient is very small
d. There is evidence of chronic heart failure

9 ___________ is/are recommended before performing an enema.
a. Abdominal radiographs
b. Abdominal palpation
c. Intravenous fluids
d. Large amounts of laxative

10 A canine blood donor should weigh no less than
a. 20 kg
b. 25 kg
c. 15 kg
d. 10 kg

BIBLIOGRAPHY

Crow SE, Walshaw SO: *Manual of clinical procedures in the dog and cat,* Philadelphia, 1997, Lippincott-Raven.

DiBartola SP: *Fluid therapy in small animal practice,* Philadelphia, 1992, WB Saunders.

Dorland's illustrated medical dictionary, ed 27, Philadelphia, 1994, WB Saunders.

Edwards NJ: *ECG manual for the veterinary technician,* Philadelphia, 1993, WB Saunders.

Heinbecker V: *Small animal blood banking,* Ontario Association of Veterinary Technicians Conference, Toronto, Ontario, February 15-17, 2001.

Kirk RW, Bistner SI, editors: *Handbook of veterinary procedures and emergency treatment,* ed 6, Philadelphia, 1995, WB Saunders.

Lane DR, Cooper B: *Veterinary nursing,* Oxford, 1994, Butterworth Heinemann.

Loncke D, Rivait P, Tighe M: *Clinical procedures handbook,* Windsor, Ontario, 2001, St Clair College of Applied Arts and Technology, Veterinary Technician Program.

Mathews KA: Fluid and electrolyte maintenance and replacement, *Veterinary emergency and critical care manual,* Guelph, 1996, Lifelearn.

McCurnin D, Bassert J: *Clinical textbook for veterinary technicians,* ed 5, Philadelphia, 2002, WB Saunders.

Meltzer LE, Pinneo R, Kitchell JR: *Intensive coronary care: a manual for nurses,* ed 4, Bowie, MD, Robert J. Brady Co, a Prentice-Hall Publishing and Communications Company.

Muir MW, DiBartola SP: *Fluid therapy, current veterinary therapy VIII,* Philadelphia, 1983, WB Saunders.

O'Grady MR: *ECG Interpretation Workshop,* Winter Conference, Toronto, Ontario, 1995, Ontario Association of Veterinary Technicians.

Pratt PW, editor: *Principles and practice of veterinary technology,* St Louis, 1998, Mosby.

Shaw D, Ihle S: *The national veterinary series, small animal internal medicine,* Baltimore, 1997, Williams & Wilkins.

CHAPTER 24

Equine Nursing and Surgery

Susan Cornwell *Kim Healey*

OUTLINE

LEARNING OUTCOMES

After reading this chapter you should be able to:

1. Recognize normal values for adult horses.
2. Understand medication treatment routes.
3. Have an understanding of disease, illnesses, and the technician's role in the animal's care.
4. Be familiar with important preoperative and postoperative care.
5. Be familiar with common vaccines.
6. Be familiar with bandaging techniques.

As veterinary technicians, we play a very large role in the day-to-day care of animals. Veterinarians rely on our instincts, knowledge, and observational skills to assist and/or alert them to the progression (or deterioration) of the animal's state of health.

PHYSICAL EXAMINATION AND NORMAL VALUES

I. Temperature: 37° to 38.5° C (98.6° to 101.3° F)
II. Pulse: 28 to 45 beats per minute
 A. Auscultate heart with stethoscope
  1. Heart sounds
   a. Four heart sounds may be heard, but often only two or three
   b. Normal sequence of sounds in cardiac cycle is S_4, S_1, S_2, S_3
   c. Loudest and most obvious sounds are S_1 and S_2
    (1) S_1 is the first sound and is due to ventricular contraction
    (2) S_2 is the second sound and is due to closure of semilunar valves
    (3) S_3 is very faint and caused by blood rushing into the ventricles
    (4) Rarely audible S_4 is caused by atrial contraction
  2. Cardiac rhythm
   a. A variety of rhythms are normal
   b. Note heart rate, rhythm, intensity, extra sounds, absence of normal sounds
   c. Abnormal rhythms
    (1) Arrhythmias: absence of rhythm
    (2) Dysrhythmia: disturbance of rhythm
    (3) Tachycardia: dysrhythmia associated with heart rates greater than 50 beats per minute
    (4) Bradycardia: dysrhythmia associated with heart rates lower than 20 beats per minute
     (a) Can occur due to hypocalcemia

d. Atrioventricular (AV) block
   (1) May occur regularly or irregularly
   (2) First degree, second degree, or third degree (complete heart block)
   (3) During second-degree block there is no S_1 or S_2 and no arterial pulse
   (4) Second-degree heart block may be present in horses that are not fit
      (a) Not always indicative of heart disease
3. Heart murmurs
   a. Turbulent flow causes vibrations that are audible during normally quiet periods of the cardiac cycle

B. Electrocardiographic (ECG) monitor
   1. A portable ECG monitor is used on the horse while it is standing quietly at rest
   2. Used for a definitive diagnosis of arrhythmias/dysrhythmias

C. Facial artery
   1. Located on medial aspect of mandible
   2. Use to assess, by palpation, blood pressure during anesthesia
   3. Use to determine if manual palpation of pulse matches the ECG

D. Coccygeal artery
   1. Located in groove on dorsal aspect of tail
   2. Use for blood pressure with a Doppler pressure monitor

III. Respiration: 8 to 20 breaths per minute
   A. Observe by watching horse flanks and nostrils
   B. Use stethoscope to listen to abnormal respiratory sounds
      1. Place on trachea
      2. Place on left and right lung fields
   C. Horse must be relaxed in a quiet environment for assessment
   D. Rhythm is important
      1. Normal horse
         a. Inspiration and expiration are followed by a pause
      2. Abnormal or excited horse
         a. Inspiration will be slightly longer than expiration
   E. Signs of respiratory problems
      1. Coughing or other abnormal respiratory sounds during rest or exercise
      2. Nasal discharge
      3. Epistaxis
         a. The presence of blood in upper airway or nose as a result of
            (1) Guttural pouch infections
            (2) Exercise-induced pulmonary hemorrhage (EIPH)
      4. Hyperpnea
         a. Increased rate and depth of respiration
      5. Dyspnea
         a. Labored breathing causing distress
   F. Pharynx and trachea examined with endoscopy

IV. Mucous membrane should be a healthy pink color

V. Capillary refill time: 1 to 2 seconds

VI. Gastrointestinal motility (borborygmus)
   A. Bubbling
   B. Gurgling
   C. Rumbling (not unlike the sound of distant thunder)
   D. Cecum is heard on the right side and no sound is cause for concern
   E. Recording of gut sounds
      1. By upper and lower quadrants on the left and right side
      2. 0 is absence of sound
      3. + (one plus) is hypomotile, ++ (two plus) is normal, and +++ (three plus) is hypermotile

VII. Digital pulses: none to slight

VIII. Fecal output
   A. Color varies with diet
   B. Should be well-formed moist balls that break easily when they hit the ground
   C. Frequency: approximately 8 to 10 times daily

IX. Urine
   A. Colorless to yellow
   B. Can be thick or turbid due to high content of mucous and calcium carbonate crystals

DENTAL FORMULA AND CARE

Dental Formula

I. Foal has 24 temporary teeth

II. Adult has 40 to 42 permanent teeth
   A. For a stallion, the dental formula is 2 × (I 3/3, C 1/1, P 3/3, M, 3/3)
   B. Mares usually do not have canine teeth
   C. Equine canine teeth are also called tushes

Dental Care

I. Wolf teeth or first premolar (P1) are located in the upper jaw
   A. If wolf teeth do not fall out on their own, the veterinarian will have to extract them because they can interfere with the bit

II. Anatomically the horse's upper jaw is wider than the lower jaw
   A. When a horse eats, it grinds food in a side-to-side motion
   B. This creates sharp edges on the buccal surface of the upper teeth and on the lingual surface of the lower teeth
   C. Floating the teeth refers to the rasping down of these sharp edges

D. A veterinarian should check the horse's teeth at least annually to determine whether teeth need floating
   1. Signs that animal's teeth need floating include
      a. Halitosis
      b. Lacerations of oral cavity
      c. Difficulty eating (tend to drop feed)
      d. Head tilt (especially when a bit is placed in their mouth)
      e. Undigested food in feces

ROUTES OF ADMINISTRATION

I. Oral route
   A. Powders
   B. Pastes (i.e., phenylbutazone, anthelmintics)
   C. Boluses
   D. Pills
   E. Liquids
   F. All of the above may be added to food (some after being dissolved in water) or dosed using a syringe
II. Nasogastric tube
   A. Tube is passed into the esophagus, usually by a veterinarian due to risk of placing the tube in trachea
   B. Common route for administering Strongid (often double dosed), mineral oil, and antigas medicine as well as refluxing the stomach contents when assessing colic
   C. Nasogastric tube may be seen or felt on the left side of the neck when being passed by placing pressure above and below the tube, at the jugular groove and blowing air into the tube
III. Intravenous (IV) injection
   A. Always swab injection site with alcohol before injecting
      1. Makes vein more pronounced and disinfects skin
   B. Common sites
      1. Jugular vein is most common
      2. For small volumes the thoracic, cephalic, or saphenous veins can be used if jugular vein not accessible
   C. Use to produce rapid onset of drug action
   D. Use to administer large volumes of fluids
   E. Use for blood collection
   F. Before injecting, ensure placement in vein by getting blood flow back from needle (catheter) or aspirated in syringe
   G. Catheter placement
      1. Commonly sewn or glued in place, then secured with tape and Elastoplast
      2. Placement will depend on surgical recumbency (commonly on the nonrecumbent side)
      3. Short-term placement (several hours): Angiocath
      4. Long-term placement (several days): Mila catheters with butterfly extensions
   H. Normal needle gauges range from 14 g (catheters) to 16 g (jugulars) to 25 or 27 g (some local anesthetic agents)
   I. Important to know properties of drugs before administering
   J. Route of administration is IV only for some drugs
   K. Incorrect route of administration could destroy the vein or cause anaphylactic reaction
   L. Administer some drugs, such as calcium, slowly to not adversely affect heart rate
   M. Administer some drugs as a bolus for effect (e.g., glycopyrrolate during anesthesia to regulate heart rate)
   N. Perivascular administration of some drugs can irreparably damage tissue
   O. Phenylbutazone (Bute) is the most common drug administered to horses and the most damaging to the vein perivascularly
IV. Intramuscular (IM) administration
   A. Swab injection site with alcohol to disinfect and make skin veins visible so they can be avoided
   B. Common sites
      1. Neck (Viborg triangle below nuchal ligament and above cervical vertebrae proximal to shoulder)
      2. Semitendinosus muscle
      3. Gluteus muscle
      4. Pectoralis descendens (chest)
   C. Avoid injecting in proximity to joints, blood vessels, or large fat deposits
   D. IM route used to prolong drug action
   E. Only safe route of administration for certain drugs
      1. To ensure that the needle is not in a blood vessel draw back on plunger of syringe to check that no blood is pulled into the syringe before injecting
      2. Procaine penicillin will cause an adverse reaction if administered into the bloodstream
      3. Mild reactions may take a few minutes to present themselves, whereas severe reactions occur immediately
      4. Reactions include restlessness, head tossing, snorting, rolling of the eyes, violent thrashing, and dropping to the ground
         a. Treat with dexamethasone (a corticosteroid) and flunixin meglumine (Banamine) (a nonsteroidal anti-inflammatory drug [NSAID])

b. Treatment should be administered IV, but one may not get close enough to inject into the vein if the animal's reaction is too violent
5. A horse that has a reaction should never be given the drug again

V. Subcutaneous (SC) administration
   A. Swab skin with alcohol as for IM injection
   B. Administer drug by pinching a loose fold of skin and placing needle tip into space
   C. Normally injected into neck
   D. Will normally leave bump due to close attachment of skin to underlying muscle
   E. Always draw back on plunger to ensure no blood is in syringe before injecting

VI. Intranasal route
   A. Catheter is placed in the medial dorsal nasal cavity for administration of drugs
      1. Vaccination against strangles *(Streptococcus equi)*
      2. Vaccination for the influenza virus (only available in the United States at present)
      3. Laryngeal/pharyngeal washes
   B. The advantage to this route is direct application of the drug to the primary area of concern

VII. Inhalation route
   A. Nebulizers and Aeromasks used to deliver microdroplets of a drug
      1. Mask is loosely fitted over muzzle
   B. Aerosol inhalants

VIII. Topical route
   A. Substances applied to skin, eyes, mucous membranes, and hooves
   B. Eye creams and ointments must be placed onto the eye or into conjunctival sacs
      1. Multiple applications of liquids may require a special catheter placed into the eyelid and braided through the mane

VACCINATIONS (Table 24-1)

I. Vaccinations routinely given IM aseptically

II. Intranasal vaccine available for strangles and influenza

III. Vaccines are made from a killed (KV) or modified live virus (MLV), bacteria or toxin (antigen)

IV. Routine vaccines depend on geographical area, prevalence of a disease in a specific area, and the animal's risk of exposure

V. In Ontario, Canada, horses are routinely vaccinated for
   A. Rabies
   B. Tetanus
   C. Rhinopneumonitis (EHV-4/1)

VI. Horses traveling outside Canada are routinely vaccinated for
   A. Encephalomyelitis, Eastern and Western strains
   B. Strangles (a few outbreaks were isolated in Ontario recently)
   C. Potomac horse fever (equine monocytic ehrlichiosis)

VII. In the United States
   A. Depending on the area, most horses are vaccinated for Eastern and Western encephalomyelitis, tetanus, and influenza annually
   B. Rhinopneumonitis is recommended if there are yearlings
   C. Strangles vaccine is common in many areas, with intranasal administration becoming more popular
   D. Rabies vaccination is recommended in most areas
   E. Administration of both West Nile virus and Potomac horse fever vaccine is being recommended as part of the vaccination protocol, in both high- and low-risk areas

VIII. Side effects of vaccinations
   A. At 24 to 48 hours after injection
      1. Generalized muscle pain
      2. Mild lethargy
      3. Mild appetite loss
      4. Mild fever
      5. If symptoms persist for longer, other causes should be examined
   B. Irritation, swelling, or abscess at injection site
   C. Anaphylactic reaction, although rare
      1. Treat with epinephrine

IX. Primary immunization

X. Important to read directions for each specific brand of vaccine

XI. Protocols for vaccination are described in Table 24-1
   A. For further information, see the description under the particular vaccinations

GASTROINTESTINAL AILMENTS

The management of all ailments and diseases is at the discretion of a veterinarian.

Common Clinical Signs

I. Restlessness, anxiety, or agitation
II. Pawing, pacing/stall walking
III. Flank watching and possible biting at flank
IV. Kicking at abdomen
V. Sweating
VI. Getting up and down in stall

Table 24-1 Equine vaccinations

Vaccine	Product	Foal	Brood mare (BM) healthy horse (HH)	Wounds
Tetanus (toxoid)	1. Tetanus toxoid 2. Supertet with Havlogen 3. Encevac TC 4 4. Fluvac EWT Plus 5. Equine EWTF	1. 3 months 2. 4 weeks later Antibody titers usually occur 2 weeks after second initial dose Annual	BM: 4 to 6 weeks before foaling	1. If booster more than 6 months earlier 2. Prior to surgery being performed
May be given as an individual vaccine or combined with another vaccine by certain manufacturers. If unknown vaccination history or vaccine not previously given, treat with the tetanus antitoxin vaccine. Administer separately and make sure the injection sites are not in close proximity to each other on the horse.				
Tetanus antitoxin	1. Tetanus antitoxin 1500 IU	1. Shortly after birth if mare unvaccinated		1. Minimum dose of 1500 IU within 24 hours of exposure to tetanus toxin
Administer SC, IV, or intraperitoneally (IP). Given to treat cases of tetanus. Massive initial doses are better than repeated smaller doses to effect a cure. If the horse has a wound, increase the dose relative to time of exposure to 30,000 to 100,000 units.				
Rabies	1. Imrab 3 2. Imrab Bovine Plus 3. Rabvac 3 4. Equine Potomavac + Imrab	1. 3 months of age and older	HH: annual booster	
Inject a 2-mL dose IM. Revaccinate annually.				
Rhinopneumonit is EHV-1, EHV-4 (equine herpes virus)	1. Fluvac EHV-4/1 Plus 2. Prestige II with Havlogen 3. Pneumabort K+1b 4. Prodigy with Havlogen	1. 3 months of age, 3 to 4 weeks later, then 6 months	BM: at months 5, 7, and 9 of gestation HH: primary vaccination at 6 to 9 months, second dose in 2 to 4 or 4 to 6 weeks, then annually	1. High-risk horses: every 3 months
Both modified live and inactivated vaccine are available. Vaccines are specifically labeled for respiration or abortion. Vaccines do not claim any protective properties for the neurological syndrome caused by this virus.				

Continued

Table 24-1 Equine vaccinations—cont'd

Vaccine	Product	Foal	Brood mare (BM) healthy horse (HH)	Wounds
Influenza	1. Flu Avert I.N. 2. Fluvac Plus 3. Fluvac EHV-4/1 Plus 4. Fluvac EWT Plus 5. Prestige II with Havlogen 6. Encevac TC 4 7. Equine EWTF	1. Controversial 2. After 3 months (maternal antibodies from the vaccinated mare may interfere with the vaccine for up to 6 months of age) OR 3. After 6 months 4. At 1 month of age if mare unvaccinated	HH: primary dose of IM vaccine 9 months and older with second dose in 2 to 4 or 3 to 6 weeks, then 6-month booster, then annually In a high-risk area, a third dose may be given within that 6-month period Older horses: every 9 to 12 months if in a low-risk, closed environment Show horses: do not vaccinate within 7 to 10 days of a show due to possible side effects	1. Booster with vaccine containing tetanus
Vaccination rarely prevents infection; it can reduce the severity of disease and decrease its spread only. Side effects include fever, depression, muscle stiffness, and reaction at injection site. Blood serum tests will show antibody titer levels. Vaccines have commonly been IM injections of a killed virus. An intranasal vaccine is available in the United States (Flu Avert I.N.) that is a modified live virus; it has a rapid immune response at the primary infection site; Administer 1-mL dose into nostril. Recommended administration twice a year, and more often in areas of high risk of exposure. The Canadian Food Inspection Agency has granted approval for the vaccine to be sold in Canada.				
Equine encephalomyelitis: Eastern (EEE), Western (WEE), and Venezuelan (VEE)	1. Encevac T 2. Encevac TC 4 3. Equine EWTF 4. Fluvac EWT Plus 5. Equiloid	1. 3 months 2. 6 months if adequate colostrum received	BM: 4 to 6 weeks before foaling HH: primary immunity, with second dose at 3 to 4 or 4 to 8 weeks, then annually (titers last 6 to 8 months) Vaccinate if there is an outbreak	1. If during first 2 months or if booster more than 12 months earlier, administer minimum 1500 IU tetanus antitoxin
Vaccinate against EEE and WEE in Canada and the United States. Vaccinate against VEE for states that border on Mexico. In cool climates, administer the vaccine in the spring when increased exposure to other horses and mosquitoes is more likely. In warm climates, biannual vaccination is recommended.				

Streptococcus equi (strangles)	1. Pinnacle I.N. 2. Strepguard	1. Before 4 months of age	BM: 4 to 6 weeks before foaling (Strepguard)	1. If during first 2 months or if booster more than 12 months earlier, administer minimum 1500 IU tetanus antitoxin
Vaccine is available as whole-cell bacteria and M-protein extract for IM injection. Vaccination is usually limited to horses at risk due to muscle soreness and incomplete protection. Available as modified live vaccine in intranasal form (Pinnacle I.N.). Two doses are given, 2 to 3 weeks apart, and then annual boosters. IM route: two or three doses 2 to 4 weeks apart and then annually. Not recommended for infected animals.				
Ehrlichia risticii (Potomac horse fever)	1. Equine Potomavac + Imrab 2. Equine Potomavac 3. Mystique 4. Potomacguard	1. In high-risk areas, at 4 months for 3 doses 1 month apart 2. In low-risk areas, treat as for healthy horses	HH: 3 months of age and older, then 3 to 4 weeks later, then annually Vaccination has a short duration of activity	
Documented in most of the United States. Vaccinations are generally limited to areas of high prevalence: Eastern and Midwest United States during mid summer to fall. In California, during the fall to spring.				
West Nile virus	West Nile Virus Vaccine	1. Nonvaccinated mare in high-risk area: 6 to 8 weeks of age, 3 doses 3 to 4 weeks apart 2. Nonvaccinated mare in low-risk area: 3 to 5 months of age, 3 doses 3 to 4 weeks apart 3. Vaccinated mare in high-risk area: give as for No. 2 (3 to 5 months) with 2 or 3 repeat doses 4. Vaccinated mare in low-risk area: 5 to 7 months old, give 2 doses 3 to 4 weeks apart 5. Foals a few days old have been vaccinated with no adverse affect	1. Administer 1 ml IM followed by second dose in 3 to 6 weeks 2. Revaccinate annually	
Is a killed virus. Horses may develop IgG and/or IgM antibodies to the West Nile virus that would affect their ability to be exported.				

VII. Rolling
VIII. Grinding teeth
IX. Distended abdomen
X. Increased heart rate and respiration rate
XI. Mucous membranes can be pale, bright or brick red, or cyanotic
XII. Toxic line (red or blue) on gums just above teeth may be present
XIII. Increased capillary refill time (CRT)
XIV. Gastrointestinal motility may be hypermotile, hypomotile, or absent
XV. Digital pulses bounding with increased heat in hoof wall
XVI. Fecal output can be absent, small amounts of hard dry balls, or cow patty form to diarrhea
XVII. Sawhorse stance (standing stretched out) or dog sitting
XVIII. Decreased appetite
XIX. Reflux, via nasogastric tube, is often present (can be absent or up to 15 L (3.5 gal) in an average-size horse)

Rule Outs of Gastrointestinal Ailments

I. Colic
  A. Refers to abdominal pain
    1. Most commonly seen ailment
  B. Gastrointestinal causes include
    1. Excessive gas
    2. Spasmodic colic
    3. Ileus (cessation of peristalsis)
    4. Parasitic infestations
    5. Volvulus (torsion of small or large intestine)
    6. Intussusception (telescoping of adjoining bowl [ileum to cecum])
    7. Impactions
    8. Obstructions
    9. Displacement
    10. Inguinal hernias
    11. Ulcers
  C. Symptoms vary with the severity of the colic and disposition of the horse
  D. Not all of these clinical signs will necessarily be seen in each case.
  E. Management of colic consists of
    1. Fluid therapy
    2. Anti-inflammatory drugs
    3. Mineral oil
    4. Anti-flatulence medication
    5. Monitoring
    6. Anti-ulcer medications
  F. Monitoring includes
    1. Vital signs
    2. Gut sounds (motility)
    3. Fecal output
    4. Hydration status (packed cell volume [PCV] and total protein [TP])
    5. Obtaining nasogastric reflux (recording of how much, if any)
    6. Walking
    7. Gradual introduction of food to the animal
  G. In cases where surgery has been performed or toxemia occurred, digital pulses are also extremely important to monitor because laminitis is always a concern
II. Colitis
  A. Acute inflammatory process of the large colon and cecum
  B. In most cases of acute colitis a cause is unknown
  C. Several possibilities include
    1. Dietary change
    2. Carbohydrate overload (eating too much grain)
    3. *Salmonella* spp.
    4. *Clostridium perfringens* (colitis X)
    5. *Clostridium difficile*
    6. Potomac horse fever
    7. Antibiotic therapy
    8. Overuse of NSAIDs
  D. Clinically, horses present with
    1. Inappetance
    2. Dull/depressed
    3. Abdominal pain
    4. Gastric motility can be either hypermotile (increased) or hypomotile (decreased)
    5. Increased heart and respiration rates
    6. Mucous membranes can be brick/dark red, muddy, or cyanotic
    7. CRT is increased (3 to 4 seconds)
    8. Diarrhea (varying from cow patty to profuse watery diarrhea)
    9. Dehydration
    10. Hypoproteinemia
    11. Electrolyte imbalances (hyponatremia, hypokalemia, hypocalcemia)
    12. Metabolic acidosis (severe cases)
    13. In severe cases, shock due to endotoxemia
  E. Management of colitis
    1. Fluid therapy with a balanced electrolyte solution (e.g., lactated Ringer's solution [LRS])
    2. If needed, addition of potassium chloride and calcium to LRS
    3. Sodium bicarbonate to correct metabolic acidosis
    4. Plasma transfusion if total protein low (<4.0 g/dL)

5. Anti-inflammatory drugs
6. Nitroglycerin (vasodilator) applied to the medial and lateral digital arteries

F. Monitoring
1. Vital signs
2. PCV and TP
3. Blood gas and electrolytes
4. Digital pulses and heat (signs of laminitis) in hooves

G. Usually free choice grass hay is offered, but grain is withheld

H. Horses with diarrhea are kept isolated because of the possibility of salmonella

I. When a horse is on IV fluids, it is vital that the indwelling catheter be monitored for
1. Heat
2. Swelling
3. Pain

J. This is very important because horses with colitis are prone to develop thrombosis of the jugular vein

III. Salmonellosis

A. A very serious problem due to zoonotic potential and high incidence of contagion to other horses
1. Horses may naturally carry salmonella as part of their intestinal flora

B. Causes include
1. Stressful situations, such as transport in a trailer
2. Sudden changes in feeding
3. Antibiotic use
4. Sickness
5. Surgery
6. Immunosuppression

C. Clinically, horses present with
1. Signs similar to those of colitis
2. Acute, profuse, watery, foul-smelling diarrhea
3. Pyrexia
4. Anorexia

D. Management is extremely important
1. The horse should be isolated
2. Handling the animal should be kept to one person to prevent the possibility of cross-contamination
3. Anyone handling the horse should be gowned and gloved and wear protective boot covers
4. When leaving the isolated animal, hands should be thoroughly washed and boots should be dipped in a foot bath containing a bactericidal solution
5. Fluid therapy with a balanced electrolyte solution is very important because hydration status is the number one concern
6. Plasma transfusion may be required if hypoproteinemia is present

E. Monitor vital signs, as with any other case of diarrhea

F. Horse is fed free choice hay; grain is withheld

IV. Intestinal clostridial infections

A. An acute inflammatory process of the bowel

B. Colitis X is the most common form and is diagnosed on postmortem examination

C. Clinically, horses present with
1. Signs similar to those of colitis
2. Often no initial diarrhea
3. Severe abdominal pain
4. Increased gut motility (hypermotility)
5. Diarrhea within a matter of hours

D. Management is the same as for colitis and salmonellosis

E. The antibiotic bacitracin, given orally, may be effective in some cases

V. Potomac horse fever (PHF) (monocytic ehrlichiosis)

A. *Ehrlichia risticii* is the cause of PHF

B. This rickittsia-like organism is thought to be transmitted by snails

C. In northeastern United States, the peak time for PHF is June through August

D. Horses can be tested for PHF with an ELISA and an indirect immunofluorescent antibody (IFA) test

E. Clinically, horses present with
1. Depression
2. Anorexia
3. Pyrexia
4. Decreased gut sounds
5. Some horses exhibit abdominal pain and diarrhea

F. Management of PHF
1. Oxytetracycline
2. Aggressive fluid therapy with a balanced electrolyte solution

G. As with cases of salmonella and colitis, the same monitoring and strict isolation procedures are applied

H. Laminitis is a major concern with PHF and should be monitored closely

I. Vaccines are available for PHF, but they are less then 100% effective

VI. Antibiotic and NSAID therapy

A. Overuse of antibiotics and NSAIDs can cause diarrhea

B. Clinically, horses present with
1. Loss of appetite
2. Depression
3. Some abdominal pain
4. Protein loss due to ulceration of the bowel or stomach

- C. Some antibiotics can cause diarrhea as a side effect
- D. Management
  1. Fluid therapy such as LRS and plasma
  2. Monitoring patient's vital signs
- E. Antibiotics and NSAIDs should be discontinued
- F. Gastroscopy can be performed to determine ulcerations
- G. Treatment with antiulcer medication can then be initiated if needed

VII. Anterior enteritis
- A. The cause is idiopathic; however, *Clostridium* spp. have been implicated
- B. There is severe inflammation of the upper portion of the small intestine
- C. Clinically, horses present with
  1. Severe colic
  2. Increased heart and respiration rates
  3. Possible pyrexia
  4. Gastric reflux obtained when a nasogastric tube is placed
- D. Signs are often the same as with an obstruction of the bowel
- E. Diagnosis is made by the veterinarian performing a rectal examination
- F. In the case of anterior enteritis, colic signs decrease when nasogastric reflux is obtained. With an obstruction, colic signs usually do not decrease. The horse will then become depressed
- G. Management
  1. Passage of a nasogastric tube and frequent siphoning to empty fluid buildup in the stomach
  2. Fluid therapy is important to replace fluid loss from the nasogastric reflux
- H. Monitoring is the same as with colic, although particular attention is paid to temperature, mucous membranes, CRT, and digital pulses as toxemia is a concern

VIII. Hyperkalemic periodic paralysis (HYPP)
- A. This disease originally resulted in a genetic mutation that has been traced back to a quarterhorse sire
- B. Clinically, horses present with any of the following
  1. Muscle fasciculations
  2. Colic-like episodes
  3. Sweating
  4. Respiratory distress
  5. Prolapsed third eye lid
  6. Loose feces
  7. Ataxia
- C. A DNA blood test has been developed and can determine
  1. If a horse is a homozygous affected animal
  2. A heterozygous carrier
  3. A normal horse
- D. If the test is positive, breeding should be discouraged and owners should be made aware that it can be dangerous to ride these horses
- E. Management of HYPP consists of
  1. A low potassium diet
  2. Grass or oat hay (no alfalfa hay)
  3. Plenty of fresh water
  4. Minimizing stress in these affected horses is beneficial

NEUROMUSCULAR DISORDERS

Common Clinical Signs

I. Ataxia
II. Depression
III. Circling
IV. Head tilt
V. Head pressing
VI. Nystagmus
VII. Facial paralysis, drooling
VIII. Incoordination, limb knuckling, and toe dragging
IX. Muscle wasting
X. Prolapsed third eyelid
XI. Seizures
XII. Altered behavior

Rule Outs of Neuromuscular Disorders

I. Tetanus (lockjaw)
- A. Caused by the bacterium *Clostridium tetani*
- B. *C. tetani* is found in the soil and infects horses through puncture wounds
- C. The bacteria produce neurotoxins, which affect the horse's nervous system
- D. Clinically, horses present with
  1. Muscle stiffness (sawhorse stance)
  2. Decreased feed and water intake
  3. Sensitivity to light and sound
  4. Muscle fasciculations
- E. Management of tetanus should begin with the infected horse receiving a booster of tetanus antitoxin
  1. This is given because the antitoxin will bind to any circulating tetanus toxins
- F. Wound treatment
  1. Cleaning
  2. Draining
  3. Local infiltration of penicillin to the site of the wound

G. Systemically, the horse should be given IV penicillin
H. The horse should be kept in a dark, quiet stall
I. IV fluids may be needed, especially if the horse is dysphagic
J. Vaccination of horses annually with tetanus toxoid to help stimulate the immune system is a preventive measure

II. Rabies
A. Caused by the rhabdovirus, which attacks the central nervous system
B. This virus most commonly is passed by a bite from an infected animal
C. Because the virus is found in large quantities in saliva, domestic animals, including humans, can become infected through open wounds and across mucous membranes
D. Clinically, horses present with the above signs, as well as the following
    1. Extreme aggression (in some cases)
    2. Dysphagia
    3. Hydrophobia
    4. Self-inflicted wounds
E. Clinical signs are always progressive
F. Management of rabies
    1. The suspected horse must be quarantined
    2. Anyone handling the horse should wear protective clothing and gloves due to rabies zoonotic potential
G. Unfortunately, if rabies is highly suspected, the horse must be euthanized because of the threat to human life and because there is no cure
H. A definitive diagnosis can be made only at postmortem
I. An annual rabies vaccine should be given as a preventive measure

III. Equine protozoal myeloencephalitis (EPM)
A. Affects the central nervous system
B. The protozoa *Sarcocystis neurona* is the causative agent
    1. The protozoa encysts in the muscle of birds
    2. Opossums eat the infected birds
    3. Opossum's feces contaminate the horse's feed and water supply
C. Symptoms depend on location of lesion
D. Locations of lesions from the protozoa
    1. Brain stem
    2. Spinal cord
    3. Peripheral nerves
E. Clinically, horses may present with any of the following
    1. Ataxia
    2. Facial paralysis
    3. Head tilt
    4. Depression
    5. Blindness
    6. Dysphagia
    7. Circling
    8. Hind end weakness and ataxia
    9. Gluteal, tongue, and masticatory muscle wasting
    10. Incontinence
    11. In some cases recumbency
F. EPM is diagnosed by performing a cerebrospinal fluid (CSF) tap
G. The spinal fluid is then analyzed for
    1. Antibodies to *Sarcocystis neurona*
    2. Protozoal DNA
H. Management of EPM consists of long-term antibiotic and antiprotozoal therapy, which usually includes trimethoprim-sulfadiazine and pyrimethamine
    1. Other antiprotozoal medications are being tested: Ponazuril (toltrazuril sulfone) and Diclazuril
I. Unfortunately, affected animals often do not recover completely and post-therapeutic relapses are common

IV. Equine herpes virus 1 (EHV-1)
A. Also known as viral rhinopneumonitis
B. This strain affects the nervous system
    1. It is transmitted via direct contact or aerosols
    2. Clinically, horses with EHV-1 can
        a. Be uncoordinated
        b. Be incontinent
        c. Be ataxic in hind limbs
        d. Have loss of tail tone
        e. In extreme cases, hind limb paralysis leads to dog-sitting posture or recumbency
C. Abortion can occur in pregnant mares
    1. Vaccinate with Pneumabort K +1b during months 5, 7, and 9 of pregnancy
D. If affected late in gestation, abortion may not occur; however, foals are infected in utero and may be born dead or die shortly after birth
E. Management of EHV-1 depends on the severity of the disease and treatment includes
    1. Antibiotics
    2. Anti-inflammatory drugs
    3. Corticosteroids
F. Vaccination of horses is a preventive measure but may not be effective against abortions or neurological diseases

V. Equine encephalomyelitides (sleeping sickness)
A. Three strains of this alphavirus
    1. Eastern (EEE)
    2. Western (WEE)

3. Venezuelan (VEE)
B. Most common to Canada and the United States: Eastern (EEE) and Western (WEE) strains
C. Transmitted by mosquitoes, outbreaks tend to occur late in the summer
D. One- to 3-week incubation period
E. Is communicable to humans (zoonotic)
F. Clinically, horses present with the following initial signs
   1. Pyrexia
   2. Anorexia
   3. Depression
   4. Increased heart rate
G. Nervous signs develop later and are mostly due to EEE
   1. Anxiousness, excitement, and restlessness
   2. Exaggerated response to touch
   3. Head pressing, circling in the stall
   4. Seizures
   5. Paralysis
   6. Incoordination
   7. Loss of consciousness
H. Death is common
I. Management
   1. Anti-inflammatory drugs
   2. Fluid therapy
   3. Corticosteroids
   4. Anticonvulsants
   5. Emphasis on supportive nursing care
J. Vaccination of horses against this disease is an effective preventive measure
K. Control disease by identifying and destroying or segregating affected individuals

VI. West Nile virus
A. This alphavirus first appeared late in 1999 in the United States
B. The virus is transmitted by mosquitoes
   1. Mosquitoes get the virus from infected birds
   2. Horses and humans are dead end hosts
C. Outbreaks tend to occur late summer and in the fall
D. In 2001 the first reported death was in north central Indiana
E. Especially at risk are the very young, elderly, and sick
   1. Horses do not necessarily die from this virus; some recover fully
   2. Deaths have been reported
F. Clinically, horses can present with some or all of the following
   1. Pyrexia
   2. Front end or hind end weakness
   3. Toe dragging
   4. Ataxia
   5. Head and neck tremors
   6. Sensitive to touch
   7. Aggression
   8. Circling
   9. Seizuring
   10. Coma
G. Management
   1. Anti-inflammatory drugs
   2. Short-acting corticosteroids
   3. Fluids (LRS)
   4. May use dimethyl sulfoxide (DMSO) in fluids

RESPIRATORY DISEASES

Common Clinical Signs

I. Coughing
II. Clear runny nasal discharge
III. Secondary bacterial infection causes purulent (pus-like) discharge
IV. Depression
V. Anorexia
VI. Dyspnea, tachypnea
VII. Pyrexic

Rule Outs of Respiratory Diseases

I. Strangles
A. A very contagious upper respiratory tract disease
   1. Caused by the bacterium *S. equi*
B. It is spread by the infected animal's secretions or by fomites
C. Another bacteria that creates similar clinical signs but is not contagious is *S. zooepidemicus*
D. Horses develop swelling of the lymph nodes
   1. Under the mandible
   2. In the guttural pouches
   3. In the throat area
E. These abscesses can be quite painful and eventually rupture
F. Management
   1. Infected horse isolated to prevent cross-contamination
   2. Abscesses hot packed (to speed maturation) or lanced to encourage proper drainage
   3. Fluids and feed slurries given if the horse is dysphagic
   4. Horse kept warm with plenty of fresh water available
   5. Possible use of antipyretics and antibiotics
   6. Anything that comes into contact with the infected horse should be well disinfected or burned if possible

7. Currently available vaccines may lessen the severity of the disease but will not prevent an infection
8. Intranasal vaccine now the route of choice

II. Equine herpes virus (EHV-4) (rhinopneumonitis)
  A. This virus is prevalent worldwide
  B. As with EHV-1 (see Neuromuscular Disorders), this virus is also spread via direct contact or aerosols
    1. This strain of virus attacks the upper respiratory tract
  C. As well as the above clinical signs, horses will have
    1. Increased lung sounds
    2. Possible swelling of the lymph nodes
  D. Management
    1. Isolate the infected animal to prevent cross-contamination
    2. Keep the horse warm in a well-ventilated stall
    3. Have plenty of fresh water available
    4. Avoid stressful situations (i.e., transport in a trailer)
    5. Exercise for brief periods to keep blood and lymph circulating
  E. A vaccine is available; although it is questionable as to prevention of the disease, it does seem to lessen the severity of it

III. Equine influenza (flu)
  A. An extremely contagious virus that attacks the upper respiratory tract
  B. Two subtypes: influenza A/equine/1 and influenza A/equine/2
  C. Is worldwide except for Australia and New Zealand
  D. Affects horses, donkeys, mules, and zebras
  E. Usually affects animals between 1 and 3 years of age
  F. It is spread very quickly in areas of extensive horse populations such as
    1. Horse shows
    2. Race tracks
    3. Barns where horses are constantly moving in and out
  G. Infection is more frequent in winter and spring due to low temperatures and humidity, but can occur all year
  H. Like the other respiratory viruses, the influenza virus also is spread by direct contact and by aerosols
  I. Clinical signs may include
    1. Lethargy/depression
    2. Pyrexia
    3. Severe dry cough
    4. Increased lung sounds (in some cases)
    5. Watery nasal discharge
    6. Loss of appetite
    7. Constipation
    8. Some muscle soreness
  J. Management is the same as EHV-4
  K. Currently available vaccines may lessen the severity of the disease but will not prevent an infection

BLOOD DISORDER

I. Equine infectious anemia (EIA)
  A. Also known as swamp fever
  B. The virus is found in
    1. Blood
    2. Semen
    3. Tissues
  C. It is transmitted by
    1. Arthropods (most commonly biting flies)
    2. Blood transfusion
    3. Dirty needles
  D. Clinically, horses will be
    1. Pyretic
    2. Depressed
    3. Anorexic and show weight loss
    4. Anemic
  E. Coggins test is used to diagnose EIA
    1. A blood sample is taken and the serum is analyzed for antibodies
    2. This test is required for
      a. Any horse that is traveling across borders
      b. Racehorses
      c. Show horses
      d. Horses that are being sold
  F. There is no cure or prevention for this disease
  G. Infected horses will always be carriers of this virus but may be asymptomatic
  H. Euthanasia depends on
    1. State regulations
    2. Provincial regulations
    3. Federal regulations
  I. If horse is not euthanized, it must be isolated for the rest of its life

FOOT AILMENTS

I. Laminitis (founder)
  A. Inflammation of the sensitive laminae of the feet
    1. Most commonly occurs in the front feet, but can occur in the hind feet
  B. Caused by
    1. Grain overload
    2. Ingestion of large amounts of cold water (water founder)
    3. Endotoxemia

4. Concussion (road founder)
5. Hormonal influences
6. Post viral respiratory diseases
7. Post administration of drugs
8. Overeating lush pastures, particularly in the spring

C. Clinically, horses will
1. Be reluctant to move
2. Be anxious (in extreme cases)
3. Toe point
4. Rock back on the heal to relieve the pressure on the toe
5. Be pyrexic
6. Be depressed
7. Be off feed
8. Have increased heat in the hoof wall and bounding digital pulses as a result of increased blood flow
9. Be sensitive to hoof testers

D. In extreme cases the coffin bone rotates and can come through the sole of the foot
E. Radiographs are used to determine degree of rotation
F. Management
1. Anti-inflammatory drugs
2. Isoxsuprine hydrochloride (vasodilator)
3. Nitroglycerin applied to the medial and lateral digital arteries (vasodilator)
4. Acepromazine
5. Fluids (LRS)
6. Grass hay free choice, no grain
7. Corrective hoof trimming
8. Cold hosing and icing feet may also be done; however, this treatment is controversial

II. Navicular syndrome
A. Degeneration of the navicular bone
B. Exact cause unknown
C. Clinically, horses may
1. Stumble
2. Have a shortened stride
3. Be intermittently lame

D. When pressure is applied over the sole of the foot with hoof testers, a horse with navicular disease will react by pulling the foot away in response to pain
E. To further diagnose navicular syndrome, the following is performed
1. Flexion tests
2. Nerve blocking
3. Radiographs

F. Management
1. Anti-inflammatory drugs
2. Vasodilator (isoxsuprine hydrochloride)
3. Corrective foot trimming and shoeing
4. Last resort: surgically performing a neurectomy

LAMENESS

I. Etiology
A. Wounds/trauma
B. Bone changes
1. Congenital (e.g., osteochondrosis dessicans)
2. Chip fragments in joints due to excessive force

C. Soft tissue damage
1. Tendon injuries
2. Suspensory ligament injuries
3. Tendon sheath and joint capsule tears

D. Neurological (e.g., EPM)
E. Circulatory disorders (e.g., laminitis)

II. Detailed medical history important
A. Duration of lameness
B. Chronic versus acute
C. Working or stall rested while lame
D. Warms out of lameness
E. Stumbling
F. Previous medication
G. Alteration in the presentation of lameness while on medication

III. Methods of diagnosing lameness
A. Visual examination
1. At rest, walk, and trot

B. Flexion testing to assess joint specific lameness
C. Palpation of tendons and suspensories to assess soft tissue lameness
D. Local anesthetics
1. Carbocaine-V 2% injected into soft tissue or intraarticularly
2. Alcohol or antiseptic scrub applied before blocking the area
3. Intraarticular blocks are evaluated after 30 minutes
4. Nonarticular blocks are evaluated after 5 to 15 minutes
5. Ensure horse is properly restrained before veterinarian injects the anesthetic
6. Horse not sedated for this procedure to accurately diagnose an effect
7. Horse is assessed at walk and trot before and after blocking, preferably with the same person handling the horse
8. For an excited, difficult-to-handle horse, acepromazine may be injected intravenously without masking the lameness

E. Radiographic examination
1. Proper holding of the plate is essential, but radiation safety is to be considered
2. Plate held parallel to the leg, with the leg standing squarely under the horse

3. Lead aprons with thyroid protectors and lead gloves must be worn
4. Dosimeters measure radiation exposure levels
5. Views include
   a. Lateral
   b. Oblique: medial and laterals
   c. Anterior-posterior
      (1) Often referred to as dorsal to palmar for front limb and dorsal to plantar for hind limb
         (a) Views distal to and including the carpus
      (2) Proximal to the carpus or tarsus, views often named cranial to caudal
   d. Flexed for fetlock and carpus
   e. Skyline of the carpus
   f. Extra views are taken of the feet with the horse standing on a cassette covered by a strong Plexiglas shield
6. Portable units used to x-ray feet, fetlocks, carpus, and hocks
7. Larger stationary units with higher mAs and kVp used for shoulder, stifle, and head
8. For pelvic radiographs, horse needs to be anesthetized and have radiographs taken in dorsal recumbency

F. Ultrasound diagnosis
1. Tendons: superficial and deep digital flexor tendons
2. Ligaments: check main suspensory, medial, and lateral branches of the suspensory

G. Nuclear scintigraphy
1. A radioactive isotope, technetium, is injected IV into the horse; 2 hours later the body is scanned for "hot spots," or areas of uptake
2. Soft tissue of the lower limbs is scanned 20 minutes from injection
3. The horse is radioactive for 24 to 36 hours, and contact is restricted to feeding and watering
4. Hind end scans involve withholding water so the bladder does not obscure the pelvis views
5. Lasix parental, a diuretic, is injected to help minimize bladder size
6. Common uses
   a. Lameness that does not block out
   b. Suspected stress fractures that do not always show on radiography
      (1) Tibial stress fracture
      (2) Condylar fracture
      (3) Pelvis
      (4) Carpus and hock
   c. Suspected suspensory and tendon injuries

H. Extracorporeal shock wave therapy (ESWT)
1. Ultrasound-guided shock wave therapy
2. Speeds up healing time by increasing blood flow to the area
3. Used on ligaments, shin saucer fractures, bucked shins, and some bone fractures
4. Beginning to be used on navicular
5. Has not proved to be successful in treating tendons
6. Only a few machines in North America because of the expense

IV. Common lameness
A. Laminitis
B. Navicular
C. Fractured splint bones
D. Bucked shins
E. Cortical stress fractures of shins (saucer fractures)
F. Chip fractures in joints
G. Condylar or P1 (first pastern bone) fractures
H. Hoof abscesses
I. Bowed tendons
J. Torn suspensories

EQUINE SURGERY

I. Presurgical preparations
A. Take horse off feed 12 hours before surgery. Water can remain
B. TPR is performed
C. Groom horse to rid excess dirt and dander; pull shoes
D. Clip and aseptically prep jugular vein; place an IV catheter
E. Placement will depend on recumbency
F. Throat operations require placement lower than normal
G. PCV and TP, blood gas, and electrolyte analysis if available
H. Rinse out horse's mouth before induction
I. After horse is induced, the veterinarian will
   1. Direct positioning of the horse on the surgery table
   2. Indicate the area that needs to be clipped and prepped
J. Horse's feet should be covered with gloves or plastic (i.e., rectal sleeves) to prevent contamination to the surgery suite

II. Positioning of horse
A. The following surgeries are performed in dorsal recumbency
   1. All abdominal surgeries (e.g., colic, exploratory, cesarean, laryngeal ventriculectomy, umbilical and inguinal hernia repair)
   2. Castrations
      a. Cryptorchid (bilateral or unilateral)

b. Routine castrations
3. Arthroscopies
a. Hock
b. Stifle
c. Carpus: surgeon preference
4. Neurectomy: surgeon preference

B. When positioning a horse in dorsal recumbency, particular attention must be paid to
1. The padding underneath the shoulder and gluteal muscles
2. If padding is not sufficient, myositis can develop

C. The following operations are performed in lateral recumbency
1. Eye surgery
2. Tooth extractions
3. Mandible fracture repair (wiring)
4. Laryngotomy
5. Laryngoplasty
6. Arthroscopies
a. Carpus
b. Fetlocks
c. Shoulders
7. Periosteal strips
8. Splint fracture removal
9. Neurectomy: if more than one branch
10. Condyle fracture repair

D. When positioning a horse in lateral recumbency
1. Pay particular attention so that there is no pressure on the down elbow
2. The down foreleg should be pulled forward to enhance circulation and protect against radial nerve paralysis
3. The contralateral limbs should be supported with pads or leg supports, to keep the weight off the down legs
4. The head should have padding between the halter and the face when dropping and recovering
5. The head should be well padded while recumbent to protect the facial nerve from paralysis
6. Halter is removed during surgery

E. The following can be performed when a sedated horse is standing
1. Extraction of wolf teeth (first premolar)
2. Rectovaginal tears using an epidural
3. Caslick's (suturing a small portion of mare's vulva to prevent air entering the vagina, commonly known as wind sucking)
4. Perianal lacerations using an epidural
5. Uncomplicated ovariectomies
6. Tendon splitting
7. Castration
8. Neurectomy: of a single branch

III. Preparation of surgical site
A. After surgical site is clipped and vacuumed, caps and masks should be worn
B. Arthroscopic surgeries may have the instrument portal sites shaved with a razor
C. Prepping
1. Clean area with a bacteriostatic agent such as chlorhexidine or an iodine-based soap
2. Minimum 7-minute scrub
3. After site is clean, apply alcohol to defat the skin
a. Do not use alcohol as a final prep for eye surgeries or castrations
4. Move horse inside the surgical suite, where a final germicidal prep solution of tincture of Savlon or iodine is used
D. Prepping for eye surgeries
1. Clip hair around eye, including eyelashes. Take care to prevent hair from getting into eyes
2. If the eye is being enucleated (removed), the eyelids are sutured closed
3. Bacteriostatic agents should be avoided because they irritate the sensitive tissue around the eye and can damage the eyeball
4. A very dilute solution of povidone-iodine and saline can be used to clean skin around the eye
5. When flushing out the eye, saline is often used

IV. In surgery
A. Be aware of sterility zones
B. Assist veterinarians with their gowns and draping of horse
C. Assist with intraoperative radiographs for fracture repair surgeries
D. May assist anesthetist with blood pressure readings, depending on type of monitoring equipment
E. Values to be aware of
1. Blood pressure
a. Systolic blood pressure should be above 80 mm Hg
b. Dobutamine used to increase blood pressure; side effect is to lower heart rate

V. Recovery
A. Recover in same recumbency as during surgery
B. Padding is placed between the halter and the face and a recovery helmet is worn
C. Legs are wrapped for protection
D. Endotracheal (ET) tube is tied in place
E. When in dorsal recumbency for surgery
1. Left lateral recumbency is preferred to right recumbency
F. Assisted recovery: ET tube is pulled when horse swallows

G. Unassisted recovery: ET tube is pulled once horse is standing

VI. Postoperative care
   A. After the horse recovers and is stable, it can be moved back to its stall
   B. Horse should be kept warm and quiet
   C. Feeding regimen is clinic specific and determined by the type of surgery
   D. Monitoring horse's feces is very important: ileus is always a risk with any general anesthetic
   E. Horse's vital signs, including gastrointestinal motility, are monitored twice daily
   F. After horse passes feces, soft food such as a small bran mash can be introduced. A few hours later, a small amount of hay can be fed
   G. If horse passes more feces and vital signs are normal, horse's regular feeding schedule can be slowly introduced, beginning with gradually increasing amount of hay fed
   H. If horse does not pass any feces, a veterinarian will perform a rectal examination to determine if horse is impacted
   I. If impacted
      1. A nasogastric tube is passed, and mineral oil and warm water is introduced into the stomach to help break down the impaction
      2. Food is withheld from the horse
      3. Horse may be placed on intravenous fluids (LRS) until horse is passing feces
      4. Frequent hand walking (if surgery allows)
      5. Monitor vital signs
      6. Particular attention is paid to gastrointestinal motility (gut sounds)
      7. Horse is monitored four times daily until impaction has passed
   J. In cases of arthroscopic surgery
      1. Bandage is monitored for any discharge
      2. Leg is monitored for any unusual heat, swelling, or pain
      3. Usually 24 hours after the surgery, hand walking for 5 minutes is introduced
   K. In cases of fracture repair
      1. The cast is monitored for softness caused by discharge leaking from the fracture site
      2. Note any unusual smell or any unusual swelling above the cast
      3. On recovery, the cast may be replaced by a firm standing bandage with lots of support
         a. This will depend on the severity of the fracture

BANDAGING

I. Much damage can be done with a poor bandage

II. Principles of bandaging
   A. Smooth and wrinkle free with no bunching of material
   B. Adequate thickness of wrap under the bandage is necessary
   C. If too loose and it slips, may constrict the back of the tendon and cause bowed tendons
   D. If too tight, can constrict blood supply to the wound or area below the bandage or cause bowed tendons
   E. Usually three layers to a bandage
      1. Primary bandage or the layer right next to the skin
      2. Secondary layer mainly used for absorption of fluid
      3. Tertiary or outer layer that protects the bandage

III. Bandage uses
   A. Wound protection
   B. Fracture support
   C. Shipping
   D. Protection when dropping for surgery
   E. Riding
   F. Keeping foot medications in place

IV. Types of wounds and wound bandages
   A. Open wounds
      1. Adherent dressing as first layer
      2. Acts to debride wound when removed
      3. As wound closes and granulation bed fills in, switch to a nonadherent dressing as the primary layer
   B. Closed wounds
      1. Medicated gauze, usually until first bandage change, depending on whether discharge present
      2. Next layer is absorbent padding, evenly and smoothly applied to the area being bandaged and secured with conform-type bandage
      3. Depending on area being bandaged, the tertiary layer is Elastoplast, Vetrap, or a cotton and bandage

V. Postoperative bandages
   A. As for closed wounds
   B. When bandaging the carpus and hock
      1. A figure-eight pattern with Elastoplast adhering to the hair above and below
      2. Keep the accessory carpal bone and point of the hock uncovered to avoid pressure sores
      3. A small incision is cut into the bandage over the tendon to prevent a bandage bow
      4. A standing bandage may be placed below the carpus or hock to keep it from slipping

VI. Cast
  A. Medicated gauze and absorbent layer held in place with conform bandage
  B. A sterile non-pervious stockinette covers the leg from toe to above the length of the cast
  C. Vetcast plaster roll is saturated in warm water and wrapped horizontally and vertically for strength
  D. For short-term casts: "Gigli" wire is placed between the non-pervious stockinette and the cast for removal once the horse is standing
  E. For long-term casts: felt is wrapped at the top of the cast in attempt to prevent rubbing
  F. Long-term casts are removed with a cast-cutting saw or cast spreaders
  G. Horses vary in tolerance and reaction to a cast and must be monitored daily
  H. Duration of time in a cast depends on the severity of the fracture

VII. Foot bandage
  A. Used to keep medication or poultice in place
  B. Animal Lintex is a manufactured bandage poultice
  C. Often left on overnight, but are replaced daily
  D. Puncture wounds and abscesses are most common reasons for a foot bandage

ACKNOWLEDGMENT

The editors and authors recognize and appreciate the original contribution of Colleen Hill.

Glossary

anorexia Lack of appetite for food
arthroscopy Ability to look inside a joint through the aid of a fiberoptic scope
asymptomatic Carrier of a disease that does not show any symptoms
ataxia Muscle incoordination or irregular muscle action
borborygmus Bubbling and gurgling sounds as a result of gas moving through the gastrointestinal tract
dysphagia Difficulty swallowing
dyspnea Difficulty breathing
endotoxemia Endotoxins present in the blood
fasciculations Involuntary muscle contractions
fecal impaction Hardened feces in the rectum
floating Filing down of points of teeth
guttural pouch Air-filled sacs, found only in the horse, that are an extension of the eustachian tubes, closed by cartilage flaps on the side of the pharyngeal wall
halitosis Offensive breath odor
hydrophobia Fear of water; rabies
ileus Cessation of intestinal motility, which leads to impactions/obstructions
in utero In the uterus
laminitis Inflammation of the sensitive laminae of the foot
laryngoplasty Surgical procedure that ties back the arytenoid cartilage that is partially or completely paralyzed because of damage by the recurrent laryngeal nerve
laryngotomy Incision of the larynx
myositis Inflammation of the muscle that results when blood flow is interrupted. This results with uneven or inadequate padding. Muscles can become damaged, and it is an extremely painful condition
nasogastric Long tube placed through horse's nose into the stomach
neurectomy Cutting the palmar digital nerves at back of the pastern to desensitize the foot to pain
nystagmus Involuntary rapid eye movement seen during anesthesia; a sign of lightness and reaction to pain
periosteal strips Surgical procedure to correct angular limb deformity in foals by incising and lifting the periosteum to accelerate growth on one side of the bone
purulent Containing or forming pus
pyrexia Presence of fever
tachypnea Very rapid respiration
thrombosis Presence of a fibrin clot in vessels
thrombus Fibrin blood clot that remains where it is formed; can affect blood flow if it obstructs the vessels
tushes Canine teeth
vasodilator Agent that causes dilatation of the blood vessels
volvulus Torsion of a loop of intestine, causing obstruction
wolf teeth Small tooth that may be present in front of each first molar

Review Questions

1 Which of these are zoonotic?
  a. *Ehrlichia risticii* and *Clostridium* spp.
  b. *Sarcocystis neurona* and *Streptococcus equi*
  c. *Salmonella* spp. and rabies
  d. *Escherichia coli* and *Klebsiella* spp.

2 Common signs of neuromuscular disease include
  a. Restlessness, anxiousness, or agitation
  b. Anorexia, pyrexia, or depression
  c. Grinding teeth and sweating
  d. Muscle wasting, head pressing, or ataxia

3 The etiological agent for strangles is
  a. *Streptococcus equi*
  b. *Streptococcus zooepidemicus*
  c. *Clostridium* spp.
  d. *Sarcocystis neurona*

4 Coggins is the test for
  a. Equine infectious anemia
  b. Equine protozoal myeloencephalitis
  c. Potomac horse fever
  d. Hyperkalemic periodic paralysis

5 What is very important when positioning a horse in dorsal recumbency for surgery?
  a. Pulling the front legs cranially
  b. Position of the head
  c. Exposure of jugular vein for intravenous access
  d. Sufficient padding for shoulders and gluteal muscles

6 When prepping a surgical site, alcohol is used as what type of agent?
   a. Bacteriostatic
   b. Defatting
   c. Germicidal
   d. Bactericidal
7 Myositis is a result of
   a. Improper padding
   b. Improper prepping
   c. Horse not taken off feed before surgery
   d. Feeding horse too soon after surgery
8 A cessation of gastrointestinal motility is referred to as
   a. Peristalsis
   b. Ileus
   c. Volvulus
   d. Intussusception
9 With a casted leg it is important
   a. Not to move them
   b. To watch for signs of colic
   c. To monitor for any discharge and unusual smell or swelling
   d. To hand walk slowly for 5 minutes
10 A caslick prevents
   a. The passing of feces
   b. Air from entering the mare's vagina
   c. Rectovaginal tears
   d. Behavioral problems

BIBLIOGRAPHY

Anderson DM, editor: *Dorland's pocket medical dictionary,* ed 24, Philadelphia, 1989, WB Saunders.

Ball MA: Bandaging, *The Horse* June 1997.

Ball MA: The ins and outs of vaccination, *The Horse* September 1996.

Brown CM, Bertone J: *The 5-minute veterinary consult equine,* Baltimore, 2002, Lippincott Williams & Wilkins.

Compendium of veterinary products, ed 7, Hensall, Ontario, Canada, 2001, Adrian J. Bayley Publisher.

Fraser CM et al, editors: *The Merck veterinary manual,* ed 8, Rahway, NJ, 1995, Merck & Co, Inc.

Hayes MH: *Veterinary notes for horse owners,* ed 17, New York, 1987, Arco Publ.

Knecht CD et al: *Fundamental techniques in veterinary surgery,* ed 3, Philadelphia, 1987, WB Saunders.

McCurnin DM, Bassert JM: *Clinical textbook for veterinary technicians,* ed 5, St Louis, 2002, WB Saunders.

Reed SM, Bayly WM: *Equine internal medicine,* Philadelphia, 1998, WB Saunders.

Riegel RJ, Hakola SE: *Illustrated atlas of clinical equine anatomy and common disorders of the horse,* Vol 1, Marysville, OH, 1996, Equistar Publications, Limited.

Rose RJ, Hodgson DR: *Manual of equine practice,* Philadelphia, 1993, WB Saunders.

Siegal M, editor: *Book of horses: a complete medical reference guide for horses and foals,* ed 1, New York, 1996, HarperCollins.

Speirs VC: *Clinical examination of horses,* Toronto, 1997, WB Saunders.

Stashak TS: *Horse owner's guide to lameness,* Philadelphia, 1996, Lea & Febiger.

FROM THE INTERNET

Church SL: West Nile virus vaccine released, The horse interactive: Upfront: News and Notes, September 2001, www.thehorse.com

Franczek R: West Nile firsthand, The horse interactive, January 2001, www.thehorse.com

Graetz KS: EPM Special Report, The horse interactive, March 2001, www.thehorse.com

Graetz KS: Viewpoint: are you ready for West Nile?" The horse interactive, August 2001, www.thehorse.com

CHAPTER 25

Ruminant and Pig Nursing, Surgery, and Anesthesia

Shirley Sandoval

OUTLINE

LEARNING OUTCOMES

After reading this chapter you should be able to:

1. Know techniques for administering medications and collecting samples in agricultural animals.
2. Know some of the common diseases of cattle, small ruminants, and pigs.
3. Recognize some of the preventable (by vaccination) diseases of agricultural animals.
4. Know some of the common surgical procedures of agricultural animals.
5. Know some of the species differences regarding surgical procedures.
6. Understand the difference between local and regional anesthesia.
7. Know the various methods of regional anesthesia in agricultural animals.
8. Know the considerations for each species with respect to anesthesia in agricultural animals.
9. Know monitoring techniques for general anesthesia in agricultural animals.

Technicians in large animal practice must be familiar with common diagnostic and therapeutic techniques, as well as various diseases, available biologicals, surgical procedures, and anesthetic principles, for all domestic species. For more in-depth information, refer to the many excellent references that are available.

RUMINANT AND PIG NURSING

The Physical Examination

I. Observations
   A. Use all senses when performing a physical examination
   B. Before entering a stall or pen, helpful information can be obtained by observation
      1. Note the animal's eyes, its stance and carriage, body condition, urine and manure output, and food and water intake
      2. Know the "normals" for each type of animal. For instance, if you are used to observing beef animals, a dairy cow may look underconditioned when in fact her weight may be optimum for her

II. Physical examination
   A. The physical examination should be consistent from patient to patient

B. Proceed from nose to tail, listening to heart, lungs, and abdomen on both sides of the animal
C. Take note of swellings, abrasions, discharges, etc.
D. Temperature, pulse, and respiration (TPR) should fall within normal ranges (see Appendix E)
E. Rumen contractions should be noted by listening with a stethoscope at the left paralumbar fossa
   1. Normal rumen motility is 1 to 3 contractions per minute
F. Palpate over the ribs, vertebral column, and pelvis of fiber animals. What may appear to be a well-muscled to overweight animal may actually be a malnourished, emaciated animal hidden under the fiber

Administering Medication and Sample Collection

I. Oral dosing
   A. Balling gun
      1. Boluses, capsules, and magnets can be administered using this device, which may be made of plastic or metal
      2. With ruminants, the animal should be secured and the head well restrained
         a. Hold the animal around the bridge of the nose, place your fingers in the interdental space, and apply pressure to the hard palate
         b. This will force the animal to open its mouth so you can introduce the balling gun at the interdental space
         c. Position it so the medication will be deposited at the base of the tongue
         d. The head should be stabilized and held horizontally
      3. In pigs, a bar speculum can be introduced into the animal's mouth to hold the jaws open so that the balling gun can be used to deposit boluses or capsules at the base of the tongue
   B. Stomach tube
      1. For delivering large amounts of liquid medication, oral fluids, or anthelmintics or for transfaunation
         a. This technique is also used to retrieve a rumen fluid sample to examine for protozoa and pH
      2. Frick speculum
         a. Hollow, stainless steel tube that is used in cattle; it is inserted similarly to the balling gun
            (1) It is also used as a guide in introducing a stomach tube to prevent the tube from being damaged
         b. In sheep, goats, and camelids, a tape roll or appropriately sized, smooth-ended syringe case can be used
      3. Measure the distance from the nose to the rumen at approximately the thirteenth rib and insert the tube through the speculum up to the mark
         a. You may detect the odor of rumen gas to let you know you are in the correct place or have someone listen over the rumen at the paralumbar fossa with a stethoscope as you blow air into the tube
            (1) A "gurgling" sound will be heard
         b. After you verify correct placement, the liquid can be administered
         c. Always kink off the tube or occlude the end before removing it to prevent the animal from aspirating any of the contents
      4. Rumen fluid sampling
         a. Pass the tube as above and siphon fluid out of the rumen by attaching a dose syringe to the end of the stomach tube
            (1) Alternatively, while the tube is in the rumen, move the tube quickly in and out a few times, about 8 to 10 inches, and occlude the end before removing the tube
            (2) This process may have to be repeated to obtain an adequate sample
         b. Pour your sample into a clean specimen container from the fluted end of the stomach tube
            (1) Passing your sample through the end of the tube that is contaminated with saliva will change the pH of your sample
   C. Drench
      1. Small amounts of liquid medication can be given via drench
      2. A dose-syringe or unbreakable bottle is placed in the interdental space (ruminants) or at the commissure of the mouth (pigs)
         a. The head is tilted slightly so the nose is level with the eye
         b. The liquid should be given at a slow rate to allow the animal to swallow

Venipuncture

I. Cattle
   A. Jugular vein is for sampling and administering large volumes of fluids
      1. Head is restrained in a head catch and drawn upward to the opposite side
      2. Injection site is cleansed with 70% alcohol and occluded
      3. A 16- or 18-gauge, 3¾- to 7½-cm (1½- to 3-inch) needle is used and pushed with one sharp motion through the skin at a 45- to 90-degree angle

a. The larger bore and needle length are used for administration of fluids

B. Tail vein (ventral coccygeal) is for sampling and injecting small volumes
1. Confine animal to an area to prevent sideways movement and bend the tail directly forward at the base
2. Cleanse with 70% alcohol
3. Use an 18- to 20-gauge, 2½- to 3¾-cm (1- to 1½-inch) needle inserted at a 90-degree angle on the midline between the hemal arches of the fourth to seventh coccygeal vertebrae

C. Milk vein (subcutaneous abdominal) forms hematomas easily and is under pressure. Use caution
1. Occlusion is not necessary before entering with a 14-gauge, 5- to 7½-cm (2- to 3-inch) needle
2. Digital pressure applied for several minutes is necessary but a hematoma may still form

II. Sheep and goat
A. Jugular vein is almost always used
1. Direct an 18- or 20-gauge, 2½-cm (1-inch) needle into the jugular furrow at about a 30- to 45-degree angle
2. Cephalic vein is uncommon
3. Femoral vein is uncommon

III. Pigs
A. Cranial vena cava for a large volume (right side preferred because the phrenic nerve and thoracic duct are found near the left external jugular vein)
1. An 18- or 20-gauge, 7½- to 10-cm (3- to 4-inch) needle is used for adult pigs
2. The jugular fossa near the manubrium sterni, a bony projection just lateral to the ventral midline and cranial to the forelegs, is used as a guideline
3. The needle is inserted perpendicular to the plane of the neck and toward the left shoulder

B. Caudal auricular (ear) for small volumes
1. An 18- or 22-gauge, 2½- to 3¾-cm (1-to 1½-inch) needle is usually used with slight negative pressure maintained on the syringe
2. A 19- or 21-gauge butterfly is commonly used for intravenous administration

Injections

Intramuscular

Where possible, this route should be avoided in meat-producing animals. If the drug must be administered via this route, it should be placed cranial to the shoulder in the muscles of the neck because the blemished tissues can be easily trimmed and discarded if necessary. Current studies have shown increased therapeutic levels of the pharmaceuticals that are administered in this area.

I. Cattle
A. The location is in the lateral cervical muscles
B. Needle commonly used for adults is 16, 18, or 20 gauge, 3¾ to 5 cm (1½ to 2 inch) with 15 to 20 mL maximum volume of medication per site
C. Smaller gauge used for calves and up to 10 or 15 mL, depending on the size of the calf
D. When giving intramuscular injections to cattle, it is customary to place the needle before attaching the syringe
1. A couple of slaps with the flat part of the fist before inserting the needle tends to desensitize the area and allows the animal to steady itself before the needle is inserted

II. Sheep and goats
A. Give in the lateral cervical muscles
1. Use 18- to 20-gauge, 3¾-cm (1½-inch) needle for adults and 20- to 22-gauge needle for young animals
2. Depending on the size of the animal, the average volume for adults is 5 to 10 mL with a maximum of 15 mL

III. Pigs
A. Dorsolateral neck muscles are best for pigs
B. For adult pigs, use 18- to 20-gauge, 3¾-cm (1½-inch) needle
C. Depending on the size of the pig(let), a maximum of 1 to 15 mL should be given

Subcutaneous

As concerns for meat quality assurance increase, this route is becoming increasingly popular with agricultural animal producers for pharmaceutical administration. There has also been a marked increase in the variety of pharmaceuticals approved for subcutaneous administration in food-producing animals.

I. Cattle
A. Site of administration is cranial to the shoulder and the lateral neck
B. Use a 16- to 18-gauge, 3¾-cm (1½-inch) needle
C. Volume depends on the personal preference of the veterinarian; however, a good guideline is up to 250 mL/site in adults and up to 50 mL/site in calves

II. Small ruminants
A. Site of administration is cranial to the shoulder and lateral neck area
B. Use an 18- to 20-gauge, 2½-cm (1-inch) needle
C. Inject 5 mL maximum/site

III. Pigs
A. Site of administration is the lateral side of the neck, close to the base of the ear

B. Use a 16- to 18-gauge, 2½- to 3¾-cm (1- to 1½-inch) needle
C. Depending on the size to the pig(let), 1 to 3 mL/site maximum

Intraperitoneal

I. Cattle
A. Use a 14- to 16-gauge, 3¾- to 5-cm (1½- to 2-inch) needle
B. Antibiotics usually given in conjunction with rehydration fluids
C. Injection site is the right flank, midway between the last rib and the tuber coxae
1. Go at least 10 cm (4 in) below the lateral processes of the vertebrae to prevent retroperitoneal or perirenal injection
II. Small ruminants (neonates)
A. Use a 20-gauge, 2½-cm (1-inch) needle
B. Hold the neonate by the forelimbs
C. Place the needle to the left of the umbilicus, aspirate to ensure proper needle placement (not in a vein or bowel), administer medication/fluids
III. Pigs
A. Use a 16- to 18-gauge, 1¼- to 2½-cm (½- to 1-inch) needle in neonates and a 16- to 18-gauge, 7½-cm (3-inch) needle in adults
B. Hold the piglet by the rear legs
C. Place the needle between the midline and the flank, aspirate to ensure proper needle placement, and administer medication/fluids
D. Administration in adult pigs can be performed with pig in a standing position

Intradermal

I. Used primarily for tuberculin testing
A. Cattle
1. Use a 22-gauge, 2½-cm (1-inch) needle
2. Tuberculin testing requires 0.1 mL of tuberculin to be injected into the dermis of the caudal tail fold
B. Sheep and goats
1. Use a 25-gauge, 1½-cm (⅝-inch) needle
2. Tuberculin testing requires 0.1 mL of tuberculin to be injected into the dermis of the caudal tail fold
C. Camelids
1. Use a 25-gauge, 1½-cm (⅝-inch) needle
2. Tuberculin testing requires 0.1 mL of tuberculin to be injected into the dermis of the axillary region

Milk Sampling

I. An important aspect of dairy herd health is early detection and treatment of mastitis. Because of rising laboratory costs, milk sampling (for culture) is often done on a herd basis
A. Quarters are sampled into one tube and individual quarter sampling is done on only those animals that test positive on the herd testing
B. Sampling should be done before routine milking or at least 6 hours after milking
C. Each teat should be washed, wiped with an alcohol swab, and allowed to dry
1. Clean in the order of far to near
2. The first part of the stream should be discarded into a strip cup, and a midstream sample is taken horizontally and directed into the sample vial, which is held horizontally out from under the near side of the animal
3. Sampling is done from the nearest side first
II. Determination of subclinical mastitis and a rough estimate of somatic cell count can be done using an on-site procedure called the California Mastitis Test (CMT)
A. The test consists of a paddle with four shallow cups and a reagent containing a pH indicator
B. A small amount of milk is mixed with an equal amount of CMT reagent
C. The paddle is gently rotated, and an interpretation is made based on the amount of precipitation
D. The amount of precipitate formed is given a 0-to-4 rating

DISEASES OF RUMINANTS AND PIGS

Metabolic

I. Hypocalcemic parturient paresis (milk fever)
A. Incidence
1. The incidence of milk fever in cattle increases in high-performing animals at 5 to 9 years of age
a. Greater in Channel Island breeds (Jersey)
b. Usually occurs at 48 to 72 hours postpartum
2. Milk fever in sheep is most common in late pregnancy but can occur in early lactation
3. The condition is rare in sows but may occur within a few hours of farrowing
B. Serum calcium level is decreased; serum magnesium level may be increased (flaccid paralysis) or decreased (tetany)
1. Low serum phosphorus may be a contributing factor
C. Clinical signs initially include muscle tremors, weakness, and staggering gait
1. Classic signs include sternal recumbency, head turned into flank, anorexia, dry muzzle, atonic rumen, increased heart rate (with decreased intensity of heart sound),

mydriasis, myositis, and nerve damage if animal is down too long
2. If left untreated, depression of the circulatory system and bloat as a result of lateral recumbency will be fatal

D. Characteristically, a quick positive response is obtained with treatment consisting of intravenous calcium borogluconate
1. Careful attention must be paid to the heart during infusion because calcium salts affect the heart muscle

E. Animals should be fed a ration high in phosphorus and low in calcium during the later stages of pregnancy

II. Ketosis (acetonemia in cattle; pregnancy toxemia in ewes)
A. Can occur in the period from just after calving until peak lactation in the cow (2 to 6 weeks after calving)
B. Generally occurs in the last trimester of pregnancy in ewes
C. As a result of increased demand for glucose for the production of milk in high-producing cows and the demands of the developing fetus (or foeti), the dam is in a negative energy balance
1. Body fat is mobilized to provide energy
2. Ketone bodies are produced in excess of tissue needs and clinical ketosis results
D. Ketosis may be secondary to any underlying disease that causes inappetance
E. There is a characteristic acetone odor to the breath, milk, and urine
F. Two forms of the disease may manifest: the wasting and the nervous forms
1. Wasting form: more common
a. The cow may begin by being off grain alone, then silage, but may continue to eat hay
b. Weight loss exceeds what one might expect from loss of appetite alone
c. Milk production declines
2. Nervous form: presents acutely with head pressing, delirium, teeth grinding, and staggering
a. In ewes and does, signs of the disease are more like the nervous form, and ketones may be detected on the breath
G. Treatment
1. Intravenous infusion of glucose (dextrose) is usually successful in cows, although it often needs to be repeated
2. Oral doses of propylene glycol and hormonal therapy may be useful
3. The same treatment in ewes is less satisfactory
4. Lambs may have to be removed by cesarean section to save the ewe
H. Most incidences of ketosis can be prevented by adhering to a careful management and ration plan

III. White muscle disease (nutritional myodegeneration)
A. Vitamin E and selenium deficiency is seen in young, rapidly growing calves, sheep, and goats
B. Most commonly, these animals are from dams that were on selenium-deficient diets during their pregnancy
C. It manifests in two forms: cardiac and skeletal
1. The cardiac form presents with severe debilitation or sudden death
2. Clinical signs include depression, respiratory distress, pulmonary edema, foaming at the mouth, and weakness
3. The skeletal form presents with weakness or muscle stiffness; the animal may be recumbent. Muscle groups in the limbs may become hard and painful to palpation
4. For prevention of this disease, give injection of vitamin E and selenium

Alimentary

I. Displaced abomasum
A. Left displaced abomasum (LDA)
1. Occurs when the abomasum is displaced from its normal position on the abdominal floor to the left side of the abdomen between the rumen and the abdominal wall
B. Occurs most commonly in large, high-producing, mature dairy cows immediately after calving
1. Clinical signs are decreased appetite, lower milk production, decreased rumen motility, intermittent diarrhea, secondary ketosis, and the presence of an auscultable "ping" in the left flank caused by the entrapment of gas
2. Surgical correction is performed using a left paralumbar (abomasopexy or omentopexy), right paralumbar (omentoabomasopexy or omentopexy), or ventral paramedian (abomasopexy-open or abomasopexy-toggle) approach

II. Right displaced abomasum (RDA)
A. Occurs within a few weeks of calving and may be complicated by right-sided torsion of the abomasum (RDA)
B. Less common than LDA but clinical signs are similar

1. Abomasal torsion will present with acute, severe abdominal pain and acute signs of toxicity; death may occur without a timely correction
2. Surgical correction is made using right flank (omentoabomasopexy or omentopexy) or ventral paramedian (abomasopexy-open) laparotomy

C. There is an increased incidence of displaced abomasum in cows fed a high-grain diet (zero grazing) in conjunction with confined housing

III. Vagus indigestion

A. Vagus indigestion is a common disease in cattle; uncommon in sheep
   1. Characterized by anorexia, decreased movement of ingesta through the stomachs, and distention

B. Most common cause: hardware disease (traumatic reticuloperitonitis)
   1. Hardware disease usually results from perforation of the reticulum and sometimes the rumen by an ingested foreign object
   2. Clinical signs are a sudden decrease in milk, anorexia, "hunching," and groaning
   3. Often the cow will grunt if pressure is applied over the xiphoid ("grunt test")
   4. Rumen becomes atonic, fecal output is decreased, and ketosis often occurs
   5. Treatment includes antibiotics and placing a magnet into the reticulum
   6. If unsuccessful, a rumenotomy may be performed
   7. Because dairy cattle are most often affected, most cases can be prevented by the administration of a bar magnet to all heifers at 6 months of age and careful adherence to debris-free forage

C. Actinobacillosis of the rumen also can cause vagal indigestion in cattle

D. In sheep the cause may be peritonitis due to *Sarcosporidia*

IV. Ruminal tympany (bloat)

A. Bloat is an acute overdistention of the rumen in the form of free gas or froth mixed with ingesta
   1. Frothy bloat occurs in cattle on legume pasture and on high-grain diets
      a. The froth produced prevents the escape of normal gases during eructation
   2. Gas bloat is caused by a physical obstruction of the gases and a failure of eructation

B. If the bloat is not life threatening, the passage of a large-bore tube into the rumen to allow the escape of gas may be sufficient

C. If the bloat is severe, the distention causes compression of the diaphragm and the animal is unable to breathe
   1. An emergency rumenotomy may be necessary to save the animal
   2. The left paralumbar fossa can be incised using a sharp knife or a trocar and cannula
   3. Antifermentive and antifrothing agents are usually administered

D. Frothy bloat can be controlled to some degree by careful pasture and feed management

V. Rumen acidosis (grain overload)

A. Grain overload is an accumulation of excessive quantities of highly fermentive carbohydrates that produce lactic acid in the rumen
   1. As lactic acid increases, rumen pH may drop below 5.0 and metabolic acidosis occurs
   2. Cattle and sheep are affected
   3. Usually occurs due to accidental access to large quantities of grain

B. Clinical signs include severe toxemia, weakness, dehydration, fluid-filled static rumen, incoordination, and recumbency, leading to death

C. Principles of treatment include decreasing fermentation and acid production in the rumen using antimicrobials, neutralizing metabolic acidosis, and rehydrating the animal using intravenous fluids with sodium bicarbonate

VI. Neonatal diarrhea

A. An important disease of farm animals with multiple infectious and noninfectious causes
   1. Stresses such as cold weather, changes in diet or housing, weaning, and failure of passive transfer of gamma globulins from colostrum predispose the neonate to infection
   2. Absorption of IgG occurs optimally in calves within the first 6 to 8 hours of life but may occur up to 24 hours
      a. Goats up to 4 days
      b. Lambs, maximally to 15 hours but up to 24 to 48 hours
      c. Piglets up to 12 to 24 hours
   3. Dietary diarrhea also can be due to ingestion of increased quantities of milk or inferior milk replacers

B. Diarrhea is characterized by profuse, watery, yellow feces, dehydration, metabolic acidosis, shock, and death

C. Successful treatment of diarrhea depends on cause and duration
   1. Replacing fluid and electrolytes lost and correcting metabolic acidosis should be the main objectives

D. Infectious causes of neonatal diarrhea can be controlled with a vaccination regimen and provision of good-quality colostrum

E. Cattle

1. *Escherichia coli* diarrhea
   a. Clinical signs include dehydration, acidosis, weakness, and death
   b. Treatable if caught early
   c. Vaccine available

F. Sheep and goats

1. Rotavirus
   a. Causes mild diarrhea
   b. Recovery usually in a few days
   c. Mortality rate increases when animal is also infected with *E. coli*

G. Pigs

1. Swine dysentery *(Treponema hyodysenteriae)*
   a. Causes depression, weakness, anorexia, hemorrhagic diarrhea, and sometimes death
   b. Can be treated, but may return after initial treatment is discontinued
   c. Effective vaccines are not available, but there is current research for the development of biological protection for this disease
2. Transmissible gastroenteritis (TGE) (porcine rotavirus)
   a. Common viral disease in pigs
   b. High morbidity and mortality rates in piglets younger than 10 days
   c. Clinical signs include diarrhea, vomiting, anorexia, dehydration, and death
   d. Vaccination available

Reproductive

I. Cattle

A. Mastitis

1. An inflammation of the mammary gland that can occur in all species, although it assumes economic importance only in species used for milk
2. A large proportion of cases are subclinical and can be detected only by screening tests based on the leukocyte count
3. Clinical mastitis is characterized by heat, pain, and swelling of the gland and marked changes in the milk such as discoloration and clots
4. A few of the major bacteria involved are *Staphylococcus aureus, Streptococcus agalactiae,* and some of the coliform bacteria
5. Treatment must include removal of infection from the quarter and returning the milk to its normal composition
6. Several treatments are available and depend on the severity of infection
   a. Includes frequent milking out of the infected quarter (stripping), udder infusions, systemic antibiotics, and perhaps drying off of the infected quarter (i.e., not milking it)
7. Prevention of mastitis through a prophylactic routine of regular screening, proper milking technique, maintenance of milking equipment, and early recognition and treatment of subclinical cases is the best course

B. Vibriosis (*Campylobacter fetus* ssp. *venerealis*)

1. A zoonotic disease
2. Causes infertility and a prolonged diestrus period
3. Periodic abortion
4. Vaccine available

C. Brucellosis *(Brucella abortus)*

1. A zoonotic disease
2. Cows
   a. Causes mid- to late-term abortions (5+ months)
   b. Subsequent pregnancies may be term or end with abortions
   c. Metritis (uterine inflammation)
   d. Retained placenta
   e. Bacterin available for calfhood vaccination
3. Bulls
   a. Orchitis (inflammation of the testis)
   b. Epididymitis (inflammation of the epididymis)
   c. Infertility

D. Leptospirosis *(Leptospira pomona)*

1. A zoonotic disease
2. Clinical signs in adult cattle include fever, anorexia, agalactia, abortion, and mastitis
3. Clinical signs in calves include septicemia, pyrexia, anorexia, depression, hemolytic anemia, and dyspnea
4. Bacterin available

E. Listeriosis *(Listeria monocytogenes)*

1. Zoonotic
2. Most commonly found in ruminants
3. Clinical signs in adults include abortion in the last trimester, ophthalmitis (inflammation of the eyeball), and uveitis (inflammation of the uvea)
4. Bacterin available

II. Sheep

A. Vibriosis *(Vibrio fetus)* (*Campylobacter fetus* ssp. *fetus*)

1. A zoonotic disease
2. Clinical signs include abortion, which occurs in the last 6 weeks of gestation
3. Also may see stillbirths and weak lambs

4. Ewes usually survive, but the viability of the ewe decreases with complications such as retention of fetuses, peritonitis, and metritis

B. Brucellosis *(Brucella ovis)*
   1. Ewes (clinical signs include abortion, stillbirths, and weak lambs)
   2. Rams (infertility due to poor-quality semen and epididymitis)

C. Listeriosis *(Listeria monocytogenes)*
   1. Also known as "circling disease," it is classified into three forms: neurologic disease, abortion, and septicemia
   2. The most common form in sheep is neurologic disease. *L. monocytogenes* are gram positive, nonsporing coccobacilli
   3. Clinical signs include nasal discharge, conjunctivitis, depression, disorientation, circling, and facial paralysis
   4. Pregnant ewes develop placentitis and abort during the third trimester of gestation, usually exhibiting no other clinical signs
   5. Septicemia in lamb is characterized by depression, anorexia, pyrexia, and diarrhea. They may die in 24 hours
   6. In adults, depression, diarrhea, and slight elevation in temperature (39° to 41.5° C) (102.2° to 106.7° F)

D. Enzootic abortion in ewes (EAE) *(Chlamydia psittaci)*
   1. A major cause of abortion in sheep and goats, EAE is characterized by abortions in the last trimester
      a. Also stillbirths and placentitis
   2. The infectious organism is present in the fluids, tissues, and fetuses at the time of parturition
   3. The main transmission of the disease is via ingestion; therefore removal of the infected tissue is important to prevent spread of the disease
   4. Pregnant women should not handle these tissues or the infected animals

III. Porcine

A. Leptospirosis *(Leptospira pomona)*
   1. A zoonotic disease
   2. Stillbirths or abortion in the last 2 to 4 weeks of gestation
   3. Term piglets may be dead or weak and die shortly after birth
   4. In its acute form, it may also cause septicemia in piglets

Respiratory

I. Cattle

A. Bovine respiratory disease complex
   1. Infectious bovine rhinotracheitis (IBR) (viral), also known as "red nose"
      a. Caused by bovine herpesvirus 1
      b. It affects cattle of all ages, but predominantly young feedlot cattle
      c. Clinical signs include upper respiratory disease, second-degree pneumonia, enteric disease (<3-week-old calves), abortion, encephalitis, and infectious pustular vulvuovaginitis (IPV)
   2. Bovine viral diarrhea virus (BVDV)
      a. Caused by a Pestivirus
      b. May present with bovine viral diarrhea (BVD), which includes these clinical signs: gastroenteritis, diarrhea, respiratory disease, oral lesions, and abortion
         (1) Affects cattle 6 to 24 months old
      c. May present with mucosal disease (MD), which includes these clinical signs: oral erosions, lameness, cachexia, and diarrheae
         (1) MD affects all ages but mostly young feedlot cattle
         (2) Transplacental infection of MD will have clinical signs that include calves born with curly hair coat, "weak calf" syndrome, and persistently infected animals
   3. Parainfluenza III (PI3) (viral)
      a. Caused by a Paramyxovirus
      b. Affects all ages of cattle
      c. Clinical signs include coughing, fever, nasal discharge, and second-degree pneumonia
   4. Bovine respiratory syncytial virus (BSRV)
      a. Caused by a Paramyxovirus
      b. It is most common in 6- to 8-month-old cattle
      c. Clinical signs include cough, nasal discharge, anorexia, and fever
      d. BSRV pneumonia causes dyspnea, polypnea, mouth breathing, and interstitial emphysema
   5. *Haemophilus somnus*
      a. Affects 6- to 8-month-old feedlot calves
      b. Treatment is often nonresponsive
      c. Clinical signs include bronchopneumonia, central nervous system disease—depression ataxia, paralysis, recumbency, septic arthritis, myocarditis
   6. *Pasteurella haemolytica* ("shipping fever")
      a. Affects young animals stressed by weaning or transport
      b. Clinical signs include acute toxemic bronchopneumonia, dyspnea, increased lung sounds, cough, and pleuritis

II. Sheep
   A. Bluetongue (viral)
      1. Transmitted by a midge vector of the *Culicoides* sp.
      2. Bluetongue is most commonly found in sheep; less common in cattle and goats
      3. A seasonal disease, it presents in the late summer and fall
      4. Initial clinical signs include a transient fever with a temperature of 41° C+ (106° F+), facial edema (including lips, muzzle, and ears), hyperemic mucous membranes, cyanotic tongue, excessive salivation, and nasal discharge. This is followed by crusty lesions of the nose and muzzle and lesions in the oral cavity such as petechial hemorrhage, erosions, and ulcerations
      5. This progresses to lameness, cardiac myopathy, and commonly bronchopneumonia
         a. This infection can also cause the sloughing of hooves, wool break, diarrhea, and death

III. Pigs
   A. Porcine reproductive and respiratory syndrome (PRRS, or mystery swine disease)
      1. A new disease in North America, making its appearance in the 1980s
      2. Characterized by reproductive failure and increased mortality rates in farrowing and nursery room pigs
      3. Reproductive problems include return to estrus, abortion, and delivery of mummified, stillborn, or poorly viable piglets
      4. Increased mortality in piglets is associated with a "thumping" respiration with severe interstitial pneumonia and several secondary infectious diseases such as diarrhea and septicemia
      5. PRRS appears to be spread by movement of pigs between farms and by airborne dispersion over distances of less than 3 km (1.8 miles)
      6. Recent development of a vaccine has proved encouraging
   B. Atrophic rhinitis *(Bordetella bronchiseptica, Pasteurella multocida)*
      1. Atrophic rhinitis is an upper respiratory disease of young pigs
      2. The nonprogressive form does not include infection from toxogenic *Pasteurella multocida*
         a. A less severe disease that is slight to severe with no transient turbinate atrophy and no clinical signs
      3. The progressive form of this disease includes infection with *P. multocida,* which causes sneezing, nasal discharge, shortening or distortion of the nose, and epistaxis
      4. Acute cases affect piglets from 3 to 9 weeks of age
         a. Severe nasal and maxillary distortion can result in occlusion of the nasal passages and inability to masticate, resulting in reduced growth rates
   C. *Actinobacillus pleuropneumoniae*
      1. This disease has a sudden onset
         a. Discovery of dead pigs without previous illness, severe respiratory distress, and a temperature of 41° C (105.8° F) is common
      2. Anorexia, weakness, labored breathing with frothy discharge from mouth and nose
      3. Can cause abortion in sows

Clostridial Diseases With Available Biologicals

The following discussion includes only the diseases for which a vaccine is available.

I. Cattle
   A. Blackleg *(Clostridium chauvoei)*
      1. Clostridial myositis
      2. Clinical signs include severe lameness, depression, anorexia, temperature of 41° C (106° F), increased pulse of 100 to 120 beats per minute, and acute edema, hot and painful, that becomes cold and painless with emphysema as the disease progresses
      3. Death occurs in 12 to 36 hours
   B. Malignant edema (*Clostridium septicum* and *Clostridium sordellii*)
      1. Gas gangrene
      2. Clinical signs include lesion with painful swelling, with or without emphysema, temperature of 41° to 42° C (106° to 107° F), depressed, weak, muscle tremor, lame, or stiff
      3. Death occurs in 24 to 48 hours
   C. Infectious necrotic hepatitis (*Clostridium novyi* type B)
      1. Black disease
      2. Initiated by damage to the liver
      3. Causes severe depression and an initial fever followed by subnormal temperatures, rumen atony, and abdominal pain, which may last 1 to 2 days
      4. Animals tend to separate from the rest of the herd
   D. Bacillary hemoglobinuria *(Clostridium haemolyticum)*
      1. Initiated by damage to the liver
      2. Clinical signs include fever, rumen atony, anorexia, abdominal pain, toxemia, arched posture, and dark-red urine ("red water")
      3. Death occurs in 12 to 96 hours

E. Pulpy kidney (*Clostridium perfringens* type D)
  1. Affects calves 1 to 4 months old
    a. Calves with peracute disease are found dead
    b. Calves with acute disease exhibit bellowing, mania, convulsions, and death in 1 to 2 hours
    c. Calves with subacute disease appear quite, docile, and adypsic and may appear blind
      (1) Signs may last 2 to 3 days
      (2) Quick, complete recovery
  2. Occurs in the summer and fall in endemic areas where fields may be irrigated

F. Hemorrhagic enterotoxemia *(Clostridium perfringens)*
  1. It mainly affects calves up to 10 days of age
  2. Clinical signs include diarrhea, acute abdominal pain, and nervous signs
  3. May result in sudden death or a slow recovery in 10 to 14 days

G. Tetanus *(Clostridium tetani)*
  1. The neurotoxins that are produced by this bacteria affect the central nervous system
  2. Clinical signs include bloat, prolapse of the third eyelid, muscle stiffness, muscle spasm, increase response to sound and tactile stimuli, and muscular rigidity ("sawhorse" stance)

II. Sheep and goats

A. Blackleg *(Clostridium chauvoei)*
  1. Clinical signs include lameness, high fever, anorexia, depression, and death

B. Malignant edema (*Clostridium septicum* and *Clostridium sordellii*)
  1. Organisms are transmitted from the soil to the animals through open cuts, wounds, surgical incisions, and the umbilicus
  2. May occur after lambing, shearing, or castration/tail docking
  3. "Swelled head"
    a. Occurs when young rams are housed together, butt heads, and create wounds for the organisms to enter the body

C. Infectious necrotic hepatitis (*Clostridium novyi* type B)
  1. Black disease
  2. Initiated by damage to the liver
  3. Causes severe depression and an initial fever followed by subnormal temperatures
    a. Clinical signs are not usually observed because death is rapid
    b. Animals usually die during the night

D. Bacillary hemoglobinuria *(Clostridium haemolyticum)*
  1. Initiated by damage to the liver
  2. Clinical signs include rumen atony, anorexia, abdominal pain, arched posture, and dark-red urine ("red water")
  3. Death occurs in 12 to 96 hours

E. Pulpy kidney (*Clostridium perfringens* type D)
  1. Lambs with peracute disease present with sudden death
  2. Lambs with acute disease (<2 hours) present with depression, clonic convulsions, diarrhea, opisthotonus, and death
  3. Adults may live up to 24 hours, lag behind, and show staggers, knuckling, and a rapid, shallow respiration
  4. Goats with peracute disease present with fever, abdominal pain, dysentery, and convulsions
    a. Death occurs in 4 to 36 hours
  5. Goats with acute disease present with abdominal pain and diarrhea
    a. May recover in 2 to 4 days or die

F. Hemorrhagic enterotoxemia *(Clostridium perfringens)*
  1. Affects lambs at 1 to 4 days of age
    a. The peracute form of the disease causes sudden death
    b. The acute form of the disease causes diarrhea, anorexia, and severe abdominal pain
      (1) Death occurs in 24 hours
  2. Adult sheep
    a. "Struck:" sudden death

G. Tetanus *(Clostridium tetani)*
  1. It is most commonly found in sheep after shearing or tail docking
  2. Clinical signs include prolapse of the third eyelid, erect ears, muscle stiffness, muscle spasms, an increased response to sound and tactile stimuli, and muscular rigidity ("sawhorse" stance), followed by convulsions, respiratory arrest, and death
  3. Can give antitoxin when processing animals

III. Porcine

A. Enteric disease in piglets (*Clostridium perfringens* type C)
  1. Causes peracute, acute, subacute, or chronic disease in piglets
    a. Peracute and acute disease each shows varying degrees of hemorrhagic diarrhea and death within 2 days
    b. Subacute disease produces diarrhea, which can last 7 days and produces a dehydrated piglet, resulting in death in 5 to 7 days
    c. Chronic infections result in diarrhea, with chronic ill thrift and sometimes death
  2. Vaccination available

Other

I. Cattle
   A. Anthrax *(Bacillus anthracis)*
      1. A zoonotic disease
      2. Causes peracute and acute disease
         a. Peracute disease causes sudden death
         b. Acute disease exhibits staggers, convulsions, and death
   B. Anaplasmosis *(Anaplasma marginale)*
      1. A rickettsial organism
         a. Transmitted from animal to animal mainly via insect vectors
         b. Also transmitted to animals by arthropod vectors, mainly ticks
      2. Calves usually get a subacute form
         a. Clinical signs include bouts of anorexia and intermittent fever and may end in death; survivors are emaciated with compromised fertility
      3. Adults manifest the subacute, acute, and peracute forms of the disease
         a. Subacute is as described earlier
         b. Acute disease causes anemia, weakness, pale mucous membranes, and abortion. These animals may become aggressive and attack caretakers before death
         c. Animals with peracute cases usually die within 24 hours. They initially present with fever, anemia, and respiratory distress
      4. Vaccination available
         a. The killed vaccine is not preventative but decreases the severity of the disease
         b. Immunity is considered short in duration, at least 5 months
         c. Vaccination of breeding cows may predispose calves to neonatal isoerythrolysis

II. Ovine
   A. Contagious foot rot
      1. *Bacteroides nodosus* synergists with *Fusobacterium necrophorum* as the causative agents
         a. *B. nodosus* is a gram-negative, anaerobic rod
         b. *F. necrophorum* is a gram-negative, anaerobic coccobacillary rod
         c. Clinical signs include varying degrees of lameness in one or more feet, walking on the knees, or recumbency
            (1) The interdigital skin becomes inflamed, and there is slight undermining of the sole
            (2) Removal of the loose hoof emits a distinct foul odor
         d. Treatment includes trimming the feet close, exposing the anaerobic bacteria to air and copper sulfate foot baths or topical 10% formalin
         e. Bacterin available
      2. Contagious ecthyma, soremouth, orf (viral)
         a. A zoonotic disease of sheep and goats
         b. Affects all ages but most common in young animals
         c. Animals present with crusty lesions on the lips, nose, and gums
         d. Older animals usually present with lesions on the udder, external genitalia, coronary band, eyelids, conjunctiva
         e. Recovery is dependent on complications that may arise from the initial insult
            (1) Complications include second-degree bacterial infection, mastitis, screwworm infestation, pneumonia, anorexia, and death
         f. Bacterin available

III. Porcine
   A. Erysipelas *(Erysipelothrix rhusiopathiae)*
      1. A zoonotic disease
      2. This bacterial infection of pigs can manifest in an acute or a chronic form
         a. The acute form presents with fever, anorexia, and diamond-shaped skin lesions
         b. The chronic form manifests as arthritis or vegetative endocarditis
         c. There are decreased incidents in swine-rearing operations where the animals are housed off soil
            (1) Most commonly affects unvaccinated pigs at 3 months to adulthood
            (2) In specific pathogen-free herds, the first signs of disease may be abortion storms and septicemic death in suckling pigs
   B. Meningitis *(Streptococcus suis)*
      1. A zoonotic disease
      2. This bacterial infection occurs in pigs younger than 12 weeks old
      3. Initial clinical signs include fever, anorexia, depression, stiff gait, blindness, muscular tremors, and ataxia
         a. Followed by recumbency, paddling, and death
      4. A more acute disease presents with sudden death
   C. Pseudorabies (Aujeszky's disease [viral])
      1. Caused by suid herpesvirus-1
      2. It is transmitted via oronasal contact with infected pigs

3. The nervous system is the primary site of infection
4. Clinical signs include fever, depression, vomiting, hindlimb ataxia, muscle tremors, paddling, recumbency, coughing, sneezing, and death within 12 hours in young pigs
5. In adult pigs, the disease can cause abortion, still births, and mummified fetuses
6. Vaccination available

RUMINANT AND PIG ANESTHESIA

Local and Regional Anesthesia (Analgesia)

Local and regional anesthetics are commonly used in large animal practice because they are often safer and more convenient than general anesthetics. Local anesthesia is the desensitization of the tissues of the surgical site by the infiltration of an anesthetic agent. Regional anesthesia is desensitization of the surgical site by blocking the nerves to the region.

I. Cattle: regional anesthesia in cattle is commonly used for standing laparotomy. The following techniques (or a variation) are frequently performed. In every case, the animal is adequately restrained, the area is clipped and prepped, and attention is paid to aseptic technique
   A. Inverted L block
      1. Nerves supplying the paralumbar fossa travel in a ventral-caudal direction from the spine
      2. Local anesthetic is infiltrated in a horizontal line just ventral to the transverse processes of the lumbar vertebrae and a vertical line just caudal to the last rib
         a. In this way the nerves supplying the incision site are blocked
      3. A variation of this technique is used for regional analgesia for a ventral midline approach
   B. Paralumbar block (Cornell block)
      1. Local anesthetic is injected below the lateral edges of the transverse processes of the first four lumbar vertebrae
         a. The needle is placed horizontally below each process directed toward the midline
         b. Twenty to 25 mL of local anesthetic is injected at each site, using an 18-gauge, 3½-inch needle
      2. In this way the branches of T13, L1, and L2 (and L3), which supply the surgical site, are blocked
   C. Paravertebral block
      1. The nerves are blocked as they come off the spinal column (T13, L1, L2, and L3)
         a. At a position about 4 cm (1½ inch) off the midline, using a long (4- to 6-inch) needle, local anesthetic is injected at the caudal edges of L1, L2, and L3
      2. Muscle relaxation and desensitization of the skin and deeper tissues will result if the block is successful
   D. Epidural block
      1. Indications for use
         a. To stop straining for obstetrical manipulations
         b. To facilitate the reduction of rectal and vaginal prolapses
         c. Perineal surgery, udder surgery
         d. To stop straining during laparotomies and cesareans
         e. Urethrostomies
      2. It is achieved by injecting a small quantity of anesthetic agent in the epidural space between the first and second coccygeal vertebrae (cranial epidural) or the sacrococcygeal junction (caudal epidural)
         a. The area blocked includes the anus, vulva, perineum, and caudal aspects of the thighs
      3. If a larger quantity of local is used (high epidural), it may provide 2 to 4 hours of analgesia for laparotomy, limb surgery, teat surgery, etc.
      4. The animal will not remain standing in the latter case
   E. Cornual nerve block: used to provide anesthesia for dehorning
      1. The cornual nerve runs along the frontal crest from the lateral canthus of the eye to the horn
      2. The head must be firmly secured, and the area clipped and prepped
      3. Five to 10 mL of local is injected about halfway along the nerve at the lateral border of the frontal crest
   F. Peterson eye block: for eye enucleation
      1. First a skin bleb is made at the point where the supraorbital process meets the zygomatic arch
         a. A 14-gauge, 2½-cm (1-inch) needle is inserted in the bleb as a cannula
         b. An 18-gauge, 12½-cm (5-inch) needle is inserted through the cannula and directed past the rostral border of the coronoid process to the pterygopalatine fossa. Approximately 8.75 to 10 cm (3½ to 4 inches) in depth
         c. Deposit 15 mL of 2% lidocaine at this site
      2. Second, local anesthetic is injected subcutaneously lateral to the zygomatic arch
         a. This technique will desensitize the globe and surrounding tissues of the eye for enucleation

G. Retrobulbar (four-point) block: local anesthetic is injected into the dorsal and ventral eyelids and at the medial and lateral canthi
   1. Then approximately 30 to 40 mL of local anesthetic is directed to the nerves at the apex of the orbit with a curved needle
   2. Both block techniques can be used for enucleation or extirpation of the eye

H. Ring block
   1. Local anesthetic agent is deposited subcutaneously and deep into the tissues completely around the surgical site, as in teat surgery, dehorning, claw amputation, etc.

I. Vascular infusion for anesthesia of the distal limb
   1. Used for digit amputation, hoof/sole surgery, corn removal, and laceration repair
   2. Place a tourniquet mid metatarsal or metacarpal region
   3. Clip and prep injection site, identify a surface vein
   4. Using a 19- to 20-gauge, 2½-cm (1-inch) needle or butterfly catheter, insert the needle intravenously. Aspirate to ensure proper placement
   5. Infuse 10 to 30 mL of 2% lidocaine slowly
   6. Remove the needle and apply pressure to the insertion site to prevent leakage and hematoma
   7. Remove tourniquet at the end of the procedure

II. Sheep and goats
   A. Regional anesthesia such as paravertebrals and epidurals can be used in sheep and goats
   B. Goats have a low pain threshold and require sedation
   C. Cornual and infratrochlear nerve blocks are used for dehorning goats
      1. The corneal nerve is blocked at the caudal ridge of the supraorbital process, 1 to 1½ cm deep, with 2 to 3 mL of 2% lidocaine (in adults)
         a. The infratrochlear nerve is blocked by inserting a needle ½ cm through the skin at the dorsomedial margin of the orbit
         b. The nerve may be palpated in some animals
      2. A total dose of 10 mg/kg (½ mL of 2% solution/kg) must not be exceeded because of the toxicity potential

III. Pig
   A. The most commonly used regional anesthetic techniques in tranquilized pigs are infiltration, lumbosacral epidural injection, and intratesticular injection
   B. Lumbosacral epidural is used for cesarean section, claw amputation, prolapsed rectum repair, scrotal and inguinal hernia repair, and testectomy
   C. A surgical prep is performed at the injection site
   D. Depending on the size of the pig, a 16- to 18-gauge, 3- to 6-inch needle is inserted into the lumbosacral space
   E. The pigs should be recovered in a quiet area, away from other pigs, until they are fully awake and aware of their surroundings

General Anesthesia

I. Cattle
   A. Bloat and regurgitation of rumen contents, respiratory depression, apnea, and poor oxygenation are problems associated with general anesthesia in cattle
      1. Feed should be withheld from cattle before general anesthesia
      2. Withhold roughage for 48 hours, grain and concentrates for 24 hours, and water for 12 hours
      3. Withhold feed for 2 to 4 hours in preruminant calves
   B. Tranquilizers are not usually administered as a preanesthetic because they do not work well to calm fractious cattle and violent recoveries are not a problem in cattle
   C. Intravenous catheter should be placed in the jugular vein
      1. Use 14-gauge, 5½-inch needle
   D. Anesthesia can be induced with a number of drugs, including, but not limited to, the following
      1. Thiamylal sodium
      2. Thiopental sodium
         a. Induction is not as prolonged as with thiamylal sodium and may cause transient apnea
      3. Guaifenesin with 2 g of a thiobarbiturate
      4. Ketamine and xylazine intramuscularly
      5. A mixture of 5% guaifenesin containing 1 mg/mL ketamine and 0.1 mg/mL xylazine
      6. Masking with isoflurane or halothane
   E. In a recumbent cow, bloat and aspiration of regurgitated rumen contents are concerns
      1. If possible, position so that the animal is in right lateral recumbency, which keeps up the rumen
         a. Elevate the neck so head is downward. Position so upper front and hind limbs are parallel to the table surface, pull lower forelimb forward to help prevent radial nerve paralysis
      2. Position in sternal recumbency as soon as possible

3. It is suggested to extubate with the cuff inflated
F. An endotracheal tube with inflated cuff should be placed even if inhalants are not used. Also use a stomach tube for the escape of rumen gases
1. On induction, a mouth speculum is inserted to aid in the introduction of the endotracheal tube
G. The surgical table should be covered with protective padding to prevent postanesthetic complications due to nerve paralysis
H. Halothane or isoflurane is usually used when inhalation anesthesia is chosen
1. At surgical plane, the cattle will have slow regular breathing, a slight palpebral reflex, and anal reflex
2. The pupil is centered between the upper and lower lids
3. The eye is rotated ventrally and the pupil is rotated medially below the lower lid when the animal is in a light plane of anesthesia
4. Oxygen should be continued 5 to 10 minutes after anesthetic delivery
5. The cuff should remain inflated during extubation
6. A stomach tube should be available to decompress the rumen in the event of bloat
I. The technician should monitor heart rate, pulse strength, muscle relaxation, respiratory rate, mucous membranes, capillary refill time, and blood pressure

II. Sheep and goats
A. Injectable anesthesia regimens and the use of halothane or isoflurane for general anesthesia are similar to those outlined for cattle
B. Intravenous catheter placement: 16- to 14-gauge, 3- to 5½-inch catheters in adults and 18- to 14-gauge, 2- to 3-inch catheters in young animals
C. Withhold feed for 24 hours and water for 12 hours in adults
1. Withhold feed for 2 to 4 hours in preruminant animals
D. Small ruminants should be intubated to prevent aspiration from regurgitation
E. Oxygen should be continued 5 to 10 minutes after anesthetic delivery
F. The cuff should remain inflated during extubation
G. A stomach tube should be available to decompress the rumen in the event of bloat
H. Eye position as a measurement of anesthetic depth is not as accurate in small ruminants as in cattle

III. Pig
A. Some concerns when anesthetizing pig
1. A higher incidence of malignant hyperthermia
2. Fewer accessible superficial veins and arteries
3. Tracheal intubation is difficult in adult pigs
a. Oral cavity is small
b. Larynx is long and mobile
c. Laryngeal spasm is common
d. Pharyngeal diverticulum
4. Withhold food 8 to 12 hours; do not withhold water
B. Induction can be achieved using
1. Thiamylal or thiopental sodium
a. These can be used alone for short procedures
2. Ketamine can be used with thiobarbiturates or inhalants such as halothane or isoflurane
3. A mixture of guaifenesin (5% solution), ketamine (1 mg/mL), and xylazine (1 mg/mL) can be used in adult pigs
4. Halothane or isoflurane by face mask
5. Droperidol and fentanyl (Innovar-Vet) intramuscularly
6. Stresnil (Azaparone)
C. Eye reflexes and position are unreliable for monitoring pigs
D. Heart rate, respiratory rate, muscle relaxation, and pulse strength (if possible) should be monitored
E. As with ruminants, continue oxygen 5 to 10 minutes after inhalation and position the animal in sternal recumbency as soon as possible
F. Unless there is evidence of regurgitation, extubate with the cuff deflated
a. Keep the animal away from other pigs until well recovered

RUMINANT AND PIG SURGERY

I. Laparotomy (cattle)
A. A laparotomy for diagnostic purposes or for surgical intervention of a condition such as LDA or RDA or for cesarean section or rumenotomy is routinely performed with the animal standing in a chute or stocks using local anesthetic
B. The incision is made in the paralumbar fossa, and the area to be prepped includes a wide margin surrounding the incision site
C. The hair is clipped, any gross debris is removed, and a surgical prep is performed over the entire clipped area
D. The tail should be tied to the animal's hind leg or attached by rope to her halter, to keep her from swinging it into the incision
1. Never tie a cow's tail to a post or rail because she can easily amputate her tail
E. Sutures should be removed 2 to 3 weeks after surgery

- F. On occasion the surgeon may elect to perform a paramedian or ventral midline celiotomy for an RDA or a cesarean
  1. The cow is cast with ropes and placed in dorsal recumbency

II. Digit amputation (cattle)
- A. The cow is placed in lateral recumbency with the affected claw up
- B. The claw and interdigital space are thoroughly cleaned of manure and debris
- C. The area is clipped from mid metacarpus to the hoof and prepped in a routine manner
- D. Anesthesia is achieved with a ring block or intravenous local using rubber tubing as a tourniquet distal to the carpus or hock
- E. Obstetrical or Gigli wire is used to amputate the claw
- F. After surgery, the foot is bandaged for 2 to 3 weeks (unless complicated by infection) and may need to be changed frequently

III. Teat laceration repair (cattle and goat)
- A. This surgery may be performed with the cow standing or in dorsal recumbency
- B. A ring block is used on the affected teat, and a complete surgical prep is performed
  1. Rubber tubing used as a tourniquet will control bleeding and milk leakage
  2. A teat prosthesis may be inserted at the time of repair
- C. Postoperatively, the insert will allow the affected teat to drain while the other quarters are being milked
- D. Hand milking should not be done because it may interfere with the suture line
- E. Sutures are removed in about 2 weeks
- F. Similar surgical technique is used on the doe

IV. Eye enucleation (cattle)
- A. The cow will have to be restrained in a chute while a halter secures its head to one side
- B. Regional anesthesia is done with a Peterson eye block or a four-point retrobulbar block
- C. Usually the eyelids are sewn together; then the area is clipped and surgically prepped
- D. Typically, the prep is complicated by necrotic and contaminated tissue
- E. Postoperative care will include antibiotics and perhaps a wound spray on the surgical site

V. Castration
- A. Cattle
  1. Calves are usually castrated at from 1 to 4 weeks of age
  2. No anesthesia or surgical prep is generally used, for financial reasons
  3. For "open" castration, an incision is made in the scrotum and an emasculator is used to sever and crush the spermatic cord
  4. Calves should be vaccinated for clostridial infections before or at the time of castration
  5. An emasculatome is used for "closed" castration
     - a. This device crushes and severs the spermatic cord without having to incise the skin of the scrotum
  6. Calves are sometimes castrated using an elastrator, or elastic band, around the testicles
     - a. This procedure is preferably performed within the first few weeks of life; however, it can be successfully performed in older animals
- B. Small ruminants
  1. Lambs (if used for wool) are castrated within the first 1 to 2 weeks of life using an elastrator and are tail-docked at the same time, also using an elastic or rubber band
  2. Sometimes an "open" or closed method of castration is used, as described for calves earlier
  3. Lambs destined for meat are usually only tail docked and are often not castrated because they reach market weight before sexual maturity
  4. Kids are castrated within the first 1 to 3 weeks of life using methods as described earlier
  5. Other procedures performed at this time include vaccination against clostridial infection and injection of vitamin E and selenium
- C. Pig
  1. Pigs are usually castrated at 1 to 2 weeks of age using an open technique
  2. Other procedures performed before or at this time are iron dextran injection to prevent anemia, tail docking to prevent cannibalism in confined housing, and clipping of milk or needle teeth (canines and third incisors) to prevent injury to the sow
  3. Frequently, inguinal hernias are discovered in the piglet at the time of castration
     - a. The skin of the inguinal area should be prepped with an antiseptic solution before repair
     - b. Piglets should be placed in a clean, warm pen until recovered

VI. Dehorning
- A. Calves: dehorning in cattle is done to prevent injury from fighting
  1. It is preferable to disbud calves at 1 to 2 weeks of age using an electric dehorner
     - a. Caustic pastes should be avoided

2. If the horn buds are 1 to 2 cm (½ to 1 inch) long, a gouge-type dehorner (Barnes) can be used
3. Mature horns can be removed with a Keystone dehorner, a hardback saw, or a wire saw
4. Local analgesia for dehorning can be achieved with a cornual nerve block or ring block
5. Considerations are control of pain and hemorrhage and protection against fly strike in the dehorn wound

B. Goats
1. Goats should be dehorned using an electric dehorner as soon as the horn buds are palpable
2. Goats are very susceptible to pain and can die of shock and fright, so analgesia is often provided
3. Brain tissue is superficial in young goats and may be damaged if the iron is left on too long

ACKNOWLEDGMENT

The editors and author recognize and appreciate the original contributions of Sandy Agla, on which this chapter is based.

Glossary

abomasopexy Abomasum is fixed to the abdominal wall using a permanent suture. The technique is used to correct a displacement of the abomasum

abomasopexy–toggle Via a dorsal approach, the abomasum is attached to the ventral body wall with a toggle suture (bar suture). Used when open surgical intervention is too costly, compared with the animal's value, and animal is being salvaged for meat

atonic Lacking in tone

balling gun Instrument used for the administration of boluses to cattle, horses, sheep, and goats

bolus A large, ready to be swallowed mass of medication. Formed into an oblong tablet or gel

cachexia Emaciated, malnourished

capsule Usually administered with a balling gun

celiotomy Incision into the abdominal cavity

clonic convulsions Seizures characterized by alternation of relaxation with jerking and flexing of muscles

commissure of the mouth Angled area at the most lateral portion of the mouth where the upper and lower lips meet

drench To give liquid medications by mouth

emasculatome Instrument for bloodless castration in cattle and sheep. It crushes the spermatic cord without incising into the scrotum

emasculator Instrument used to cut and crush the spermatic cord in an open castration

endemic Present in an animal community at all times

enucleation Surgical removal of the globe of the eye

epistaxis Nasal bleeding

eructation Expelling of gas from the rumen via the oral cavity; part of the normal digestive process in ruminants

extirpation Surgical removal of everything within the orbit of the eye, including globe, muscles, adipose tissue, and lacrimal gland

flaccid paralysis Loss of voluntary movement and decreased tone of limb muscles

fly strike Infestation of fly larvae in the cutaneous tissues. Usually in wool or hair contaminated with feces or urine; also in skin wounds. Also called cutaneous myiasis

grunt test In cattle, the test is performed to detect reticuloperitonitis. It can be accomplished by a withers pinch or placing a board under the cow at the sternum, just behind the elbow. A positive test will elicit a grunt

mydriasis Dilation of the pupil

myositis Voluntary muscle inflammation

omentoabomasopexy Right paralumbar approach in which the abomasum is sutured in place through the ventral body wall separate from but in addition to a basic omentopexy

omentopexy Omentum is anchored to the abdominal wall similar to an abomasopexy, usually in the case of right-sided torsion of the abomasum

opisthotonus Involuntary posture in which the head and tail are bent upward and flexed over the back while the abdomen is bowed downward. It is an indicator of medulla, pons, and midbrain disease

paralumbar fossa Area in the flank bordered dorsally by the spinous processes of the lumbar vertebrae, cranially by the last rib, and caudally by the tuber coxae. It provides a flank approach to the abdomen for laparotomy

paramedian Off midline

peracute Duration of a few hours, very acute

petechial hemorrhage Small (pinpoint) round, red spots. They are not raised; may be intradermal or submucosal

prophylactic Prevention of disease by treatment or vaccination

ring block Injection of a local anesthetic in a circle around the circumference of a teat, or a lower limb, to facilitate closure of lacerations or to help in the diagnosis of lameness

rumenotomy Surgical procedure for evacuation of the rumen. A left flank approach is used. A rumenotomy is indicated under the following conditions: removal of metallic foreign bodies (traumatic reticuloperitonitis), rumen overload, obstructing foreign bodies, and rumen impaction

somatic cells Cells of the body other than germ cells

speculum (Frick) Instrument used to facilitate the passage of an orogastric tube by protecting the tube from damage by the animal's teeth

subacute Duration of disease process that is between acute and chronic. Considered to be about 1 week

subclinical Disease process that is not detectable by physical examination, or very mild case of disease process

tetany Condition in which localized spasmodic contraction of the muscle takes place. It results from a decreased level of blood calcium

transfaunation Reconstitution of the rumen flora through the use of cud transfer

uvea Structure made up of the iris, ciliary body, and choroids

zero grazing Animal husbandry technique in which animals are raised in confinement, on a dry lot, such as dairy cattle. Their daily feed rations are harvested plant material, concentrates, and/or grains

Review Questions

1 The most dangerous defense strategy of cattle is
   a. Herding
   b. Charging
   c. Biting
   d. Kicking

2 Starting at the esophagus and going to the duodenum, the order of the ruminant's compartments is
   a. Reticulum, rumen, omasum, abomasum
   b. Abomasum, omasum, reticulum, rumen
   c. Rumen, reticulum, omasum, abomasum
   d. Omasum, abomasum, rumen, reticulum

3 To auscult the rumen, place the stethoscope over the
   a. Right paralumbar fossa
   b. Left paralumbar fossa
   c. Animal's left side just below the point of the elbow
   d. Animal's right side just below the point of the elbow

4 Screening for subclinical mastitis can be done by
   a. Monitoring milk output
   b. CMT
   c. Observation
   d. Palpating the udder for heat and pain

5 Parturient paresis is commonly known as
   a. Milk fever
   b. Hardware disease
   c. Pizzle rot
   d. Mastitis

6 A common clinical sign in LDA is
   a. Toxemia
   b. Auscultable ping
   c. Hunching
   d. Head pressing

7 Gas bloat is caused by
   a. Increased amounts of lactic acid in the rumen
   b. Ingestion of too much grain
   c. A physical obstruction to eructation
   d. A negative energy balance

8 Blackleg is a disease of ruminants caused by
   a. *Pasteurella haemolytica*
   b. *E. coli*
   c. Anthrax
   d. *Clostridium chauvoei*

9 Which of the following veins should be used with caution when taking a blood sample from a cow?
   a. Jugular
   b. Lateral thoracic
   c. Milk
   d. Coccygeal

10 Which of the following is not a part of bovine respiratory disease complex?
   a. Leptospirosis
   b. *Haemophilus somnus*
   c. Bovine viral diarrhea
   d. IBR

BIBLIOGRAPHY

McCurnin DM, Bassert JM: *Clinical textbook for veterinary technicians,* ed 5, Philadelphia, 2002, WB Saunders.

Muir WW III, Hubbell, JAE et al: *Handbook of veterinary anesthesia,* ed 3, St Louis, 2001, Mosby.

Noordsy JL: *Food animal surgery,* ed 3, Trenton, NJ, 1994, Veterinary Learning Systems Co, Inc.

Pratt PW: *Medical, surgical and anesthetic nursing for veterinary technicians,* ed 2, Goleta, CA, 1994, American Veterinary Publications.

Radositis OM et al: *Veterinary medicine: a textbook of the diseases of cattle, sheep, pigs, goats and horses,* ed 9, London, 2000, Bailliere Tindall.

Reibold TW, Geiser DR, Goble DO: *Large animal anesthesia: principles and techniques,* Ames, 1995, Iowa State University Press.

The Merck veterinary manual, ed 8, Rahway, NJ, 1998, Merck and Co, Inc.

CHAPTER 26

Veterinary Dentistry

Barbara Donaldson

OUTLINE

LEARNING OUTCOMES

After reading this chapter you should be able to:

1. Recognize normal and abnormal dental structures, conditions, and lesions.
2. Identify teeth by means of the Anatomical and Triadan Numbering Systems.
3. Use dental terminology to accurately chart dental morphology.
4. Recognize and correctly use, care for, and sharpen dental hand instruments.
5. List the steps to perform a complete dental prophylaxis.
6. Describe the causes and stages of gingivitis and periodontitis.
7. Perform dental radiography.
8. Recommend a dental home care program.

It is estimated that 85% of all dogs and cats over the age of 2 years have periodontal disease. Periodontal disease is a progressive condition that affects the supporting tissues of the teeth. Bacterial plaque is the initial cause of periodontitis; it can lead to tooth loss and infections of the heart, liver, and kidney. Proper dental consideration is a vital part of the veterinary care necessary to ensure a healthy and happy pet.

ANATOMY OF THE TOOTH

I. Tooth structure (Figure 26-1)
   A. Enamel
      1. Outer covering of the crown composed of hydroxyapatite
      2. Formed by ameloblasts during tooth development. Production stops once the tooth erupts
      3. Acts as an effective barrier to bacteria
      4. Has no sensory capacity
      5. In hypsodont teeth (long crown) of herbivores such as horses, the enamel is also invaginated into longitudinal grooves and infundibula (cups) of the teeth
   B. Dentin
      1. Composes the bulk of the tooth
      2. Formed by odontoblasts in a tubular fashion
      3. As hard as bone, much softer than enamel
      4. Composed of roughly 72% mineral, 18% organic matter (mostly collagen), and 10% water by weight
      5. Sensitive to heat, cold, touch, and variations in osmotic pressure. All stimuli are felt as pain
      6. Capable of repair by producing tertiary dentin
   C. Pulp
      1. Occupies the interior cavity
      2. In the root it is called the root canal

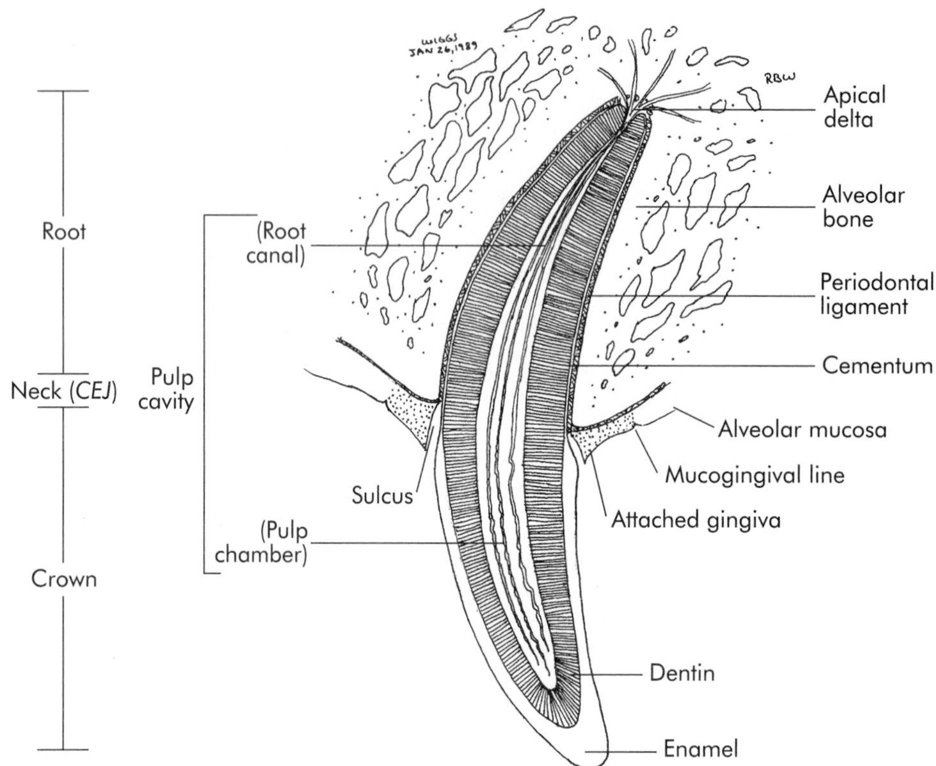

Figure 26-1 Anatomy of a tooth and supporting structures. *CEJ*, Cementoenamel junction. (From Pratt PW: *Principles and Practice of Veterinary Technology*, St Louis, 2001, Mosby.)

3. Rich with blood vessels, nerves, and lymphatics
4. Composed of odontoblasts, fibroblasts, and other cells
5. Enters the tooth through many tiny openings in the root apex and is known as the apical delta
6. Registers pain and quickly becomes contaminated, inflamed, and necrotic if exposed

D. Cementum
1. A type of bone that covers the root of the tooth
2. Attached by the periodontal ligament fibers
3. Inorganic content: 45% to 50% hydroxyapatite
4. Organic content: mainly collagen fibers and Sharpey's fibers
5. Constantly undergoing resorption and repair

E. Cementoenamel junction (CEJ)
1. Junction between crown and root

II. Tooth-supporting structure

A. Periodontal ligament
1. Holds the tooth in the alveolus (socket) by attaching the tooth to the alveolar bone
2. Composed of collagen with some elastic fibers, blood vessels, nerves, and lymphatics
3. Main components are the principal fibers, which are embedded in cementum and alveolar bone: termed Sharpey's fibers
4. Absorbs shock of impact
5. Protects vessels and nerves in the periodontal space
6. Contains sensory nerve endings, which register pain and tactile pressure

B. Alveolar bone
1. Surrounds and supports the teeth
2. Constantly remodeling internally, yet remains constant throughout adult life as deposition and resorption occur
3. Sharpey's fibers are embedded deeply into alveolar bone

C. Gingiva
1. Soft tissue providing epithelial attachment
2. First line of defense
3. Divided into three regions: marginal gingiva, attached gingiva, and interdental gingiva

D. Gingival sulcus
1. Space between the gingiva and the tooth
2. Normal depth in dogs is 1 to 3 mm; in cats, 0.5 to 1 mm

E. Sulcular fluid
1. Secreted from the gingival connective tissue, passes through sulcar epithelium

2. Flushes the sulcus
3. Rich in immunoglobulins and other antimicrobial properties

DENTITION

I. Dogs
  A. Deciduous teeth: 28
  B. Permanent teeth: 42
    1. Formula is 2 × (I 3/3, C 1/1, P 4/4, M 2/3)
II. Cats
  A. Deciduous teeth: 26
  B. Permanent teeth: 30
    1. Formula is 2 × (I 3/3, C 1/1, P 3/2, M 1/1)
    2. The three upper premolars are numbered 2, 3, and 4, and the lower premolars are numbered 3 and 4
      a. Anatomists conclude that the first upper premolar and the lower first and second premolars are missing
III. Horse
  A. Deciduous teeth: 24
  B. Permanent teeth: 40 to 42 (stallion); 30 to 36 (mare)
    1. Formula is 2 × (I 3/3, C 1/1, P 3/3, M 3/3)
      a. Mares often do not have the canine teeth
IV. Swine
  A. Deciduous teeth: 32
  B. Permanent teeth: 44
    1. Formula is 2 × (I 3/3, C 1/1, P 4/4, M 3/3)
V. Ruminants (e.g., sheep, cattle)
  A. Deciduous teeth: 20
  B. Permanent teeth: 32
    1. Formula is 2 × (I 0/4, C 0/0, P 3/3, M 3/3)
VI. Hamsters, gerbils, mice, and rats
  A. Permanent teeth: 16
    1. Formula is 2 × (I 1/1, C 0/0, P 0/0, M 3/3)
VII. Guinea pigs
  A. Permanent teeth: 20
    1. Formula is 2 × (I 1/1, C 0/0, P 1/1, M 3/3)
VIII. Rabbits
  A. Permanent teeth: 28
    1. Formula is 2 × (I 2/1, C 0/0, P 3/2, M 3/3)

TOOTH SURFACES

I. Crown
  A. Above the gum line
II. Root
  A. Below the gum line
III. Buccal
  A. Surface toward the cheek
IV. Lingual
  A. Surface toward the tongue
V. Labial
  A. Surface toward the lips
VI. Palatal
  A. Surface toward the soft palate
VII. Mesial
  A. Surface toward the rostral end or front of the mouth
  B. Incisor is the edge closest to the midline
VIII. Distal
  A. Surface toward the back of the tooth
IX. Rostral
  A. Surface facing the nose of the animal
X. Occlusal
  A. Chewing surface
XI. Furcation
  A. The space between two roots where they meet the crown

TOOTH ROOTS

I. Dogs
  A. One root: incisors, canines, first premolars, third molar of lower jaw
  B. Two roots: second and third premolars, fourth premolars of lower jaw, first and second molars of lower jaw, possibly third molars of lower jaw
  C. Three roots: fourth premolars of upper jaw, first and second molars of upper jaw
II. Cats
  A. One root: incisors, canines, first premolars of upper jaw, and first molars of upper jaw
  B. Two roots: second premolars of upper jaw, two premolars of lower jaw, and lower molars
  C. Three roots: third premolars of upper jaw

TOOTH FUNCTION

I. Incisors
  A. Cutting, nibbling
II. Canines
  A. Holding, tearing
III. Premolars
  A. Cutting, shearing, holding
IV. Molars
  A. Grinding
V. Carnassial teeth
  A. Largest cutting teeth
  B. Dogs: upper fourth premolars and lower first molars
  C. Cats: upper fourth premolars and lower molars

NUMBERING TEETH

I. Anatomical system
  A. Uppercase letters: permanent teeth
  B. Lowercase letters: deciduous teeth (primary)
  C. Superscript right: upper right teeth
  D. Subscript right: lower right teeth

E. Examples
1. I_2: second permanent incisor, lower right
2. ^1c: primary canine, upper left
3. Sp^1: supernumerary first primary premolar, upper right

II. Triadan system
A. Uses quadrants with three-digit numbers
B. First number indicates the quadrant in which the tooth is found and the type of tooth
C. Permanent teeth begin with the numbers 1, 2, 3, and 4
D. Deciduous (primary) teeth begin with the numbers 5, 6, 7, and 8

Upper right quadrant	Upper left quadrant
1 if permanent tooth 5 if deciduous tooth	2 if permanent tooth 6 if deciduous tooth
Lower right quadrant	Lower left quadrant
4 if permanent tooth 8 if deciduous tooth	3 if permanent tooth 7 if deciduous tooth

E. The second and third numbers refer to the specific tooth in each quadrant, always beginning from the midline of the mouth
F. Examples
1. 103: upper right third permanent incisor
2. 308: lower left last permanent premolar
G. Cats are missing teeth 105, 205, 305, 306, 405, 406
H. Cats

(101-103)	104	(106-108)	109	Upper right
I	C	P	M	
(401-403)	404	(407-408)	409	Lower right

I. Dogs

(101-103)	104	(105-108)	(109-110)	Upper right
I	C	P	M	
(401-403)	404	(405-408)	(409-411)	Lower right

DENTAL INSTRUMENTS

I. Hand instruments
A. Three parts: handle, shank, and working end
B. Instruments are held in a modified pen grasp
C. Use a finger rest for more stability
D. Sickle scaler
1. Has a sharp pointed tip with two sharp sides
2. Used for supragingival calculus
3. Always pull away from the gum line
E. Curette scaler
1. Has a U-shaped tip with one sharp side
2. Used for subgingival calculus and root planing
3. Place the cutting edge against the tooth. The handle is held parallel to the tooth root. Pull the instrument away from the root in a series of overlapping strokes to remove the calculus until the tooth root is glassy smooth
F. Periodontal probe
1. Has no sharp sides
2. Used to measure the depth of the gingival sulcus
3. Measured in millimeters with a light touch
4. Insert the probe between the gingiva and tooth root surface, parallel to the long axis of the tooth. Walk the probe along the circumference of each tooth in at least four locations. Chart any abnormal sulcus depths
G. Shepherd's hook or explorer
1. Has a sharp tip only. Use a light touch to avoid gingival trauma
2. Used to detect subgingival calculus and tooth mobility
3. Used to detect feline external odontoclastic resorptive lesions (FEORs)
4. Used to detect cavities and broken teeth

II. Mechanical scalers
A. Ultrasonic scaler
1. Magnetostrictive: tip vibrates in an elliptical motion, 18,000 to 29,000 cycles per second
a. Use the back or sides of the distal $\frac{1}{16}$th inch lightly
2. Piezoelectric: tip vibrates in a linear motion, 40,000 cycles per second
a. Least traumatic due to cool operation and linear vibration
3. Sonic: tip vibrates in an elliptical motion, up to 18,000 cycles per second
a. No heat buildup in these units; some units are more efficient than others
4. Used for gross calculus above the gum line
a. Cooling water cannot reach the tip if it is used below the gum line; damage to the tooth will likely result
5. Used lightly on the teeth to avoid heat buildup and pitting of the enamel with possible pulpal damage
6. Maximum of 5 seconds per tooth (it does depend on the unit)
7. The scaler tip will wear with time; as it becomes shorter, its resonance frequency changes and it becomes less efficient
a. Tips should be replaced periodically
8. Use a lot of water to cool teeth
a. Distilled or filtered water will prevent a mineral buildup in the tubing of the dental unit
b. If you use a water bottle, rinse it with disinfectant such as 0.12% chlorhexidine solution
B. Roto-pro burs
1. Spins at 300,000 to 400,000 rpm
2. Used to remove tartar and calculus
3. Can easily damage the enamel, dentin, and soft tissue

C. Air-driven units
   1. Basic units come with low-speed handpiece, high-speed handpiece, and a three-way air/water syringe
   2. More elaborate units have piezoelectric scaler or outlet for sonic scaler, suction, fiberoptic illumination, extra electrical outlets, electrosurgical outlets, and a variety of other options
   3. Air is provided by compressors or compressed gas in bulk tanks
   4. Compressors are either oil cooled or oil free
      a. Very quiet oil-cooled compressors are available
      b. Oil-free dental compressors tend to be noisier and more expensive
   5. The oil level of the oil-cooled compressors must be checked weekly to ensure the level of oil is adequate
      a. The oil should be changed every 6 months

III. Sharpening hand instruments
   A. Sharpen after each use before sterilization
   B. Use an acrylic stick to test for sharpness
   C. If light reflects from the cutting edge, the instrument is dull
   D. Sharpening stones vary from coarse to fine
      1. Ruby stone: coarse; water lubricant
      2. Arkansas stone: fine; oil lubricant
      3. India stone: fine or medium; oil lubricant
      4. Carborundum stone: coarse; water lubricant
      5. Ceramic stone: fine or medium; water or dry lubricant
   E. Information on sharpening can be found in sharpening guide booklet and video "It's About Time" (published by Hu Friedy, available from Ash Temple 1-800-223-3300)

DENTAL PROPHY

I. Examine the patient, beginning with the history
   A. Look for symmetry of the head and face
   B. Look for nasal or ocular discharges or swellings
   C. Examine lips, mouth, and tongue
   D. Examine teeth and gums
   E. Measure the gingival sulcus all the way around each tooth
      1. May be measured after the prophy
      2. Normal sulcus depth for dogs, 1 to 3 mm; for cats, less than 1 mm
   F. Scale the teeth above and below the gum line
      1. Use proper method and equipment as discussed previously
      2. Remove gross calculus with dental extractors
      3. Remove supragingival calculus and plaque with a mechanical power scaler
      4. Remove subgingival calculus with hand curettes
   G. Polish to remove microscopic grooves left by the scaling process and to remove plaque
      1. Keep prophy cup moving to avoid heating of the tooth, maximum 5 seconds per tooth
      2. Use plenty of paste
      3. Wet teeth with water to cool them
      4. Use a light touch but sufficient pressure to flare the cup
      5. Polish the enamel in the sulcus
      6. Use a medium or fine paste
      7. Set the polisher below 3000 rpm
   H. Flush the gingival sulcus with 0.12% chlorhexidine
   I. Wipe and air dry the teeth
   J. Can use a disclosing solution to reveal any remaining plaque (solution may stain hair or clothing)
   K. Apply fluoride and leave on 1 to 4 minutes
      1. Serves as an antibacterial agent
      2. Desensitizes the teeth
      3. Strengthens the enamel
      4. May not be necessary if fluoride is found in the prophy paste, but many believe that the teeth must be dry for fluoride to be effective
      5. Wipe off the fluoride
   L. Charting
      1. Each hospital should select a dental charting system
      2. Becomes part of the patient's medical file
      3. Should be such that each tooth and tooth surface can be depicted
      4. Should allow space to record calculus, caries, fractures, gingivitis index, periodontal index, mobility index, malocclusions, resorptive lesions, and oral lesions
      5. Dates when dental procedures were performed, what was done, treatment, and prognosis
      6. Accurate charting will allow for an accurate assessment at future dental appointments
   M. Animal positioning
      1. Always turn the animal sternally to avoid gastric torsion
      2. To minimize the number of times required to turn the animal, include the labial surfaces, followed by the opposite palatal and lingual surfaces
         a. Then turn the animal and complete the scaling/polishing on the remaining labial, palatal, and lingual surfaces
         b. Work is completed first on one half of the mouth, the animal is turned, and then work is completed on the second half of the mouth

SAFETY

I. In animals, dentistry involves oral and environmental bacteria. Sterilization and bacterial control are essential to protect cross-contamination of patients and personnel
   A. Use sterile and well-maintained instruments and equipment
      1. At the end of every procedure, wash, rinse, and wipe off gross debris
      2. Use ultrasonic instrument bath with a detergent solution, with the lid on
      3. Use surgical milk for hinged and sharp instruments
      4. Sharpen instruments before sterilization
      5. Most dental instruments can be sterilized in an autoclave
      6. To reduce the length of time to achieve sterilization, package in autoclave film or envelopes
      7. Can also use autoclavable instrument trays
      8. For equipment that is not autoclavable, use disposable, plastic infection barriers such as tray sleeves

Note: Read the manufacturer's recommendations for sterilization procedures.

   B. Use an appropriately sized mouth gag to avoid problems in the temporomandibular joints
   C. Use a cuffed endotracheal tube
   D. Place gauze sponges in the back of the throat as a protection against excessive water and debris
   E. Keep the patient's head downward
   F. Cover the patient's eyes
   G. Roll the patient with the sternum under, especially in large breed dogs
   H. Maintain the patient's body temperature to prevent hypothermia

II. Humans
   A. Wear a surgical mask, glasses, and gloves to protect against oral bacteria
   B. May help to spray the patient's mouth with 0.12% chlorhexidine to reduce the bacterial load
   C. Work comfortably seated on a stool at a proper height
   D. Support the working hand on a surface in the same quadrant you are working
   E. Use adequate light source such as one worn on the head

DENTAL RADIOGRAPHY

I. Purpose
   A. Ascertain condition of teeth and gingival sulcus
   B. Identify cavities and resorptive lesions
   C. Identify retained roots
   D. Identify bone and root system of the teeth
   E. Help evaluate intraoral neoplasia
   F. Identify number of teeth in the mouth
   G. Identify periapical abscesses

II. Recommendations
   A. Obtain routine dental radiographs in young animals to identify the permanent dentition
   B. In the treatment of periodontal disease, obtain radiographs every 12 to 24 months
   C. Use radiographs before extractions to determine condition of the roots and number of teeth and roots involved
   D. Perform radiography during endodontic procedures to confirm the procedure
   E. Obtain radiographs as follow-up to root canal procedure to check the file depth

III. Equipment
   A. Intraoral film for detail
      1. Comes in a variety of sizes: common sizes used in dogs and cats are 0, 2, and 4
         a. Size 0 works well in cat
         b. Size 2 works well in dog and cat
         c. Size 4 is necessary in dog to radiograph the incisors and canines
            (1) Called occlusal film
         d. Size 2 is the least expensive because it is the size used routinely in human dentistry and therefore is produced in quantity
      2. Available in D and E (faster) speeds
   B. Chair side darkroom to free up the main dark room
      1. Rapid processing solutions
   C. Dental x-ray machine with a lead-lined cone to achieve greater detail and versatility
   D. Protective shielding, film-holding devices, finger-ring dosimeter badges

IV. Positioning
   A. Routine dental survey of six films

Quadrant and teeth	No. of films	Technique	Position
Mandibular canines and incisors	1	Bisecting angle	Dorsal or lateral
Mandibular premolars and molars	2	Parallel lateral oblique	Dorsal
Maxillary canines	1 each	Bisecting angle	Lateral or rostrocaudal oblique
Maxillary incisors	1	Bisecting angle	Sternal or lateral
Maxillary premolars and molars	2	Bisecting angle Rostrocaudal or caudorostral oblique	Sternal or lateral

V. Techniques
   A. If possible, use
      1. Twelve-inch source image distance (SID) for dental films and 30 inches for standard screens
      2. Nonscreen film, which gives high detail
      3. Small focal spot
      4. Collimate as much as possible
   B. Parallel (Figure 26-2)
      1. For mandibular molars and premolars
      2. Place the dental film parallel to the end of the x-ray tube and the long axis of the tooth
      3. The central ray will be perpendicular to the teeth and the film
      4. Place folded gauze between the top edge of the film and the occlusal surfaces of the teeth to securely push the film down into the bottom of the mouth
   C. Bisecting angle (Figure 26-3)
      1. Place the film inside the animal's mouth behind the affected tooth
      2. Direct the central ray perpendicular to the line that bisects the angle formed by the film and the long axis of the tooth
      3. This technique will reduce the artifact of foreshortening or elongation
         a. Foreshortening makes the tooth appear shorter than it is
            (1) Occurs when the x-ray beam is more perpendicular to the film
         b. Elongation makes the tooth appear much longer
            (1) Occurs when the x-ray beam is more perpendicular to the tooth axis
      4. Can be used for intraoral and extraoral films
      5. Can apply the tube shift technique to better visualize structures
         a. Also called buccal object rule or SLOB rule
         b. Acronym means same, lingual; opposite, buccal
         c. Objects (e.g., roots) that are lingual to a reference point will appear to shift in the same direction in which the tube head has been moved
         d. Objects that seem to move in the opposite direction to the tube head will be on the buccal side

HOME CARE

I. Goal: to control plaque and tartar buildup
II. Daily brushing with veterinary products
III. May involve use of antibacterial and fluoride products
IV. Feed hard food that does not stick to the teeth as well as other products
V. Use chew toys to provide an abrasive action, to strengthen the periodontal ligaments, and to increase crevicular flushing
   A. Use toys that are softer than the teeth to avoid fractures and chronic trauma
   B. Do not feed dried hooves, which may cause slab fractures
   C. Nylon chew bones can cause slab fractures
   D. Nylon rope toys should be avoided because they can cause gingival trauma when the fine nylon threads slice the gingiva
   E. Dense rubber toys are safer and work the jaw bones well
   F. Rawhide strips reduce plaque and calculus and are unlikely to cause fractures
      1. They absorb saliva, become mushy, and are squished between the teeth to remove debris
      2. If swallowed in small pieces, they are digestible

OCCLUSION

I. Normal bite
   A. Scissor bite

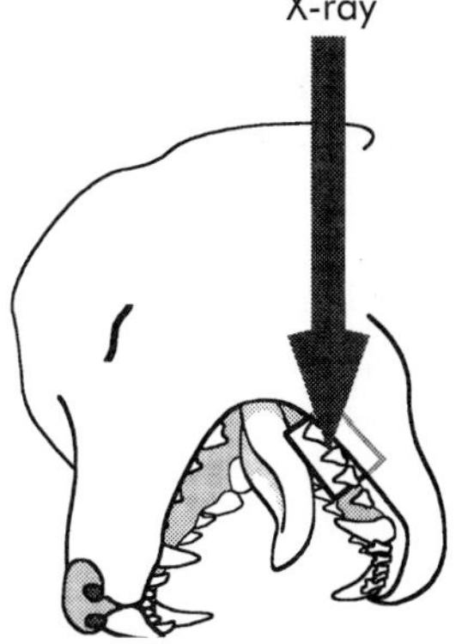

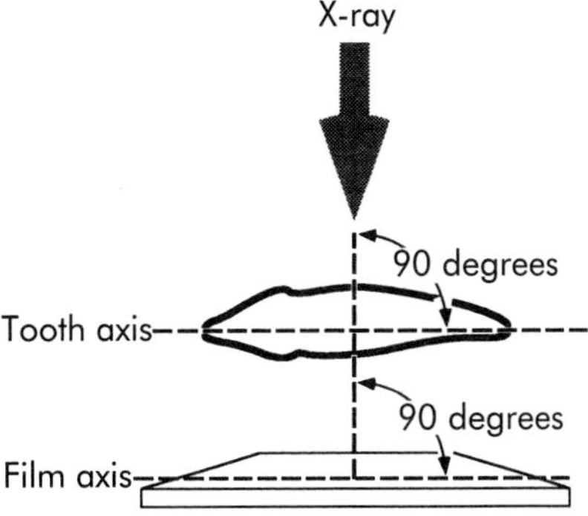

Figure 26-2 Parallel position technique for dental radiographs of the mandibular premolar teeth. (From Harvey CE, Emily PE: *Small animal dentistry,* St Louis, 2001, Mosby.)

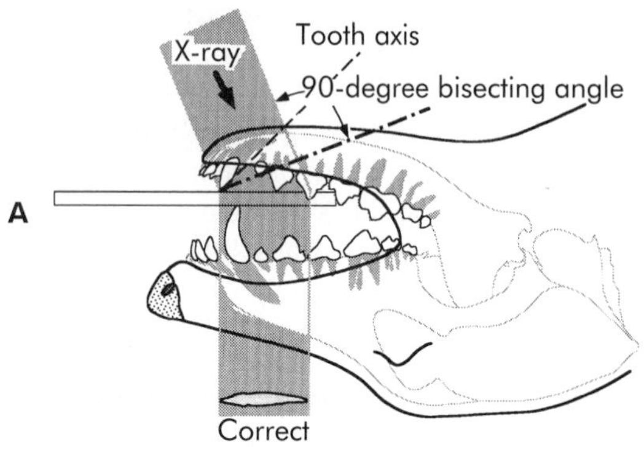

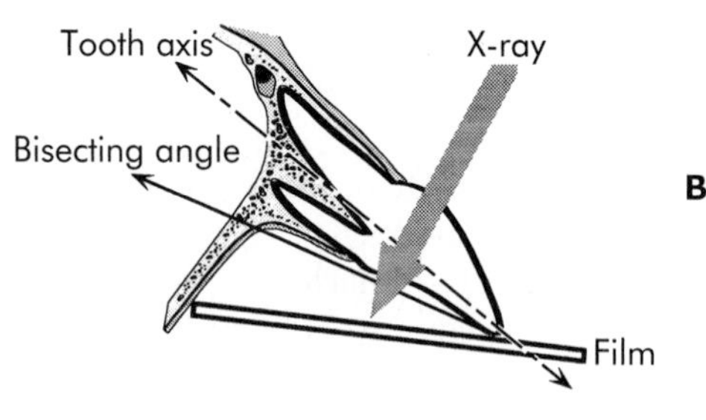

Figure 26-3 Bisecting angle technique for dental radiographs. **A,** Lower canine tooth. **B,** Carnassial tooth. (From Harvey CE, Emily PE: *Small animal dentistry,* St Louis, 2001, Mosby.)

B. The upper incisors close just in front of the lower incisors
C. The lower canines lie between the upper incisors and canines without touching either
D. The lower first premolars are the most rostral with the upper arcade fitting into the spaces between the lower premolars forming a zigzag pattern
E. The upper fourth premolars overlap the lower first molars, forming the carnassial teeth in dogs
F. In cats the upper third and fourth premolars tightly overlap the lower fourth premolars, as well as the first molars. The upper fourth premolars and lower molars are the feline carnassial teeth

II. Malocclusions
  A. Prognathism
    1. Undershot jaw
    2. Mandible longer than maxilla
    3. Normal for brachycephalic breeds
    4. Often associated with anterior crossbite
  B. Brachygnathism
    1. Overshot jaw or parrot mouth
    2. Maxilla longer than mandible
  C. Level bite
    1. End-to-end bite of the incisors
    2. Genetically a degree of prognathism
  D. Wry mouth
    1. Genetically only affects one side of the head
    2. One half of the head is longer than the other half
  E. Posterior crossbite
    1. Mandible is wider than the maxilla in the area of the premolars
    2. Occurs occasionally in boxers and long nosed breeds
  F. Oligodontia
    1. Fewer teeth than normal
  G. Anodontia
    1. Missing teeth
  H. Polydontia
    1. More teeth than normal
  I. Dental interlock
    1. Deciduous teeth that erupt in an abnormal pattern
    2. The upper deciduous canine teeth are pushed rostral to the lower canine teeth, which prevents the forward growth of the mandible
  J. Retained deciduous teeth
    1. Permanent teeth erupt lingually to the deciduous teeth (except the upper canine teeth)
    2. Common in toy breed dogs

ORAL LESIONS

I. Malignant tumors
  A. Melanoma
    1. Most common in dog; rare in cat
    2. Spreads slowly, invades bone
  B. Squamous cell carcinoma
    1. Second most common tumor in dog; most common in cat
    2. Spreads slowly, invades bone
  C. Fibrosarcoma
    1. Third most common tumor in dog
    2. Guarded prognosis
II. Nonmalignant tumors
  A. Epulis (an oral mass: osseous or fibromatous lesion)
    1. Requires biopsy to differentiate
    2. Three classifications: fibromatous, ossifying, acanthomatous
    3. Involves the periodontal ligament
    4. Can be locally invasive to bone
III. Gingival hyperplasia

A. Thickening of gingiva as a result of chronic inflammation

IV. Stomatitis
   A. Inflammation of soft tissue of the oral cavity
   B. Can be caused by foreign bodies or chemical or electrical burns, or can be immune related

V. Contact ulcers
   A. Lesions caused when a tooth makes contact with the mucosa

VI. Eosinophilic ulcers
   A. Rodent ulcers that occur on the lip of cats, benign

FURTHER DENTAL PROBLEMS

I. Gemini
   A. One root with two crowns

II. Fusion
   A. Two tooth buds grow together to form one larger tooth

III. Enamel hypoplasia
   A. Known as "distemper teeth" where sections of enamel are reduced or missing

IV. Misdirected teeth
   A. Teeth that erupt in an abnormal direction

V. Retained deciduous
   A. Retained primary teeth

VI. Tetracycline staining
   A. Yellow stain due to the administration of tetracycline to a pregnant dog or to young pups

VII. Impaction
   A. The inability of the tooth to erupt through the gum

VIII. Abscessed teeth
   A. Advanced periodontal disease may result in root abscesses
   B. Most commonly seen abscessed tooth in dogs is the upper fourth premolar

IX. Oronasal fistula
   A. Caused by an abscess of the maxillary canine and can show clinical signs of nasal discharge and/or swelling over the root

X. Caries
   A. True coronal caries not a common problem in carnivores compared with humans
   B. If present are often multiple advanced lesions affecting several teeth
   C. Upper first and second molars and lower first molar are most commonly affected

XI. Worn teeth
   A. Exhibit a brown center but do not allow access by an explorer

XII. Trauma
   A. Caused by chewing hard objects or by blows to the head

GUM DISEASE

I. Gingivitis
   A. Inflammation of the gingiva. If treated properly, is entirely reversible
   B. If not treated will advance to periodontal disease
   C. Nonmotile, aerobic, gram-positive rods and cocci predominate
   D. Gingivitis Index: designates the degree of inflammation
      1. GI0: normal, healthy gingiva, shrimp colored, normal gingival sulcus depth, no odor
      2. GI1: marginal gingivitis, mild inflammation, slight edema, no bleeding on probing, no increase in gingival sulcus depth
      3. GI2: moderate gingivitis, increased hyperemia, edema, bleeds on gentle probing, normal sulcar depth
      4. GI3: advanced gingivitis, inflammation, edema, hyperemia, tendency to bleed spontaneously, may have attachment loss

II. Periodontal disease
   A. Inflammation of the supporting structures of the teeth
   B. Progressive, usually nonregenerative and incurable. If treated properly can be managed
   C. Bacterial flora changes to motile, anaerobic, gram-negative rods and filamentous organisms that produce endotoxins and exotoxins
   D. Periodontal Index: amount of periodontal attachment loss as a percentage of the periodontal support that has been destroyed by the disease
      1. Measured with a periodontal probe in millimeters from the CEJ to apex of the defect
      2. PI0: healthy gingiva, deeper structures, no clinical disease
      3. PI1: gingivitis only with no attachment loss
      4. PI2: less than 25% attachment loss
      5. PI3: 25% to 50% attachment loss
      6. PI4: greater than 50% attachment loss
   E. Mobility Index helps to assess the prognosis for a tooth
      1. M0: no tooth mobility
      2. M1: slight mobility, less than 1 mm laterally with no apical mobility

3. M2: moderate tooth mobility, 1 to 2 mm laterally, no apical mobility
4. M3: both lateral and apical mobility, requires extraction

III. Causes
A. Lack of daily dental care
B. Accumulation of plaque, which is composed of bacteria
C. Formation of calculus, which is mineralized plaque
1. Plaque can form within 6 hours
2. Plaque can mineralize within 24 to 48 hours
D. Systemic factors such as hormonal changes play a secondary role by exaggerating the tissue response

IV. Classification of gum disease
A. Healthy
1. Sharp gingival margin
2. Shrimp color
3. No odor
B. Grade I
1. Marginal gingivitis
2. Slight redness, not swollen, mild odor
3. Gram-positive aerobic cocci and rods
C. Grade II
1. Moderate gingivitis
2. Swelling begins, ruby red, plaque
3. Bleeding on probing
D. Grade III
1. Severe gingivitis, early periodontitis
2. Red and purple margins, beginning of pocket formation with swelling and bleeding on probing
3. No tooth mobility
E. To this point, conditions are reversible.
F. Grade IV
1. Moderate periodontitis
2. Severe inflammation and swelling with deep pockets
3. Slight tooth mobility
G. Grade V
1. Severe periodontitis
2. Tooth mobility and loss
3. Lots of pus, 50% bone loss
4. Anaerobic gram-negative rods

V. Treatment
A. Depends on disease classification and discretion of the veterinarian
1. Complete prophy
2. Root planing
3. Antibiotics
4. Possible gum surgery
5. Possible tooth extraction
6. Home care
7. Dry food
8. Chew toys

FELINE EXTERNAL ODONTOCLASTIC RESORPTIVE LESIONS (FEORs)

I. Also called feline cervical neck lesions, neck lesions, enamel erosions

II. Etiology involves many facets, including
A. Nutritional hyperparathyroidism
B. Chronic calici virus
C. Viral infection at the time of tooth development
D. Chronic hair balls
E. Low-pH diets
F. Genetics: higher incidence in Persians, Abyssinians, Siamese, Russian blue, Scottish fold, and Oriental shorthairs

III. Periodontal disease is the most consistent factor associated with neck lesions

IV. Usually starts at CEJ

V. Not the result of bacterial digestion of teeth such as in human caries

VI. Lesions are filled with granulation tissue high in odontoclasts that actively resorb dentin and enamel

VII. Lesions spread in all directions
A. Once it reaches the pulp, it spreads quickly
B. The crown may look normal, but the tooth may have very little or no root left

VIII. Neck lesions create excruciating pain

IX. Advanced lesions require extraction

X. Teeth with suspected neck lesions must be radiographed to assess the amount of damage

XI. Graded from class I to V (the most advanced)

LYMPHOCYTIC/PLASMACYTIC STOMATITIS

I. Seen commonly in cats

II. Very inflamed gums, often with minor calculus accumulation

III. Many cats have underlying disease that interferes with cat's local immunity in the gingiva

IV. Cats should be screened for diseases

V. Complete intolerance to dental plaque

VI. Higher incidence in highly bred cats, Siamese, Himalayans, Abyssinians

VII. Thoroughly clean teeth, antibiotics, oral antiseptic, daily brushing with antibacterial solution, hard diet, and monthly rechecks

VIII. If the condition recurs, extract all premolars, molars and retained roots
A. Clean canines and incisors
B. If problem still recurs, remove the remaining teeth

Glossary

alveolar bone Cancellous bone adjacent to tooth roots
ameloblast Enamel-producing cells
anodontia Absence of teeth
apex Bottom of the root
apical Toward the apex
attached gingival Gingiva from the free gingival groove to the mucogingival line
brachygnathism Overshot jaw
buccal Tooth surface nearest the cheek
calculus Mineralized plaque
canine tooth Large single-rooted tooth used to grasp and tear
caries Cavities
carnassial tooth Upper fourth premolar and lower first molar used to shear
caudorostral oblique Tube head is at the back of the head and aimed toward the nose at about 45-degree angle from the lateral position
cementoenamel junction Where the enamel meets the cementum
cementum Bony tissue covering the dentin of the root
collagen Produced by fibroblasts; found in gingiva and cementum
coronal Toward the crown
crevicular fluid Secreted from the gingiva
crown Portion of the tooth covered by enamel
cusp Tip of the crown
deciduous teeth Baby or primary teeth
dental quadrant Half of an arch when divided by the midline
dentin Bulk of the tooth covered by cementum in the root and enamel in the crown
distal Away from the midline
enamel Hydroxyapatite covering of the crown
epulis Fibrous tumor of the gum
erosion Loss of tooth structure by chemical means not involving bacteria
free gingival Portion of gingiva not attached to the tooth
free gingival margin Free edge of the gingiva on the tooth
furcation Space between two roots where they join the crown
gingival Soft tissue surrounding the teeth
gingival hyperplasia Increase in the amount of gingival tissue
gingival sulcus Space between the free gingiva and the tooth
hydroxyapatite Inorganic crystals found in enamel and cementum
hyperemia Excess bleeding
incisal Biting surface of the anterior teeth
interdental Area between the proximal surfaces of adjacent teeth in the same arch
labial Surface of the incisors nearest the lips
lingual Surface of the mandibular teeth nearest the tongue
malocclusion Deviation from the normal bite
mandible Bone of the lower jaw
maxilla Bone of the upper jaw
mesial Toward the midline of the dental arch; can also be the surface or edge of the tooth closest to the rostral end (front of the mouth)
molar Large multicusped tooth used for grinding
mucogingival line Line where the gingiva meets the alveolar mucosa
neck Cementoenamel junction
occlusal Chewing surface of the posterior teeth
odontoblasts Cell in the pulp that produces dentin
oligodontia Fewer teeth than normal
oronasal fistula Abnormal opening between the nasal and oral cavities
palatal Surface of the maxillary teeth nearest the palate
palate Structure separating the oral and nasal cavities
periapical abscess Abscess at the apex of the tooth
periodontal ligament Network of fibers connecting the tooth to the bone
periodontium Supporting structures of the teeth
plaque Thin film covering the teeth composed of bacteria, saliva, food, and epithelial cells
premolars Teeth between the canines and the molars used for shearing
***primary* teeth** First teeth to erupt
prognathism Undershot jaw
proximal Surface of the tooth adjacent to another tooth
pulp Soft tissue inside the tooth composed of blood vessels, nerves, lymphatics, and connective tissue
resorption Loss of substance by a physiological or pathological process
root Part of the tooth covered by cementum
root canal Part of the tooth containing the pulp
root planing Scaling of the tooth root
rostral Toward the nose of the animal
rostrocaudal oblique Tube head is at the nose and aimed towards the back of the head at about a 45-degree angle from the lateral position
saliva Secretions from the salivary glands, containing enzymes
Sharpey's fibers Terminal portions of collagen fibers of the periodontal ligament
subgingival curettage Removal of plaque and calculus from the gingiva below the gum line

Review Questions

1 The normal depth of the gingival sulcus in a dog is
a. 0.5 to 1 mm
b. 1 to 2 mm
c. 1 to 3 mm
d. 4 to 6 mm

2 Severe inflammation and swelling with deep gingival pockets and slight tooth mobility occur in periodontal disease at stage
a. II
b. III
c. IV
d. V

3 The teeth that are radiographed using standard parallel technique are the
a. Maxillary incisors
b. Mandibular canines
c. Maxillary premolars
d. Mandibular molars

4 The recommended chew toys for dogs are
a. Nylon chew bones
b. Rawhide strips
c. Dried hooves
d. Nylon rope toys

5 Lymphocytic/plasmacytic stomatitis in cats is
a. A complete intolerance to dental plaque
b. Caused by underlying disease
c. Associated with calculus accumulation
d. Is easily treated by a dental prophy

6 Sharpey's fibers connect the
a. Gingiva to the cementum
b. Tooth to the alveolar bone
c. Cementum to the enamel
d. Dentin to the enamel

7 Pain is not felt in the
a. Enamel
b. Dentin
c. Pulp
d. Root

8 Dentin is formed by
a. Ameloblasts
b. Hydroxyapatite
c. Fibroblasts
d. Odontoblasts

9 The lubricant to use on an Arkansas stone is
a. Water
b. Oil
c. Silicone
d. None required

10 Plaque will form on a clean tooth surface within
a. Seconds
b. Minutes
c. Hours
d. Days

BIBLIOGRAPHY

Bellows J: *Home study course,* Venice, FL, 1995, American Society of Veterinary Dental Technicians.

Burns S: *It's about time: longer life for dental instruments,* Chicago, 1995, Hu-Friedy.

Emily P, Penman S: *Handbook of small animal dentistry,* Toronto, 1993, Pergamon Press.

Frost P: *Canine dentistry,* ed 5, Vero Beach, FL, 1995, JH Day Communications Inc.

Hale F: *Veterinary dental services,* lecture notes, Fergus, Ontario, September 1997.

Harvey CE: *Small animal dentistry,* St Louis, 2001, Mosby.

Hawkins J: *Waltham applied dentistry for veterinary hospital staff,* Vernon, CA, 1993, Veterinary Learning Systems Co.

Miller B, Harvey C: Sharpening of dental instruments, *Vet Tech* 15:29, 1994.

Piasentin W: Techniques of veterinary dental radiography, *Vet Tech* 17:419, 1996.

CHAPTER 27

Emergency Medicine

Sally Powell   Elisa A Petrollini

OUTLINE

LEARNING OUTCOMES

After reading this chapter you should be able to:

1. Describe triage and the guidelines for executing triage.
2. Describe how to monitor respiratory, cardiovascular, renal and neurological status of the emergency patient.
3. Describe the clinical signs, treatment, and monitoring of patients with respiratory, cardiovascular, central nervous system, renal, and reproductive system emergencies.
4. Describe emergencies caused by the ingestion of toxic substances by defining the clinical signs and treatment.
5. Describe cardiopulmonary cerebral resuscitation (CPCR).
6. List equipment and supplies that may be needed to perform first aid and CPCR.

Clinical evaluation of the emergency patient should initially focus on four major organ systems: respiratory, cardiovascular, central nervous, and renal. It is essential for the veterinary technician to understand how to rapidly evaluate each system to provide emergency care and monitor the critically ill patient. This chapter describes CPCR, first aid and discusses guidelines for triage (initial evaluation). It also outlines in chart form the common disease processes that affect the four major organ systems, including clinical signs, initial treatment, and parameters that should be monitored.

CARDIOPULMONARY CEREBRAL RESUSCITATION

Cardiopulmonary cerebral resuscitation (CPCR) can only be performed by a team, and therefore the first step should always be to alert the veterinarian and other technicians of an emergency situation involving cardiac arrest.

I. A common memory cue for the steps to perform CPCR is ABCD
   A Airway   C Cardiac
   B Breathing   D Drugs
   A. Airway
      1. Establish and secure a patent airway
         a. Endotracheal intubation
         b. Tracheostomy if unable to intubate
   B. Breathing
      1. Resuscitation bag connected to oxygen supply or anesthesia machine 30 to 60 breaths per minute
         a. Maximum of 20 cm of H_2O pressure for dog (if using anesthetic machine)
         b. Maximum of 15 cm of H_2O pressure for cat (if using anesthetic machine)

2. Mouth to endotracheal tube if there is no oxygen supply
3. Mouth to muzzle if needed

C. Circulation
1. Continuous electrocardiographic monitoring
2. Chest compressions (external cardiac massage)
a. Animal should be in right lateral recumbency except for large round-chested dogs and cats
(1) Cats should be in dorsal recumbency
(2) Large round-chested dogs should be in right lateral or dorsal recumbency
b. Count four to six rib spaces or use point of the elbow to locate the heart
c. Using two hands in large dogs, press down on the chest with heal of the lower hand
(1) For cats and small dogs, squeezing the chest between the index finger and thumb is adequate
(2) Compress the chest for 1 second and release for 1 second
(3) A ventilation rate of 1 ventilation to 1 chest compression is recommended
3. Volume replacement
a. Isotonic crystalloids
b. Blood components
c. Synthetic colloids

D. Drugs
1. Intravenous access
2. Intravenous drugs
a. Atropine sulfate: increases heart rate
b. Epinephrine: increases heart rate and force of contraction
c. Lidocaine: used in occasional arrest situations as an antiarrhythmic
d. Sodium bicarbonate: used in occasional arrest situations to correct metabolic acidosis
3. Intratracheal drugs
a. When venous access can not be obtained immediately, the following drugs should be administered via endotracheal tube
(1) Using a syringe, inject the drug down the tube and forcefully blow air through the tube
(2) Epinephrine
(3) Atropine
4. Intracardiac drugs
a. *Only to be used as a last resort: this route is not recommended*
b. Use lower dose of drug, place needle in the area where the heart would be anatomically, aspirate checking for blood, administer drug
c. Epinephrine
d. Isoproterenol

II. Hints for successful CPCR
A. An arrest station or special area to conduct CPCR is ideal; however, many practices have "crash carts" to allow for all necessary supplies to be readily available
B. Necessary supplies include
1. Oxygen
a. S-bag or anesthesia machine
2. Crash cart or emergency kit
a. Endotracheal tubes
b. Laryngoscope
c. Intravenous catheters, fluids, administration sets, tape, syringes, needles, tourniquet
(1) Venous cutdown supplies: scalpel blades, catheter introducers, suture material
d. Drugs
e. Chart of dose rates for all drugs in the kit
f. Clippers
g. Electrocardiographic monitor
h. Defibrillator
i. Suction and suction tips

TRIAGE

I. Definitions
A. An emergency can be described as any situation that arises suddenly and unexpectedly resulting in a sudden need for action
B. Triage is the initial assessment of the emergency patient
1. Triage is performed immediately on presentation and should take less than 5 minutes
2. Triage is the evaluation of the four major organ systems (cardiovascular, respiratory, neurological, and renal systems) while simultaneously obtaining a capsule history
a. Acquiring the history can be the most difficult step
b. Conversation should be limited to salient points only, avoiding irrelevant details
c. The history should include the primary complaint, duration of the problem, and any current drug therapy

II. After triage the patient is categorized as stable or unstable, allowing appropriate prioritization of care
A. A stable patient is *not* in a life-threatening condition
B. An unstable or an emergent patient is in life-threatening circumstances and requires quick judgment and prompt action

III. There are several different classification systems for triage; however, every case is unique and classifications do not cover every scenario

IV. If a patient is critical, a primary survey should be performed by a veterinarian with the assistance of a veterinary technician

SYSTEMIC APPROACH TO TRIAGE

Respiratory System

I. Airway: determine patency of airway
  A. Normal (patent/clear breath sounds)
  B. Upper airway noise (stridor/stertor)
  C. Distress with inspiration associated with stridor

II. Breathing
  A. Assess respiratory rate
    1. Normal: cat, 24 to 42; dog, 10 to 30 respirations per minute
    2. Tachypnea: increased respiratory rate
    3. Apnea: no respirations
    4. Cheyne-Stokes: tachypnea interspersed with apnea
  B. Assess respiratory effort
    1. Normal: there should no effort
    2. Labored inspiration
    3. Labored expiration
    4. Labored inspiration and expiration
    5. Paradoxical respiration: chest wall and abdominal wall do not move synchronously
  C. Postural adaptations of dyspnea
    1. Normal: patient should not be posturing to breath
    2. Orthopnea
      a. Stand rather than sit
      b. Abduct elbows
    3. Abdominal movement
    4. Extended neck, open mouth, head lifted

Cardiovascular System

I. Mucous membrane color
  A. Pink: normal
  B. Muddy or gray: poor perfusion
  C. Pale or white: anemia or poor perfusion
  D. Brick red (hyperemic): septic shock (not to be confused with severe gingivitis)
  E. Dark blue (cyanosis): hypoxia
  F. Yellow (jaundice): hepatic dysfunction, hemolysis or biliary obstruction
  G. Brown: methemoglobinemia (most commonly seen with acetaminophen toxicity)

II. Capillary refill time (CRT)
  A. Normal: 1 to 2 seconds
  B. Prolonged: greater than 2 seconds; indicates poor perfusion
  C. Rapid: less than one second; indicates hyperdynamic state or hemoconcentration

III. Normal pulse rate
  A. Dog: 70 to 160 beats per minute (bpm)
    1. Less than 70 bpm: bradycardia
    2. Greater than 160 bpm: tachycardia
  B. Cat: 150 to 210 bpm
    1. Less than 150 bpm: bradycardia
    2. Greater than 210 bpm: tachycardia

IV. Pulse quality
  A. Normal: strong and synchronous with heart rate
  B. Weak: indicates poor perfusion
  C. Hyperdynamic: anemia or sepsis
    1. ECG appears either
      a. Snappy (tall and thin)
      b. Bounding (tall and wide)

Central Nervous System

The following should be assessed on triage. Their severity will determine the stability of the patient.

I. Gait
  A. Ataxia/weakness
  B. Loss of motor function

II. Muscular twitching
  A. Hypocalcemia (i.e., eclampsia)
  B. Pyrethrin toxicity

III. Head trauma

IV. Nystagmus: rapid eye movement

V. Head tilt

VI. Level of consciousness
  A. Alert
  B. Depressed
    1. Quiet, unwilling to perform normally; responds to environmental stimuli
  C. Delirium/dementia: responds abnormally to environmental stimuli
  D. Stuporous: unresponsive to environmental stimuli; responds to painful stimuli
  E. Comatose: no response to environmental and painful stimuli

Renal System

On triage, the renal system is assessed with abdominal palpation when urinary blockage is suspected. Other emergencies affecting the renal system are identified while assessing the patient's cardiovascular status.

I. Acute renal failure

II. Chronic end-stage renal failure

III. Disruption of the urinary tract
  A. Ruptured ureter
  B. Ruptured bladder
  C. Ruptured urethra

IV. Urinary obstruction

Life-Threatening Wounds

I. Open or penetrating chest wounds
II. Wounds to upper airway
III. Open or penetrating abdominal wounds
IV. Wounds affecting major blood vessels

MONITORING STATUS OF EMERGENCY PATIENTS

Frequent and perceptive evaluation of physical examination parameters is the fundamental basis of emergency and critical care monitoring. The four major organ systems should be closely monitored at all times. The status of the emergent patient can rapidly change; therefore it is essential that the emergency technician is capable of noticing slight changes in the patient's physical parameters. If changes occur in the patient's status, the veterinarian should be notified immediately. The following sections will not discuss normal parameters; only abnormal parameters will be addressed.

Respiratory System

Patients in respiratory distress are often very unstable; minimizing stress to the animal is extremely important. Physical examination, diagnostics, and treatments are performed in stages to allow the patient to rest and breathe in an oxygen-enriched environment. It may be necessary to rule out primary heart disease before sedation in some cases.

Patient monitoring should include respiratory status, cardiovascular status, renal status, and temperature (Table 27-1, pp. 442-443).

I. Postural adaptations of dyspnea
 A. Orthopnea
  1. Patient would rather stand than sit or lie sternally
  2. Abducted elbows
II. Respiratory rate
 A. Tachypnea: increased respiratory rate
 B. Apnea: no respiratory rate
 C. Cheyne-Stokes: tachypnea interspersed with apnea
III. Respiratory effort
 A. Labored inspiration
  1. Upper airway disorders
   a. Collapsing trachea
   b. Laryngeal paralysis
   c. Foreign body
   d. Soft tissue swelling
   e. Brachycephalic occlusive syndrome
 B. Labored expiration
  1. Feline asthma
 C. Labored inspiration and expiration
  1. Parenchymal disorders
   a. Pneumonia
   b. Contusions
   c. Pulmonary edema
   d. Neoplasia
 D. Short inspiration and expiration
  1. Pneumothorax
  2. Pleural effusion
  3. Diaphragmatic rupture
 E. Paradoxical respiration: chest wall and abdominal wall do not move synchronously
IV. Auscultation of lungs
 A. Dull lung sounds ventrally
  1. Indicates a pneumothorax
 B. Dull lung sounds dorsally
  1. Indicates a pleural effusion
 C. Harsh lung sounds
  1. Indicates parenchymal disorders
   a. Pneumonia
   b. Pulmonary contusions
   c. Pulmonary edema
   d. Neoplasia
 D. Rales
  1. Parenchymal disorders
   a. Cardiogenic
    (1) Right-side heart failure
   b. Noncardiogenic
    (1) Fluid overload
    (2) Strangulation
    (3) Electrocution
V. Oxygenation status
 A. Arterial blood gas is more invasive and more accurate
  1. It requires placement of an arterial line (most commonly placed in the metatarsal artery) or obtaining sample via a blood gas syringe
  2. PaO_2 (partial pressure of oxygen in the arterial blood) less than 80 mm Hg: may require oxygen supplementation or mechanical ventilation
  3. $PaCO_2$ (partial pressure of carbon dioxide in the arterial blood) greater than 45 mm Hg: may require mechanical ventilation
 B. SaO_2 (percentage of available hemoglobin that is saturated with oxygen) reading
  1. Less invasive and potentially less accurate
  2. Readings can be falsely high or low because of equipment failure, heart arrhythmias, human error, motion, and patient's pigmentation
  3. Requires a pulse oximeter
  4. Less then 92% indicates hypoxia

Cardiovascular System

Emergencies affecting the cardiovascular system result from failure of the heart to pump blood throughout the body or from an inappropriately low blood volume. The mainstay of therapy for hypovolemic, septic, neurogenic, and anaphylactic shock is aggressive volume replacement. In contrast, volume replacement can be fatal in the patient with heart failure; therefore it is essential to differentiate between these conditions. Monitoring devices such as direct and indirect blood pressure are necessary; however, physical examination parameters are most important.

Patient monitoring should include respiratory status, cardiovascular status, neurological status, renal status, and temperature. Serial evaluations of an emergency blood screen are an integral part of patient monitoring (Table 27-2, p. 444).

I. Mucous membrane color
II. Capillary refill time
III. Pulse rate
IV. Pulse quality
V. Blood pressure reading
   A. Direct arterial pressure readings
   B. Indirect pressure readings by
      1. Oscillometric pressure monitor
      2. Doppler
VI. Electrocardiography

Central Nervous System

Emergencies of the central nervous system (CNS) may affect the brain and/or the spinal cord. It is important to rule out hypoglycemia as a cause of seizures in patients presenting with continuous seizure activity. Behavior, pupillary reflexes, pupil size, and eye movement are used to evaluate the brain. The spinal cord is assessed by noting conscious proprioception, voluntary motor function, and superficial and deep pain (Table 27-3, p. 444).

The causes of seizures include congenital/hereditary factors; inflammatory disease processes; viral, bacterial, fungal, protozoal, or rickettsial organisms; metabolic or nutritional deficiencies; trauma; a central vascular system breakdown; neoplasia; epilepsy; and toxicity.

I. Level of consciousness
   A. Alert: normal
   B. Depressed: quiet, unwilling to perform normally; responds to environmental stimuli
   C. Delirium/dementia: responds abnormally to environmental stimuli
   D. Stuporous: unresponsive to environmental stimuli; responds to painful stimuli
   E. Comatose: no response to environmental and painful stimuli
II. Pupillary reflexes
   A. Blink
   B. Menace
   C. Pupillary light response
      1. Direct
      2. Consensual
III. Pupil size
   A. Miosis: pinpoint
   B. Anisocoria: asymmetrical or unequal
   C. Mydriasis: dilated
IV. Eye movement/position
   A. Nystagmus
      1. Horizontal eye movement
      2. Vertical eye movement
   B. Strabismus: abnormal eye position
V. Evaluate spinal cord compression by
   A. Conscious proprioception
   B. Voluntary motor function
   C. Superficial pain
   D. Deep pain

Renal System

The causes of renal system emergencies include acute and chronic renal failure, urethral obstructions, ruptured ureter/bladder, and urethral tears. Patients with renal disease should be monitored by measuring urine production, serum, creatinine, blood urea nitrogen (BUN), electrolytes (sodium, potassium, phosphorus, calcium), and acid-base parameters on a pretreatment basis and throughout the patient's treatment. Patient monitoring should include respiratory status, cardiovascular status, neurological status, temperature, and serial emergency blood screen readings (Table 27-4, p. 445).

I. Urination
   A. Monitor urination
   B. Measure urine output
      1. Indwelling urinary catheter with closed collection system
      2. Normal values are 1 to 2 mL/kg/hr
   C. Central venous pressure: evaluates ability of the right ventricle to handle fluid therapy
      1. An early indicator of fluid overload
      2. Used when aggressive fluid therapy is indicated to treat renal failure
II. Temperature
   A. Hypothermia because of poor perfusion, anesthesia, exposure to cold
   B. Hyperthermia because of infection, sepsis, heat prostration, malignant hyperthermia, seizures, upper airway obstruction
III. Fluid losses should be assessed and recorded
   A. Vomiting
   B. Diarrhea
   C. Blood loss
   D. Effusions
   E. Edema
   F. Respiratory losses: excessive panting
IV. Emergency blood screen
   A. Packed cell volume/total solids
   B. Blood urea nitrogen and glucose analysis
   C. Electrolyte analysis
      1. Sodium
      2. Potassium
      3. Chloride
      4. Calcium
      5. Magnesium

D. Acid-base analysis
   1. pH
   2. Po_2
   3. Pco_2
   4. HCO_3^-

ENDOCRINE AND METABOLIC EMERGENCIES

The treatment for a patient with an endocrine and/or metabolic emergency includes correcting dehydration, electrolyte abnormalities, and metabolic abnormalities and providing appropriate drug therapy. Metabolic disorders are always associated with a primary disease process.

Patient monitoring should include respiratory status, cardiovascular status, renal status, temperature, and serial emergency blood screen analysis (Table 27-5, pp. 445-446).

GASTROINTESTINAL EMERGENCIES

Patient monitoring should include respiratory status, cardiovascular status, renal status, and serial emergency blood screen readings. For gastric dilation, serial measurement of abdominal girth may be performed. A patient with severe vomiting and diarrhea can be classified as emergent because of the cardiovascular effects of fluid loss (Table 27-6, pp. 446-447).

REPRODUCTIVE SYSTEM EMERGENCIES

Patient monitoring should include respiratory status, cardiovascular status, renal status, and temperature. Note vomiting/diarrhea, serial database readings, and serial emergency blood screen analysis. The female patient should also be closely observed for active contractions, vaginal discharge, and delivery. Reproductive emergencies affecting the male often require prompt surgical intervention (Table 27-7, p. 447).

TOXIC SUBSTANCE EMERGENCIES

Because of the wide variety of effects caused by toxins, it can be difficult to recognize an intoxicated patient without a detailed history. A local poison control center can often give treatment options to the veterinarian. There are a variety of plants that may potentially be toxic to animals. If plant toxicity is suspect, refer to a plant toxicity reference or contact poison control. Patient monitoring should include respiratory status, cardiovascular status (electrocardiogram), renal status, vomiting/diarrhea, coagulopathy, and neurological status. See Table 27-8, pp. 448-449 for the most common toxins.

OCULAR EMERGENCIES

Ocular emergencies can be caused by trauma, primary medical problems, penetrating foreign objects, or increased intraocular pressure. It is essential that the eye(s) be rechecked frequently so progress can be monitored. More complicated ophthalmic emergencies require the expertise of an ophthalmologist. Misdiagnosis and improper treatment can lead to the loss of vision (Table 27-9, p. 449).

Table 27-1 Respiratory emergencies

Clinical signs	Treatment
COLLAPSING TRACHEA (most commonly seen in small breed dogs)	
Loud goose honk cough with expiration, ± postural indications of dyspnea, ± hyperthermia	Supply oxygen, calm with sedation when necessary (rule out primary heart disease before sedation), ± surgical intervention
LARYNGEAL PARALYSIS (most commonly seen in large breed dogs)	
Noisy breathing, distress with inspiration, postural adaptations of dyspnea	Supply oxygen, calm with sedation, endotracheal intubation, ± surgical intervention, ± tracheostomy
FOREIGN BODY	
Noisy breathing, distress with inspiration, acute onset of gagging with severe respiratory distress, postural adaptations of dyspnea, ± hyperthermia	Supply oxygen, remove obstruction
SOFT TISSUE SWELLING: ALLERGIC REACTION	
Facial swelling, ± generalized urticaria (hives) ± noisy breathing, ± distress with inspiration, ± postural indications of dyspnea	Dexamethasone sodium phosphate (anti-inflammatory agent), diphenhydramine HCl (inhibits histamine release)

Table 27-1 Respiratory emergencies—cont'd

Clinical signs	Treatment
SOFT TISSUE SWELLING—TUMOR	
Noisy breathing, distress with inspiration, postural adaptations of dyspnea, ± hyperthermia	Supply oxygen, calm with sedation, ± intubation, ± tracheostomy, ± surgical intervention
BRACHYCEPHALIC OCCLUSIVE SYNDROME (elongated soft palate, stenotic nares, hypoplastic trachea, everted laryngeal saccule)	
Upper airway stertor, distress with inspiration, postural adaptations of dyspnea, ± hyperthermia	Supply oxygen, calm with sedation, ± intubation, ± surgical intervention, ± tracheostomy
SMALL AIRWAY DISEASE: FELINE ASTHMA	
Dyspnea (prolonged expiration), postural indications of dyspnea, expiratory wheeze	Supply oxygen, bronchodilator, corticosteroids
PNEUMONIA	
Tachypnea, dyspnea (inspiration and expiration), postural indications of dyspnea, ± pyrexia, ± cyanosis, lung auscultation (harsh sounds), ± rales	Supply oxygen (100% initially), 40% oxygen is suggested for long-term therapy (100% oxygen for more than 12 hours can result in pulmonary oxygen toxicity), appropriate antibiotic therapy, nebulize, coupage, ± positive pressure ventilation
CONTUSIONS	
Tachypnea, dyspnea, postural indications of dyspnea, evidence of recent trauma, ± shock, ± cyanosis, ± hemoptysis, lung auscultation (harsh lung sounds), ± rales	Supply oxygen, ± fluid therapy, ± positive pressure ventilation
PULMONARY EDEMA	
Tachypnea, dyspnea, postural adaptations of dyspnea, ± cyanosis, ± burns in mouth (suggestive of electric shock), ongoing fluid therapy (suggestive of fluid overload), harsh lung sounds, ± rales, ± heart murmur	Supply oxygen, diuretics, ± positive pressure ventilation
PULMONARY NEOPLASIA	
Tachypnea, dyspnea, ± cyanosis, harsh lung sounds, ± rales	Supply oxygen, ± positive pressure ventilation
PNEUMOTHORAX	
Tachypnea, dyspnea, (rapid and short inspirations and expirations), ± cyanosis, postural indications of dyspnea, decreased/muffled lung sounds dorsally, evidence of recent trauma	Supply oxygen, evacuate air (thoracocentesis), ± chest tube (placed when negative pressure is not achieved or when it is necessary to tap chest repeatedly)
PLEURAL EFFUSION (hemothorax, pyothorax, chylothorax, and serous effusion)	
Tachypnea, dyspnea, postural adaptations of dyspnea, ± cyanosis, decreased muffled lung sounds ventrally	Supply oxygen, evacuate fluid (chest tap), ± chest tube
DIAPHRAGMATIC RUPTURE	
Tachypnea, dyspnea (paradoxical abdominal movement), postural adaptations of dyspnea, ± cyanosis, ± evidence of trauma, ± auscultate borborygmi in thorax, decreased/muffled lung sounds, cardiac displacement	Supply oxygen, surgical correction

Table 27-2 Cardiovascular emergencies

Clinical signs	Treatment
HYPOVOLEMIC SHOCK	
Pale, gray, or muddy mucous membrane color; prolonged capillary refill time; rapid pulse rate, weak pulse quality; ± evidence of acute blood loss; ± evidence of fluid loss (vomiting, diarrhea); ± evidence of fluid sequestration	Shock fluid therapy (isotonic crystalloid, hypertonic crystalloids, blood products, artificial colloid), ± oxygen supplementation
SEPTIC, NEUROGENIC, OR ANAPHYLACTIC SHOCK	
Brick red mucous membrane color, hyperdynamic, rapid capillary refill time (less than 1 second), tachycardia, bounding pulse quality, ± hyperthermia, ± hypoglycemia	Shock fluid therapy, ± blood culture (for septic shock), ± antibiotics for septic shock, ± corticosteroids for anaphylactic shock, ± diphenhydramine for anaphylactic shock
CARDIOGENIC SHOCK: CONGESTIVE HEART FAILURE, PERICARDIAL TAMPONADE	
Pale or muddy mucous membrane color, prolonged capillary refill time, rapid pulse rate, weak pulse quality, ± tachypnea/dyspnea, ± postural indications of dyspnea, ± cyanosis, ± evidence of trauma	*Congestive heart failure:* oxygen supplementation, diuretics, inotropes, vasodilators, ± fluid therapy (very conservative, minimize stress levels) *Cardiac tamponade:* oxygen supplementation, pericardiocentesis, ± fluid therapy (very conservative, minimize stress levels)

Table 27-3 Central nervous system emergencies

Clinical signs	Monitoring	Treatment
EPILEPSY		
Hyperthermia, hyperdynamic state, ± nystagmus/strabismus, ± pupillary changes (miosis, mydriasis, anisocoria)	Respiratory status (potential for aspiration during seizure); cardiovascular status; neurological status (mental status: alert and responsive; depressed, stupor, coma, and pupillary light response); renal status, body temperature	Diazepam (good anticonvulsant activity, must give to effect), phenobarbital, pentobarbital (heavy anesthesia)
HEAD TRAUMA		
Depression, ± stupor, ± coma, ± convulsions, ± pupillary changes (miosis, mydriasis, anisocoria), ± nystagmus/strabismus, ± blood in aural canal, ± hyphema, ± scleral hemorrhage, ± skull/facial fractures	Respiratory status (trauma to the brain stem can cause altered ventilatory status, important to keep carbon dioxide levels normal to low, increased carbon dioxide will cause increased intracranial pressure), cardiovascular status, neurological status, renal status	Corticosteroids, ± mannitol (osmotic agent, can decrease intracranial pressure through its osmotic effects), elevate head (place patient on flat board and elevate board to approx. 30 degrees in attempt to decrease intracranial pressure), ± ventilation (to decrease carbon dioxide levels)
ACUTE PARESIS/PARALYSIS		
Loss of conscious proprioception, loss of voluntary motor function, loss of superficial pain, loss of deep pain	Respiratory status (patients with tetraparesis can experience loss of function to intercostal muscles), cardiovascular status, neurological status (conscious proprioception, voluntary motor activity, superficial pain, deep pain), renal status (upper motor neuron: hypertonic sphincter), (lower motor neuron: bladder hypotonia)	Conservative (commonly used when voluntary motor function is still present), corticosteroids, strict cage rest, surgical intervention (myelogram, laminectomy)

Table 27-4 Renal system emergencies

Clinical signs	Treatment
ACUTE RENAL FAILURE	
Vomiting, diarrhea, dehydration, ± evidence of exposure to toxins (e.g., ethylene glycol or gentamicin)	Pretreatment, emergency blood screen and creatinine and phosphorus, fluid therapy (isotonic crystalloid solutions, measure urine output, diuretics after rehydration), ± peritoneal dialysis, gastrointestinal protectants
CHRONIC END-STAGE RENAL FAILURE	
Weight loss, vomiting, anorexia, dehydration, anemia, lethargy	Fluid therapy, electrolyte replacement (i.e., potassium, ± blood transfusion, measure urine output
FELINE URETHRAL OBSTRUCTION	
Dysuria, ± hematuria, vomiting, vocalizing, painful abdomen, distended bladder on abdominal palpation, ± hyperkalemia, ± hypocalcemia	Fluid therapy, ECG, treat arrhythmias with calcium gluconate, emergency blood screen, treat hyperkalemia because it can cause life-threatening arrhythmias
URETER/BLADDER RUPTURE	
Vomiting, diarrhea, ± hematuria, ± evidence of trauma, ± abdominal effusion, ± RBC in urine, abdominal pain, ± hypovolemic shock, ± decreased urine output	Radiographs, urinary catheter, ± excretory urogram, ± retrograde urethrography/cystography, surgical intervention, ± abdominocentesis
URETHRAL TEARS	
± Vomiting, ± dysuria/hematuria, ± anuria, ± abdominal effusion, ± SQ edema of hind limbs and ventral abdomen, ± hypovolemic shock, ± hyperkalemia	± Urinary catheter, ± surgical intervention, ± abdominocentesis

Table 27-5 Endocrine and metabolic emergencies

Clinical signs	Treatment
ADDISONIAN CRISIS (hypoadrenocorticism)	
Hyponatremia, hyperkalemia (causing bradycardia), ± hypovolemic shock, hypoglycemia, hypercalcemia, vomiting, diarrhea, PU/PD	Fluid therapy: normal saline, glucocorticoid (dexamethasone most commonly used) will not interfere with ACTH stimulation test, correct acidosis (if severe give sodium bicarbonate, supply oxygen)
DIABETIC KETOACIDOSIS	
PU/PD, vomiting, diarrhea, dehydration, ± hypovolemic shock, hyperglycemia, glucosuria, ketonuria, acidemia, tachypnea	IV fluid therapy, insulin therapy, ± KCl replacement, ± phosphorus replacement
HYPOGLYCEMIA	
Depressed, weakness, ataxia, stupor, blindness, seizure activity, coma	Supplement with dextrose; a dextrose bolus must be diluted 1:4 with a crystalloid to prevent phlebitis
HYPERGLYCEMIA	
Vary depending on underlying disease process	When diabetes is suspected, insulin therapy will be initiated
HYPERCALCEMIA	
Vary depending on cause of hypercalcemia	Hypercalcemia is a medical emergency because of its effects on the kidney. Fluid therapy with 0.9% NaCl for rehydration and increased calcium excretion. Find underlying cause of increased calcium

Continued

Table 27-5 Endocrine and metabolic emergencies—cont'd

Clinical signs	Treatment
HYPOCALCEMIA	
Increased neuromuscular excitability (muscular twitching), generalized muscle tremors, seizures, hyperthermia	Calcium supplementation. Must be given slowly with continuous ECG monitoring. If arrhythmias or bradycardia occur, calcium administration should be discontinued
HYPERNATREMIA	
Dehydration, neurological signs	Slowly correct dehydration and gradually lower sodium levels
HYPONATREMIA	
Protracted vomiting and diarrhea, lethargy, coma	Electrolyte replacement, correction of dehydration
HYPERKALEMIA	
ECG: increased amplitude of T wave with decreased amplitude of R wave and prolonged PR interval, then bradycardia with widening of QRS complex are eventually seen; cardiac arrest	Restore potassium balance; fluid therapy, administration of intravenous regular insulin followed by dextrose administration is used to lower potassium levels. Ongoing fluid therapy with dextrose supplementation. Administer calcium gluconate to protect myocardium and reverse arrhythmias
HYPOKALEMIA	
Severe muscle weakness, ventroflexion of neck, stilted forelimb gait	Potassium supplementation via intravenous fluid administration. If giving shock bolus of fluid, do not use fluids that have been supplemented with potassium

Table 27-6 Gastrointestinal emergencies

Clinical signs	Treatment
GASTRIC DILATION AND/OR VOLVULUS	
Abdominal distention; nonproductive retching; pale; muddy, or gray mucous membrane color; prolonged capillary refill time; tachycardia; weak pulse; ± tachypnea; dyspnea	Fluid therapy (rapid IV bolus), decompression (trocharization or gastric intubation/lavage), corticosteroids, abdominal radiographs (right lateral most important), surgical intervention if torsion
GASTROINTESTINAL OBSTRUCTION (foreign body, intussusception, tumor)	
Vomiting; diarrhea; red, pale, gray, or muddy mucous membrane color; fast or prolonged capillary refill time; abdominal pain, ± pale mucous membranes; prolonged capillary refill time; tachycardia; weak pulse quality; dehydration; tachypnea; dyspnea	Fluid therapy, ± endoscopy, ± surgical intervention, abdominal radiographs, ± upper GI study, ± abdominal ultrasound
PERITONITIS (gastrointestinal perforation, ruptured prostatic abscess)	
Hyperemic; brick-red mucous membrane, rapid capillary refill time, tachycardia, bounding pulse quality, hyperthermia, ± hypoglycemia, abdominal pain	Fluid therapy, appropriate antibiotics, abdominocentesis (obtain sample for cytology), ± diagnostic peritoneal lavage, surgical intervention
PARVOVIRUS INFECTION	
Vomiting; diarrhea; pale, gray, or muddy mucous membrane color; prolonged capillary refill time; tachycardia; weak pulse quality; dehydration; ± hypoglycemia; ± hypokalemia; ± leukopenia	Fluid therapy, antibiotics to prevent secondary bacterial infection, correct hypoglycemia, correct hypokalemia, ± antiemetics, abdominal palpation to rule out intussusception

Table 27-6 Gastrointestinal emergencies—cont'd

Clinical signs	Treatment
LIVER FAILURE	
Vomiting; ± hematemesis; diarrhea; ± melena; PU/PD; ± dementia; ± seizures; ± jaundice; ± anemia; ± coagulopathy; hypoalbuminemia; hypoglycemia; hyperbilirubinemia; hypocholesterolemia; low BUN	Fluid therapy, gastrointestinal protectants, ± lactulose, vitamin K_1, ± antibiotics, ± fresh frozen plasma
HEMORRHAGIC GASTROENTERITIS	
Hematochezia, vomiting, dehydration, lethargy, anorexia	Fluid therapy, ± colloid replacement, gastrointestinal protectants
PANCREATITIS	
Vomiting, diarrhea, lethargy, anorexia, painful abdomen, pyrexia	Fluid therapy, ± colloid therapy, ± antibiotic therapy, ± pain medication

Table 27-7 Emergencies of the reproductive system

Clinical signs	Treatment
PYOMETRA	
PU/PD, recent estrus, vomiting, ± hyperthermia, ± vaginal discharge (depends on whether the cervix is open or closed), ± abdominal distention	Fluid therapy (isotonic crystalloid), antibiotic therapy, surgical intervention
ECLAMPSIA	
Muscle tremors, evidence of whelping and lactation usually 2 to 3 weeks before, brick-red mucous membranes (hyperemic), tachycardia, bounding pulse quality, hyperthermia, hypocalcemia	Calcium gluconate (slow IV bolus), fluid therapy (when hyperthermia, isotonic crystalloid solution), oral calcium throughout lactation, ECG while administering calcium gluconate. If bradycardia, arrhythmia, or vomiting occurs, stop treatment
DYSTOCIA	
Active contractions for more than 30 minutes, more than 2 hours between deliveries, green discharge with no delivery of fetus	Rule out obstructive dystocia (digital examination, abdominal radiographs), oxytocin, ± calcium gluconate, ± glucose, ± surgical intervention

Table 27-8 Emergencies caused by toxic substances

Clinical signs	Treatment
ACETAMINOPHEN (Tylenol) TOXICOSIS	
One to 2 hours postingestion (salivation, vomiting, tachypnea, brown or cyanotic mucous membrane color, dark or chocolate colored blood, edema of face)	Induce emesis if less than 1 hour postingestion (not performed if showing signs of tachypnea), acetylcysteine, ascorbic acid, fluid therapy (isotonic crystalloid), supply oxygen
ANTICOAGULANT RODENTICIDE TOXICITY	
No clinical signs: ingested recently, dyspnea, hematuria, hematemesis, epistaxis, melena, hemothorax	Induce emesis (if recently ingested, activated charcoal, vitamin K_1), prothrombin time analysis 2 days postingestion, then prothrombin time analysis 2 days after vitamin K_1 finished, fresh whole blood or fresh frozen plasma if coagulopathy is present
CHOCOLATE TOXICOSIS (methylxanthine) (active ingredient theobromine) (LD_{50}: 100 mg/kg)	
Vomiting, diarrhea, hyperactivity, muscle tremors, tachycardia, arrhythmia, hypertension, ± seizures	Induce emesis, ± gastric lavage, activated charcoal, cathartics, fluid therapy (isotonic crystalloid), ± oxygen supplementation
ETHYLENE GLYCOL TOXICITY (LD_{50}: dog, 4 to 6 mL/kg; cat, 1.5 mL/kg)	
Vomiting, PU/PD, tachypnea, tachycardia, azotemia, increased serum osmolality, metabolic acidosis, hypocalcemia, oliguria, ataxia, seizures, stupor, coma	Gastric lavage, cathartics, fluid therapy (isotonic crystalloid), ethanol (7%), peritoneal dialysis, ± methylpyrazole test for ethylene glycol within 12 hours of ingestion; if patient is exhibiting seizure activity, obtain blood for ethylene glycol test before administration of diazepam (propylene glycol in diazepam can make ethylene glycol test falsely positive)
LEAD POISONING	
Vomiting, diarrhea, lethargy, abdominal pain, ataxia, blindness, seizures, evidence of nucleated RBC on blood smear with no evidence of anemia	Remove lead from gastrointestinal tract, enema, emetic, surgical intervention, remove lead from tissues and blood, calcium EDTA, penicillin, control seizures
NONSTEROIDAL ANTI-INFLAMMATORY DRUGS (NSAIDs)	
Vomiting, diarrhea, gastrointestinal bleeding (hematemesis, melena)	Fluid therapy (isotonic crystalloid, isotonic colloid, blood products, artificial colloid), gastrointestinal protectants (sucralfate, cimetidine HCl)
ORGANOPHOSPHATE TOXICITY	
Acronym: DUMBELS = Diarrhea, Urination, Miosis, Bradycardia, Emesis, Lacrimation, Salivation; dyspnea, fasciculation, vomiting, diarrhea, seizures	Remove toxin (bathe with soap and water), atropine sulfate, diphenhydramine, ± pralidoxime (2 Pam), fluid therapy (isotonic crystalloid), control fasciculation/convulsions (diazepam or pentobarbital)
PYRETHRINS	
CNS signs, severe muscular twitching, ± hypothermia, ± hyperthermia, ± dyspnea	Bathe patient immediately, initially administer diazepam IV to effect, methocarbimal IV p.r.n. to effect (do not exceed 330 mg/kg/day), ± fluid therapy
PHILODENDRON/DUMBCANE (insoluble calcium oxalate)	
Pain and burning of throat, oral mucosa and lips. Mucosal edema and dyspnea can occur if severe	Will resolve without treatment
MARIJUANA (Tetrahydrocannabinol)	
Depression, ataxia, animal appears anxious, abnormal vocalization, ± vomiting	Induce vomiting, ± gastric lavage, activated charcoal, place animal in a quiet environment

Table 27-8 Emergencies caused by toxic substances—cont'd

Clinical signs	Treatment
EASTER AND TIGER LILIES (unknown poison)	
Anorexia, vomiting, renal failure	Treat for acute renal failure (see Table 27-4)
RHODODENDRON AZALEA (andromedotoxins)	
Salivation, diarrhea, vomiting, muscle weakness, bradycardia, hypotension, coma, and convulsions	Induce vomiting, ± gastric lavage, activated charcoal, ECG, fluid therapy, treat bradycardia

Table 27-9 Ocular emergencies

Clinical signs	Treatment
GLAUCOMA	
Enlarged eyeball, dilated pupil, negative menace response, absent papillary light response, corneal edema and pain. Diagnosis is determined by measuring intraocular ocular pressure (IOP). IOP is measured by the use of a Schiotz or electronic tonometer	Medically treating the IOP by drawing fluid out the vitreous chamber by the use of drugs such as mannitol and pilocarpine
CORNEAL FOREIGN BODIES AND LACERATIONS	
Blepharospasm, ocular discharge, photophobia as a result of pain	*Corneal foreign body:* gentle irrigation with sterile saline to dislodge foreign object, ± surgical intervention *Laceration:* surgical intervention, topical antibiotics and atropine sulfate, oral antibiotics
HYPHEMA	
Hemorrhage in anterior chamber	Treat underlying cause (trauma, infection ± uveitis, neoplasia ± uveitis, coagulopathy)
UVEITIS	
Painful, red, inflamed iris; blepharospasm; miotic pupil; prolapsed nictitans; decreased IOP; ± hypopyon; ± hyphema	Topical atropine; if secondary glaucoma is present, use adrenaline (epinephrine), topical corticosteroids
PROPTOSIS	
Proptosis of eye	First note severity of proptosis: ± enucleation, ± replacement of eye
CORNEAL ULCERS	
Blepharospasm, ocular discharge, photophobia as a result of pain	*Superficialulcers:* topical antibiotics, ± atropine sulfate *Indolent ulcers (Boxer ulcers):* debride edges of ulcer, keratectomy, topical antibiotics *Deep ulcer:* avoid excessive restraint—may lead to perforation, topical antibiotics, topical atropine sulfate, patients with melting or infected ulcers need topical anticollagenase (autologous serum administered every hour for the first day of treatment, ± Elizabethan collar to prevent patient scratching of eye)
DESCEMETOCELE	
Descement's membrane penetrated through ulcer, looks transparent; cornea is in danger of penetration	Surgical intervention, topical antibiotics

Glossary

abducted To draw away from an axis or a median plane
acidemia Abnormal acidity of the blood
acidosis State characterized by actual or relative decrease of alkali in body fluids in relation to acid content
ACTH Adrenocorticotropic hormone
anaphylactic Serious reaction (shock) brought about by hypersensitivity to an allergen such as a drug or protein (anaphylaxis)
anisocoria Unequal or asymmetrical pupil size
anticollagenase Drug that is used to prevent the body from breaking down collagen
anuria No urine production
apnea No respirations
ataxia Incoordination of limb movement
auscultation Listening for sounds produced within the body
autologous The self
azotemia Retention of renal excretory products
blepharospasm Spasm of the eyelid
borborygmi Rumbling or gurgling noises produced by movement of gas in the gastrointestinal tract
cardiac tamponade Reduction of venous return to the heart because of increased volume of fluid in the pericardium
cathartics Agent that increases gastrointestinal flow
chylothorax Accumulation of milky chylous fluid in the pleural space, usually on the left side
coagulopathy Any disorder of blood coagulation
colloid Solution containing large molecules that can not pass out of blood vessels
coma State of unconsciousness with no response to external stimuli
coupage Striking the thoracic area to aid in the removal of secretions
crystalloid Solution containing small molecules that can pass out of blood vessels
cyanosis Bluish discoloration of skin and mucous membranes
cystography Radiography of the urinary bladder using a contrast medium
descemetocoele Herniation of Descemet's membrane, usually through a corneal ulcer
Descemet's membrane Posterior portion of the cornea; a membrane
diuretic Agent that promotes excretion of urine
Doppler Device for measuring blood flow that transmits sound for measurement
dyspnea Difficulty breathing
dysuria Difficult urination
ecchymosis Large area of nonelevated bruising in the skin or mucous membranes
edema Accumulation of an excessive amount of watery fluid in cells, tissues, or serous cavities
effusion Escape of fluid from blood vessels or lymphatics into tissues or cavities
encephalitis Inflammation of the brain
epistaxis Nasal hemorrhage; nosebleed
fasciculation Localized involuntary muscular contraction
hematemesis Vomiting blood
hematochezia Blood in feces
hematuria Blood in urine
hemoptysis Coughing blood
hemothorax Blood in the pleural cavity
hydrocephalus Condition marked by an excessive accumulation of fluid in the brain
hyperdynamic Excessive muscular activity
hyperkalemic Abnormally high potassium levels
hypernatremia Increased sodium in the blood
hyperthermia Increased body temperature
hyphema Blood in the anterior chamber of the eye
hyponatremia Deficiency of sodium in the blood
hypoplasti Underdevelopment of an organ or tissue
hypopyon Pus in the anterior chamber of the eye
hypothermia Decreased body temperature
hypoxia Decrease in oxygen
indwelling (catheter) Catheter that is designed to stay in the urethra to drain urine from the bladder
intussusception Infolding of one segment of the intestine into another
IOP Intraocular pressure
isotonic Of similar osmolality to normal plasma
laminectomy Surgical excision of the dorsal arch of a vertebra
lavage Washing out or irrigating the intestinal tract or stomach
LD_{50} Dose that will kill 50% of the tested population
menace reflex* or *menace response Reflex assessed by stabbing a finger toward an eye. Positive response is closing of the eyelids; absence of response could indicate paralysis of the eyelids or serious depression of consciousness
methemoglobinemia Presence of methemoglobin in the circulating blood
miosis Contraction of the pupil
mydriasis Dilation of the pupil
myelogram Graphic representation of cells found in a bone marrow sample
nebulization Treatment by a spray
neoplasia Pathological process that results in the formation and growth of a tumor
neurogenic Originating in the nervous system
nystagmus Rhythmic involuntary movement of the eyeballs in a vertical, horizontal, or rotary direction
occlusive State of being closed; an obstruction or a closing
oliguria Reduced daily output of urine
orthopnea Discomfort in breathing aggravated by lying flat: minimizing chest wall compression by standing or sternal recumbency with elbows abducted
osmolality Concentration of a solution in terms of osmoles or solutes per kilogram of solvent
paralysis Loss of power of voluntary movement in a muscle
paraphimosis Inability to retract the penis
parenchyma Distinguishing or specific cells of a gland or organ, contained in and supported by the connective tissue framework
paresis Incomplete voluntary movement
perfusion Passage of fluid through the vessels of an organ
pericardiocentesis Passage into the pericardium with a needle or hollow instrument for the purpose of removing fluid
periodontitis Inflammation of the area surrounding a tooth or the periodontium
pleura Serous membrane enveloping the lungs and lining the walls of the pleural cavity
pneumothorax Presence of air or gas in the pleural cavity
postural Pertaining to position or posture
prolapsed nictitans Proplapsed third eyelid. When the eye is depressed within the socket because of dehydration or emaciation and the third eyelid is moved across the eye

proprioceptive Capable of receiving stimuli originating in muscles, tendons, and other internal tissues

protectant Agent that promotes defense immunity against a harmful substance

PU/PD Polyuria/polydipsia

pyothorax Empyema (pus) in the pleural cavity

pyrexia Fever

rales Commonly used to denote crackling sounds heard on lung auscultation

septic Pertaining to sepsis; the presence of toxins in the blood or other tissues

sequestration Abnormal separation of a part or a whole portion by a disease process

serous Relating to, containing or producing, or a substance having a watery consistency

shock Stage in which the body is unable to adequately deliver oxygen to tissues

status epilepticus Repeated seizure or a seizure prolonged for at least 30 minutes

stenotic Abnormal narrowing or constriction

stertor Snoring; a noisy inspiration sometimes because of obstruction of the larynx or upper airway

strabismus Change in the visual axis; examples: wandering eye, walleye, cross eye, squint

stridor High-pitched, noisy respiration sometimes because of obstruction of the larynx or upper airway

stupor State of impaired consciousness with response to noxious stimuli

tachypnea Rapid respirations

tetraparesis Muscular weakness affecting all four extremities

thoracocentesis Passage into the pleural cavity with a needle or hollow instrument for the purpose of removing fluid or air

tonometer Instrument for measuring intraocular tension or pressure

torsion Act of twisting

ventroflexion Flexion of the cervical spine with movement of the head towards the ventral surface

urogram Radiography of any part of the urinary tract

urticaria Vascular reaction of the skin that is a response to direct exposure to a chemical or an immunological response; wheals or hives

Review Questions

1 What are the four major organ systems that are immediately evaluated in an emergency situation?
- a. Renal, gastrointestinal, cardiovascular, respiratory
- b. Endocrine, central nervous, gastrointestinal, renal
- c. Musculoskeletal, gastrointestinal, endocrine, renal
- d. Respiratory, cardiovascular, renal, central nervous

2 What are the postural adaptations for dyspnea?
- a. Coughing, tachypnea, extended neck, upper airway noise
- b. Lay rather than sit, labored expiration, abdominal movement
- c. Stand rather than sit, abducted elbows, abdominal movement, extended neck
- d. Dyspnea, stertor, extended neck, abdominal movement

3 Forty percent oxygen is suggested for long-term therapy; 100% oxygen for more than _________ can result in pulmonary oxygen toxicity.
- a. 6 Hours
- b. 8 Hours
- c. 12 Hours
- d. 24 Hours

4 What disease process requires nebulization as a treatment?
- a. Contusions
- b. Pulmonary edema
- c. Laryngeal paralysis
- d. Parenchymal lung problems

5 A capillary refill time of greater than 2 seconds is indicative of
- a. Hyperdynamic state
- b. Liver problems
- c. Cerebral edema
- d. Poor perfusion

6 Emergency situations treated with vitamin K_1 include
- a. Liver and anticoagulant rodenticide toxicity
- b. Chocolate toxicity and NSAID toxicity
- c. Acute paresis and acute renal failure
- d. Ethylene glycol and lead toxicities

7 Initial treatment for a patient in respiratory distress is
- a. Electrocardiogram
- b. Chest radiographs
- c. Diuretics
- d. Oxygen supplementation

8 Dull lung sounds ventrally on auscultation indicate
- a. Pneumonia
- b. Pleural effusion
- c. Pulmonary edema
- d. Pneumothorax

9 The clinical signs of anaphylactic shock are
- a. Brick-red mucous membranes, CRT of 1 second, and tachycardia
- b. Pale mucous membranes, CRT of 1 second, and bradycardia
- c. Muddy colored mucous membranes, prolonged CRT, and weak pulse
- d. Pale mucous membranes, CRT of 1 second, and tachycardia

10 Clinical signs for eclampsia are caused by
- a. Hypoglycemia
- b. Hyperkalemia
- c. Hypocalcemia
- d. Hypernatremia

BIBLIOGRAPHY

Hensyl WR, editor: *Stedman's medical dictionary,* ed 27, Baltimore, 2000, Williams & Wilkins.

King L, Hammond R, editor: *Manual of canine and feline emergency and critical care,* Shurdington, Cheltenham, UK, 1999, British Small Animal Veterinary Association.

Kirby R et al, editor: *The Veterinary Clinics of North America: small animal medicine,* vol 2(6), *Emergency Medicine,* Philadelphia, 1994, WB Saunders.

Kirk RW et al: *Current veterinary therapy,* ed 13, Philadelphia, 2000, WB Saunders.

Murtaugh et al: *Veterinary emergency and critical care medicine,* St Louis, 1992, Mosby.

Plunkett SJ: *Emergency procedures for the small animal veterinarian,* Philadelphia, 2001, WB Saunders.

CHAPTER 28

Zoonoses

Kisha L. White-Farrar

OUTLINE

LEARNING OUTCOMES

After reading this chapter you should be able to:

1. Define bacterial, rickettsial, viral, parasitic, mycotic, and other miscellaneous zoonotic diseases.
2. Recognize etiology, symptoms (human and animal), transmission, diagnosis, treatment, prevention, and control of various zoonotic diseases.

Zoonoses are infections or parasitic diseases that can be transmitted between humans and animals. It is beyond the scope of this chapter to address all of the known zoonoses, but descriptions of many important or commonly encountered diseases are presented. Any ill or infected animal represents a potential source of zoonotic infection, but with the use of proper precautions the chances of disease transmission can be greatly reduced. People who are immunocompromised (e.g., the very young, the aged, those on chemotherapeutic regimens), splenectomized individuals, and those who are immunodeficient should avoid contact with sick animals because most pathogenic organisms can "set up shop" in atypical host species if an individual has greatly lowered (or absent) body defenses.

The practice of epidemiology analyzes factors that influence the incidence, distribution, and control of infectious disease. By understanding how to recognize the symptoms, transmission, diagnosis, treatment, and control of transmitable diseases, the incidence of serious illness in humans and animals can be reduced (Tables 28-1 to 28-5).

Table 28-1 Bacterial zoonosis

Zoonosis/etiology	Symptoms—human	Symptoms—animal	Transmission	Diagnosis	Treatment	Prevention control
Bacillus anthracis: susceptible species; all mammals, most birds	Three clinical presentations: cutaneous, intestinal, pulmonary; disseminated septicemia and/or meningitis may occur; disseminated septicemia is rapidly fatal if untreated	Three clinical presentations; peracute, acute, subacute/chronic	Direct contact with infected animal or animal products; insect vectors and contaminated water possible	Culture/isolation, microscopic identification	Human: AB* therapy Animal: AB therapy (effective early in disease)	Vaccines available for humans and animals; disinfection/sterilization of animal products; do not perform necropsy on suspected cases; incinerate or deep-bury and cover carcass with quicklime
Brucellosis (Bang's disease, undulant fever): *Brucella* spp.; susceptible species: most mammals; common in cattle, dog	Clinical presentation, from latent to chronic, may include flulike symptoms, fatigue, weight loss, depression, meningitis, encephalitis, endocarditis; common in vocationally high-risk persons	Varied, may include abortion, retained placenta, mastitis, fistulous withers, arthritis, orchitis, lymphadenopathy, sterility	Direct contact with infected animals or animal products; humans are always accidental hosts	Culture/isolation, serum agglutination, ELISA, CF (most reliable)	AB therapy	Test/slaughter, vaccinate cows and calves, protective clothing, good sanitation/hygiene, proper food handling
Campylobacteriosis (vibriosis): *Campylobacter* spp.; susceptible species: most species, common in birds	May include: abdominal pain, acute (possibly bloody) diarrhea for 3 to 5 days; spontaneous recovery is common, without AB therapy latent carriers may result	May include: 3 to 7 days of watery, mucoid, or bloody diarrhea, anorexia, abortions; spontaneous recovery with or without AB therapy, may become latent carriers	Fecal-oral, contaminated water, infected food products (animal and vegetable)	Culture/isolation, cytological examination of feces	AB therapy—does not shorten clinical course of disease, but eliminates carrier state	Primarily good sanitation/hygiene

Continued

Table 28-1 Bacterial zoonosis—cont'd

Zoonosis/etiology	Symptoms—human	Symptoms—animal	Transmission	Diagnosis	Treatment	Prevention control
Avian chlamydiosis (psittacosis, parrot fever, ornithosis); *Chlamydia psittaci:* susceptible species: primary reservoirs are birds (common in psittacines, pigeons, sea/shore birds, poultry, waterfowl)	Severity ranges from mild flulike illness to death; may include flulike symptoms, pneumonitis, pneumonia, myocarditis, encephalitis, thrombophlebitis	Acute or latent carriers (intermittently shedding infective organisms); stress induces disease/ shedding; may include depression, anorexia, ocular/nasal discharge, dyspnea, diarrhea (green color)	Fecal-oral route; inhalation/ingestion of infected aerosolized fecal matter	Cloacal/fecal culture/isolation, serological testing (collected 2 weeks apart)	AB therapy	Quarantine/detection/treatment of infected animals, protective clothing, dampen cage floor before cleaning (to reduce aerosolization)
Capnocytophaga canimorsus; susceptible species: primarily dog and cat	Can be asymptomatic or self-limiting, but may present as nonspecific febrile illness that frequently progresses to a severe septicemia; DIC, cellulitis, endocarditis, renal failure and gangrene may occur	No signs in animals. *C. canimorsus* may be a commensal organism in dog and cat	Directly, or indirectly transmitted by domestic dogs through bites or scratches; domestic cats have also been indicated in transmission	Clinical presentation/appropriate history, culture/isolation, serology, cytological identification	AB therapy (usually penicillin)	Prevention of bites and scratches through cleaning/irrigation of all bites, immediate medical attention if fever or cellulitis develops
Cat scratch disease: multiple bacterial species have been implicated; EXAMPLES: *Afipia felis, Bartonella henselae, Pasteurella multocida*; susceptible species: primarily cat	Primarily in children <12 years; may include identifiable primary innoculatory lesion, regional lymphadenopathy, flulike symptoms, anorexia osteolytic lesions, oculoglandular syndrome	Cats display few, if any, clinical signs; endocarditis, usually self-limiting with no recurrence in recovered patients	Directly or indirectly transmitted by domestic cats (bacilli may be normal oral flora—transmitted to claws during grooming), usually transmitted through bite/scratch; some evidence of flea vector	Clinical presentation/appropriate history, primary innoculatory lesion, positive Hangar-Rose skin test, culture/isolation Most commonly from male, intact cats (<1 year), with fleas, not declawed, and indoor/outdoor access	Usually self-resolving but may require AB therapy	Declaw young cats; do not allow cats to lick open wounds; good sanitation/hygiene, handle cats gently to prevent bites/scratches

Erysipelothrix infection; *Erysipelothrix rhusiopathiae;* susceptible species: pig wild and domestic fowl	Cutaneous infection known as erysipeloid on fingers and hands; raised lesions accompanied by severe pain and swelling	Acute, subacute or chronic; septicemia; raised, reddish purple, rhomboidal lesions (diamond skin disease) Chronic may cause arthritis, endocarditis, and death	Occupational exposure via scratches, abrasions, or puncture wound	Culture/isolation	AB therapy	Good sanitation/hygiene
Leptospirosis (Weil's disease, Ft. Bragg fever): *Leptospira* spp.; susceptible species: wide variety mammals/reptiles but rodents are a primary reservoir	Incubation 1 to 2 weeks, duration 1 to 7 days; may include flulike symptoms, jaundice, anuria, rash, conjunctivitis, liver/kidney failure, death	Three clinical presentations: acute hemorrhagic, subacute, subclinical; may include (acute/subacute) high fever, septicemia, anorexia, depression, icterus, hemolytic anemia, endotoxemia, abortion, mastitis, infertility	Contact with infective urine, contaminated water/soil, direct contact with infected animals	Culture/isolation (blood, urine), microagglutination and macroagglutination, ELISA	AB therapy: treatment or prophylactic	Protective clothing, rodent control, good sanitation/hygiene, avoid contaminated water sources, vaccinate (moderately effective)
Listerosis: *Listeria* spp.; susceptible species: many species of mammals, fowl, fish (common in ruminants)	Several clinical presentations: depends on route of infection; may include dermal lesions, enteritis, septicemia, encephalitis, abortion/stillbirth, birth of infected neonates	May include diarrhea, flulike symptoms, excessive salivation, mastitis, monocytosis, septicemia, purulent/necrotic lesions of visceral organs/lymph nodes, abortion/stillbirth, encephalitis	Exposure to infected animal/bird products, contaminated silage/vegetables	Culture/isolation	AB therapy	Good sanitation/hygiene, protective clothing

Continued

Table 28-1 Bacterial zoonosis—cont'd

Zoonosis/etiology	Symptoms—human	Symptoms—animal	Transmission	Diagnosis	Treatment	Prevention control
Plague: *Yersinia* spp.; susceptible species: chief reservoirs—rodents, birds, lagomorphs; also common in carnivores	Three main clinical presentations: bubonic (acute), septicemic, pneumonic; may include acute fever, painful lymphadenitis, anorexia, flulike symptoms, dyspnea, fatigue	May include: fever, lymphadenitis/abscess formation; some species may show high mortality rates	Flea bites, direct contact with infected animals, inhalation of aerosolized contaminants	Culture/isolation, IFA, serological testing	AB therapy	Rodent/flea control, protective clothing, good sanitation/hygiene
Q fever (coxiellosis) *Coxiella burnetii*; susceptible species: cattle, sheep, goat, many other mammals can be carriers	Acute febrile disease, respiratory involvement, flulike symptoms, pneumonia, meningoencephalitis and cardiac involvement; most cases are mild and self-limiting; if left untreated causes fatal endocarditis	Asymptomatic, although sometimes causes abortion	Inhalation of aerosol spores from infected birth fluid and ruminant placentae; wool or hides; unpasteurized milk from infected animals can lead to human infection	Serological testing	AB therapy	Avoid contact with infected animals
Salmonellosis (enteric fever): *Salmonella* spp.; susceptible species: almost all species (especially prevalent in reptiles)	Incubation: 6 to 72 hours; primarily presents as acute gastroenteritis; may also include focal infections, chronic rheumatoid conditions, colitis, autoimmune disorders, chronic enteric hyperplastic/inflammatory conditions; shedding of infected organisms occurs for days to weeks	Four clinical presentations: subclinical, acute enteritis, subacute enteritis, chronic enteritis Acute: may include high fever, explosive diarrhea (possibly bloody), depression, death within 48 hours; Chronic: may include mild symptoms, low-moderate fever, soft feces/mild diarrhea, abortion	Primarily fecal-oral route; commonly found in beef and poultry products; unthrifty appearance—stress can induce shedding of infective organisms	Clinical presentation/appropriate history, culture/isolation	AB therapy	Good sanitation/hygiene; proper cooking/handling of beef/poultry products; do not bathe animals or wash cage items in kitchen or bathroom sink

Tuberculosis (TB) *Mycobacteria* spp.; susceptible species: most species	Two clinical signs: acute, chronic Acute: may include acute miliary TB meningitis, secondary infections Chronic: may include pulmonary/bone/joint lesions, meningitis, genitourinary infections, cervical lymphadenitis	May include lymphadenopathy, lesions/granulomas of organs, anorexia, weakness, weight loss, coughing/ dyspnea, pleural pneumonia, death; latent carrier state is common	Primarily fecal-oral route; ingestion of contaminated food products; contact with/infected tissues/animal products	Reaction to interdermal tuberculin test(s), culture/isolation	Human: anti-TB drug therapy/prophylaxis (for known exposure)	Intradermal tuberculin testing (animals and vocationally high-risk persons), animal test/cull programs, proper preparation/ handling of food
Tularemia (rabbit fever) *Francisella tularensis* sp.; susceptible species: many species of vertebrates/invertebrates	Incubation 2 to 3 days; several clinical presentations—depend on route of infection: ulceroglandular, typhoidal, oculoglandular, glandular, tularemic pneumonia	Usually manifests as septicemia (may show high mortality rates), heavy tick infestation may be concurrent	Blood/tissue of infected animals, fluids/feces of infected ticks, bites from infected ticks	Culture/isolation, FA testing, serology (later in disease)	AB therapy	Protective clothing, tick control, sanitation/hygiene

*Antibiotic therapy.

Table 28-2 Rickettsial zoonosis

Zoonosis/etiology	Symptoms—human	Symptoms—animal	Transmission	Diagnosis	Treatment	Prevention control
Ehrlichiosis: *Ehrlichia* spp.	May include: acute fever, flulike symptoms, leukopenia; primarily canids	Three clinical presentations: acute, subacute, chronic thrombocytopenia, elevated hepatic enzyme activity (especially AST, ALT) May include fever, anorexia, depression, lymphadopathy, thrombocytopenia, "fading puppy syndrome"	Primarily bite from an infected tick, also oral (splashed, infective urine), placental transmission	Clinical presentation/appropriate history, IFA, isolation from tissues	AB therapy	Use of protected clothing, tick repellents, prevention of prolonged tick attachment, environmental tick treatment, treatment of pets for ticks. Vaccine available
Lyme borreliosis (Lyme disease): *Borrelia burgdorferi;* susceptible species: variety of wild/domestic animals	Three stages First stage: "bull's eye" red lesion (usually at site of tick bite), maculopapular/petechial/vesicular rashes, flulike symptoms	May include: fever, arthralgia, arthritis, lameness, CNS involvement, encephalitis, abortion	Primarily bite from an infected tick, also oral (splashed, infective urine), placental transmission	Clinical presentation/history of tick exposure, culture/isolation, IFA and EIA available but false positive/negative results have been reported	AB therapy	Use of protected clothing, tick repellents, prevention of prolonged tick attachment, environmental tick treatment, treatment of pets for ticks. Vaccine available

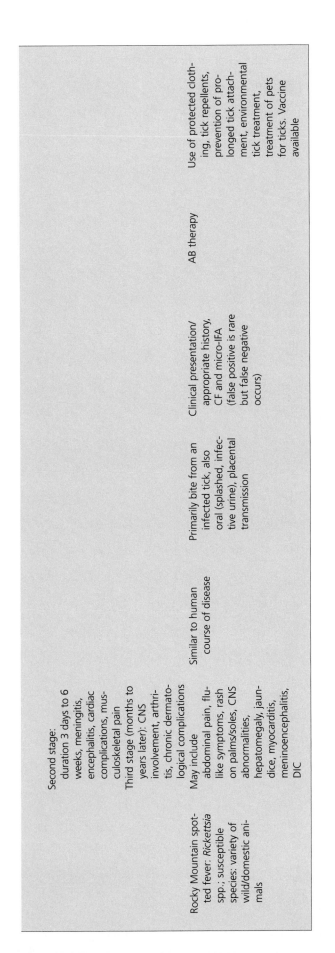

	Second stage: duration 3 days to 6 weeks, meningitis, encephalitis, cardiac complications, musculoskeletal pain Third stage (months to years later): CNS involvement, arthritis, chronic dermatological complications					
Rocky Mountain spotted fever: *Rickettsia* spp.; susceptible species: variety of wild/domestic animals	May include abdominal pain, flu-like symptoms, rash on palms/soles, CNS abnormalities, hepatomegaly, jaundice, myocarditis, meninoencephalitis, DIC	Similar to human course of disease	Primarily bite from an infected tick, also oral (splashed, infective urine), placental transmission	Clinical presentation/ appropriate history, CF and micro-IFA (false positive is rare but false negative occurs)	AB therapy	Use of protected clothing, tick repellents, prevention of prolonged tick attachment, environmental tick treatment, treatment of pets for ticks. Vaccine available

Table 28-3 Viral zoonosis

Zoonosis/etiology	Symptoms—human	Symptoms—animal	Transmission	Diagnosis	Treatment	Prevention control
Arboviral encephalitis (sleeping sickness): *Arboviridae* spp.; EXAMPLES: EEE, WEE, VEE, St. Louis; susceptible species: many bird/wild animals (primarily rodent) reservoirs, common in equines	Usually biphasic First phase may include headache/high fever, which may abate before disease progresses Second phase (encephalitic): cervical stiffness, nausea/vomiting, disorientation, frequent progression to coma/convulsions	Symptoms vary but may include fever, depression, impaired vision, irregular gait, wandering, incoordination, slowed reflexes, facial/general paralysis, death	Viral reservoir is maintained by mosquito vectors	Culture/isolation, serological testing	AB therapy and antiviral therapy in humans	Avoid bite of mosquitoes; use protective screening/clothing; liberal use of insect repellent; use of vaccines
Herpes B viral infection: *Herpesvirus simiae;* susceptible species: primarily macaque species (principally Rhesus)	Causes an ascending encephalitis that is usually fatal—those who survive often have severe, permanent neurological damage; symptoms usually occur within 30 days of exposure; may include vesicular skin lesions, localized neurological symptoms, regional lymphadenopathy, fever, headaches, ataxia, encephalitis, death—usually 2 to 3 days after onset of clinical signs	Chiefly gingivostomatitis with buccal mucosal lesions; asymptomatic infection is believed to be common	Primarily by exposure to infected monkey saliva/tissues	Culture/isolation, serological testing	Thoroughly clean/disinfect all primate bite/scratch wounds; immediately report any rash/itching/numbness at wound site; evidence suggests that early administration of acylovir may aid recovery	Thoroughly clean/disinfect all bites/scratches; use protective clothing, liberal use of chemical/mechanical restraint

Newcastle disease: an RNA virus, paramyxovirus, especially susceptible species: primarily poultry, also wild birds	Conjunctivitis, swelling of subconjunctival tissues; occasionally systemic—flulike symptoms, lymphadenitis of the lymph nodes in front of the ear	Respiratory: gasping, coughing CNS: drooping wings, twisted neck, paralysis, depression, anorexia Viserotropic: acute watery, green diarrhea, facial edema, tracheal exudate, necrosis of intestinal mucosa, high mortality rate associated with this type	Virus can be aerosolized or passed in feces; improper handling/use of vaccine	Viral isolation—tracheal exudate, lung or spleen, serological testing	Usually self-resolving in humans	Good hygiene, vaccinate flocks with a live lentogenic vaccine; use care when handling live vaccine, use mask/eye protection, avoid creating aerosols when cleaning or when handling vaccine
Poxviral disease (contagious ecthyma, bovine papular stomatitis, pseudopox): *Poxviridae* spp.	Usually progressive, localized skin lesions, may progress to cellular proliferation/ necrosis	Same course as human	Direct contact (usually through dermal abrasion)	Clinical presentation/ appro-priate history, culture/isolation, CF, IFA	AB therapy for secondary bacterial infection	Use of protective clothing, use of vaccines
Rabies (hydrophobia, "mad" dog disease); a rhabidovirus; susceptible species: all mammalian species (common in skunk, bat, dog, cat, horse)	Incubation 9 days to 2+ years, clinical course usually 2 to 8 days; may include anxiety, hyperesthesia, hyperactivity, aerobia, increased salivation, laryngopharyngeal muscular spasms, convulsions, coma, and ultimately death	Two stages First stage: duration 1 to 6 days, may include behavioral changes (unusual friendliness/aggression), excitability, altered vocalizations Second stage: duration 1 to 4 days, progressive paralysis and death	Primarily contamination of a wound (bite, abrasion) by infected saliva; ingestion/ mucosal contact with infected saliva	Clinical presentation/ appropriate history, IFA (optimal recovery from hippocampus, brain stem, cerebellum)	Practice prophylactic treatment	Immunization of applicable species, preexposure prophylaxis to vocationally high-risk persons
West Nile virus: a flavivirus; susceptible species: wild birds—especially crows, jays, geese, domestic equids, possibly domestic dog and cat	Most are asymptomatic; fever, headaches, and myalgia, often with something rash and regional lymphadenitis, severe encephalic infection may show high fever, cervical stiffness, disorientation, convulsions, paralysis, coma, or death (3% to 15%)	Many are asymptomatic, acute illness, fever, convulsions, paralysis, and death	Viral reservoirs maintained by mosquito vectors, ticks have been found infected with virus, but their role in disease maintenance and transmission is uncertain	Culture/isolation, serological testing (HI) histopathology, PCR (tissues)	There is no specific therapy, intensive supportive therapy, AB therapy—prevent secondary infection, good nursing care	Avoid mosquito bites, use protective screening/clothing, liberal use of insect repellant, wear gloves when handling/cleaning game birds, cook wild game thoroughly, conditional vaccine for domestic equine use

Table 28-4 Parasitic zoonosis

Zoonosis/etiology	Symptoms—human	Symptoms—animal	Transmission	Diagnosis	Treatment	Prevention control
Ancylostomiasis (hookworm disease) (cutaneous larval migrans); many species of hook-worms may infect man and animals; susceptible species: most species	May include bloody diarrhea, anemia (which may lead to tachycardia, heart failure, hypopro-teinemia, ascites), cutaneous infection, dermatitis, genera-lized edema, regional lymphadenitis, pneu-monitis, corneal opacities	May include anemia, dark/tarry stools, dehydration, emaciation; fatalities are common in young animals	Fecal-oral route, cutaneous penetra-tion by larvae	Ova on fecal flotation, clinical presenta-tion/appropriate history	Anthelmintic therapy	Good sanitation/ hygiene; treat infected animals; cover sandboxes; use protective clothing
Cryptosporidiosis: *Cryptosporidium parvum* (coccidian protozoan parasite) susceptible species: cattle, cat, and other domestic animals	Profuse, watery diarrhea with abdominal cramps, symptoms may recur, but is often self-limiting; resolution usually occurs within 30 days, but can be fatal	Often subclinical in adult animals, newborns/juveniles usually demonstrate profuse diarrhea	Primarily fecal-oral route	Detection of oocysts from feces, histopathology, ELISA, and an immunofluorescence test	No specific therapy, supportive therapy and nursing care	Good sanitation and hygiene, thorough disinfection procedures
Sarcoptic mange (scabies): *Sarcoptes scabei* mite; susceptible species: many species	Intensely pruritic dermal lesions, may develop alopecia/skin crusting/skin thickening, peripheral lymphadenopathy	(Same as human)	Direct contact with infested animal	Visualization of mites/ova from skin scraping	Anthelmintic therapy	Treat infected animals, protective clothing, regular washing/ changing of animal bedding, prophy-lactic ivermectin

Tapeworm infection (low pathogenicity): multiple species: *Dypilidiae* spp., *Taeniae* spp., *Hymenolipiae* spp.; susceptible species: most species	Common in very young children, symptoms usually mild; may include abdominal discomfort, diarrhea, pruritus, anemia, weight loss	Migrating proglottids may cause anal irritation; may include weight loss, unthrifty appearance	Ingesting infected fleas or proglottids/ova	Primarily by presence of proglottids on feces/perianally (rarely observed on fecal flotation)	Anthelmintic therapy	Flea control; treat infected animals; good sanitation/ hygiene
Tapeworm infection (high pathogenicity): *Echinococcus* spp.; susceptible species: many species (common in dog, cat, rodents) Predator-prey cycle: predator species are the definitive hosts, prey species are intermediate hosts, human is (accidental) intermediate host	Alveolar hydatid disease; progressive onset of symptoms may include epigastric pain, malaise, progressive jaundice, hepato-megaly, hepatic cysts	(see Tapeworm infection—low pathogenicity)	(see Tapeworm infection—low pathogenicity)	Due to small size of proglottids very difficult to detect on or in feces, indistin-guishable ova (from other cestodes)	Animals: anthelmintic therapy Humans: surgical excision of cysts	(see Tapeworm infection—low pathogenicity)
Toxocariasis (visceral larval migrans [VLM], ocular larval migrans [OLM]); *Toxocara* spp.; susceptible species: most species	VLM: larval migration through somatic tissues; may include fever, hepatomegaly, bronchiolitis, asthma, pneumonitis, CNS	Usually inapparent in adults (larval incystation in tissues); in young may include diar-rhea, dehydration, intestinal disten-tion/obstruction, exaggerated immunological response OLM: larva enter into orbit of the eye, usually no other signs	Fecal-oral (2-week incubation period)	Ova found on fecal flotation, clinical presentation/appro-priate history, ELISA	Anthelmintic therapy	Good sanitation/ hygiene, treat infected animals

Continued

Table 28-4 Parasitic zoonosis—cont'd

Zoonosis/etiology	Symptoms—human	Symptoms—animal	Transmission	Diagnosis	Treatment	Prevention control
Toxoplasmosis: *Toxoplasma gondii;* susceptible spp.: most species but cat is definitive and intermediate host	Most adults show subclinical symptoms, but may include flulike symptoms, transient cervical lymphadenopathy, myocarditis, splenomegaly, hepatomegaly, encephalitis, retinochoroiditis; congenital infections may manifest a subclinical or clinical presentation of variable severity; fatalities do occur	Most are subclinical but may include (same as human and possibly icterus, granulomatous panuveitis)	Fecal-oral, ingestion of improperly cooked meats; congenital transplacental transmission	Leukocytosis, eosinophilia, observation/isolation of tachyzoites from blood/tissues, Sabin Feldman dye test, IFA, CF, ELISA, oocyst identification from fecal flotation (requires sporulation)	Anticoccidial anthelmintic therapy	Proper handling/preparation of food, keep pet cats indoors (reduce hunting opportunities), clean litterbox regularly (ova require 3+ days incubation before infective), good sanitation/hygiene, gloves when cleaning litterbox/gardening, cover sandboxes

Table 28-5 Mycotic zoonosis

Zoonosis/etiology	Symptoms—human	Symptoms—animal	Transmission	Diagnosis	Treatment	Prevention control
Dermatophytosis: (ringworm, dermatomycosis); most common: *Microsporum* spp., *Trichophyton* sp.; susceptible species: most common in young mammals	Incubation 1 to 2 weeks; superficial infections of skin/hair/nails; acute inflammatory reaction; lesions usually papulosquamous with circular/reddened borders (but may be dry/alopecic or moist/eczematous lesions)	Lesions are usually circular/crusty with or without redness/alopecia	Direct contact with an infected animal (or its hair, skin, leashes/brushes) equipment, or contaminated soil	Dermatophyte/mycological culture/isolation, ultraviolet fluorescence (Wood's lamp), biopsy/cytology	Topical/oral antifungal therapy, vaccine (limited use)	Protective clothing, good sanitation/hygiene, treat infected animals
Systemic mycoses; most common: *Histoplasmae* spp., *Coccidiodae* spp., *Blastomycae* spp., *Cryptoccae* spp.; susceptible species: most species	Usually begin as pulmonary infection with fever/myalgia/congestion; may progress into chronic/granulomatous pneumonia or disseminate to other organs; may develop into subacute or chronic meningoencephalitis	Similar to course of disease in human	Usually aerosolized organisms (fecal/infective soil)	Culture/isolation, ELISA	Antifungal therapy	Protective clothing (when handling infected animals or cleaning their pens/supplies)

Glossary

acute Having severe signs of a short duration, such as 12 to 24 hours

anthelmentic Chemical agent that destroys, kills, or expels parasites

CF Complement fixation (test)

chronic Disease that persists longer than 1 week

clinical Showing signs

commensal Two nonparasitic organisms that live together; one benefits from the association while the other is neither benefited nor harmed

ELISA Enzyme-linked immunosorbent assay (test)

epidemiology Scientific study of the factors that influence the incidence, distribution, and control of infectious diseases

FA Fluorescent antibody assay (test)

flulike symptoms Usually sudden onset of fever, shivering, headache, myalgia, and malaise

IFA Indirect fluorescent antibody assay (test)

latent carrier State where disease-causing organisms are present but clinical disease symptoms are not manifested

lentogenic vaccine Only marginally virulent

miliary TB Disseminated tuberculosis, usually manifested by small, millet seed–sized nodules

myalgia Muscle pain

mycotic Relating to fungi or vegetating microorganisms

peracute Very acute, a duration of a few hours

petechial Minute, pinpoint hemorrhaging

proglottids Cestode segments that contain fertile, infective oocytes

reservoir Alternative host or a pathogenic agent

subacute Between acute and chronic in duration: approximately 1 week

subclinical Without clinical manifestations; the early signs or stages of a mild form of a disease

typhoidal Symptoms marked by sustained high fever, severe headache, and a rash

undulant To fluctuate in wavelike patterns

vector Carrier, usually an arthropod, that transfers an infective agent from one host to another

VLM Visceral larval migrans

Review Questions

1 Most infectious organisms have certain species that are preferred hosts. Which statement is most true about infectious organisms?
   a. They will always invade any animal, regardless of the immune status of that individual
   b. They will never invade outside their preferred host species
   c. They may invade outside their normally preferred hosts if an individual is sufficiently immunocompromised
   d. If an individual is immunocompromised, an infectious organism will always invade the preferred host

2 The rhabidovirus that causes "hydrophobia" is not capable of infecting a/an __________ patient.
   a. Canine
   b. Equine
   c. Avian
   d. Feline

3 Antibiotic therapy would be indicated for a patient who has
   a. Visceral larval migrans
   b. Rabies
   c. Salmonellosis
   d. Toxoplasmosis

4 Echinococcal
   a. Proglottids are identical to the *Taenia* ssp. proglottids
   b. Ova are indistinguishable from those of other species of cestodes
   c. Human infestations are treated with anthelmintic therapy
   d. Infection in humans is considered benign

5 Ringworm infection
   a. Is caused by a small parasite
   b. Affects only cats
   c. Commonly occurs in healthy, adult animals
   d. Is treated with a regimen of antifungal agents (topical and/or oral)

6 Cat scratch disease can be prevented in part by
   a. Allowing a cat to lick open wounds, thus raising antibody levels
   b. Administering a vaccine to cats
   c. Administering a vaccine to humans
   d. Declawing young cats and handling them gently

7 Salmonellosis
   a. Is transmitted by flea bites
   b. Can be prevented with yearly vaccination
   c. Is not commonly shed by latent carriers
   d. Can be transmitted in food products such as chicken or eggs

8 In humans, the first stage of Lyme disease can be diagnosed on the basis of a characteristic lesion. The lesion is similar to a/an
   a. Bull's eye
   b. Mosquito bite
   c. Red rash
   d. Area of petechiae

9 Psittacosis can be contracted only from __________ species.
   a. Bovine
   b. Avian
   c. Ovine
   d. Equine

10 A preventive flea program is an important factor in controlling __________ infestations.
   a. Toxascaris
   b. Toxoplasmosis
   c. *Sarcoptes* spp.
   d. *Taenia* spp.

BIBLIOGRAPHY

August JR: *Zoonosis updates,* ed 2, Schaumberg, IL, 1995, American Veterinary Medical Association.

Benenson AS: Cryptococcosis. In Benenson AS, editor: *Control of communicable diseases manual,* Washington, DC, 1995, American Public Health Association.

Bonagura J, editor: *Kirk's current veterinary therapy, XIII: small animal practice,* Philadelphia, 1999, WB Saunders.

Bowman DD: *Georgi's parasitology for veterinarians,* ed 6, Philadelphia, 1995, WB Saunders.

Clark WH, Dawkins B, Audin JH, editors: *Zoonosis updates,* Schaumberg, IL, 1990, American Veterinary Medical Association.

Fowler ME, editor: *Zoo and wild animal medicine,* ed 2, Philadelphia, 1986, WB Saunders.

Fraser CM, Mays A, editors: *The Merck manual,* ed 6, Rahway, NJ, 1986, Merck & Co, Inc.

Gillespie JH, Timoney JF: *Hagan and Bruner's infectious diseases of domestic animals,* ed 8, Ithaca, NY, 1988, Cornell University Press.

Hendrix CM, editor: *Laboratory procedures for veterinary technicians,* ed 4, St Louis, 2002, Mosby.

Howard JL, Smith R (eds): *Current veterinary therapy: food animal practice,* ed 4, Philadelphia, 1998, WB Saunders.

Hugh-Jones ME, Hubbert WT, Hagstad HV: Newcastle disease. In *Zoonosis: recognition, control and prevention,* Ames, 1995, Iowa State University Press.

Kirk RW, editor: *Kirk's veterinary therapy, small animal practice,* ed 7, Philadelphia, 1995, WB Saunders.

McCurnin DM, Bassert JM, editors: *Clinical textbook for veterinary technicians,* ed 5, St Louis, 2001, WB Saunders.

Mills L, Robison NE, editors: *Current veterinary therapy in equine medicine,* ed 4, Philadelphia, 1997, WB Saunders.

Rakel RE, Bope ET, editors: *Conn's current therapy, 2001: latest approved methods of treatment for the practicing physician,* Philadelphia, 2001, WB Saunders.

Sasaki DM, Katz AR, Middleton CR: *Capnocytophaga* and related infections. In Beran GW, Steele JH, editors: *Handbook of zoonoses,* ed 2, Boca Raton, FL, 1994, CRC Press.

PART VI

Practice Management and Self-Management

CHAPTER 29

Personal and Professional Management Skills

Carlene A. Decker *A. Patrick Navarre*

OUTLINE

LEARNING OUTCOMES

After reading this chapter you should be able to:

1. Describe the elements of communication, including verbal, written, and electronic.
2. Describe techniques that can increase client communication and communication in the workplace.
3. Understand basic management and business principles for hospital managers and employees.
4. List personal management techniques.
5. List career management techniques and personal growth strategies.
6. Describe internal and external marketing strategies.

The work environment for many veterinary technicians has changed over the past decade. Now veterinary technicians must be skilled in the medical and technical aspects of veterinary medicine and may also take on responsibility for many of the business decisions that occur in the workplace. For this reason, communication skills, management skills, and marketing have become important tools for the veterinary technician. These skills are also important for personal career planning and professional advancement.

COMMUNICATION

Overview

Communication is the process individuals or organizations use to create meaning with others.

I. Components of communication
   A. Sender: the sender develops a message or thought that will be conveyed
      1. The message will determine the channel
   B. Receiver: individual who receives the sender's message
   C. Message: thoughts or ideas expressed by the sender
   D. Feedback: response by the receiver as perceived by the sender
      1. Feedback enables the sender to determine how much of the message was accurately understood and interpreted by the receiver
   E. Channels: mechanisms for communication based on the five senses of sight, sound, smell, touch, and taste, including verbal, written, and electronic channels
   F. Interference: any interruption (external or internal) that enters the communication loop

            1. Interruptions can include physical noise, receiver interpretation, incorrect grammar, electronic failure, and body language
        G. Listening: a crucial element of verbal communication
    II. Flow of communication
        A. Communication within an organization travels in at least three directions: downward, upward, and horizontal
            1. Downward: information from figures of authority to subordinates, providing instructions related to the task at hand
            2. Upward: information from subordinates to authority figures
            3. Horizontal: communication that takes place among individuals with the same status

Verbal Communication

Verbal communication is involved in many types of conversations that take place on a daily basis. Effective communication also includes nonverbal elements.

Nonverbal Communication

The unspoken elements that replace, reinforce, or contradict verbal communication; they include visual, temporal, vocal, and spatial.

- I. Visual cues include posture, facial expressions, eye contact, and hand gestures, among others
    - A. Posture communicates mood of the sender
        - 1. Upright posture can imply confidence
        - 2. Slouched posture can indicate insecurity, sadness
    - B. Facial expressions are good indicators of how messages are received
    - C. Direct eye contact between sender and receiver indicates an open communication channel
        - 1. Indirect eye contact can imply uneasiness in or a closure of the communication process
    - D. Hand gestures such as a handshake or a touch on the arm add meaning to communication
- II. Temporal cues are in relation to time of day
    - A. Receiving a message the first thing after arriving at work indicates urgency
    - B. A message sent at the end of the day with a "see me at your convenience tomorrow" does not indicate the same level of urgency
    - C. Timely response indicates a commitment to the message and sender
    - D. A failure to respond indicates a lack of interest
- III. Vocal cues are voice qualities that qualify verbal messages. Some vocal cues include pitch, rate, and volume
    - A. Voice pitch ranges from low to high
        - 1. Monotone can imply disinterest in the topic
        - 2. Varied range or pitch implies enthusiasm and commitment to the topic
        - 3. A voice pitch inconsistent with the message may indicate incongruence
    - B. Rate of speech
        - 1. Normal speech is 125 to 150 words per minute
        - 2. Both rapid and slow speech may lose the receiver
    - C. Volume of voice
        - 1. Lack of volume can indicate tension, insecurity, lack of commitment to message
            - a. A designed lack of volume can better illustrate a point by forcing the receiver(s) to listen more intently
        - 2. Too much volume can indicate enthusiasm and excitement but also tension and insecurity
- IV. Spatial cues refer to the use of space often determined by culture, which significantly affects communication
    - A. Personal space is the area around oneself, known as the comfort zone
        - 1. Intrusion into the receiver's personal space can create interference in the message being sent
        - 2. If a person is leaning away from you as you are speaking, you are probably in his or her space
        - 3. It is best to be on the same level plane as the person to whom you are speaking (e.g., both standing, both sitting)
        - 4. The generally recognized area of "personal space" is approximately 46 cm to 1.2 m (18 inches to 4 feet)
    - B. Office space often dictates a professional tone of a communication
        - 1. If the sender is separated from the receiver by a desk, there is an implied message of an authority/subordinate relationship
        - 2. This set-up should be reserved for formal conversations, reprimands, and negotiations
        - 3. Informal conversations are best held in a neutral setting within the office such as around a small work table or sitting in chairs next to one another

Listening

Effective communication requires listening capabilities of the sender and the receiver.

- I. The listening process requires total concentration on the message being sent
- II. Active listening implies that you are aware of both the speaker's words and feelings on a subject. Being attentive to both gives the listener an advantage in

truly understanding the message. There are basic principles to active listening

A. Using words and expressions to encourage the speaker to share information with you freely (being sincere is the key to making the speaker feel he or she can share with you)
B. Repeating the speaker's message will give him or her confidence that you understand what was said and will encourage him or her to share more
    1. Often referred to as paraphrasing
C. Perform periodic checks of the message by asking short questions that will clarify a point
D. Make sure you capture the feelings that are presented along with the message; to make sure you understand, question the speaker by asking, "You are excited about this opportunity?" etc.

III. Barriers to effective listening can be avoided by
    A. Concentrating on the message being sent with a clear, undivided mind
    B. Avoiding judgment of the message sender. Do not let personal and emotional opinions distort the message
    C. Understanding
        1. The mind can process information faster than *the words* can be spoken
            a. To effectively listen, do not get ahead of the message being sent
    D. Presenting a communication from a supervisor in such a way as to encourage feedback from subordinates

IV. Better listening requires practice of the following
    A. Do not interrupt the sender while the message is being delivered
    B. Ask for clarification of the message if necessary
    C. Ignore distractions in the environment
    D. Respond to the message; provide feedback
    E. Observe the sender's body language to uncover other meanings in the message
    F. Do not place personal opinions or preconceived opinions into the message

SPECIAL COMMUNICATION SITUATIONS

Client Communication

Clients are the most important person in any practice. Effective communication is essential. Communication with clients takes place in different ways, such as client education, information gathering, grief counseling, emergency situations, telephone conversations, and dealing with angry/hostile clients.

I. Client education is a vital component of the veterinary technician's role in the hospital
    A. Technicians communicate with the client by describing routine procedures performed on pets using terminology understood by the client
    B. To assist in this communication the technician often develops visual tools, including diagrams, charts, specimens, and newsletters
    C. Special explanations for children can be developed to assist them in understanding procedures performed on their pets
    D. Technicians may be responsible for obtaining information from clients
        1. If detailed answers are required, use open-ended questions
            a. Begin with "What?" "When?" "Where?" "Who?" and "How?"
        2. Ask leading questions only if a yes or no answer is desired
            a. Include "Did it...?" or "Was it...?"
            b. Avoid because client may feel the need to answer yes or no, even if not sure of the answer
        3. Use active listening techniques

II. Grief counseling is an important communication tool used to help clients deal with grief and emotional pain resulting from the loss of a pet
    A. Listening skills are an essential component of grief counseling
    B. Elizabeth Kübler-Ross, MD, was the first to identify the stages in the grieving process
    C. The six stages of grief a client may experience at various times (not necessarily in order)
        1. Denial—usually the first stage the body goes through to prepare for emotional trauma. During this stage, the client refuses to deal with the pet's condition
            a. The client needs support, understanding, and permission to grieve
            b. Communicate clearly and listen actively, rephrase if necessary and avoid medical jargon
            c. Remain nonjudgmental; give client time to move out of the denial stage at his or her own pace
            d. Allow client to feel a sense of closure such as viewing the body or saying goodbye
        2. Bargaining—often an irrational attempt to reverse or control a situation and may include negotiation with a higher being for the health/life of the pet
            a. This phase is not seen as often in pet loss as in the loss of a human
            b. It is important not to become defensive and to patiently answer any questions or concerns
        3. Anger—often follows denial. The veterinary technician or the veterinarian may be the target of that anger as the client places the

blame for the death of the pet on the ones who were entrusted with its medical care
   a. It is particularly important not to become defensive or to mirror the anger
   b. Give the client permission to vent anger
   c. Listen actively by mirroring, maintaining eye contact, using empathetic statements
4. Guilt—often accompanies this stage so relieve it by assuring the client that the best decision was made. Guilt inhibits progress toward resolution. Dealing with the guilt is key in moving on
5. Depression—sadness that follows after anger subsides
   a. This phase begins and ends at different times for each client
   b. Allow clients to express feelings and follow up after the death of the pet
   c. Listen actively and empathetically; a touch on the forearm or shoulder may convey compassion
   d. Validate normalcy of the client's feelings
   e. This may be a good time to encourage memoralization of the pet such as planting a tree, starting a scrapbook
6. Resolution—when the pet owner accepts the fate of the pet
   a. Memories become a comfort rather than a source of sorrow
   b. It is during this phase that clients may consider getting another pet

III. Emergency situations require quick assessment and response to patient needs
   A. The first key to successfully handling an emergency is to be familiar with the hospital's policies for such situations
      1. Know the first aid protocols that the hospital follows
      2. Be familiar with the standard recommendations to the clients that the veterinarians prefer that you use
      3. You must be prepared technically to be able to respond with a sense of "taking charge"
   B. Assessing the needs of the animal and/or client is the first step once an actual emergency has taken place. This assessment requires that appropriate instructions be given to the client for management of the emergency
      1. To determine if you understand the situation, summarize and repeat the client's situation
      2. Once you have given directions, ask the client to repeat the instructions back to you and ask if he or she has any questions
   C. Clients under stress may not have appropriate listening capabilities so communications must be short, concise, and without emotion in the technician's voice tones

IV. Telephone conversations with clients are an important means of communication. Telephone etiquette includes
   A. Professional greetings, name of the business, and name of the person answering the telephone
   B. The ability to assess the caller's needs (i.e., an emergency, etc.)
   C. Appropriate voice tones
   D. Following rules associated with length of time to keep a client "on hold"
   E. Answering the telephone before a predetermined number of rings, usually a maximum of three
   F. Appropriate use of voice mail systems
   G. Protocol for taking and returning messages

V. Communication with angry/hostile clients requires recognizing the potentially hostile situation before it escalates. Considerations include
   A. A proper place for conversation with an angry client
   B. Disassociation of the problem from the person so that solutions might be more easily seen
   C. One of the best ways to diffuse a hostile situation is to use active listening skills
      1. Appearing to agree may diffuse the problem
   D. Never argue with a dissatisfied client because the client is always right, even when wrong
   E. Use conflict resolution techniques. The steps include
      1. Recognize and define each piece of the problem
      2. Generate ideas to develop a resolution plan
      3. Make and implement a decision where everyone wins
      4. Evaluate the outcome
   F. If the client seems unreasonable, ask the veterinarian to handle the problem as quickly as possible
   G. People on drugs or alcohol could become violent and uncontrollable: be careful
      1. Law enforcement officials may have to be called if substances are used in excess

Co-worker Communication

Communication with coworkers is the key to success of the team. Positive idea exchange, the act of providing and receiving constructive criticism, is essential.

I. Types of co-worker communication
   A. Supervisor and employee

B. Employee and supervisor
C. Employee and employee

II. Mechanisms of positive idea exchange
   A. Communication on work-related issues should focus on identifying the issue with the end result being to identify a solution
      1. The work environment should be conducive and support exchange of information and ideas
   B. Staff meetings provide an open forum for exchange of ideas and should be scheduled regularly
   C. Goals of the practice provide all staff members with a clear understanding of the direction in which the organization is heading
   D. New techniques learned at continuing education meetings or seminars should be shared
   E. Clearly worded manuals containing written policies and protocols, including job responsibilities, should be available

III. Conflict resolution: handling of conflict through appropriate channels within the workplace is essential for dealing with conflict. The following are further pertinent elements of conflict resolution
   A. Face-to-face conversation about a problem allows all parties an opportunity to air opinions
   B. A mediated session can be held where a neutral party is identified and serves as an intermediary to observe, listen, and keep the discussion focused on issues, not individuals
   C. A written grievance can be filed, following steps accepted by the hospital
   D. Staff meetings can be a good source for conflict resolution because all variables surrounding a conflict can be discussed openly
   E. Conflict can result in positive change in the work environment in the form of constructive criticism or critique of current protocols, techniques
   F. Conflict should be resolved immediately
      1. Waiting provides an opportunity for conflict to build up into a larger problem
      2. Immediate handling allows clear memory of the situation by those involved
      3. Waiting too long to address a conflict gives the "injured party" a sense that the problem is not important

Written Communication

I. Definition: communication through messages delivered in written form. Good writing skills are essential for the veterinary technician

II. The technician will have to communicate in writing with co-workers and other professionals in the form of letters, memos, and reports

III. The technician will communicate with clients and the general public via client information handouts, written take-home directions, hospital newsletters, public education information in newspapers, etc.

IV. Main components of business communications
   A. Audience should be identified and materials tailored to educational/knowledge level
   B. Correct grammar and punctuation are a must
   C. Pitfalls to avoid
      1. Wordiness
      2. Slang terms or expressions
      3. Long words, medical terminology not familiar to the reader
      4. Vague expressions: be concise and direct
      5. Condescending statements
      6. Sexist language
      7. Negative expressions
   D. All written communication should be printed on good-quality paper with attention to appearance of the final document
      1. Typographical errors must be eliminated by repeated proofreading

Electronic Communication

Also known as telecommunications, electronic communication is a means to transmit voice, data, and images from one location to another through the use of a host of electronic equipment.

I. Computers have become vital in most veterinary practices for the management of information and communication
   A. Patient records, data, financial management, inventory of medical supplies, and communication with colleagues are now performed with computers
   B. Software packages specifically designed for veterinary hospitals allow word processing, database management, ordering, and inventory control
   C. Electronic communication, known as e-mail, has become popular because of its speed and ease of use
      1. Messages are posted in the receiver's electronic mailbox in a fraction of the time of conventional methods
      2. E-mail should not take the place of talking about a problem and listening to coworkers about concerns
      3. Tips for being a responsible e-mail user include keeping the message short and concise, always using respect for the person to whom you are sending the message, refraining from using derogatory terms and inappropriate language, identifying the purpose and receiver of the e-mail and drafting

the message accordingly, and using humor sparingly (some people do not appreciate the same humor as you do)
4. Remember that e-mail provides a written record of your thoughts and ideas

D. The Internet has revolutionized the way information is disseminated. This has affected veterinary medicine by connecting a once fragmented community. The latest political and scientific information is now as close as your nearest computer
1. Latest information on veterinary related subjects is provided
2. Online discussion or chats also provide continuing education opportunities and the opportunity to network with colleagues thousands of miles away
3. Many places of employment have their own Web pages that clients access

II. Telephone systems using multiple telephone systems and features allow better communication with the client
A. On-hold message feature: allows client while on hold to listen to messages developed by the veterinary hospital describing services or facilities that are available
B. Call waiting feature: signals when another call is coming in and can ensure a quicker response to a client's inquiry
C. Conference call option: allows multiple individuals to be included simultaneously in a conversation
D. Cellular telephones: send messages by using radio transmitters. These telephones allow greater mobility and portability for individuals
1. Can be used to keep communication lines open between the hospital and individuals traveling to clients by vehicle
2. Also allow access to computer on-line networks for consultations, drug formulas, and new information regarding medical issues in combination with portable computers while in the field

MANAGEMENT

Organizational Management

I. Definition: working with and through people to accomplish organizational goals

II. Within a veterinary hospital, managerial tasks may be delegated to a practice manager, who may be a veterinary technician. The practice manager is involved with four functions
A. Planning: thinking through and making decisions about goals and actions in advance so that objectives can be defined and procedures established
B. Organization: the next step after planning, so that human and material resources of a practice will achieve goals of the organization
C. Leadership: directing and influencing the practice's employees to carry out the organization's objectives
D. Control: monitoring and evaluating performance

III. The understanding of certain management principles will facilitate efficiency and harmony among the employees. These include, but are not limited to, the following concepts
A. Teamwork: the result of all members of an organization understanding their roles and working together to accomplish the goals of an organization
1. Teamwork is an essential component of the organizational structure
a. Each position should have specified tasks based on education and legal limits of the practice
b. More efficiency will result if the task is given to the lowest paid qualified worker
B. Supervisory skills: involve the ability to direct a co-worker or subordinate's work to meet goals of the organization
1. An effective supervisor motivates, provides constructive criticism, and evaluates performance
C. Delegating: formally assigning responsibility for completion of a given task to a subordinate. For delegation to be effective the following rules apply:
1. Carefully consider who should be given the assignment and which tasks can and should be delegated
2. Provide all pertinent information about the responsibility at the time of delegation
3. Provide a system for feedback

IV. Consistency can be facilitated by making commonly performed procedures and policies accessible to every employee
A. Policy manual: provides a written record of organization policies and includes policies that govern organization-wide actions and those that cover the actions of individuals
1. Organization-wide activities include history, the organization's purposes and goals, mission statement, policies on community affairs, etc.
2. Individual activities or what the employee needs to know

a. Policies on personnel guidelines, job descriptions of all team members, scheduling, absenteeism, tardiness, injury on the job, impairment on the job, etc.

B. Procedures manual
1. Outlines protocols for various procedures performed within an organization such as surgery, laboratory, or radiology protocols and safety procedures
2. Helps ensure that all employees adhere to the standards of the organization
   a. Written clearly and provides suggestions on the efficient completion of tasks
   b. Highlighted government rules and regulations and quality control measures

Business Management

I. Definition: practices required for the successful financial operation of a facility

II. Time is often a limiting factor but without proper business policies there would be no practice

III. Various aspects of business include

A. Records
1. Involved in all aspects of hospital operation
2. Many formats available, but whatever format is used, there must not be complete obliteration or erasure
   a. Handwritten records must be legible, accurate, and written in permanent ink
   b. Any errors should be crossed out with a single line, corrections made, dated, and initialed by the person making the entry
3. Some records and consent forms may require client's signature
   a. A minor cannot legally enter into a contract
4. Ownership
   a. The veterinary practice, not the client, owns the records
   b. Original records are a legal document and must be retained by the practice
   c. Any release of information is at the discretion of the veterinarian or practice
   d. A request for transfer should be made in writing; best to mail prepared records directly to referring or new veterinarian
5. Information contained in all medical records is confidential and should not be discussed with outside parties without client's written permission
   a. Exception is the reporting of certain contagious and zoonotic diseases
6. Statute of limitations requires that records be legally retained for a certain length of time, usually 5 to 7 years (depending on the state or province) from the date of last visit or discharge
7. Many record filing systems are available; most medical records arranged alphabetically by the owner's last name
8. Any lost records should be explained to the client and a new record begun immediately
9. Medical records include
   a. Log books: contain entries of services provided and include controlled drugs (required by law), radiography, surgery, euthanasia, laboratory, and necropsy logs
   b. Animal records: must be individualized and contain certain information such as signalment (owner's name, address, and telephone; patient's name, sex, species, age, breed, and color), as well as date seen, chief complaint, history, clinical signs, diagnosis, prognosis, authorization records, radiographic data, laboratory reports, and vaccination and surgical records
   c. Financial information may be included in medical records, but separate billing is becoming more common practice
10. Basic formats include
   a. Chronological or conventional method: events are entered as they occur
   b. Problem-oriented method includes separating out the problems, database, comprehensive history and physical examination, and progress notes
      (1) Progress notes are divided into SOAP
         (a) S = Subjective data
         (b) O = Objective data
         (c) A = Assessment
         (d) P = Procedure for diagnosis and treatment
11. Vaccination and spaying/neutering certificates need to be accurate
12. Authorization or consent forms are not legal requirements but protect the veterinarian and ensure that the client understands all treatments and procedures
   a. Includes treatment, surgery, fee estimate, euthanasia, and necropsy
   b. Should be part of permanent record
   c. Euthanasia authorization essential
13. Medication labels must be complete and accurate

B. Credit and collection policies
1. Policies should be written and strictly adhered to

2. A written estimate should always be used
3. Accounts receivable should be kept to a minimum

C. Inventory control
   1. Two goals
      a. Have items on hand when needed
      b. Minimize expense of keeping supplies in stock
   2. Turnover rate should be six to eight times per year depending on the product
      a. Calculated by: yearly inventory expense ÷ average cost of inventory on hand
      b. Inventory turned over close to once a month so items used up before the bills are due
      c. Turnover rate can be calculated on the 80:20 rule whereby 20% of items stocked account for 75% to 85% of the expenditures
   3. Elements of a good inventory system include
      a. Good record keeping that includes a reorder log, purchase order records, individual inventory records, inventory master list, and vendor files
      b. Effective use of inventory control cards or computer control
      c. Appropriate arrangement and storage of inventory
      d. Effective monitoring of inventory levels and expiration dates
      e. Smart purchasing policies, including knowledge of products

D. Accounts payable should be paid close to the due date to maximize use of capital
   1. Arrange for discounts for prompt payment
   2. Do not allow accounts to proceed beyond due date (credit rating may drop)

E. Consider use of a computer if the practice does not already have one
   1. Much of the hospital operation can be provided by the computer, including inventory control, medical records management, client communication and information analysis, vaccination reminders, and accounting
   2. Many well-designed programs are available
   3. Research particular needs so that the proper system can be purchased

F. A fax (facsimile) is an efficient rapid mode of communication
   1. Strict confidentiality must be maintained

G. Monthly analysis should be completed to establish trends, make comparisons of past months and past years, note immediate changes, and review fees, inventory comparisons, and credit policies

Personal Management

I. Definition: skills and techniques required of each individual member of an organization to make the team function most efficiently

II. Personal management skills allow the veterinary technician to manage within the team to the benefit of the team. Components of personal management are time management, goal setting, decision making, stress management, coping with burnout, and negotiating

Time Management

I. Effectively using available time during the workday maximizes productivity for the employee and helps alleviate stress

II. Time is a unique resource in that it cannot be accumulated and each person has the same amount

III. Time management is a personal process and must fit into one's lifestyle and circumstances

IV. The following suggestions can be applied to almost everyone to help manage time and reduce stress
   A. Make a daily "to do" list
   B. Develop daily, weekly, and yearly lists of goals
   C. Learn to say "no:" gain control of what takes up your time
   D. Establish priorities
   E. Use technology to acquire more efficiency: computer, calculator, and new laboratory equipment
   F. Never handle a piece of paper more than twice
   G. Learn to skim what you read
   H. Keep procrastination to a minimum
   I. Work at meeting deadlines
   J. Exercise at least 20 minutes per day to help you focus

Goals

I. Life offers a series of choices and decisions that need to be made

II. Establishing goals allows an individual to have a choice in the course of action required to accomplish a certain task and help lead in this direction

III. Set effective goals
   A. Identify possible needs in areas such as career, personal life, financial concerns, physical fitness, community involvement, leisure time
   B. Set a goal for each identified need by describing the result
   C. Prioritize

D. Define objectives required to achieve the goal (steps to be done to achieve the goal)
E. Select activity to complete each objective
F. Indicate time frame for implementation
G. Evaluate and monitor accomplishments

IV. As much as possible, make sure the objectives set for achieving the goals are measurable, clear, realistic, and stated as required results

V. Greater success will be achieved if one
A. Prioritizes
B. Draws up written plans to help achieve goals
C. Breaks goals into smaller sequential steps that can be achieved one at a time
D. Begins now

Decision Making

I. The process of identifying and selecting a course of action for a specific problem or situation

II. Indecision or making no choice paralyzes the ability of an organization or an individual to move forward

III. Key components to making a decision are similar to problem-solving techniques and include
A. Listing options
B. Evaluating options (thinking it over)
C. Factoring in personal feelings
D. Evaluating how the decision will affect priorities already set
E. Making the decision and discarding other options
F. Committing to the decision (mentally not looking back)
G. Doing everything possible to make the decision work

Stress Management

I. Stress is the feeling of tension and pressure that results when a demand cannot be readily dealt with or there is a perceived threat

II. Stress is response to a force that upsets one's equilibrium; strain is the adverse effects of stress on an individual's mind, body, and actions

III. Stressor: a force that brings about stress

IV. The body's physiological and chemical changes react to the fight-or-flight response and include an increase in heart rate, blood pressure, blood glucose, and blood clotting

V. Short-term physiological changes and prolonged stress can lead to annoying and life-threatening conditions and a weakening of the immune system

VI. Due to lack of control, job pressures create stress for many people

VII. Not all stress is bad; some stress leads to achieving goals and meeting or exceeding personal potential
A. Referred to as eustress

VIII. Stress management is individual and varies from highly specific techniques to a change in lifestyle
A. Identify stress signals
B. As much as possible, eliminate or modify stressors
C. Improve work habits
D. Physical exercise reduces tension and keeps one in good condition and more resistant to fatigue
E. Stress can be managed through mental relaxation techniques, including relaxation response, biofeedback training, muscle monitoring, and concentration techniques

Coping with Burnout

I. Burnout is closely related to stress and is defined as a state of exhaustion (physical, mental, and emotional) caused by involvement in situations that are demanding

II. Burnout is a set of behaviors that result from strain

III. Persons suffering from burnout exhibit many symptoms—some physical, some emotional

IV. Employer role: reduce the amount of burnout
A. Jobs should be clearly defined and provide the employee with a sense of purpose and opportunities for growth

V. Employee role: find significance in something other than work
A. Develop new interests that provide satisfaction outside the workplace
B. Time management and goal setting might also be effective

VI. Counseling and support are needed for recovery from burnout

Negotiating/Conflict Resolution

I. Differences of opinion or situations of conflict frequently arise

II. A win-win solution is a key to being a valuable team member

III. To prepare for negotiation
A. Always separate the person from the problem
B. Focus on the interest at hand, not the position taken
C. Identify options for a viable solution
D. Discuss options after clearly weighing all possible solutions

Career Management

I. Make career decisions that move one closer to self-fulfillment

II. Key components to finding the right job opportunity include personal finance, job search, and interview

Personal Finance

I. Step 1 in career planning is to determine the type of income that will be required to meet financial obligations
   A. Prepare a budget that will allow you to view your obligations and make correct important career decisions
      1. Budget is defined as a statement of resources allocated for specific activities over a certain period of time
      2. All income, which includes salary, return on investments, and interest income, is projected and should be listed
      3. List all expected expenses
         a. Housing, utilities, telephone, property tax, all types of insurance, automobile expenses (including loan payments, gas, and maintenance), other outstanding loan payments (including credit cards), food, household repairs, clothing, entertainment, travel, and miscellaneous expenses
      4. The goal is to have more income than expenses
         a. If there are more expenses, one of the categories will have to be adjusted
         b. It is wise not to accept a job that will not allow you to meet current financial obligations

Job Search

I. Career choices and options for veterinary technicians are not limited to practice settings
   A. Opportunities also exist in biomedical research, specialty practice, education, universities, industry, zoos, animal husbandry related areas, military service, and humane societies
   B. Research each of the areas that interest you and note pros and cons
   C. A career choice is not necessarily a long-term decision because changing career paths is not uncommon

II. Seek job notices in placement services, classified advertisements, and through networking
   A. Resume, cover letter, references
      1. Resume
         a. Summarizes your background, qualifications, and accomplishments
         b. Key components of a resume
            (1) Personal identification, including name, address, and telephone number where you can be reached
            (2) Career objective defines what type of job you are seeking
               (a) State clearly what you hope to achieve in your professional career
            (3) Traditionally, work history is in reverse chronological order
               (a) Accomplishments highlight pertinent achievements at each job
            (4) Traditionally, education is also in reverse chronological order
            (5) Personal interests are optional
               (a) May be best to include job-related activities only
            (6) The traditional chronological resume, functional resume, or a combined format can be used
      2. Cover letter
         a. Usually read before the resume, its goal is to get you to the interview stage
         b. Key components
            (1) The letter should be one page in length with approximately three paragraphs
               (a) First paragraph: introduces yourself and identifies the position for which you are applying
               (b) Second paragraph: lists accomplishments that would be beneficial for the business
               (c) Third paragraph: serves as a closing and indicates your next step, which is usually a telephone call in a few days
         c. Rules governing cover letter and resume
            (1) Always use premium paper and matching envelopes
            (2) Check very carefully for typographical errors, including spelling and punctuation
            (3) Make sure the appropriate person at the prospective place of employment is addressed
            (4) Keep copies of all documents you send out and a list to whom they were sent
            (5) Do not include photographs or mention your race, color, creed, or political affiliation
            (6) Proofread all materials several times
      3. References
         a. Provided by former employers, college instructors, and clients (check with an individual before using them as a reference)

b. Provide prospective employers with a telephone number where a reference can be contacted
c. If a written reference is required, provide references with the correct address and background information

Interview

I. Provides a personal opportunity to impress a potential employer
II. Research your potential employer. Obtain
  A. Detailed job description
  B. Background on the business, including type of practice and number of owners
  C. Contact employees of the business and or company representatives
  D. Gather information from the Chamber of Commerce or a local newspaper on the community in which the business is located
  E. Make a list of questions you have about the job
  F. Estimate the wages you will need to earn (as indicated by your budget) to take the job
  G. Prepare a list of potential questions the interviewer may ask and format your responses
III. During the interview your objective is to gather information, as well as provide the potential employer with knowledge about you
  A. In less than 10 seconds you will make a first impression on the interviewer, and in less than 4 minutes the interviewer will acquire a lasting impression of you
  B. Personal appearance for the interview is very important
    1. Your appearance should convey a clean, conservative, and professional person
  C. Be punctual
  D. Relax
  E. Listen to and answer questions carefully
  F. Ask questions you have about the potential employment
  G. Stress your strengths as well as what you can offer
  H. Encourage the employer to make you an offer. A decision can be made later on whether to accept or not
IV. Certain questions do not have to be answered during an interview. These involve marital status, child care, plans for having a family, arrest record, and age
  A. These are questions that can be construed as prejudicial
V. Be prepared to negotiate salary and benefit packages
  A. Best to have offer presented in writing
  B. Consider the entire package, not just salary
    1. A lower salary with health insurance, life insurance, and paid vacation may be better
  C. Benefits are a vital portion of any job offer and add to value of the job. Benefits that may be offered include, but are not limited to
    1. Health insurance/dental insurance
    2. Life insurance
    3. Bonuses
    4. Discounted pet care and uniforms
    5. Paid vacation
    6. Paid sick days
    7. Expenses for continuing education, including registration, time off, travel, lodging, and per diem expenses
    8. Professional association dues
VI. It is important to personally thank each person who was involved in your interview process at the conclusion of the interview
  A. The thank you may also be sent in writing 24 hours after the interview is complete
VII. Wait at least 1 day before accepting any offer to allow time to compare all propositions

PROFESSIONAL OBLIGATIONS

I. Definitions
  A. Profession: a vocation or occupation requiring advanced education and training, and involving intellectual skills
  B. Professional: engaged in or worthy of the high standards of a profession

Professional Organizations (see Appendix F)

Professional organizations for veterinary technicians provide members with the opportunity for career advancement by supporting groups who work to advance the entire profession.

I. During their careers, technicians have obligations to their profession and professional organization, as well as to themselves
II. National/international organizations
  A. Organizations that deal with issues affecting a broad range of topics, including public image of the veterinary technician, laws and legislation governing the profession, and effective use of the veterinary technician within the veterinary health care team
  B. These organizations actively interact with other organizations, looking for ways that a collaborative effort might benefit the entire health care team
    1. Career building and professionalism are important goals of these types of associations
III. State/provincial/local organizations

A. Provide members with information pertinent to the profession on a local level
B. Become actively involved in laws pertinent to their specific location, providing information to residents of their area and updating members on local issues

Community Involvement

The veterinary technician has an obligation to provide information about his or her career to the general public, coworkers, and peers as a means of promoting the profession and their own career.

Professionalism

Professionalism includes demeanor, appearance at work and in the community, and ethics.

I. The perception of the entire profession can be affected
II. Key components of professionalism
  A. Demeanor: outward behavior or conduct should always reflect positively on you, your employer, and the profession
    1. A professional will always project a proper image to those around them
III. Dress: clothing, hairstyle, jewelry, etc. worn during the workday and in the community reflect a person's level of professionalism
  A. Workplace: clothing should be appropriate for the job
    1. Uniforms with a name tag identifying you as a veterinary technician are appropriate for a practice setting
      a. The uniforms should be changed if soiled
    2. Business casual clothing is most appropriate for continuing education seminars, workshops, or presentations
      a. T-shirts, jeans, and shorts are generally not acceptable and do not portray a sense of professionalism
  B. Speech: words used to communicate with the public, clients, co-workers, and even patients reflect a level of professionalism
    1. Avoid personal problems, gossip, health, controversial social issues, politics, religion, sex, and slang phrases
    2. Maintaining confidentiality is essential when dealing with business matters. Office situations, clients, and their pets should not be discussed socially or in the presence of the general public
    3. Jokes and terminology that may be offensive to those of a certain sex, physical appearance, or ethnic origin should be avoided
  C. Ethics: rules established by organizations to set guidelines for and influence behavior and actions of the group
    1. As legal agents for veterinary employers, technicians must "accept [their] obligations to practice [their] profession conscientiously and with sensitivity, adhering to the profession's Code of Ethics" (from the North American Veterinary Technician Association [NAVTA]) (see Chapter 30)
      a. Veterinarians are held liable for the actions of veterinary technicians
    2. Veterinary technicians are under supervision and control of a veterinarian and must never engage in practices reserved for the veterinarian
      a. These include diagnosing, prognosing, performing surgery, and prescribing medication
      b. Technicians must never complain about veterinarians or other employees to or in the presence of a client
    3. As professionals the actions of technicians must be based on the best interests of patients and clients
    4. The veterinary technician code of ethics
      a. Communicates the profession's ideals to the public and members of the profession
      b. Is a general guide for professional ethical conduct
      c. Provides disciplinary procedures to members who are not operating at an acceptable level of conduct

Education

The veterinary technician has an obligation to remain current and up to date on technical information that pertains to the job. This involves a commitment to continuing education and lifelong learning and may even require higher-level education for advancement.

I. Continuing education comes in various forms, including advanced, review, and new information
  A. Registration requirements in certain areas demand proof of attendance
  B. Lifelong learning shows a commitment to growth
II. Advanced degrees
  A. Most veterinary technicians' education consists of a 2-year program in the field of veterinary technology
  B. As career plans change and job opportunities become available a bachelors or masters degree may become important
  C. Investigate all options for degrees, including those offered through computer access and

special programs set up for the employed adult learner

MARKETING

I. Definition: communication to others about goods or services that are offered
   A. In veterinary medicine, marketing is the process of educating the client/public on services that can be provided for quality care
   B. Marketing consists of all activities employed to promote goods and services
   C. Veterinary technicians have an important role in these activities
   D. Marketing in a veterinary hospital can be divided into two distinctly different areas: internal marketing and external marketing

Internal Marketing

The process of marketing veterinary services to clients and potential clients. The following are areas of the veterinary hospital suited to internal marketing.

I. Outward appearances: the initial visual image that a client/potential client sees when approaching and entering the veterinary hospital
   A. Exterior of building, parking lot, and grounds should all be well kept
   B. First impressions of the inside of the building and waiting room are important, including cleanliness and freedom from odor
   C. Consider equipment, including availability of modern equipment and computers
   D. Professional appearing staff, clean uniforms, name tags
   E. A sense of order
II. A caring attitude should be displayed by ALL staff members at all times
   A. The staff should be positive and enthusiastic and not display anger or dissatisfaction with their jobs
III. Client needs must be evaluated in any marketing plan, consider
   A. Location of the practice
      1. Clients in rural areas will require different services than those in a strictly urban environment
         a. Goods and services should be provided accordingly
   B. The time commitment made by your client in coming to your practice. Do not minimize
      1. Today's consumer should be greeted with fast, courteous service
   C. Conveying the importance of clients and their pets will make them more eager to return to your practice for future veterinary care
   D. Client needs can be evaluated by focus groups, questionnaires, and listening to complaints
IV. Marketing tangible products to the client can be done most effectively by identifying a need of a client and/or pet and finding a product within the hospital to fill it
   A. The veterinary technician must be knowledgeable about the products being sold to clients
   B. Improper information about a product can be hazardous to the pet and to the confidence the client has in the practice
   C. The veterinary/client/patient relationship must be considered when dispensing products
      1. This relationship means the client's animal has had contact with the veterinarian within a specified period of time
   D. Over-the-counter products versus professional products should be handled accordingly
V. Tangible items that can be used to market goods or services include
   A. Client reminders—a simple postcard reminder to the client of routine vaccinations and dental and heartworm checks can go a long way to keeping clients coming back year after year. This is also seen as an extension of the caring veterinary hospital
   B. Commercial handouts—many companies provide materials that are available to describe their product and its benefits to the client and pet when used
      1. These materials provide excellent marketing of goods without expense of preparation
   C. Practice newsletters and health bulletins keep the client in contact with the practice throughout the year
      1. They can provide valuable information on seasonal needs of pets, special promotions being run by the practice, and updates on new or common diseases
      2. All newsletters must clearly indicate the hospital, be printed in a professional appropriate manner, and be free of typographical errors
   D. Sympathy communication—a very personal and caring message is sent (through a card or letter from the practice staff) when client's grief at the loss of a pet is recognized
   E. Sales point displays—often corporations will provide displays for their products for use in the clinic's waiting area
      1. Display products in a visually appealing manner
      2. Only use such displays for marketable products

F. Animal care talks—the practice that provides puppy and kitten talks, behavior classes, etc. has opened another avenue for marketing its goods and services and for showing care

VI. Intangible items such as services cannot be overlooked even though results are not often visually beneficial. Preventive health care programs fall into this category and may or may not be equated with veterinary care

External Marketing

External marketing activities are aimed at expanding current client activity within the practice and increasing the exposure of goods and services to those who are currently not clients.

I. External marketing usually involves advertising and can be done in some of the following ways
   A. External visual signs promoting the practice include use of hospital signs and distribution of business cards for the veterinarian and the veterinary technician
   B. Media routes for advertising services include telephone directories, newspaper articles or advertisements, and radio and television commercials
   C. Direct mail provides information to a targeted audience via the postal service
      1. Primarily to acquaint nonclients with services

II. Community activities can be seen as gestures of good will and can be accomplished by talking to community groups about good quality pet care, by promoting the veterinary technology profession, and by participating in community service such as volunteering to judge children's animal projects at a local fair
   A. The veterinarian and the veterinary technician should volunteer their expertise to the community

Glossary

accounts payable Money owed by one business to another

accounts receivable Money owed to a business, usually owed by the clients

burnout State of emotional, mental, and physical exhaustion in response to prolonged stress

career development Planned approach to achieving growth and satisfaction in work experiences

chronological resume Job resume that presents education, work experience, interests, and accomplishments in reverse chronological order

communication Sending, receiving, and interpretation of messages

conflict Situation in which there is disagreement, incompatibility, or mutual exclusiveness

counseling Formal discussion method, usually with a professional, in which an individual is encouraged to overcome a problem or improve his or her potential

ethics Rules established by an organization to influence actions and behaviors of the group, not enforced in a court of law

eustress Positive or good stress that rejuvenates, excites, or stimulates an individual

fight-or-flight response Body's physiological and chemical response to stressors in which the individual attempts to avoid or cope with the situation

functional resume One that organizes skills and accomplishments into the functions or tasks required for the position sought

relaxation response Lowered metabolism, heart rate, respiration, and blood pressure

stress Body's response to stressors that threaten to disturb homeostatic state

stressor Anything that causes stress

win-win conflict resolution A method of resolving conflict whereby both sides gain something of value

Review Questions

1 Feedback is from the receiver and allows the sender to
   a. Interpret the message
   b. Interpret the interference
   c. Understand how much of the message is comprehended
   d. Understand the receiver's message

2 Body language does not include
   a. A handshake
   b. Direct eye contact
   c. Slouched posture or upright posture
   d. A kind word in a low voice

3 "Good" communication techniques include all of the following skills except
   a. Concentrating on the message
   b. Processing the information too rapidly
   c. Providing feedback
   d. Avoiding judgment of the message sender

4 The six stages of grief a client may experience are
   a. Denial, bargaining, anger, depression, blame, and celebration
   b. Denial, bargaining, anger, guilt, depression, and resolution
   c. Anger, violence, sadness, bargaining, grief, and depression
   d. Anger, sadness, grief, resolution, celebration, and guilt

5 Which of the following actions diminishes a successful resolution of a problem with a staff member?
   a. A staff meeting
   b. Waiting 2 months before talking about the problem
   c. Allowing all parties to express opinions
   d. A written grievance filed with the manager

6 All of the following techniques may be used to increase a veterinary technician's time management abilities except
   a. Make a daily list of jobs to do
   b. Establish priorities
   c. Learn to say "no" to your employer
   d. Procrastinate less and meet deadlines more

7 The best personal reference for a potential position in a large progressive veterinary practice is
   a. Your childhood neighbor
   b. Your family physician
   c. Your college instructor
   d. A former client, whom you have not seen in 2 years

8 An example of a tangible internal marketing tool is
   a. An advertisement in the telephone directory
   b. An announcement of a new practice in the area
   c. A sympathy card to a client who recently lost a pet
   d. A visit to the local primary school

9 A message sent in a loud voice indicates
   a. Tension
   b. Insecurity
   c. Enthusiasm
   d. All of the above

10 The area of personal space or "comfort zone"
   a. Depends on personal preference
   b. Is approximately 4 to 6 m (13 to 19 ft)
   c. Is approximately 46 cm to 1.2 m (18 inches to 4 ft)
   d. Depends on gender of the individual

BIBLIOGRAPHY

Brock SL: *Better business writing,* Los Altos, CA, 1988, Crisp Publications.

Brounstein M: *Communicating effectively for dummies,* New York, 2001, Hungry Minds, Inc.

Dessler G: *Personnel/human resource management,* ed 8, Englewood Cliffs, NJ, 2000, Prentice-Hall.

Dubrin A: *Human relations for career and personal success,* ed 4, Englewood Cliffs, NJ, 1995, Prentice-Hall.

Haynes ME: *Personal time management,* Los Altos, CA, 1987, Crisp Publications.

McCurnin D: *Clinical textbook for veterinary technicians,* ed 5, Philadelphia, 2002, WB Saunders.

Perreault WD: *Basic marketing,* ed 13, Boston, 2000, Irwin.

Pratt PW: *Principles and practice of veterinary technology,* St Louis, 1998, Mosby.

Quible ZK: *Administrative office management,* ed 7, Englewood Cliffs, NJ, 2000, Prentice-Hall.

Rosenberg MA: *Companion animal loss and pet owner grief,* ed 2, Lehigh Valley, PA, 1993, Alpo Pet Foods, Inc.

Tannenbaum J: *Veterinary ethics: animal welfare, client relations, competition and collegiality,* ed 2, St Louis, 1995, Mosby.

CHAPTER 30

Veterinary Technician Ethics

Julie Ovington

OUTLINE

LEARNING OUTCOMES

After reading this chapter you should be able to:

1. Define ethics.
2. Differentiate between professional and personal ethics.
3. Describe why there is a need for professional ethics.
4. Define the benefits that ethics impart to a profession.
5. List the components of a code of ethics.
6. Define the definition of a profession.
7. Describe the ethics of NAVTA and CAAHTT.
8. Define the purpose of a professional association.
9. Describe and understand the role of a veterinary technician.
10. Describe the role of the veterinary state boards in veterinary technology.

HISTORY OF ETHICS

I. The word "ethics" comes from the Greek word *ethos,* which means "character"
   A. Philosophers such as Socrates, Plato, and Aristotle espoused on moral ethics, based on a man's experience and education
      1. Socrates initiated the need for definitions of "courage," "justice," "law," and "government" before we could be called good citizens
      2. Since these times social ethics or values have become very diverse based on geography and social history, including traditions and the church
      3. These morals are the principles that govern our view of "right" and "wrong"

II. The ethics that are outlined in this chapter are the study of the principles of right and wrong as they apply to our profession

PROFESSIONAL ETHICS

I. There are a number of reasons as to why a profession should have a code of ethics
   A. There are ethical expectations from employers, clients, and co-workers
   B. Members of a profession perform a special function in society
      1. That function involves special education, situations, and decisions that not all people face
      2. In most societies, it is assumed that the people in a profession understand the ethical issues that they come in contact with and can therefore construct their own rules, standards, and bylaws
   C. A code of ethics establishes a framework of professional behavior and responsibilities
      1. It promotes high standards of practice and provides a benchmark for individual evaluation
   D. Professional ethics is the middle ground between moral ethics, which each person holds

as an individual, and the social ethics, which are expected by society as a whole

1. With autonomy it is important that members of the profession maintain records and regulate themselves in a way that meets with the understanding of society
2. This is especially important with the social concern regarding the treatment of animals

E. The establishment of a code of ethics for a profession can also mark the maturity of the profession

1. The development of the ethics includes having a large number of people think through their mission and obligations as a group and as individuals with respect to society

II. A code of ethics will often have two components

A. The ideals of the organization

B. The rules or principles, which the members of the organization or profession are expected to follow

III. Ethics can also be outlined as a statement of values, a policy, or a mission statement (Box 30-1)

A. The mission statement for the National Association of Veterinary Technicians of America (NAVTA) is "Connecting veterinary technicians to one another and the profession to the world"

B. The mission statement of the Canadian Association of Veterinary Technologists and Technicians (CAAHTT) is "Dedicated to fulfilling the goal of professional recognition nationally and internationally through communication, direction, and support of the provincial AHT/VT associations"

IV. Once the professional ethics have been approved and documented, it is important to have a way to present this information and ensure it is made public both internally and externally

A. It is also important that the code of ethics values be included in the organization's policies and reviewed and revised as required by the organization

B. It is also important to define a method to enforce the code of ethics and to describe the possible results of noncompliance

Box 30-1 Professional Ethics

NATIONAL ASSOCIATION OF VETERINARY TECHNICIANS IN AMERICA (NAVTA)

CODE OF ETHICS

Veterinary Technicians shall

- Aid society and animals through providing excellent care and services for animals
- Prevent and relieve the suffering of animals
- Promote public health by assisting with the control of zoonotic diseases and informing the public about these diseases
- Assume accountability for individual professional actions and judgments
- Protect confidential information provided by clients
- Safeguard the public and the profession against individuals deficient in professional competence or ethics
- Assist with efforts to ensure conditions of employment consistent with the excellent care of animals
- Remain competent in veterinary technology through a commitment to lifelong learning
- Collaborate with members of the veterinary medical profession in an effort to ensure quality health care services for all animals

From NAVTA 2001 Resource Guide.

PROFESSIONAL ASSOCIATIONS

I. In the preamble to the Code of Ethics of NAVTA, it is stated that "Veterinary Technology includes the promotion and maintenance of good health in animals, the control of diseased and injured animals, and the control of diseases transmissible from animals to man"

A. Although a code of ethics can help with professional identity and form a foundation for an organization, there are still many other purposes and characteristics of a professional organization

1. NAVTA has stated that the association's purpose is to represent and promote the profession of veterinary technology; provide direction, education, support, and coordination for its members; and work with other allied professional organizations for the competent care and humane treatment of animals
2. The objectives of the CAAHTT are similar to those of NAVTA with the addition of promoting greater communication nationally and internationally, through direction and support of the provincial AHT/VT associations
3. Professional associations can begin to govern their members through the ethics and purpose of the association

VETERINARY TECHNOLOGY AS A PROFESSION

With the definition of the profession, there also needs to be a definition of the professional (Box 30-2).

I. This definition is based on both the description of the professional role and what is required to achieve the status of the profession

A. As a description of the role, the Ontario Association of Veterinary Technicians (OAVT) has stated that "Veterinary Technicians are

Box 30-2 Veterinary Technology as a Profession

The definition of a profession from Webster's Dictionary is "A calling requiring specialized knowledge and often long and intensive preparation including instruction in skills and methods as well as in the scientific, historical or scholarly principals underlying such skills and methods, maintaining by force of organization or concerted opinion high standards of achievement and conduct and committing its members to continued study and to a kind of work which has for its prime purpose the rendering of a public service."

From Webster's Third New International Dictionary.

Box 30-3 Accomplishments of Veterinary Technology

THE CANADIAN ASSOCIATION OF VETERINARY TECHNOLOGISTS AND TECHNICIANS

The objects of the Corporation are to:

- Establish and maintain a national standard of membership
- Promote and assist in continuing education for AHT/VTs
- Promote greater communication nationwide
- Promote the profession of AHT/VT within the animal health community and to the general public
- Be a resource regarding national and international issues

specifically trained professionals who work as an integral part of the veterinary medical team, to provide humane quality animal health care"

B. NAVTA further defines this role: "The Veterinary Technician/Technologist is educated to be the veterinarian's nurse, laboratory technician, radiography technician, anesthetist, surgical nurse and client educator." With this must also come the requirements to fulfill the role. In both statements, the words "trained" and "educated" lead the definition

II. In the United States, a veterinary technician is a graduate of a 2-year, American Veterinary Medical Association (AVMA–accredited program from a community college, college, or university)

A. A veterinary technologist is a graduate from an AVMA-accredited bachelor degree program

III. Almost every state requires a veterinary technician/technologist to pass a credentialing examination

A. The examination is a means to ensure the public that a veterinary technician has entry-level knowledge of the duties they are asked to perform in a veterinary clinic or hospital

ACCOMPLISHMENTS OF VETERINARY TECHNOLOGY

I. In the United States, the first formal academic program was started in 1961

II. "Animal technician" was the official title chosen to recognize graduates of an accredited program in 1967

A. The name was changed to "veterinary technician" in 1989 to recognize graduates of AVMA-recognized colleges

B. The first credentialing examination: the Veterinary Technician National Examination (VTNE) was administered by PES (Professional Examination Service) in 1978. The examination process was the responsibility of a committee of the American Veterinary Medical Association (AVMA) until 1995, when PES signed on with the American Association of Veterinary State Boards (AAVSB)

C. Continuing education programs for technicians have been available since the 1970s

D. Publications specific to technicians have been in print since the 1980s

III. The NAVTA Executive Board adopted a resolution in June 1993 declaring the third week in October as National Veterinary Technician Week (NVTW)

A. CAAHTT has also declared the third week of October as NVTW and continues to pursue an official proclamation

IV. In April 1970, a nucleus of Animal Health Technology graduates formed the Canadian Association of Animal Health Technicians (Box 30-3)

A. To incorporate their objects into a strong national body, representatives of the seven provincial associations founded the Canadian Association of Animal Health Technologists and Technicians (CAAHTT) in July 1989

B. In 1993 CAAHTT adopted reciprocity for the VTNE, through PES

V. In 1991 at Michigan State University, the North American Veterinary Technician Association was formed

VI. In January 2002, NAVTA changed their name to the National Association of Veterinary Technicians in America to delineate their focus

REGISTRATION, LICENSING, AND CERTIFICATION

I. In the United States, once a veterinary technician has passed the VTNE, he or she is then eligible to use one of the following designations

A. Licensed Veterinary Technician

B. Certified Veterinary Technician

C. Registered Veterinary Technician

D. The three designations, or licenses, are granted by a state agency or board

E. Each state has their own Veterinary Practice Act or rules of practice

1. Veterinary state boards write these rules and regulations
2. These regulations can include education, continuing education, and specific duties

F. At present, the following states do not have laws or regulations governing the registration of veterinary technicians
1. Delaware, District of Columbia, Hawaii, Idaho, Montana, New Hampshire, Puerto Rico, Rhode Island, Utah, Vermont, and Wyoming
2. In other states, such as California, Maryland, Michigan, Missouri, Nevada, New Mexico, New York, North Dakota, Ohio, Oregon, South Carolina, Tennessee, Virginia, Washington, and Wisconsin, tasks that can be performed only by registered, certified, or licensed technicians are identified and cannot be performed by other employees without veterinary supervision

G. Most states require a continuing education component to maintain credentialing

H. In Canada, "animal health technician" and "veterinary technician/technologist" are titles given to graduates of postsecondary programs, as approved by their provincial associations
1. To use the designation of "registered" with the graduate program title, the candidate must pass the VTNE, as well as meet any other requirements designated by the governing provincial association
2. One of these requirements may be a mandatory continuing education component to maintain registered status
   a. The Veterinary Technician National Examination (VTNE) is used by all Canadian provinces to designate "registered" status, which allows for reciprocity across Canada

I. The province of Ontario has a private members bill that restricts the use of the title "registered veterinary technician"

J. The provincial associations of Saskatchewan and Alberta are included in the provincial veterinarian's act
1. In these two provinces, a technician must be registered with the provincial association to be employed by a member of the respective veterinary associations

K. In Canada and the United States, a veterinary technician cannot perform a similar list of duties
1. The duties include diagnosing, providing a prognosis, prescribing medications or therapy, and performing major surgery

SUMMARY

I. There has been much growth and accomplishment in the field of veterinary technology
   A. It started with common goals and mission statements and the development of a code of ethics to provide a solid foundation for the profession and to continue the establishment of specialty organizations within the profession
   B. There are still many areas in which the profession can continue to expand, including continuity within the profession from state to state and internationally, improvements to self-regulation, and a clear definition of the role of veterinary technicians in practice
   C. Through participation in provincial or state professional organizations, maintaining a high quality of education, pursuing an ongoing firm belief in the goals and ethics of the profession, and continuing to improve relationships between associations and related professions, many more accomplishments will be possible in the future

BIBLIOGRAPHY

MacDonald C: www.ethicsweb.ca (accessed August 27, 2002).
Rollin BE: *Veterinary ethics, social ethics and animal welfare,* Colorado State University, 1999, OAVT Conference Proceedings.

APPENDIX A

Abbreviations and Symbols

A

Å Angstrom unit; anode; anterior
a Ampere; anterior; area; artery
āā Of each
AAHA American Animal Hospital Association
AALAS American Association for Laboratory Animal Science
AAVSB American Association of Veterinary State Boards
ab Antibody
A_2 Aortic second sound
ABO Three basic human blood groups
AC Alternating current; adrenal cortex
a.c. Before meals *(ante cibum)*
ACE Adrenocortical extract
ACh Acetylcholine
ACH Adrenocortical hormone
ACTH adrenocorticotropic hormone
ACTTSA Association Canadienne des Techniciens et Technologistes en Santé Animale
AD Right ear
ad lib As much as desired *(ad libitum)*
ADH Antidiuretic hormone
A/G; A-G ratio Albumin-globulin ratio
Ag Silver
ag Antigen
AHT Animal Health Technician
AIDS Acquired immune deficiency syndrome
AKC American Kennel Club
AL Left ear
Al Aluminum
ALAT Assistant Laboratory Animal Technician
Alb Albumin
ALT Alanine aminotransferase (formerly SGPT)
AMA American Medical Association
AMI Acute myocardial infarction
amp Ampere
ana So much of each, or āā
anat Anatomy or anatomic
ANS Autonomic nervous system
A-P; AP; A/P Anteroposterior
A.P. Anterior pituitary gland
APHIS Animal and Plant Health Inspection Service
Aq Water *(aqua)*
ARD Acute respiratory disease
As Arsenic
ASD Atrial septal defect
AST Aspartate aminotransferase (formerly SGOT)
AU Both (left and right) ears
Au Gold
A-V; AV; A/V Arteriovenous; atrioventricular
Av Average *(avoirdupois)*
AVECCT Academy of Veterinary Emergency Critical Care Technicians
AVMA American Veterinary Medical Association
AVTA Academy of Veterinary Technician Anesthetists
ax Axis

B

B Boron; bacillus
Ba Barium
Bact Bacterium
BBB Blood-brain barrier
BE Barium enema
Be Beryllium
BER Basal energy requirement
Bi Bismuth
bid; b.i.d. Twice a day *(bis in die)*
BM Bowel movement
BMR Basal metabolic rate
BP Blood pressure
bp Boiling point
BPH Benign prostatic hypertrophy
BSA Body surface area
BSP Bromsulphalein
BUN Blood urea nitrogen
BVD Bovine virus diarrhea
BW Body weight

C

C Carbon; centigrade; Celsius
c̄ With
Ca Calcium; cancer; cathode
CAAHTT Canadian Association of Animal Health Technologists and Technicians
$CaCO_3$ Calcium carbonate
Cal Large calorie
cal Small calorie
CALAS Canadian Association for Laboratory Animal Science
CBC; cbc Complete blood count
cc Cubic centimeter
CCl_4 Carbon tetrachloride
CD Canine distemper
CDCP Centers for Disease Control and Prevention
cf Compare or bring together
CFT Complement-fixation test
cg; cgm Centigram
$CHCl_3$ Chloroform
CH_3COOH Acetic acid
CHD Canine hip dysplasia
ChE Cholinesterase
CHF Congestive heart failure
$C_5H_4N_4O_3$ Uric acid

C_2H_5OH Ethyl alcohol
CH_2O Formaldehyde
CH_3OH Methyl alcohol
CKC Canadian Kennel Club
Cl Chlorine
cm Centimeter
CMT California Mastitis Test
CNS Central nervous system
CO Carbon monoxide
CO_2 Carbon dioxide
Co Cobalt
CPC Clinicopathologic conference
CRF Chronic renal failure
CRT Capillary refill time
C&S Culture and sensitivity
CSF Cerebrospinal fluid
CT; CAT Computed (axial) tomography
Cu Copper
$CuSO_4$ Copper sulfate
CVA Cerebrovascular accident
CVMA Canadian Veterinary Medical Association
CVP Central venous pressure
CVT Certified Veterinary Technician
CVTS Committee on Veterinary Technician Specialties

D

D Dose; vitamin D; right *(dextro)*
DC Direct current
DCA Deoxycorticosterone acetate
DEA Drug Enforcement Agency; dog erythrocyte antigen
Deg Degeneration; degree
DES Diethylstilbestrol
dg Decigram
diff Differential blood count
dil Dilute
dimone Half
DJD Degenerative joint disease
DLH Domestic longhair (cat)
DNA Deoxyribonucleic acid
DOA Dead on arrival
D/S Dextrose in saline
DSH Domestic shorthair (cat)
DVM Doctor of Veterinary Medicine
D_x Diagnosis

E

E Eye
ECC Emergency and critical care
ECG Electrocardiogram; electrocardiograph
ED Effective dose
ED_{50} Median effective dose
EDTA Ethylenediamine tetraacetic acid
EEG Electroencephalogram; electroencephalograph
EENT Eye, ear, nose, and throat
EFA Essential fatty acid
EIA Equine infectious anemia; enzyme immunoassay
EKG Electrocardiogram; electrocardiograph
ELISA Enzyme-linked immunosorbent assay
EMB Eosin-methylene blue
EMC Encephalomyocarditis
EMG Electromyogram
EMS Emergency medical services
ENT Ear, nose, and throat
ER Emergency room (hospital); external resistance
ESR Erythrocyte sedimentation rate
ext Extract

F

F Fahrenheit; formula
FA Fatty acid
FANA Fluorescent antinuclear antibody test
F&R Force and rhythm (pulse)
FB Foreign body
FBS Fasting blood sugar
FD Fatal dose
FDA Food and Drug Administration
Fe Iron
$FeCl_3$ Ferric chloride
FeLV Feline leukemia virus
FFD Film Focal Distance
FIP Feline infectious peritonitis
FIV Feline immunodeficiency virus
Fl Fluid
fld Fluid
fl oz; fl.oz. Fluid ounce
FLUTD Feline lower urinary tract disease
FPV Feline panleukopenia virus
FR Flocculation reaction
FSH Follicle-stimulating hormone
ft Foot
FUO Fever of undetermined origin
FUS Feline urological syndrome
Fx Fracture

G

g Gram
gal Gallon
Galv Galvanic
GB Gallbladder
GBS Gallbladder series
GDV Gastric dilatation volvulus
GFR Glomerular filtration rate
GH Growth hormone
GI Gastrointestinal
GLPs Good laboratory practices
Gm; gm; g Gram
GnRH Gonadotrophin-releasing hormone
GP General practitioner; general paresis
gr Grain(s)
GSW Gunshot wound
gt Drop *(gutta)*
GTT Glucose tolerance test
gtt Drops *(guttae)*
GU Genitourinary
Gyn Gynecology

H

h Hour
H Hydrogen
H^+ Hydrogen ion

H_x History
H&E Hematoxylin and eosin stain
Hb; Hgb Hemoglobin
HBC Hit by car
H_3BO_3 Boric acid
HC Health certificate
HCG Human chorionic gonadotropin
HCl Hydrochloric acid
HCN Hydrocyanic acid
H_2CO_3 Carbonic acid
HCT; Hct Hematocrit
HDL High-density lipoprotein
H of A Health of Animals
He Helium
Hg Mercury
HNO_3 Nitric acid
H_2O Water
H_2O_2 Hydrogen peroxide
HR Heart rate
hs At bedtime *(hora somni)*
H_2SO_4 Sulfuric acid

I

I Iodine
^{131}I Radioactive isotope of iodine (atomic weight 131)
^{132}I Radioactive isotope of iodine (atomic weight 132)
IB Inclusion body
IBR Infectious bovine rhinotracheitis
IC Intracardiac
ICF Intracellular fluid
ICH Infectious canine hepatitis
ICS; IS Intercostal space
ICSH Interstitial cell-stimulating hormone
ICU Intensive care unit
id The same *(idem)*
ID Intradermal
IM Intramuscular
IOP Intraocular pressure
IP Intraperitoneal
IT; i.t. Intratracheal
IU Immunizing unit; international unit
IV Intravenous
IVP Intravenous pyelogram
IVT Intravenous transfusion
IVU Intravenous urogram/urography

K

K_9 Canine
K Potassium
k Constant
Ka Cathode or kathode
KBr Potassium bromide
kc Kilocycle
kcal Kilocalorie
KCl Potassium chloride
kev Kiloelectron volts
Kg Kilogram
KI Potassium iodide
km Kilometer
KOH Potassium hydroxide
kV Kilovolt
kW Kilowatt

L

L Left; liter; length; lumbar; lethal
LAT Laboratory Animal Technician
LATG Laboratory Animal Technologist
lb Pound *(libra)*
LCM Left costal margin
LD Lethal dose
LD_{50} Median lethal dose
LDA Left displaced abomasum
LDL Low-density lipoprotein
LE Lupus erythematosus
LFD Least fatal dose of a toxin
LH Luteinizing hormone
Li Lithium
lig Ligament
Liq Liquor
LN Lymph node
LPF Leukocytosis-promoting factor
LRS Lactated Ringer's solution
LTH Leuteotrophic hormone
LV Left ventricle
LVT Licensed Veterinary Technician

M

M Muscle; thousand
m Meter; milli; thousand
μC Microcurie
mcg; μg Microgram
MCH Mean corpuscular hemoglobin
MCHC Mean corpuscular hemoglobin concentration
mCi; mc Millicurie
mcm; μm Micron
MCV Mean corpuscular volume
MCT Mast cell tumor
MED Minimal effective dose
MEq Milliequivalent
mEq/L Milliequivalent per liter
ME ratio Myeloid-erythroid ratio
Mg Magnesium
mg Milligram
MI Myocardial infarction; mitral insufficiency
MID Minimum infective dose
MIP Mare's immunological pregnancy test
ML Midline
mL; ml Milliliter
MLD Median or minimum lethal dose
MLV Modified live virus
MM Mucous membrane
mm Millimeter; muscles
mM Mol/L
mm Hg Millimeters of mercury
Mn Manganese
mN Millinormal
mol/liter Mole per liter
MRI Magnetic resonance imaging
MS Mitral stenosis; morphine sulfate
MT Medical Technologist
mu Mouse unit

N

N Nitrogen
n Normal
Na Sodium
NaBr Sodium bromide
NaCl Sodium chloride
$Na_2C_2O_4$ Sodium oxalate
Na_2CO_3 Sodium carbonate
NaF Sodium fluoride
$NaHCO_3$ Sodium bicarbonate
Na_2HPO_4 Sodium phosphate
NaI Sodium iodide
$NaNO_3$ Sodium nitrate
Na_2O_2 Sodium peroxide
NaOH Sodium hydroxide
Na_2SO_4 Sodium sulfate
NAVTA National Association of Veterinary Technicians in America
NAVTTC North American Veterinary Technician Testing Committee
NCC Nucleated cell count
Ne Neon
NH_3 Ammonia
Ni Nickel
NMR Nuclear magnetic resonance
non rep Do not repeat
NPL Nonpalpable lesion
NPN Nonprotein nitrogen
NPO; n.p.o. Nothing by mouth *(non per os)*
NR Not remarkable
NRBC Nucleated red blood cell
NS Normal saline
NSF No significant findings
NSR Normal sinus rhythm
NTP Normal temperature and pressure
NVL No visible lesions

O

O Oxygen; oculus
O_2 Oxygen
O_3 Ozone
OAVT Ontario Association of Veterinary Technicians
OBGYN Obstetrics and gynecology
OCD Osteochondritis dissecans
OD Right eye *(oculus dexter);* optical density; overdose
OFA Orthopedic Foundation for Animals
OHE Ovariohysterectomy
Ol Oil *(oleum)*
OR Operating room
OS Left eye *(oculus sinister)*
Os Osmium
OSA Osteosarcoma
OSHA Occupational Safety and Health Administration
OU Both eyes
oz Ounce

P

P Phosphorus; pulse; pupil
P_2 Pulmonic second sound
P-A; P/A; PA Posteroanterior
P&A Percussion and auscultation
PAB; PABA Para-aminobenzoic acid
PAC Premature atrial contraction
PAS; PASA Para-aminosalicylic acid
Pb Lead
PBI Protein-bound iodine
p.c. After meals *(post cibum)*
PCV Packed cell volume
PDA Patent ductus arteriosus
PDR *Physician's Desk Reference;* passive defense reflex
PE Physical examination; pulmonary edema
PEG Pneumoencephalography
per os Orally
PET Positron emission tomography
PFF Protein-free filtrate
PG Prostaglandin
PGA Pteroylglutamic acid (folic acid)
pH Hydrogen ion concentration (alkalinity and acidity measure)
Pharm; Phar. Pharmacy
PI Parainfluenza virus
PM Postmortem; evening
PMN Polymorphonuclear neutrophil
PMSG Pregnant mare serum gonadotrophin
PN Percussion note
PNS Parsympathetic nervous system
PO; p.o. Orally *(per os);* postoperatively
POVMR Problem-oriented veterinary medical records
PPB Parts per billion
PPD Purified protein derivative (TB test)
PPM Parts per million
PPV Porcine parvovirus
PRN; prn As required *(pro re nata)*
pro time Prothrombin time
PRRS Porcine reproductive and respiratory syndrome
PS Pulmonic stenosis
PSP Phenosulfonphthalein
Pt Platinum; patient
PT Pint
PTA Plasma thromboplastin antecedent
PTC Plasma thromboplastin component
PTH Parathyroid hormone
Pu Plutonium
PVC Premature ventricular contraction or complex
PZI Protamine zinc insulin

Q

QBC Quantitative buffy coat
q Every
qd Every day *(quaque die)*
qh Every hour *(quaque hora)*
qid; q.i.d. 4 times daily *(quater in die)*
ql As much as desired *(quantum libet)*
qns Quantity not sufficient
qod Every other day
q.p. As much as desired *(quantum placeat)*
qs Sufficient quantity
qt Quart
qv As much as you please *(quantum vis)*

R

R Respiration; right; *Rickettsia*; roentgen
R_x Take
Ra Radium
RAD Radiograph
rad Unit of measurement of the absorbed dose of ionizing radiation
RAI Radioactive iodine
RAIU Radioactive iodine uptake
RBC; rbc Red blood cell; red blood count
RDA Right displaced abomasum
RE Right eye; reticuloendothelial tissue or cell
Re Rhenium
Rect Rectified
Rep. Let it be repeated *(repetatur)*
RES Reticuloendothelial system
Rh Symbol of rhesus factor; rhodium
RHF Right heart failure
Rn Radon
RNA Ribonucleic acid
R/O Rule out
RPM; rpm Revolutions per minute
RT Radiation therapy
RVT Registered Veterinary Technician

S

S Sulfur
S. Sacral
s̄ Without *(sine)*
S-A; S/A; SA Sinoatrial
SD Skin dose
Se Selenium
Sed rate; SR Sedimentation rate
SGOT Serum glutamic oxaloacetic transaminase (see AST)
SGPT Serum glutamic pyruvic transaminase (see ALT)
Si Silicon
Sig Label; prescription
SMEDI Stillbirths, mummified, embryonic death infertility
Sn Tin
SNS Sympathetic nervous system
SOAP Subjective Objective Assessment Plan
Sol Solution
sp Species
Sp Spirit
sp. gr.; SG Specific gravity
SPCA Society for the Prevention of Cruelty to Animals
Sr Strontium
SR Suture removal
s̄s̄ One half *(semis)*
Staph *Staphylococcus*
Stat Immediately *(statum)*
STD Sexually transmitted disease
STH Somatotropic hormone
Strep *Streptococcus*
SVBT Society of Veterinary Behavior Technicians
Sx Sign or symptom
Sym Symmetrical

T

T Temperature; thoracic
t Temporal
T_3 Triiodothyronine
T_4 Thyroxine
tab Tablet
TAT Tetanus antitoxin
TB Tuberculin; tuberculosis; tubercle bacillus
TBW Total body water
TDN Total digestible nutrient
Te Tetanus
TGC Time gain compensation
TGE Transmissible gastroenteritis
Th Thorium
tid; t.i.d. 3 times daily *(ter in die)*
T-L Thoracolumbar vertebrae
Tl Thallium
TLC Tender loving care
TP Total protein
TPP Total plasma protein
TPR Temperature, pulse, and respiration
tr Tincture
TS Test solution
TSH Thyroid-stimulating hormone
TSI Triple sugar iron
TT Tetanus toxoid
Tx Treatment

U

U Uranium; unit
UA Urinalysis
ung Ointment *(unguentum)*
UO Urinary obstruction
URI Upper respiratory infection
US Ultrasonic
USDA United States Department of Agriculture
USP U.S. Pharmacopeia
Ut. dict. As directed *(ut dictum)*
UTI Urinary tract infection

V

v Vein
V Vanadium; vision
V Volt; vein
VC Vital capacity
VEE Venezuelan equine encephalomyelitis
VHD Valvular heart disease
VLDL Very low-density lipoprotein
VMD Veterinary Medical Doctor
VS Volumetric solution; vital signs
VSD Ventricular septal defect
VTA Veterinary Technician Anesthetist
VTNE Veterinary Technician National Examination
VTS Veterinary Technician Specialty
VW Vessel wall

W

w Watt
WBC; wbc White blood cell; white blood count
WEE Western equine encephalomyelitis
WL Wavelength
WNL Within normal limits
Wt; wt Weight

X

X-ray Roentgen ray
XRT Radiation therapy

Z

z Symbol for atomic number
Zn Zinc

Symbols

> greater than
< less than
♀ Female
♂ Male

APPENDIX B

The Metric System and Equivalents

The basis of measurement in science is the *Système International d'Unités* (SI), in which the main units are the meter, the gram, and the liter. Although the English system is still used in the United States, the metric system is the preferred system because of its logic and accuracy.

SI ABBREVIATIONS

The rules for writing metric units are (1) use lowercase letters for abbreviations, except for the symbol for liter (L) or if the units are named after a person; (2) symbols are never pluralized; and (3) decimals are used instead of fractions.

centimeter	cm
deciliter	dL
dekaliter	dkL
gram	g
hectoliter	hL
kilogram	kg
kilometer	km
liter	L
meter	m
microgram	mcg or μg
milliliter	mL
millimeter	mm

Units of Length

Given are metric linear decimal scale and English (U.S.) equivalents.

10 millimeters	=	1 centimeter	=	0.3937 inch
10 centimeters	=	1 decimeter	=	3.937 inches
10 decimeters	=	1 meter	=	39.37 inches (3.2808 feet)
10 meters	=	1 dekameter	=	10.936 yards
10 dekameters	=	1 hectometer	=	19.884 rods
10 hectometers	=	1 kilometer	=	0.62137 mile
10 kilometers	=	1 myriameter	=	6.2137 miles
1 inch	=	2.54 centimeters	or	25.4 millimeters
1 foot	=	3.048 decimeters	or	304.8 millimeters
1 yard	=	0.9144 meter	or	914.40 millimeters
1 rod	=	0.5029 dekameter		
1 mile	=	1.6093 kilometers		

Units of Weight

Given are metric weights and English (U.S.) equivalents.

1 milligram	=	0.001 gram	=	0.015 grain
1 centigram	=	0.01 gram	=	0.154 grain
1 decigram	=	0.10 gram	=	1.543 grains
1 gram	=	1 gram	=	0.035 ounce
1 dekagram	=	10 grams	=	0.353 ounce
1 hectogram	=	100 grams	=	3.527 ounces
1 kilogram	=	1000 grams	=	2.205 pounds
1 grain	=	0.0648 gram		
1 ounce	=	28.349 grams		
1 pound	=	0.453 kilogram		
To convert kg to lb:		lb = kg × 2.204		
To convert lb to kg:		kg = lb ÷ 2.204		

Units of Volume

Given as metric liquid measure capacity and English (U.S.) equivalents.

1 milliliter (cc)			=	16.23 minims or 0.0338 fluid ounce
1 liter			=	33.8148 fluid ounces or 2.1134 pints or 1.0567 quarts or 0.2642 gallon
1 teaspoon			=	5 mL
1 tablespoon			=	15 mL
1 fluid ounce			=	29.573 mL
1 pint	=	16 ounces	=	473.166 mL or 0.473 L
1 quart	=	2 pints	=	946.332 mL or 0.946 L
1 gallon	=	4 quarts	=	3.785 L

Temperature Equivalents

To convert Fahrenheit to Celsius: $^{\circ}C = {^{\circ}F} - 32 \times 5/9$

To convert Celsius to Fahrenheit: $^{\circ}F = {^{\circ}C} \times 9/5 + 32$

Other Equivalents

Freezing point: 0° C or 32° F at 1 atmospheric pressure

Boiling point: 100° C or 212° F at 1 atmospheric pressure

APPENDIX C

Medical Terminology

PREFIXES

a, ab, abs From; away; departing from the normal
ad Addition to; toward; nearness
amb, ambi Both; ambidextrous, having the ability to work effectively with either hand
amphi On both sides
ampho Both
an Negative; without or not
ana Upper, away from
andro Signifying man
angi Vessel
aniso Unequal
ant, anti Against
ante, antero Front; before
auto Self
bi Two
bili Pertaining to bile
brady Slow
brom, bromo A stench
broncho Relating to the bronchi
cac Bad, ill
cardi, cardio Relating to the heart
cata Down or downward
centi Hundred
cervico Relating to the neck
circa About
circum Around
co With or together
con Together with
contra Opposite; against
de Down from
deci One tenth
demi Half
di Twice
dia Through, apart, across or between
dialy To separate
dis Reversal, separation, duplication
dys Bad, difficult, disordered
en In
end, endo, ento Inward; within
ep, epi On; in addition to
eu Normal, good, well, easy
ex Out; away from
exo Without, outside of
extra Outside of; in addition to
fibro Relating to fibers
gaster, gastr, gastro Pertaining to the stomach
hecto Hundred
hemi Half
hemo Relating to the blood
hepat, hepatico, hepato Pertaining to the liver
heter, hetero Meaning other; relationship to another
homeo Denoting likeness or resemblance
homo Denoting sameness
hyal, hyalo Transparent
hyper Above; excessive; beyond
hypo Below; less than
ideo Pertaining to mental images
idio Denoting relationship to one's self or to something separate and distinct
in Not; in; inside; within; also intensive action
infra Below
inter In the midst; between
intra Within
intro In or into
iso Equal or alike
juxta Of close proximity
karyo Relating to a cell's nucleus
kilo One thousand
kypho Humped
laryngo Pertaining to the larynx
mal Illness, disease
medi Middle
micro Small
milli One thousandth
myelo Pertaining to the spinal cord or bone marrow
nano Dwarf, small size
oari, oaric Pertaining to the ovary
omni All
pan All
para Pair
per Through; by means of
peri Around; about
post Behind or after
postero Relating to the posterior
pre Before
pro Before, in front of
pseudo False
quadri Four
re Back; again (contrary)
retro Backward
semi Half
steato Fatty
sub Under; near
syn Joined together
trans Across; over
tri Three
un Not; reversal
uni One

SUFFIXES

able, ible, ble The power to be

ad Toward; in the direction of
aemia, emia Pertaining to blood
age Put in motion; to do
agra Denoting a seizure; severe pain
algia Denoting pain
ase Forms the name of an enzyme
blast Designates a cell or a structure
cele Denoting a swelling
centesis Denoting a puncture
ectasia Expansion, dilatation, distention
ectomy A cutting out
emia Condition of the blood
esthesia Denoting sensation
facient That which makes or causes
gene, genesis, genetic, genic Denoting production; origin
gog, gogue To make flow
gram A tracing; a mark
graph A writing; a record
iasis Denoting a condition or pathological state
id Denoting shape or resemblance
ism State, process or condition
ite Of the nature of
itis Denoting inflammation
logia Denoting discourse, science, or study of
lysis Dissolution
malacia Softening
megaly Enlargement
oid Denoting form or resemblance
oma Denoting a tumor
osis Denoting any morbid process
ostomosis, ostomy, stomy Denoting an outlet; to furnish with an opening or mouth
paresis Slight or incomplete paralysis
pathy Morbid condition or disease
penia Deficiency
pexy Surgical fixation
plasty Denoting molding or shaping
plegia Paralysis
rhagia Denoting a discharge; usually a bleeding
rhaphy Meaning suturing or stitching
rhea Meaning a flow or discharge
rrhexis Rupture of a blood vessel
scopy Generally an instrument for viewing
tomy Denoting a cutting operation
tripsy Crushing
trophy Denoting a relationship to nourishment

COMBINING FORMS

aer, aero Denoting air or gas
alge, algesi, algo Relating to pain
allo Other; differing from the normal
ankylo Bent, crooked, in the form of loop
anomalo Denoting irregularity
arthro Relating to a joint or joints
brevi Short
celio Denoting the abdomen
centro Center
cheil, cheilo Denoting the lip
chol, chole, cholo Relating to bile
chondr, chondri Relating to cartilage
chrom, chromo Relating to color
cole, coleo Denoting a sheath
colp, colpo Relating to the vagina
cranio Relating to the cranium of the skull
crymo, cryo Denoting cold
crypt To hide; a pit
cyano Dark blue
cyclo Pertaining to a cycle
cysto Relating to a sac or cyst
cyto Denoting a cell
dacryo Pertaining to the lacrimal glands
dactylo Relating to digits
dent, dento Relating to teeth
derma, dermat Relating to the skin
desmo Relating to a bond or ligament
dextro Right
diplo Double; twofold
dorsi, dorso Referring to the back
duodeno Relating to the duodenum
electro Relating to electricity
encephalo Denoting the brain
entero Relating to the intestines
episio Relating to the vulva
erythro Red, erythrocyte
eso Inward
esthesio Relating to feeling or sensation
facio Relating to the face
gangli, ganglio Relating to a ganglion
geno Relating to reproduction
gero, geronto Denoting old age
giganto Huge
gingivo Relating to the gingiva or gum
gloss, glosso Relating to the tongue
gluco Denoting sweetness
glyco Relating to sugar
gon Denoting a seed
grapho Denoting writing
hapt, hapte, hapto Relating to touch or a seizure
helo Relating to a nail or a callus
hist, histio, histo Relating to tissue
holo Relating to the whole
hydr, hydro Denoting water
hygro Denoting moisture
hyl, hyle, hylo Denoting matter or material
ileo, ilio Relating to the ileum
ipsi Meaning self
irido Relating to a colored circle
iso Equal
jejuno Referring to the jejunum
kerato Relating to the cornea
kino Denoting movement
labio Pertaining to the lips
lacto Relating to milk
laparo Pertaining to the loin or flank
latero Pertaining to the side
leido, leio Smooth
leuk, leuko Denoting deficiency of color
lip, lipo Pertaining to fat
litho Denoting a calculus
macr, macro Large; long

mast, mastro Relating to the breast
meg, mega Great; large
melano Black, melanin
meli Sweet
meningo Denoting membranes; covering the brain and spinal cord
micr, micro Small in size or extent
mono One
morpho Relating to form
multi Many
my, myo Relating to muscle
myc, mycet Denoting a fungus
myringo Denoting tympani or the eardrum
myx, myxo Pertaining to mucus
narco Denoting stupor
naso Relating to the nose
necro Denoting death
neo New
nephr, nephro Denoting the kidney
noci Harm, injury
normo Normal or usual
oculo Denoting the eye
odyno Denoting pain
oleo Denoting oil
onco Denoting a swelling or mass
onycho Relating to the nails
oo Denoting an egg
ophthal, ophthalmo Pertaining to the eye
opisth, opistho Backward
optico Relating to the eye or vision
orchi, orcho Relating to the testes
oro Relating to the mouth
ortho Straight; right
oscillo Denoting oscillation
osteo Relating to the bones
ot, oto Denoting an egg
palato Denoting the palate
patho Denoting disease
pedia, pedo Denoting a child
perineo A combining form for the region between the anus and scrotum or the vulva
phago Denoting a relationship to eating
pharyngo Pertaining to the pharynx
phleb, phlebo Denoting the veins
phon, phono Denoting sound
phot, photo Relating to light
phren Relating to the mind
picr, picro Bitter
pilo Denoting hair
plasmo Relating to plasma or the substance of a cell
pnea Respiration, breathing
pneuma, pneumono, pneumoto Denoting air or gas
pod, podo Meaning foot
poly Many
proct, procto Denoting the anus and rectum
psych, psycho Relating to the mind
ptyalo Denoting saliva
pubio, pubo Denoting the pubic region
pulmo Denoting the lung
pupillo Denoting the pupil
py, pyo Denoting pus
pyel, pyelo Denoting the pelvis
pyloro Relating to the pylorus
recto Denoting the rectum
rhin, rhino Denoting the nose
rrhagia Denoting abnormal discharge
salpingo Denoting a tube, specifically the fallopian tube
schizo Split
sclero Denoting hardness
scoto Relating to darkness
sero Pertaining to serum
sialo Relating to saliva or the salivary glands
sidero Denoting iron
sinistro Left
somato Denoting the body
somni Denoting sleep
spasmo Denoting a spasm
spermato, spermo Denoting sperm
sphero Denoting a sphere; round
sphygmo Denoting a pulse
splen, spleno Denoting the spleen
staphyl, staphylo Resembling a bunch of grapes
steno Narrow; short
sterco Denoting feces
steth, stetho Relating to the chest
stomato Denoting the mouth
sym, syn With; along
tacho, tachy Swift
tarso Relating to the flat of the foot
thermo Heat
thoraco Relating to the chest
thrombo Denoting a clot of blood
toxico, toxo Denoting poison
tracheo Denoting the trachea
trichi, tricho Denoting hair
ur, uro, urono Relating to urine
varico Denoting a twisting or swelling
vaso Denoting a vessel
veno Denoting a vein
ventri, ventro Denoting the abdomen
vertebro Relating to the vertebra
vesico Denoting the bladder
viscero Denoting the organs of the body
vivi Denoting alive
xantho Denoting yellow
xero Denoting dryness

TERMINOLOGY FREQUENTLY USED TO DESIGNATE BODY PARTS OR ORGANS

anus Anal, ano
arm Brachial, brachio
blood Heme, hemat
cheek Buccal
chest Thoracic, thorax
ear Auricle, oto
eye Ocular, oculo, ophthalmo
foot Pedal, ped, pod
gallbladder Chole, chol
head Cephalic, cephalo
heart Cardium, cardiac, cardio

intestines Cecum, colon, duodenum, ileum, jejunum
kidney Renal, nephric, nephro
lip Cheil, labia
liver Hepatic, hepato
lungs Pulmonary, pulmonic, pneumo
mouth Oral, os, stoma, stomat
muscle Myo
neck Cervix, cervical, cervico
penis Penile
rectum Rectal
skin Derma, integumentum
stomach Gastric, gastro
teeth Odonto, dento
testicle Orchio, orchi, orchido
tongue Lingua, glosso
urinary bladder Cysti, cysto
uterus Hystero, metra
vagina Vulvo, vaginal
viscera Splanchno, viscero

APPENDIX D

Species Names

Common name	Scientific name (generic)	Male/female terminology	Neutered male	Act of parturition	Young called
Cat	*Felis catus* (feline)	Tom/queen		Queening	Kitten
Cattle	*Bos taurus* *Bos indicus* (bovine)	Bull/cow	Steer	Calving	Calf
Chicken	*Gallus domesticus*	Rooster/hen	Capon	Laying/hatching	Chick
Chinchilla	*Chinchilla brevicaudata*	Male/female		Parturition	
Dog	*Canis familiaris* (canine)	Dog/bitch		Whelping	Puppy
Ferret	*Mustela putorius furo*	Hob/jill	Male: gib Female: sprite	Kindling	Kit
Gerbil (jird)	*Meriones unguiculatus*	Male/female		Parturition	Pup
Goat	*Capra hircus* (caprine)	Buck/doe	Wether	Kidding	Kid
Guinea pig (cavy)	*Cavia porcellus*	Boar/sow		Farrowing	Pup/piglet
Hamster	*Mesocricetus auratus*	Male/female		Parturition	Pup
Horse	*Equus caballus* (equine)	Stallion/mare	Gelding	Foaling	Foal (either sex) Colt (male) Filly (female)
Llama	*Llama glama*	Bull/cow	Gelding		Cria
Mouse	*Mus musculus*	Male/female		Parturition	Pup
Pig	*Sus scrofa* (porcine)	Boar/sow	Barrow	Farrowing	Piglet, pig
Rabbit	*Oryctolagus cuniculus*	Buck/doe	Lapin	Kindling	Bunny, nestling
Rat	*Rattus norvegicus*	Male/female		Parturition	Pup, nestling
Sheep	*Ovis aries* (ovine)	Ram/ewe	Wether	Lambing	Lamb

Modified from McBride DF: *Learning veterinary terminology*, St Louis, 1996, Mosby.

APPENDIX E

Normal Values

Species	Temperature °F	Temperature °C	Heart rate (beats/min)*	Respiratory rate (min*)	Onset of puberty (months)	Gestation (days)	Length of estrous cycle	Length of estrus
Feline	100.4 to 102.2	38 to 39	150 to 210	24 to 42	5 to 9	63 to 65	6 months	4 days
Canine	99.5 to 102.2	37.5 to 39	70 to 160	10 to 30	6 to 8	63 to 65	7 to 8 months	5 to 9 days
Equine	98.6 to 101.3	37.5 to 38.5	28 to 50	8 to 20	12 to 18	336	22 days	6 days
Porcine	100.4 to 104	38 to 40	58 to 100	8 to 18	5 to 7	114	21 days	48 to 55 hr
Bovine	100.4 to 102.2	38 to 39	40 to 80	12 to 36	9 to 10	285	21 days	18 to 24 hr
Ovine	100.4 to 104	39 to 40	60 to 120	12 to 72	6 to 7	148	17 days	10 to 30 hr
Caprine	101.3 to 104.9	38.5 to 40.5	40 to 60	12 to 20	3 to 7	149	21 days	40 hr

*These values are estimated for mature animals. In general, immature animals have slightly higher ranges for respiration and heart rate.

APPENDIX F

Additional Veterinary Technician Resources

STATE REPRESENTATIVES TO NATIONAL ASSOCIATION OF VETERINARY TECHNICIANS IN AMERICA

Alabama
Tammy Robinson
Alabama Vet. Tech. Assoc.
c/o Snead State CC
Drawer D
Boaz, AL 35957
trobison@snead.cc.al.us

Arkansas
Treva Lawson, CVT, LATG
Arkansas Vet. Tech. Assoc.
6707 Sayles Rd.
Jacksonville, AR 72076
lawsontreval@exchange.uams.edu

Arizona
Victoria Kasel, CVT
Vet. Tech. Assoc. of Arizona
9201 S. 157th Pl.
Gilbert, AZ 85234
vkasel@netscape.net

California
Cindy Alvaro
CVMA RVT Committee
230 Coy Dr. #1
San Jose, CA 95123

Connecticut
Kathy Loughman, CVT
Connecticut Assoc. of AHT
11 Hillside Dr.
East Longmeadow, MA 01028
Kloughman1@charter.net

Colorado
Tracy Wangler
Colorado Assoc. of CVT
325 E. 42nd St.
Loveland, CO 80538
deputy62@msn.com

Delaware
Patricia Kowal
121 Paladin Dr.
Wilmington, DE 19802
patricia.kowal@astrazeneca.com

Florida
Mike Patrick, CVT
1402 E. Mohawk Ave.
Tampa, FL 33604
mikecvt@pipeline.com

Iowa
Anne Conrad-Duffy, RVT
6301 Kirkwood Blvd. S.W.
Cedar Rapids, IA 52406
anneconradduffy@earthlink.net

Illinois
Crystal Brown, CVT
P.O. Box 198
Wapella, IL 61777
Critcvt@aol.com

Indiana
Jamie Schoenbeck, RVT
Lynn Hall, G-171
West Lafayette, IN 47907
jss@v.purdue.edu

Kansas
Lori Baney, BS, RVT, HT(ASCP)
Kansas Vet. Tech. Assoc.
1255 S. Range
Colby, KS 67701

Kentucky
Walter M Moore, LVT
Kentucky Vet. Tech. Assoc.
3350 Knox Ave.
Vine Groove, KY 40175-6156
mickmor@hotmail.com

Massachusetts
Christy J. Boris, CVT
Massachusetts Vet. Tech. Assoc.
272 Otter River Rd.
Templeton, MA 01468
cmboris@yahoo.com

Michigan
Matthew Mott, LVT
Michigan Assoc. of Vet. Tech.
5595 Galbraithline
Croswell, MI 48422

Minnesota
Korrine Rietfort, CVT
Minnesota Assoc. of Vet. Tech.
19 S.W. 9th Ave.
Faribault, MN 55021
korriner@hotmail.com

Missouri
Julie Holle
Missouri Vet. Tech. Assoc.
12050 Amber Ln.
Rocheport, MO 65279
hollej@missouri.edu

Mississippi
Fran Bernard
Mississippi Assoc. of CVT
3 Lakewood Ln.
Vicksburg, MS 39180
rsbernard1031@aol.com

Nebraska
Lisa Redington
Nebraska Vet. Tech. Assoc.
5522 N. 65th St.
Omaha, NE 68104

From National Association of Veterinary Technicians in America. P.O. Box 224, Battle Ground, IN 47920; Tel: 765-742-2216; Executive Director, A. Patrick Navarre, BS, RVT; Available at: http://www.navta.net

New Jersey
Robin Del Bove, RVT
New Jersey Vet. Tech. and Assist.
39 Park Ave.
Wyckoff, NJ 07481-3346
Rdelbove@aol.com

New Mexico
Lorraine Wyant
New Mexico Reg. Vet. Tech. Assoc.
6703 Prairie Rd. N.E. #723
Albuquerque, NM 87109
WyantL@express-scripts.com

New York
Kim Baldwin, LVT
New York State Assoc. of Vet. Tech.
220 Hulbert Hollow Rd.
Spencer, NY 14883
Kab28@cornell.edu

North Carolina
Meri Frances Winchester, RVT
NC Assoc. of Vet. Tech.
5017 Adder Ridge Ln.
Burlington, NC 27217
merwinch@aol.com

North Dakota
Lynn Bailey
North Dakota Vet. Tech. Assoc.
1064 E. Main
Valley City, ND 58072

Ohio
Linda Jackson, RVT
Ohio Vet. Tech. Assoc.
5969 Richardson Rd.
Conneaut, OH 44030-9733

Oklahoma
Dana Call, CVT
Oklahoma Vet. Tech. Assoc.
13160 Eastridge Dr.
Oklahoma City, OK 73170
calld@osuokc.edu

Oregon
Shireen L. Murphy
6909 Henley Rd.
Klamath Falls, OR 97603
CowTrukz@aol.com

Pennsylvania
Joy Ellwanger
437 S. Plum St.
Mount Joy, PA 17552
jle9@psu.edu

South Carolina
Janice D. Parler, RVT
907 Greenmeadow Dr.
Chapin, SC 29036
jparler@newberry.edu

South Dakota
Dennis Lively, RVT
South Dakota Assoc. of Vet. Tech.
P.O. Box 2517
Rapid City, SD 57709-2517
Dlively@rapidnet.com

Tennessee
Deanna Bayless, BS, LVT
Tennessee Vet. Tech. Assoc.
86 Henry Bayless Rd.
Ardmore, TN 38499

Texas
Renee Thornton
Texas Vet. Tech. Assoc
12807 Aste Ln.
Houston, TX 77065

Vermont
Debbie Danforth
Vermont Assoc. of Vet. Tech.
21 Village Dr.
Milton, VT 05468
duck4th@aol.com

Virginia
Melanie S. Yurczak, LVT, VDT
Virginia Assoc. of LVT
4916 Cliffony Dr.
Virginia Beach, VA 23464

Washington
Cindy Polley, RVT
WA State Assoc. of VT
209303 Bryson Brown Rd.
Kennewick, WA 99337

Wisconsin
Tamara Brantley, CVT
Wisconsin Vet.Tech. Assoc.
2817 Curry Pkwy. #D
Madison, WI 53713
Brantley@chorus.net

Wyoming
Donna Jeane Hansen
Wyoming Vet. Tech. Assoc.
15205 W. Poison Spider Rd.
Casper, WY 82604

AMERICAN STATE VETERINARY TECHNICIAN ASSOCIATIONS

Veterinary Technician Association of Arizona
http://www.geocities.com/vtaaz/

California Veterinary Technicians—California Veterinary Medical Association
http://www.cvma.org/doc.asp?ID=508

Colorado Association of Veterinary Technicians
http://www.cacvt.com

Florida Veterinary Technician Association
http://www.fvta.net

New York State Association of Veterinary Technicians
http://nysavt.org

North Carolina Veterinary Technician Association
http://triangle.citysearch.com/E/V/RDUNC/2010/47/99/3.html

North Dakota Veterinary Technician Association
http://www.ndsu.nodak.edu/instruct/devold/vetmicro/ndvta.htm

North Valley Veterinary Technician Association
http://www.angelfire.com/ca/nvvta/

Veterinary Technician Community at the Texas A and M University,
College of Veterinary Medicine and Veterinary Teaching Hospital
http://www.cvm.tamu.edu/vth-tech/

Cincinnati Vet. Tech. Association
www.geocities.com/cincivettechs

From National Association of Veterinary Technicians in America;
Available at: http://www.navta.net

AHT/VT PROVINCIAL ASSOCIATIONS OF CANADA

BRITISH COLUMBIA

AHTA of BC—Animal Health Technologists Association of B.C.
Executive Assistant—Tina Douglas
Box 275
Sicamous BC V0E 2V0
Fax/answering service: 250-836-4815, e-mail: ahtabc@sicamous.com

ALBERTA

AAAHT—The Alberta Association of Animal Health Technologists
#750 Weber Centre 5555 Calgary Trail South
Office Administrator—AVMA office staff
Edmonton AB T6H 5P9
Tel: 780-435-0486, Fax: 780-484-8311, e-mail: aaaht@telusplanet.net
Web: www.aaaht.com

SASKATCHEWAN

SAVT Inc.—Saskatchewan Association of Veterinary Technologists
Box 346 RPO University
Office Administrator—Michele Moroz
Saskatoon SK S7N 4J8
Tel: 306-373-0466, Fax: 306-477-3819, e-mail: savtinc@shaw.ca

MANITOBA

MAHTA—Manitoba Animal Health Technologists Association
Box 3025
Winnipeg MB R3C 4E5
Tel/answering service: 204-832-1394

ONTARIO

OAVT—Ontario Association of Veterinary Technicians
Executive Director—Kim Hilborn
Box 833
Guelph ON N1H 6L8
Tel: 519-836-4910, Fax: 519-836-3638, e-mail: oavt@oavt.org
Web: www.oavt.org

QUEBEC

ATSAQ—Association des Techniciens en Santé Animale du Québec
Secrétariat de l'ATSAQ
7400, boul. des Galeries d'Anjou, bur.410
Ville d'Anjou QC HIM 3M2
Tel: 514-355-9512, Fax: 514-355-4159, courriel: atsaq@spg.qc.ca

ATLANTIC PROVINCES

EVTA—Eastern Veterinarian Technician Association Ltd. of the Atlantic Provinces
Executive Director—Beverly Sutherland
146 East St.
Port Hood NS BOE 2W0
Tel/Fax: 902-787-2531, e-mail: b.sutherland@ns.sympatico.ca

CANADA

CAAHTT/ACTTSA—Canadian Association of Animal Health Technologists and Technicians
Association Canadienne Des Techniciens Et Technologistes En Santé Animale
Executive Director—Sandy Hass
Box 91 Grandora SK SOK 1V0
Tel: 306-329-4956, Fax: 306-329-4700, e-mail: s.vettech@sk.sympatico.ca
Web: http://www.caahtt-acttsa.com/

From CAAHTT/ACTTSA; Available at: http://www.caahtt-acttsa.com/

ADDITIONAL INTERNATIONAL VETERINARY NURSES AND TECHNICIAN ASSOCIATIONS

Veterinary Nurses Council of Australia, P.O. Box 2233, North Ringwood, Victoria 3134, Australia

Foreningen af Veterinaersygeplejersker I Danmark, Co. Jannie Larsen, Valdemarskrogen 36, 2860 Soborg, Denmark

"Klinikkaelainhoitajat r.y.," c/o Katarina Anhava, Tehtaankatu 7 C 20, 00140 Helsinki, Finland

Berufsverband der Artzt-, Zahnarzt- und Tierarzthelferinnen e.V., Bissenkamp 12-16, 44135 Dortmund, Germany

Secretary VEMTAG, P.O. Box A442, La Accra, Ghana

Secretary, c/o Chiharu Ishida, 33 kakezakuri-cho, Wakayama-shi, Wakayama-ken, 640, Japan

New Zealand Veterinary Nursing Association, Veterinary Clinical Sciences, Massey University, Palmerston North, New Zealand

Norwegian Veterinary Nursing Association, Post Box 8146, 8146 Dep. N-0033 Oslo, Norway

Veterinary Nurses Association of South Africa, Vice-President, c/o SAVA, P.O. Box 25033, Monument Park, 0105, South Africa

SCATAN, Region Djursjukhuset, Oskarshalls 9.6, 55303 Jonkoping, Sweden

British Veterinary Nursing Association, BVNA, Level 15 Terminus House, Terminus Street, Harlow, Essex CM20 1XA, England; Tel: 01279 450567, Fax: 01279 4208, e-mail: bvna@bvna.co.uk

From IVNTA (International Veterinary Nurses and Technicians Association); Available at: http://www.vetweb.co.uk/sites/ivna/

Registration of technicians

At the present, the following states **do not** have laws or regulations governing the registration of veterinary technicians: Delaware, District of Columbia, Hawaii, New Hampshire, Puerto Rico, Rhode Island, Utah, Vermont, and Wyoming.

Registration Responsibility	Requirements Before Registration	Examination Fee and Information	Renewal Fee and Requirements
Alabama[‡] Law, Licensed VT Executive Director, Board of Veterinary Medical Examiners, P.O. Box 1968, Decatur 35602; 256-353-3544; asbvme@mindspring.com	[†]Accredited program, VTNE	$25 application fee $100 VTNE fee	Annual renewal-$50 8 hr CE/yr
Alaska[†‡] Law and Regulation, Licensed VT Dept. of Commerce and Economic Development, Division of Occupational Licensing, Board of Veterinary Examiners, P.O. Box 110806, Juneau 99811-0806; 907-465-5470	[*]State Board has authority to license veterinary technicians; accredited program or completion of 2 years of on-the-job training under the supervision of a licensed veterinarian, VTNE	$50 nonrefundable application fee $130 VTNE $60 license fee	$60 biennial 5 hr continuing education per yr
Arizona[‡] Law, Certified VT Veterinary Medical Examining Board, Executive Director, 1400 W. Washington, Rm. 230, Phoenix 85007; 602-542-3095	Accredited program or other program approved by the Board, or 2 years with an AZ-licensed veterinarian and recommendation	$150	Biennial renewal—$50; expired certificate renewable up to 5 yr—$25 penalty for late renewal
Arkansas[‡] Law, Certified VT Executive Secretary, AR Veterinary Medical Examining Board, P.O. Box 8505, Little Rock 72215; 501-224-2836	Accredited program, recommendation by veterinarian, VTNE	$40 state application $125 VTNE fee	$25 plus $50 if delinquent 4 hr continuing education per yr
California[**] Law and Regulation, Registered VT Executive Officer, Veterinary Medical Board, 420 Howe Ave., Suite 6, Sacramento 95825; 916-263-2610	One of the following: BS or BA in animal science related field and 12 months of practical experience; graduate of approved program with no practical experience; graduate of nonapproved program plus 18 months of practical experience under veterinarian supervision; graduate of private approved program; completion of approved coursework at the post-secondary education level and 36 months of practical experience under direct supervision of CA-licensed veterinarian; or out-of-state RVTs who possess 36 months of practical experience and prior written examination,plus completed NVTE or written practical examination	$75 examination fee $25 1-yr registration period based on registrant's birth date	$50 biennially, based upon registrant's birth date

Continued

Registration of technicians—cont'd

Registration Responsibility	Requirements Before Registration	Examination Fee and Information	Renewal Fee and Requirements
Colorado[‡] Law, Identified in Practice Act, but not recognized CACVT, P.O. Box 24922, Denver 80224-0922; 303-300-4810	AVMA-accredited program or program recognized by CVMA and State Board	$160 VTNE (includes first yr membership in CACVT); offered in January and June	Renew by 8/30 of even-number yr; $80 for 2-yr renewal of certification and membership in CACVT. Test fee expected to go up in 1999; $10 late fee; 16 hr continuing education biennially
Connecticut[‡¶] Certified, but certification is VOLUNTARY Connecticut Association of AHTs (CAAHT), P.O. Box 1054, Naugatuck, CT 06770	AVMA accredited program graduate and/or 2 yr working full time as VT and performing duties as such and verification of employing veterinarian	$130 VTNE, CAAHT members $150 VTNE, nonmembers of CAAHT Write to P.O. Box address	15 hr continuing education every 2 yr, $30 biennial fee $10 late fee
Florida[‡¶] Law, Certified VT, but certification is VOLUNTARY Ms. Lynn Vannier, FVMA, 7131 Lake Ellenor Dr., Orlando 32809; 800-992-3862	Certification is voluntary; accredited program, statement of moral character, and/or current licensure in another state to sit for examination	$150 VTNE (National) Florida only FPE $50 Both together $150 (VTNE and FPE) $25 Florida practical examination only if VTNE transfers score from another state	Recertification is processed every other yr in even-numbered yr to recertify: 1/1/2002 10 CE hr required, $25 fee 1/1/2004 15 CE hr required, $25 fee
Georgia[‡] Law and Regulation, Registered VT Anita O. Martin, Executive Director, Professional Licensing Board, 237 Coliseum Dr., Macon 31217; 478-207-1686	Accredited program $50 application fee, VTNE	$50 application plus $65 VTNE	$70 for 2 yr $80 late fee
Idaho[‡] Law and Regulation, Registered VT Thomas A. Shelton, DVM, Executive Officer, Board of Veterinary Medicine, P.O. Box 7249, Boise 83707; 208-332-8588	Notorized proof of age (birth cert/ passport/drivers license) and two affidavits of moral character from personal acquaintance. Graduate of AVMA accredited veterinary technology program or other program approved by the board, or licensure in another state as an actively practicing VT; or prior to 7/1/2002, at least 2 yr employment as a veterinary assistant in the USA or Canada with a licensed veterinarian	$175 VTNE $100 state examination fee (required)	$50 Annual renewal $25 Late fee 15 CE hr required annually reported every 3 yr

Illinois‡¶** Law and Regulation, Certified VT Dept. of Prof. Regulation, 320 W. Washington, Springfield 62786; 217-782-8556	Accredited program and successful completion of the VTNE	$50 application plus VTNE fee	$50 biennially $10 late fee 10 hr CE every 2 yr beginning 1/31/97 renewal
Indiana‡ Law and Regulation, Registered VT Ms. Cindy Vaught, Health Professions Bureau, 402 W. Washington St., Rm. 041, Indianapolis 46282; 317-233-4407	Accredited program, passing score on VTNE, and IN veterinary juris prudence	A cost equal to cost of purchasing VTNE plus a fee of $30	$15 biennially; expires 1/1 even-numbered yr; renewable up to 5 yr after expiration-$15 plus $50 renewal fee; 16 hr approved CE required at renewal
Iowa‡ Law and Regulation, Registered VT Secretary, Iowa Veterinary Medical Examining Board, Wallace Bldg., 2nd Floor, Des Moines 50319; 515-281-5305	Accredited Program Passing grades VTNE and state board	$25 plus VTNE fee	Effective 1/1/93-triennial renewal $15 and 30 hr continuing education triennially
Kansas‡ Law, Registered VT Registration Board, KS Registered VTs, 1255 S. Range, Colby 67701	Accredited program and VTNE	$20 state examination and initial application $105 VTNE	4 hr continuing education $10 per yr $50 late fee
Kentucky‡ Law and Regulation, Registered AT KY Board of Veterinary Examiners, P.O. Box 1360, Frankfort 40602; 502-564-3296	Accredited program and verification of employment by state-licensed veterinarian; VTNE	$100 VTNE $25 application	Employment $30 annually 6 hr CE/yr
Louisiana‡ Certification VOLUNTARY, Regulation by Law Louisiana Board of Veterinary Medicine, 263 3rd St., Ste 104, Baton Rouge, 70801; 225-342-2176 Web site www.lsbvm.org	Accredited program, VTNE administered by Louisiana Board of Veterinary Medicine, references; $25 application fee	VTNE—$140 total ($40 plus vendor cost of examination $100) $25 application fee	$30 original fee $30 renewal fee $20 late fee
Maine‡¶ Law and Regulation, Registered VT Professional and Financial Regulations, 35 State House Station, Augusta 04333; 207-624-8620	College-level, 2-yr program or board-determined equivalent, and VTNE	VTNE examination fee is set by contract	$50 annually

Continued

Registration of technicians—cont'd

Registration Responsibility	Requirements Before Registration	Examination Fee and Information	Renewal Fee and Requirements
Maryland[‡**] Law and Regulation, RVT Paulette Holloway, Administrative Specialist, State Board of Veterinary Medical Examiners, 50 Harry S. Truman Pkwy., Rm. 203, Annapolis 21401; 410-841-5862	Accredited program or higher degree; VTNE and state examination (practical)	$50 state examination $100 VTNE	$25 for 3 yr with 24 hr continuing education
Massachusetts[‡] Certified VT Massachusetts VT Association, Joint Committee on VT Certification, c/o Angell Memorial Animal Hospital, 350 S. Huntington Ave., Rm. 208, Boston 02130; 617-522-7282, ext. 4001	Proof of successful completion of VTNE within last 5 yr and one of the following: graduation from accredited program; graduation from nonaccredited program plus 1 yr of practical experience; associate degree in animal or biological science plus 3 yr of practical experience; 5 yr of employment as VT plus 18 semester hours of college credit in animal or biological science; 8-yr employment as VT	$175 VTNE—given in January and June	12 hr continuing education per yr $40 original fee $20 renewal fee
Michigan[‡**] Law and Regulation, Licensed VT MI Board of Veterinary Medicine, Dept. of Consumer and Industry Services/BOPR, P.O. Box 30670, Lansing 48909; 517-335-0918	Accredited program, VTNE, practical	$170 includes VTNE fee	$50 every 2 yr; expires 12/31 every other yr; $20 late fee after 12/31
Minnesota[‡] VOLUNTARY, VT Certified VT VT Committee of MVMA, 393 N. Dunlap St, Ste. 400, St. Paul 55104	Verification of any of the following: accredited program, unaccredited program with committee approval	$110 VTNE $45 practical examination	10 hr continuing education every two yr; $25 renewal fee every other yr
Mississippi[§¶**] Law, AT Executive Secretary, MS Board of Veterinary Medicine, 209 S. Lafayette St., Starkville 39759; 601-324-9380	Diploma from school approved by state board, or high school diploma and 5 yr of continuous approved training as VT, a credit of 2 yr of practical training may be given by the board for a degree by an institution of higher learning, VTNE	$150 VTNE $25 state examination	Employment by veterinarian $5 per yr; 10 clock hr CE

Missouri[‡¶**] Law, Registered VT Executive Director, Missouri Veterinary Medical Board, P.O. Box 633, Jefferson City 65102; 573-751-0031	Accredited program, VTNE, state jurisprudence examination	$100 VTNE $30 state examination $50 registration $15 certificate replacement	$20 annually-active $10 annually-inactive 5 hr CE annually
Montana[‡¶] VOLUNTARY, Certified VT MVMA VT Committee 4217 2nd Ave. N., Great Falls, MT 59405	One of the following: **Accredited program and VTNE; or 5 or more consecutive years experience employed as a veterinary technician and VTNE by July 1, 2006 (grandfather clause)	$125 VTNE given in June	16 hr CE biannually $10 initial registration fee (good through 12/31 of first yr) $50 fee every 2 yr, expires 12/31 every other yr $10 late fee after 3/1
Nebraska Law, Licensed VT Director, Credentialing Division, HHSR&L, P.O. Box 94986, Lincoln, 68509-4986; 402-471-2118	Accredited program, pass the VTNE (grandfather provision exists temporarily)	$6 application fee for veterinary technician $5 application fee for veterinarian VTNE required—contact: Vicki Bumgarner, Credentialing Coordinator, HHSR&L, P.O. Box 94986, Lincoln, NE 68509-4986, 402-471-2118	$26 per yr for VT 24 hr CE every 3 yr
Nevada[‡**] Law, Licensed VT State Board of Veterinary Medical Examiners, 4600 Kietzke Ln., Bldg. O, Suite 265, Reno 89502; 775-688-1788; Fax 775-688-1808	One of the following: AVMA-accredited program, state-accredited program in state where program is located or accepted by State Board in said state, other educational and/or clinical background approved by Board	$130 VTNE and $100 state examination	5 hr continuing education annually $50 annual renewal
New Jersey[‡¶] AHT registered with JVMA NJVMA, 66 Morris Ave., Springfield 07081; 973-379-1100	One of the following: accredited program and VTNE or equivalent; certification in another state with comparable requirements; VTNE or equivalent and 3 yr of clinical experience under the supervision of a licensed veterinarian	$120 voluntary VTNE examination	$20 every 2 yr Late fee of $5 after 2/1 $25 initial registration fee 20 hr CE/2 yr
New Mexico[‡**] Law, Registered VT (permit) Director, NM Board of Veterinary Medicine, 1650 University Blvd. N.E., Suite 400 C, Albuquerque 87102; 505-841-9112	Accredited program, VTNE and state examinations	$20 state examination $100 VTNE	8 hr CE per yr $25 per yr

Continued

Registration of technicians—cont'd

Registration Responsibility	Requirements Before Registration	Examination Fee and Information	Renewal Fee and Requirements
New York[‡**] Law, Registered and Licensed VT Executive Secretary, Board for Veterinary Medicine, Education Bldg., 2nd Floor, 89 Washington Ave. Albany, NY 12234; 518-474-3817, ext 210	Accredited program and successful completion of VTNE	$279 total—covers application, first 3 yr registration, and VTNE	$80/3 yr $50 limited permit fee
North Carolina[‡] Law, Registered VT Executive Director, Veterinary Medical Board, P.O. Box 12587, Raleigh 27605; 919-733-7689	Accredited program, VTNE and state examination	$120 VTNE $50 state examination	$15 annually paid biennially 12 hr CE biennially
North Dakota[‡**] Law and Regulation, Licensed VT Board of Veterinary Medical Examiners, Office of Executive Secretary, P.O. Box 5001, Bismarck, ND 58502; 701-328-9540; Fax 701-224-0435; Web site ndbvme@state.nd.us	Examination and graduation from 2-yr VT training program	$25 application fee $100 VTNE	$10 annually 8 hr CE biennially
Ohio[**] Law and Regulation, Registered VT Executive Secretary, Veterinary Medical Licensing Board, 77 S. High St., 16th Floor, Columbus 43266-0116; 614-644-5281	Board-approved program established by rule	Voluntary VTNE offered—contact: Dr. H. Marie Suthers, CSCC VT Program, 550 E. Spring St., Columbus, OH 43216; 614-227-2632	Initial fee of $25 for even numbered yr and $35 for odd numbered yr, 10 hr continuing education biennially, $35 biennially
Oklahoma[‡] Law and Regulation, Certified VT Executive Director, Board of Veterinary Medical Examiners, 201 N.E. 38th Terr., Ste. 1, Oklahoma City 73105	School approved by State Board, VTNE and state examinations	VTNE-$100; state $60; application processing $50; certificate $20	$40 annually, 10 hr continuing education per yr

Oregon‡** Law and Regulation, Licensed VT Veterinary Medical Examining Board, 800 N.E. Oregon St., Suite 407, Portland 97232; 503-731-4051	Accredited program or 4 yr of practical training with veterinarian; currently licensed as certified technician in another state with 5 or more calendar years of clinical experience and graduated from an accredited veterinary technology college prior to 1990	$105 VTNE and first year's certification $25 VTNE only or certification only	$25 annually
Pennsylvania†**‡¶ Law and Regulation, Certified AHT State Board of Veterinary Medicine, P.O. Box 2649, Harrisburg 17105-2649; 717-783-7134	One of the following: accredited program and successful completion of VTNE; accredited program and previous completion of VTNE in other state	$155 VTNE $35 application fee	8 hr in 2 yr continuing education $60 biennial renewal fee
South Carolina‡** Law and Regulation, Certified AHT South Carolina Board of Veterinary Medical Examiners, P.O. Box 11329, Columbia 29211-1329; 803-896-4598	Accredited Program, state examination, VTNE not administered, but required	$25 plus cost of VTNE $10 temporary certificate	$20 annually 5 hr CE annually
South Dakota‡ Law, Registered VT SD Veterinary Medical Examining Board, c/o State Veterinarian, 411 S. Fort St., Pierre 57501; 605-773-3321	Accredited program, registered to veterinarian, functions under licensed veterinarian	$125 VTNE annually in June (includes state oral examination) $25 state fee for oral examination only in June $10 registration fee	Employment, re-register if employment changes, $5 renewal fee annually
Tennessee‡** Law and Regulation, Licensed VMT Mr. Eric Bloom, Executive Director, Board of Veterinary Medical Examiners, 425 5th Ave. N., Cordell Hull Bldg., Nashville 37247-1010; 615-532-5090	Accredited program, successful completion of VTNE and recommendation by TN-licensed veterinarian	$75 application fee $100 VTNE fee	12 hr CE/yr $40 biennial $10 state fee-biennial

Continued

Registration of technicians—cont'd

Registration Responsibility	Requirements Before Registration	Examination Fee and Information	Renewal Fee and Requirements
Texas‡¶ Regulation, Registered RVT State VMA, 6633 Hwy. 290 E., Suite 201, Austin 78723; 512-452-4224	Accredited program or previous certification as RVT in Texas. Successful completion of VTNE and state examinations. Texas allows technicians from other states to transfer and take the test only if graduate of AVMA-accredited program	$175 (covers both examinations and registration for first yr, $125 VTNE, $85 state). Given in January and June Both $175, VTNE $125, state $85	5 hr annual continuing education $30 per yr re-registration; after 5/31 $40 (includes $10 late fee)
Vermont, VT		Voluntary VTNE offered—contact Mr. Craig Stalnaker, President, Vermont VT Association, c/o Vermont Technical College VT Program, P.O. Box 500, Randolph Center, VT 05061; 802-728-3391	
Virginia‡** Law and Regulation, Licensed VT VA Board of Veterinary Medicine, 6606 W. Broad St., 4th Fl., Richmond 23230-1717; 804-662-9915	Accredited program, VTNE	$150 VTNE $25 application fee for licensure	$25 annually on 2/28 $15 late fee 6 hr CE/yr
Washington‡** Law and Regulation, Registered VT Dept of Health, Veterinary Board of Governors, P.O. Box 1099, Olympia 98507-1099	One of the following: accredited program, nonaccredited program plus 36 months of full-time work experience, previous registration in another state plus 36 months of full-time work as VT, completion of VT education in U.S. military, or 5 yr of full-time work experience with licensed veterinarian. Passing score on examinations	$100 VTNE $80 state board examination $60 initial registration fee	$51 and $17 penalty for late renewal

West Virginia, Law and Regulation, RVT WV Board of Veterinary Medicine, 1900 Kanawha Blvd. E., Charleston 25305-0119; 304-558-2016	Graduate of accredited program, 18 yr old, U.S. citizen or applicant, good moral character	$40 $150 VTNE $25 test material	Employment by licensed veterinarian, $25 annually, $30 if paid after 12/31 6 hr Classroom CE
Wisconsin‡¶** Law and Regulation, Certified VT Veterinary Examination Board, P.O. Box 8935, Madison 53708; 608-266-2811	Accredited program, or 2 yr with licensed veterinarian; successful completion of VTNE and state examinations	$111 VTNE $44 initial credential fee $57 state law examination $27 written examination administration fee $15 contract examination fee	Renewal-$48, plus social security number

*"State Board" refers to State Board of Veterinary Medical Examiners.
†"Accredited program" refers to accreditation by the American Veterinary Medical Association.
‡These states administer the Veterinary Technician National Examination (VTNE).
§These states offer the VTNE when requested.
¶These states offer reciprocity to technicians who are certified, registered, or licensed in another state.
**These states identify tasks that can be performed only by registered, certified, or licensed technicians and may not be performed by other employees without a veterinarian's supervision.
AHT, Animal Health Technician; *AT,* Animal Technician; *VT,* Veterinary Technician; *RVT,* Registered Veterinary Technician; *CVT,* Certified Veterinary Technician; *LVT,* Licensed Veterinary Technician.
Permission to provide the preceding information was granted from the American Veterinary Medical Association and was accurate at the time of writing.

ADDITIONAL INTERNET SITES

Web Site	Organizations/Companies
http://www.aavsb.org	American Association of State Boards Licensing requirements for VT
http://www.navta.net/	National Association of Veterinary Technicians in America
http://www.caahtt-acttsa.com/	Canadian Association of Animal Health Technologists and Technicians
http://www.avma.org/	American Veterinary Medical Association
www.avte.net	Association of Veterinary Technician Educators
http://www.cvma-acmv.org/	Canadian Veterinary Medical Association
http://www.vetweb.co.uk/sites/ivna/index.htm	International Veterinary Nurses and Technician Association
http://veccs.org/technicians/index.cfm	Academy of Veterinary Emergency Critical Care Technicians (AVECCT)
http://www.oavt.org/	Ontario Association of Veterinary Technicians
http://www.AZVT.org	Association of Zoo Veterinary Technicians
http://www.vhma.org	Veterinary Hospital Managers Association
http://www.healthypet.com/	American Animal Hospital Association for pet owners
http://www.aahanet.org/	American Animal Hospital Association for veterinary personnel
http://www.aps.uoguelph.ca/IS.OVC/services.html	University of Guelph–Animal and Poultry Science
http://www.lifelearn.com	Life Learn
http://www.us.elsevierhealth.com/	Harcourt/Mosby + links
http://www.vet.cornell.edu/	Cornell University
http://www.vetmed.ucdavis.edu/vetnet.html	University of Davis Veterinary School
http://www.vetweb.co.uk/	Royal College of Veterinary Surgeons
http://cal.vet.upenn.edu/	University of Pennsylvania
http://duke.usask.ca/~ladd/vet_libraries.html	Veterinary Medicine Libraries
http://civic.bev.net/aava/	American Association of Veterinary Anatomists
http://www.acva.org	College of Veterinary Anesthesiologists
http://veccs.org/technicians/index.cfm	Academy of Veterinary Emergency Critical Care Technicians (AVECCT)
http://www.akc.org/index.cfm	American Kennel Club—access to many publications
http://www.dogs-in-canada.com/	Canadian Kennel Club
http://www.wwwins.net.au/dog/downunder.html	Dogs Down Under—Australia site
http://www.ama-assn.org	American Medical Association
http://www.guidedogs.com	Guide dogs
http://www.erc.on.ca/	Equine Research Center
http://www.wehn.com/	Kentucky Equine Research Inc
http://gnv.ifas.ufl.edu	University of Florida Institute of Food and Agriculture
http://www.vetmed.ucdavis.edu	University of California, Davis, School of Veterinary Medicine
http://www.fda.gov/cvm/	U.S. Food and Drug Administration Center for Veterinary Medicine
http://www.aabp.org	American Association of Bovine Practitioners
http://www.aasp.org	American Association of Swine Practitioners
http://www.vet.purdue.edu	Purdue University
http://www.aaep.org	American Association of Equine Practitioners
http://www.canswine.ca/sw.html	Canadian Swine Breeders Swine health
http://www.aclam.org	American College of Laboratory Animal Medicine
http://www.aalas.org	American Association of Laboratory Animal Science Journals
http://calas-acsal.org	Canadian Association for Laboratory Animal Science
http://www.nabr.org	National Association of Biomedical Research
http://www.arav.org	Association of Reptile and Amphibian Veterinarians

http://www.fanciers.com	Cat Fanciers Association—cat-related topics
http://www.cca-afc.com	Canadian Cat Association—cat-related topics
http://www.vetinfo.com/	Veterinary Information Service—many sites
http://www.pbs.org/	Public Broadcasting Service—different sites

Anatomy

http://www.vetmedicine.about.com/health/vetmedicine/cs/anatomy/index.htm.htm	About site
http://www.hoflink.com/~house/Animal.html	Biology Web site—lots of other links
http://www2.kenyon.edu/depts/biology/heithausp/cat-tutorial/welcome.htm	Kenyon College—cat anatomy tutorial
http://www.vetgate.ac.uk/	UK Vetgate—teaching resources

Behavior and Restraint

http://www.vetmedicine.about.com/health/vetmedicine/cs/behavior/index.htm	About site—behavior
http://users.erols.com/mandtj/about.htm	University of Maryland—list of further sites
http://www.grandin.com	Dr. Temple Grandin—animal behavior and restraint
http://www.ahc.umn.edu/rar/handling.html	Research animal resources—restraint and handling of animals

Breeds

http://vetmedicine.about.com/health/vetmedicine/cs/breeds/index.htm	About site—breeds
http://www.ansi.okstate.edu/breeds	Oklahoma State—breeds of animals—virtual library
http://www.fanciers.com/breeds.html	Cat Fanciers Association breeds
http://www.akc.org/breeds/index.cfm	American Kennel Club
http://www.dogs-in-canada.com	Dogs in Canada

Basic Clinical Sciences

http://www.vetmedicine.about.com/health/vetmedicine/cs/parasites/index.htm	About site—parasites
http://www.roberth.u-net.com/horseflies.htm	Rob Hutchinson—horse flies
http://www.medvet.umontreal.ca/serv-diag/englishv/urologie_en.html	Urinalysis
http://cal.nbc.upenn.edu/dxendopar/	University of Pennsylvania—parasitology

Laboratory Animal Science

http://www4.nas.edu/cls/ilarhome.nsf	Institute for Laboratory Animal Research (ILAR)
http://www.ahc.umn.edu/rar/HANDLING.HTML	University of Minnesota—Research Animal Resources—laboratory animal restraint
http://oslovet.veths.no/norina	Norina Data Base of laboratory animal science and alternatives
http://www.ahc.umn.edu/rar/index.html	Research animal resources

Medicine

http://www-sci.lib.uci.edu/HSG/Vet.html	Martindale's Health Science Guide
http://www.vet.purdue.edu	Purdue University

Pharmacology

http://www.fda.gov/	Food and Drug Administration
http://www.vetinfo.demon.nl/	Dutch Veterinary Information Systems—electronic formulary

Additional Sites

http://www.spjc.edu/hec/vettech/vt1.html	St. Petersburg Junior College—distance education—classes
http://vetmedicine.about.com/health/vetmedicine/	About—any veterinary topic
http://www-sci.lib.uci.edu/HSG/Vet.html	Martindale's Health Science Guide
http://www.VetTeam.com	(Registration Required) Vet. Team
http://www.vetgate.ac.uk	Vetgate
http://www.vetinfonet.com	Veterinary Information Network
http://netvet.wustl.edu/	Net Vet. (Electronic Zoo) Info. on almost anything animal related
http://www.eb.com	Britannica Online
http://cancerweb.ncl.ac.uk/omd/	Online medical dictionary
http://www.netpets.com	Netpets
http://www.dogpatch.org/dogs/dogweb.cfm#A5	Dog Patch—lots of sites

Modified with permission from Association of Veterinary Technician Educators, Inc. Images for Veterinary Technician Educators.
Note: The websites listed in this table were valid at the time of writing. There is no guarantee that each site will continue to be viable. Your main technician and veterinary associations will have the most up-to-date links.

APPENDIX G

Comprehensive Test With Answer Key

This comprehensive examination is meant as a study aid only and thus covers 10 questions from each chapter. The number in parenthesis represents the chapter in which the answer can be found.

1. Which of the following is a function of bile? *(1)*
   a. Activation of pancreatic sucrase
   b. Emulsification of fat
   c. Decrease intestinal motility
   d. Cause contraction of the gallbladder
2. Which of the following chemical constituents in urine is the result of fatty acid catabolism? *(2)*
   a. Acetone
   b. Bilirubin
   c. Glucose
   d. Hemoglobin
3. A common neoplasia of cats is *(3)*
   a. Pyelonephritis
   b. Feline infectious peritonitis
   c. Mastitis
   d. Renal lymphosarcoma
4. The term "mange" means *(4)*
   a. Hair loss
   b. Infestation by mites
   c. Infestation by lice
   d. Rough hair coat
5. *Salmonella (5)*
   a. Can infect the gastrointestinal tract of humans, mammals, birds, and reptiles
   b. Is a gram-positive rod
   c. Normally inhabits the respiratory tract
   d. Are lactose fermenters on MacConkey agar
6. All the of the following are commonly used in a liver profile except *(6)*
   a. Total bilirubin
   b. Urea
   c. Total protein
   d. AP
7. Viruses may possess one of four different genomic constructs. *(7)*
   a. True
   b. False
8. Clients should be educated as to the possible adverse reactions an animal may have to a vaccination. *(8)*
   a. True
   b. False
9. To restrain a cat it is important to *(9)*
   a. Immediately apply the maximum restraint possible
   b. Make friends first and then apply the maximum restraint
   c. Make friends first and then apply least restrictive restraint
   d. Immediately apply the least restrictive restraint
10. An appropriate chemical disinfectant for stainless steel tables is *(10)*
    a. Bleach
    b. Alcohol
    c. Iodine solution
    d. Peroxide
11. The purpose of an aluminum filter in an x-ray machine is to *(11)*
    a. Limit the size of the x-ray beam
    b. Focus the x-ray beam to the focal spot
    c. Remove the long wavelength x-rays from the x-ray beam
    d. Increase the number of short wavelength x-rays in the beam
12. At which area does the ultrasound beam reach its narrowest point? *(12)*
    a. Focal point
    b. Near field
    c. Far field
    d. Reverberation point
13. The breakage of two chromosomes, resulting in repair in an abnormal arrangement is called *(13)*
    a. Deletion
    b. Anomalies
    c. Duplication
    d. Translocation
14. Which of the following statements regarding puppy classes is false? *(14)*
    a. Puppies will learn canine language through puppy class
    b. All puppies should be neutered in a puppy class
    c. Owners will learn how to prevent the most common behavior problems
    d. Veterinarians should encourage their clients to participate in a puppy class
15. Average moisture (water) content of canned food is *(15)*
    a. 25% to 40%
    b. 72% to 82%
    c. 40% to 60%
    d. 10% to 12%

16. The trace mineral that is an essential part of vitamin B_{12} is *(16)*
    a. Copper
    b. Zinc
    c. Cobalt
    d. Molybdenum
17. In an animal colony, how can you be assured that you are maintaining disease-free animals? *(17)*
    a. Absence of clinical signs
    b. Use of sentinel animals
    c. By purchasing only SPF and VAF animals
    d. By housing animals within a barrier facility
18. Suitable sites for blood collection in birds are *(18)*
    a. Jugular, cephalic, and saphenous
    b. Jugular, brachioulnar, and medial tibiotarsal
    c. Jugular, cephalic, and femoral
    d. Jugular, brachioulnar, and toenail
19. Which of the following is an indication to include an anticholinergic in preanesthetic medication? *(19)*
    a. To produce analgesia
    b. To produce sedation
    c. To prevent bradycardia
    d. To treat tachypnea
20. Many drugs used in chemotherapy can cause severe side effects. Side effects may include *(20)*
    a. Liver and kidney toxicities, low blood cell counts, vomiting and diarrhea
    b. Hemorrhage, seizures, gastroenteritis, hair loss
    c. Allergic reaction, anorexia, cardiac and nervous system toxicities
    d. All of the above
21. A patient must be given 1 L of fluids and a vitamin mixture (50 mg/mL) at the rate of 75 mg/kg. The patient weighs 35 kg. The IV line has to run for 5 hours with an administration set calibrated at 15 drops/mL. The drip rate is calculated at *(21)*
    a. 9 drops/min
    b. 0.9 drops/sec
    c. 8 drops/sec
    d. 49 drops/min
22. An ultrasonic cleaner is how many times more effective than manual cleaning of the instruments? *(22)*
    a. 3
    b. 10
    c. 16
    d. 25
23. The most common vein used for blood donation is the *(23)*
    a. Jugular
    b. Cephalic
    c. Saphenous
    d. Femoral
24. When positioning a horse in lateral recumbency, it is important to pull the *(24)*
    a. Upper foreleg forward to enhance circulation
    b. Upper hind leg forward to enhance circulation
    c. Down foreleg forward to enhance circulation
    d. Down hind leg forward to enhance circulation
25. When performing orogastric intubation in ruminants, which of the following is *false? (25)*
    a. Measure the tube length to the last rib
    b. Occlude the tube before removal
    c. Rumen gas may be detected on correct placement
    d. Visual observation of esophageal tube placement may be made on the right side of the neck
26. The percentage of dogs and cats over the age of 2 years with some form of periodontal disease has been estimated to be *(26)*
    a. 50%
    b. 65%
    c. 75%
    d. 85%
27. Which of the following signs is common in acetaminophen toxicity? *(27)*
    a. Icterus
    b. Hemolysis
    c. Methemoglobinemia
    d. Hematuria
28. A nocturnal animal foraging for food at 11:00 in the morning may be infected with *(28)*
    a. Rabies
    b. Anthrax
    c. Tularemia
    d. *Capnocytophaga canimorus*
29. Which of the following is not true of good e-mail policy? *(29)*
    a. Message should be short and concise
    b. You should never e-mail a co-worker when you are very angry
    c. E-mail is a great way to share jokes and humorous stories
    d. E-mail should not take the place of conversation
30. Which of the following cells would most likely have the largest number of mitochondria? *(1)*
    a. Osteocytes
    b. Smooth muscle cells
    c. Skeletal muscle cells
    d. Adipocytes
31. Iron deficiency is a common cause of which of the following erythrocyte findings? *(2)*
    a. Polychromasia
    b. Hypochromasia
    c. Macrocytosis
    d. Basophilic stippling
32. Infections with *Histoplasma* or *Balantidium* organisms are commonly identified using *(3)*
    a. Fine needle aspiration
    b. Intestinal biopsy
    c. Rectal mucosal scraping
    d. Fecal smear
33. The "Baermann technique" is used for the recovery of *(4)*
    a. Lungworm larvae
    b. Microfilariae
    c. Mites
    d. *Cryptosporidia* oocysts

34. *Candida albicans* is a yeast that *(5)*
    a. Can grow on some bacteriological media and can cause opportunistic infections
    b. Is found only in the gastrointestinal tract
    c. Does not produce germ tubes
    d. Is encapsulated
35. The test of choice for assessing if animals have exocrine pancreatic insufficiency is *(6)*
    a. Serum lipase
    b. Serum amylase
    c. Serum trypsin
    d. TLI
36. Samples for virology testing may include which of the following? *(7)*
    a. Frozen postmortem tissues
    b. EDTA plasma samples
    c. Frozen serum samples
    d. All of the above
37. To provide maximal immunity to the neonate, all vaccines should be given *(8)*
    a. Just before parturition
    b. According to the vaccine protocol
    c. Immediately after parturition
    d. Before the dam becomes pregnant
38. White around the eyes, sharp movements of the head and ears, trembling lips, and boisterous behavior indicate a dog is *(9)*
    a. Nervous/frightened
    b. Happy
    c. Normal acting
    d. Hostile
39. Which of the following disinfectants is toxic to cats? *(10)*
    a. Alcohols
    b. Quaternary ammonium compounds
    c. Phenols
    d. Aldehydes
40. The degree of overall blackness on a radiograph is termed *(11)*
    a. Density
    b. Contrast
    c. Radiolucent
    d. Radiopaque
41. The purpose of the time-gain compensation is to *(12)*
    a. Make tissues look alike
    b. Decrease contrast of the image
    c. Increase speed of the returning image
    d. Adjust brightness of the image
42. Colostrum is *(13)*
    a. Formed in the ovary after ovulation and produces progesterone
    b. The act of artificial insemination
    c. The period of ovulation
    d. The immunoglobulin-rich milk secreted from the mammary gland shortly after parturition
43. When using drug therapy to modify pet behavior, what should be done to obtain the maximum results? *(14)*
    a. Monitor the side effects
    b. Keep the animal in a calm and noise-free environment
    c. Combine drug therapy with a behavior modification program
    d. Combine drug therapy with an extensive physical exercise program
44. What is the best feeding method for growing puppies? *(15)*
    a. Free choice
    b. Food-restricted meal feeding
    c. Time-restricted feeding
    d. Food- and time-restricted feeding
45. Ruminants utilize non-protein nitrogen (NPN) through: *(16)*
    a. Microbial fermentation in the rumen
    b. Digestion in the omasum
    c. Digestion in the abomasum
    d. Direct absorption into the blood stream
46. What is an HEPA filter? *(17)*
    a. High Energy Particle Absorber
    b. High Efficiency Particle Absorber
    c. High Efficiency Particulate Air
    d. High Energy Particulate Air
47. In lizards and turtles, IM injections are best given in the *(18)*
    a. Rear leg
    b. Lumbar muscles
    c. Front leg
    d. Renal portal system
48. Which opioid preanesthetic agent has a higher incidence of producing vomiting and should be avoided with cases such as gastrointestinal obstruction or diaphragmatic hernia? *(19)*
    a. Butorphanol
    b. Morphine
    c. Meperidine
    d. Oxymorphone
49. Antitoxin and antiserum vaccines *(20)*
    a. Stimulate the body to create antibodies
    b. Last at least 1 year
    c. Create passive immunity
    d. Should not be given to pregnant animals
50. An animal is given 26 mg of a drug. The dose rate is 1 mL/15 kg. The concentration of the drug is 10 mg/mL. How much does this animal weigh? *(21)*
    a. 2.6 kg
    b. 3.9 kg
    c. 26 kg
    d. 39 kg
51. Which is *not* a type of sterilization monitor? *(22)*
    a. Indicator tape
    b. Chemical indicator strips
    c. Biological indicators
    d. David Bowie test
52. A constricting bandage is *not* likely to cause *(23)*
    a. Difficulty breathing
    b. Swelling or edema
    c. Coldness of the extremity
    d. Normal color of the body part
53. Twelve hours before surgery, the horse must *(24)*
    a. Be taken off feed
    b. Have water withheld
    c. Have the surgical site clipped
    d. Have the mouth rinsed out with water
54. By visual inspection, malnutrition or emaciation in cattle may be difficult to detect in *(25)*
    a. Older animals
    b. Young animals
    c. Fully haired animals
    d. Freshly shorn animals

55. The normal bite of a dog is best described as *(26)*
    a. An anterior crossbite
    b. A scissor bite
    c. A level bite
    d. A posterior bite
56. Which of the following statements is true regarding ethylene glycol toxicity? *(27)*
    a. The ethylene glycol test can be performed days postingestion
    b. Seizure activity is not commonly related to ethylene glycol toxicity
    c. Ethylene glycol toxicity causes liver failure
    d. A blood sample to test for ethylene glycol should be obtained before administering diazepam in patients with seizure activity
57. Which steps should be taken to prevent human infection with *Toxoplasma gondii? (28)*
    a. Eating rare meat
    b. Allowing pet cats the opportunity to hunt and eat prey
    c. Leaving the cover off children's sandboxes
    d. Cleaning the litterbox every 1 to 2 days
58. Active listening *(29)*
    a. Means that you interrupt the speaker to interject your thoughts
    b. Involves speaking in a loud voice with many hand jesters
    c. Implies that you are aware of the speaker's words and feelings
    d. Encourages everyone in the room to participate in the conversation
59. The vertebral column of the cat would be represented by the following *(1)*
    a. C7 T13 L7 S3 Cd 21-23
    b. C7 T18 L6 S5 Cd 16-18
    c. C7 T12 L5 S5 Cd 4-5
    d. C5 T13 L8 S3 Cd 20-23
60. Which term describes cells as having spiny projections around the margin and is often the result of slow drying of the blood film? *(2)*
    a. Target cells
    b. Acanthocyte
    c. Schistocyte
    d. Crenation
61. The presence of cells with prominent dark black granules indicates *(3)*
    a. Purulent inflammation
    b. Mast cell tumor
    c. Mesothelioma
    d. Melanoma
62. A zoonotic parasite does *not* include *(4)*
    a. *Cryptosporidia*
    b. *Toxocara canis*
    c. *Gasterophilus* spp.
    d. *Ixodes* spp.
63. *Mycobacteria* sp. are bacteria that are *(5)*
    a. Often the cause of diarrhea in many animals
    b. Gram-negative rods
    c. Easy to grow on usual bacteriological media
    d. Acid-fast negative
64. Which of the following is considered to be a very specific test for all forms of liver disease in most species? *(6)*
    a. AST
    b. ALT
    c. Bile acids
    d. AP
65. The best animals to sample for virology testing are those that are showing the severest clinical signs. *(7)*
    a. True
    b. False
66. In which of the following species can IgG antibody cross the placental barrier? *(8)*
    a. Horse
    b. Cattle
    c. Cat
    d. Pig
67. Which dog would be most likely to show aggressive behavior? *(9)*
    a. Large dog like a Newfoundland
    b. A medium-size dog like a beagle
    c. A small dog like a Chihuahua
    d. All dogs can be equally aggressive
68. The use of _____ on a contaminated open wound may result in the formation of a coagulum. *(10)*
    a. Peroxide
    b. Alcohol
    c. Iodine
    d. Quaternary ammonium compound
69. An example of positive contrast media that may be injected intravascularly is *(11)*
    a. Nonsoluble barium
    b. Water-soluble barium
    c. Water-soluble iodine
    d. Both b and c
70. The transducer needs crystals that can transform electrical energy into sound, etc. The effect exhibited by these crystals is *(12)*
    a. Electromagnetic
    b. Impedance
    c. Piezoelectric
    d. Attenuation
71. In what breed does maintenance of pregnancy depend on luteal progesterone? *(13)*
    a. Sheep
    b. Pig
    c. Goat
    d. Cat
72. Which is the least effective procedure to prevent barking? *(14)*
    a. Counterconditioning
    b. Cage training
    c. Obedience training
    d. Muzzling the dog
73. Puppies should be weighed and body condition score monitored every________ to ensure proper growth. *(15)*
    a. Week
    b. 2 Weeks
    c. Month
    d. 2 Months

74. Which of the following is the major site for roughage fermentation in the horse? *(16)*
  a. Stomach
  b. Small intestine
  c. Cecum
  d. Rectum
75. If restrained improperly, which of the following animals will have "fur slip"? *(17)*
  a. Chinchilla
  b. Degu
  c. Rabbit
  d. Mouse
76. The clinical signs of lead toxicity in a bird include *(18)*
  a. Lethargy, depression, green diarrhea, and paresis
  b. Bradycardia, pale mucous membranes, and high blood pressure
  c. Tachycardia, hyperemic membranes, and high blood pressure
  d. Hypoventilation, muddy mucous membranes, and low blood pressure
77. Which inhalation anesthetic agent has the quickest induction and recovery? *(19)*
  a. Halothane
  b. Isoflurane
  c. Methoxyflurane
  d. Pentobarbital
78. Antiulcer drugs can work in any of the following ways except *(20)*
  a. Decreasing the pH in the stomach
  b. Neutralizing stomach acid
  c. Protecting the stomach lining
  d. Stimulating mucous production
79. If a bucket holds 5 gallons, how much iodine must be added to make a concentration of 2 ppm? (1 gallon = 3785 mL) *(21)*
  a. 0.1 g
  b. 0.04 g
  c. 0.002 g
  d. 9.46 g
80. Storing sterile packs in what type of cabinet will provide the longest shelf-life? *(22)*
  a. Open
  b. Closed
  c. Perforated
  d. Does not matter
81. Anal sacs are expressed *(23)*
  a. To decrease odor caused by fecal material
  b. To increase the chances of a ruptured anal sac
  c. Due to perforation of the rectum
  d. To instill medication in diseased anal sacs
82. Parasitic infestations in horses can cause *(24)*
  a. Colic
  b. Swamp fever
  c. West Nile virus
  d. Colitis
83. Under general anesthesia, all of the following are used to judge the depth of anesthesia in small ruminants except *(25)*
  a. Heart rate
  b. Respiratory rate
  c. Pulse quality
  d. Eye signs
84. Retained deciduous teeth *(26)*
  a. Present no problems for the pet
  b. Affect larger breeds more often
  c. Cause malocclusions and gingivitis
  d. Occur commonly in a wry bite
85. Pericardiocentesis is indicated for which condition? *(27)*
  a. Pericarditis
  b. Pericardial tamponade
  c. Hemothorax
  d. Peritonitis
86. Which of the following statements is least often true regarding brucellosis? *(28)*
  a. Carried by cattle
  b. Small animal veterinarians and staff are not at risk
  c. Can cause abortions in bovids
  d. Can lead to sterility
87. The guilt phase of grieving *(29)*
  a. Is with a person forever; you never get over it but can move on to the other stages
  b. Is the first stage
  c. Inhibits progress toward resolution
  d. Is usually targeted at the veterinarian
88. Which of the following is a strong protective covering of the heart? *(1)*
  a. Epicardium
  b. Myocardium
  c. Visceral pericardium
  d. Parietal pericardium
89. Which intracellular parasite appears fairly large, paired, and teardrop shaped? *(2)*
  a. *Hemobartonella felis*
  b. *Anaplasma marginale*
  c. *Babesia canis*
  d. *Hemobartonella canis*
90. An example of a noninflammatory, nonneoplastic lesion is *(3)*
  a. TVT
  b. Hematoma
  c. Metastasis
  d. Fibroma
91. The common name for an ascarid is *(4)*
  a. Whipworm
  b. Bloodworm
  c. Roundworm
  d. Tapeworm
92. Enteral bacteria are bacteria that *(5)*
  a. Are normal flora of the gastrointestinal tract
  b. Do not cause infections
  c. Grow well on CNA agar plates
  d. Are identified using the germ tube test
93. Which of the following pairs of electrolytes have an inverse relationship in the body; that is, when the level of one increases in the body, the level of the other decreases? *(6)*
  a. Calcium and phosphorus
  b. Sodium and calcium
  c. Potassium and chloride
  d. Sodium and potassium

94. Which of the following is true about viral samples? *(7)*
    a. They should be frozen to ensure stability
    b. They survive up to 3 weeks without refrigeration
    c. They are inherently unstable and must be submitted as soon as possible
    d. Only naked virus samples can be shipped because they are very refractory
95. Which antibody class is produced during the secondary immune response? *(8)*
    a. IgM
    b. IgG
    c. IgA
    d. IgE
96. Which tool is considered the main tool(s) of restraint on a horse? *(9)*
    a. Halter and lead rope
    b. Stanchion
    c. Stocks
    d. Lariat
97. The mode of action of moist heat is *(10)*
    a. Oxidation
    b. Protein denaturation
    c. Hydrolysis
    d. Reduction
98. To increase the radiographic detail or definition *(11)*
    a. Increase the object-film distance
    b. Decrease the source-image distance
    c. Increase the source-image distance
    d. Increase the focal-spot size
99. In ultrasonography, the artifact that is exhibited posterior to a bladder stone is *(12)*
    a. Mirror image
    b. Reverberation
    c. Refraction
    d. Shadowing
100. The order of the stages of the estrous cycle is *(13)*
    a. Proestrus, estrus, metestrus, anestrus
    b. Proestrus, anestrus, metestrus, estrus
    c. Estrus proestrus, anestrus, metestrus
    d. Estrus, anestrus, proestrus, metestrus
101. Which statement best describes the advice you would give to the owner of a 3-month-old puppy who asks how to housetrain the dog? *(14)*
    a. Set up a newspaper area in each room of the house
    b. Rub the animal's nose in his feces when it eliminates in the house
    c. Set a regular routine to go outside
    d. The puppy cannot be trained before 4 months of age
102. Cats are *(15)*
    a. Omnivores
    b. Carnivores
    c. Herbivores
    d. Vegetarian
103. Pigs are not usually fed *(16)*
    a. Diets high in nonprotein nitrogen
    b. Protein supplements
    c. Ground grains
    d. Pelleted premixes
104. What type of bedding is inappropriate for use as a contact bedding for laboratory animals? *(17)*
    a. Hardwood shavings
    b. Cedar chips
    c. Corn cob bedding
    d. Aspen chips
105. The normal gastrointestinal flora of psittacines include *(18)*
    a. Predominantly gram-positive bacteria
    b. Predominantly gram-negative bacteria
    c. *Klebsiella* and *Salmonella*
    d. Predominantly anaerobic bacteria
106. How do you prevent diffusion hypoxia after discontinuation of N_2O use in general anesthesia? *(19)*
    a. Increase the O_2 flow rate for at least 5 minutes
    b. Provide intermittent positive pressure ventilation
    c. Increase the intravenous fluid rate
    d. Turn off inhalant anesthetic agent
107. A goal of antimicrobial therapy is to *(20)*
    a. Kill microorganisms in the host and restore normal flora
    b. Prevent microorganisms in the host from infecting other animals
    c. Kill microorganisms in the host without killing the host
    d. Prevent microorganisms in the host from moving to other places in the body
108. How much NaCl should be measured out to produce 500 mL of a 4.5% w/v solution? *(21)*
    a. 225 g
    b. 22.5 g
    c. 1111.1 g
    d. 111.1 g
109. What size of clipper blade should be used for patient preparation? *(22)*
    a. 10
    b. 20
    c. 30
    d. 40
110. The origin of electrical activity in the myocardium is *(23)*
    a. AV node
    b. SA node
    c. Atrium
    d. Ventricle
111. The etiological agent for tetanus is *(24)*
    a. *Clostridium difficile*
    b. *Clostridium perfringens*
    c. *Clostridium tetani*
    d. *Ehrlichia coli*
112. The vein most commonly used in ruminants for IV catheterization in large animals is *(25)*
    a. Cephalic
    b. Saphenous
    c. Jugular
    d. Mammary
113. The most common oral tumor in dogs is a(an) *(26)*
    a. Melanoma
    b. Squamous cell carcinoma
    c. Fibrosarcoma
    d. Eosinophilic ulcer

114. __________ is used for cardiac arrest and is commonly administered via the intratracheal route *(27)*
 a. Lidocaine
 b. Atropine
 c. Epinephrine
 d. Sodium bicarbonate
115. Intradermal skin testing is used to detect *(28)*
 a. Mycobacteria
 b. Rabies
 c. Cryptosporidium
 d. *Sarcoptes scabei*
116. The Internet can be used by veterinary technicians for all except *(29)*
 a. Searching for the latest information on a disease process
 b. Keeping current on the political happenings in the profession
 c. Plagiarizing assignments
 d. Sharing ideas via chat rooms
117. Which of the following contains valves? *(1)*
 a. Arteries and veins
 b. Veins and lymphatic vessels
 c. Veins and capillaries
 d. Arteries and lymphatic vessels
118. A large leukocyte with variable nuclear shape with diffuse chromatin, blue-gray cytoplasm, vacuoles, and possible fine pink granules is descriptive of a (an) *(2)*
 a. Lymphocyte
 b. NRBC
 c. Monocyte
 d. Basophil
119. An epithelial cell tumor that usually exfoliates sheets of cells is also referred to as *(3)*
 a. Sarcoma
 b. Carcinoma
 c. Lipoma
 d. Hematoma
120. The intermediate host for *Dipylidium caninum* is a (an) *(4)*
 a. Infective egg
 b. Rodent
 c. Flea
 d. Mosquito
121. The goal of streaking for isolation is to *(5)*
 a. Cover the surface of the bacterial plate as evenly as possible
 b. Sterilize the loop used for streaking
 c. Determine if a bacteria is gram positive or gram negative
 d. Obtain bacterial colonies that are isolated from each other so they can be identified
122. Which of the following enzymes is considered a liver specific enzyme in dogs and cats? *(6)*
 a. Alkaline phosphatase
 b. Aspartate aminotransferase
 c. Sorbitol dehydrogenase
 d. Alanine aminotransferase
123. Viruses are *(7)*
 a. The smallest form of life
 b. Never found outside the host
 c. Obligate intracellular parasites
 d. Always difficult to disinfect
124. Why is a second vaccine administered to elicit a secondary immune response in a patient? *(8)*
 a. To stimulate the production of more phagocytes
 b. To stimulate the production of an increased IgM antibody titer
 c. To cause the patient to produce an acquired artificial passive immunity
 d. To result in a stronger, faster immunity by causing a secondary immune response
125. A lead shank in a horse is used for all *except*, when you need *(9)*
 a. It to lift up the horse's leg
 b. More restraint
 c. A distraction technique
 d. To discipline a horse
126. Which of the following disinfectants has sporicidal activity? *(10)*
 a. Alcohols
 b. Aldehydes
 c. Phenols
 d. Peroxides
127. There is about a 1-inch clear band along one of the narrow film edges of the manually processed radiograph. This occurred because the *(11)*
 a. Developer is too low
 b. Fixer is too low
 c. Field size was collimated in too far
 d. Film edge was exposed to light
128. Ultrasound uses sound that is in what range of human hearing? *(12)*
 a. Within
 b. Below
 c. Above
 d. Equal to
129. A masking of one allele over the genes on another is called *(13)*
 a. Polygenic
 b. Epistasis
 c. Expressivity
 d. Codominance
130. Which of the following is not a cause of inappropriate urination in the house? *(14)*
 a. Diet change
 b. Separation anxiety
 c. Fear
 d. Medical condition
131. The minimum time for an elimination food trial is *(15)*
 a. 4 weeks
 b. 6 weeks
 c. 4 months
 d. 6 months
132. How many gallons of water does a lactating cow require to produce 1 gallon (3.8 L) of milk? *(16)*
 a. 1 to 2 (3.8 to 7.5 L)
 b. 3 to 5 (11.4 to 18.9 L)
 c. 8 to 10 (30.2 to 37.8 L)
 d. 12 to 15 (45.5 to 56.7 L)

133. Newborn offspring from which of the following species are precocious, with hair, erupted teeth, and open eyes? *(17)*
 a. Guinea pig, chinchilla, and degu
 b. Guinea pig, rabbit, and hedgehog
 c. Mouse, guinea pig, and rat
 d. Gerbil, hamster, and degu
134. The avian pectoral girdle is composed of *(18)*
 a. Clavicle, scapula, and humerus
 b. Clavicle, coracoid, and scapula
 c. Humerus, radius, and ulna
 d. Femur, tibia, and fibula
135. To reduce the amount of rebreathing during the use of a rebreathing system, which of the following would you do? *(19)*
 a. Increase the total fresh gas flow rate
 b. Decrease the total fresh gas flow rate
 c. Increase percent of inhalant anesthetic gas
 d. Decrease percent of inhalant anesthetic gas
136. Which class of reproductive drug can be potentially dangerous to pregnant females who come into contact with it? *(20)*
 a. Gonadotropins such as hCG
 b. Prostaglandins such as dinoprost (Lutalyse)
 c. Estrogens such as estradiol cypionate (ECP)
 d. Progestins such as megestrol acetate (Ovaban)
137. There is a client on the telephone trying to figure out an old prescription. She reads to you the following: "Put 2 drops O.S. q.4h for 3 days then q.8h for 3 days until finished. Not for p.o. use." What does this label mean? *(21)*
 a. Put 2 drops on the mouth every 4 hours for 3 days, then every 8 hours for 3 days until finished
 b. Put 2 drops in the right eye about 4 times a day for 3 days, then about every 8 hours for 3 days until finished. Before meals
 c. Put 2 drops in the left eye about 3 times a day for 3 days, then about 4 times a day for 3 days until finished. Not for oral use
 d. Put 2 drops in left eye every 4 hours for 3 days, then every 8 hours for 3 days until finished. Not for oral use
138. What is not a standard method of gloving when preparing for surgery? *(22)*
 a. Open gloving
 b. Open cuffed gloving
 c. Closed gloving
 d. Closed hand gloving
139. What is not represented on an ECG tracing? *(23)*
 a. Ventricular systole
 b. Atrial systole
 c. Ventricular repolarization
 d. Atrial repolarization
140. Potomac horse fever is transmitted by *(24)*
 a. Mosquitoes
 b. Ticks
 c. Flies
 d. Snails
141. All of the following are zoonotic except *(25)*
 a. Orf
 b. Blue tongue
 c. Leptospirosis
 d. Erysipelas
142. The lesion that occurs at the neck of the tooth in cats is called a (an) *(26)*
 a. Epulis lesion
 b. Crevicular lesion
 c. Root cavity
 d. External odontoclastic resorption (EOR)
143. What are the clinical signs of dystocia? *(27)*
 a. Active contractions for more than 30 minutes
 b. More than 2 hours between deliveries
 c. Green discharge with no delivery of fetus
 d. All of the above
144. *Capnocytophaga canimrsus* causes which of the following in canids? *(28)*
 a. Profuse, watery diarrhea
 b. Abortions
 c. No symptoms
 d. Eating of feces
145. A good supervisor will *(29)*
 a. Tell people what to do at the start of each day
 b. Delegate only those things that they do not want to do
 c. Motivate and provide constructive criticism
 d. Control employees' activities so the job is done correctly
146. The four primary body tissues are *(1)*
 a. Dense, muscle, nervous, bone
 b. Epithelial, bone, muscle, aerolar
 c. Nervous, cartilage, connective, reticular
 d. Muscle, nervous, epithelial, connective
147. Staining urine sediment can be easily accomplished by using which of the following? *(2)*
 a. Papanicolaou stain
 b. Sedi-stain
 c. Gram stain
 d. Wright-Giemsa
148. A mesenchymal cell tumor that usually exfoliates single cells may be referred to as *(3)*
 a. Sarcoma
 b. Carcinoma
 c. Lipoma
 d. Hematoma
149. *Taenia* spp. ova are *(4)*
 a. Dark brown and nearly spherical with striations evident
 b. Different colors compared with other ova
 c. Larger than *Toxascaris leonina* ova
 d. Indistinguishable from other ova
150. Salmonella-Shigella agar do all of the following *except (5)*
 a. Select pathogenic enteric bacteria
 b. Select gram-positive bacteria
 c. Differentiate on the basis of lactose fermentation
 d. Differentiate on the basis of hydrogen sulfide production
151. The anticoagulant of choice for collecting samples for electrolyte determination is *(6)*
 a. Heparin
 b. EDTA
 c. Sodium fluoride
 d. Sodium citrate

152. A latent infection is *(7)*
    a. One that never causes clinical signs
    b. Often dormant until the host is stressed
    c. Caused by a cancer-causing oncogenic virus
    d. One against which the animal is vaccinated
153. Ingestion of colostrum is an example of *(8)*
    a. Acquired artificial passive immunity
    b. Acquired natural active immunity
    c. Acquired natural passive immunity
    d. Innate immunity
154. Where is the safest place to stand when you are next to a cow? *(9)*
    a. Slightly in front and to the left of the head
    b. Slightly in front of the shoulder
    c. Next to the abdomen
    d. Slightly in front of the back leg
155. Liquids to be autoclaved must be placed in a container at least ______ time(s) the size as the liquid volume. *(10)*
    a. One
    b. Two
    c. Three
    d. Six
156. Which of the following will give you 20 mAs *(11)*
    a. 100 mA and $\frac{1}{10}$ second
    b. 100 mA and $\frac{1}{20}$ second
    c. 200 mA and $\frac{1}{10}$ second
    d. 300 mA and $\frac{1}{20}$ second
157. A mechanical sector scanner consists of one or more crystals mechanically moved to produce what type of image? *(12)*
    a. Rectangular
    b. Pie-shaped
    c. Square
    d. Linear
158. In which animal is the age of puberty directly related to body weight? *(13)*
    a. Cat
    b. Dog
    c. Cattle
    d. Goat
159. The owner of a two-cat household complains about feces found outside of the litterbox. Which statement is the least correct to resolve the problem? *(14)*
    a. Provide a second litterbox
    b. Clean the litterboxes more frequently
    c. Avoid perfumed litter substrate
    d. Confine both cats in the same room as the litterbox
160. The most common nutrient of concern in adverse food reactions is *(15)*
    a. Carbohydrate
    b. Protein
    c. Vitamins
    d. Fat
161. A disease that is associated with a lack of usable carbohydrates during late gestation in sheep or early lactation in cattle is *(16)*
    a. Milk fever
    b. White muscle disease
    c. Rickets
    d. Ketosis
162. Normal rabbit urine is *(17)*
    a. Clear and brown
    b. Clear and orange
    c. Cloudy and thick
    d. Blood-tinged
163. When restraining a bird, it is important to *(18)*
    a. Not restrict movement of the sternum
    b. Cover their eyes
    c. Use large leather gloves
    d. Hold them by their wings
164. During a surgical plane of anesthesia, where will the eye position be *(19)*
    a. Ventral-medial
    b. Dorsal-medial
    c. Lateral
    d. Central
165. Why is it important to know the cause of vomiting before giving an antiemetic? *(20)*
    a. Different drugs work on different emetic centers
    b. Giving an inappropriate drug could make the problem worse
    c. In some cases vomiting should be encouraged
    d. All of the above
166. A patient needs to receive 1.2 L of lactated Ringer's solution at the drip rate of 50 drops/min using a 15 drops/mL administration set. How long will it take for the fluids to be administered? *(21)*
    a. 4 hours
    b. 3 hours
    c. 6 hours
    d. 120 minutes
167. Which style of surgical mask allows the least amount of air to escape? *(22)*
    a. Molded
    b. Hooded
    c. Flat pleated
    d. See through
168. What would be evident in a lightly tranquilized dog if an orogastric tube has been placed in the patient's trachea? *(23)*
    a. Dyspnea and coughing occur
    b. Popping and gurgling sounds are coming from the tube
    c. After palpation, there appears to be two tubes in the neck region
    d. Vomiting occurs
169. Which of the following is transmitted by mosquitoes? *(24)*
    a. *Clostridium difficile* and *Salmonella* spp.
    b. *Ehrlichia risticii* and colitis
    c. *Equine encephalmyelitides* and West Nile virus
    d. HYPP and EPM
170. In cattle undergoing general anesthesia, which of the following will not assist in the prevention of bloat in the patient? *(25)*
    a. An orogastric tube should be placed
    b. They should be placed in sternal recumbency for recovery
    c. Withhold feed 24 to 48 hours
    d. Deflate cuff before extubation

171. The bulk of the tooth is composed of *(26)*
   a. Enamel
   b. Dentin
   c. Cementum
   d. Pulp
172. How is hyperkalemia treated if a cat has a urinary obstruction? *(27)*
   a. Insulin/dextrose
   b. Calcium gluconate
   c. Lidocaine
   d. Sodium bicarbonate
173. Leptospirosis is mainly passed through contact with *(28)*
   a. Skin of infected animal
   b. Infective urine
   c. Aerosolized discharges
   d. Fomites
174. Greater success in achieving goals can be realized if *(29)*
   a. Priorities are set
   b. You wait to start to determine if the goal will change —you never know
   c. Give all responsibility for completing the goal to someone else who is faster
   d. Use procrastination to your advantage
175. The receptors for hearing are part of the ________ within the ________________ *(1)*
   a. Stapes/cochlea
   b. Cochlea/middle ear
   c. Organ of Corti/inner ear
   d. Organ of Corti/middle ear
176. The presence of intact RBCs in the urine is referred to as *(2)*
   a. Oliguria
   b. Pollakiuria
   c. Azotemia
   d. Hematuria
177. A stain used specifically for staining of nuclei, mast cells, or infectious agents is *(3)*
   a. Romanovsky
   b. Giemsa
   c. New methylene blue
   d. Gram stain
178. *Giardia* spp. have *(4)*
   a. Undulating membrane
   b. Long flagella from the anterior end
   c. Bipolar plugs
   d. An operculum
179. Which of the following CANNOT be used to sterilize a bacteriology loop *(5)*
   a. An electric heating element
   b. An incubator
   c. A Bunsen burner
   d. An alcohol lamp
180. Many of the electrolytes act closely with other electrolytes. Which of the following combinations of electrolytes are closely related? *(6)*
   a. Sodium, potassium, and hydrogen
   b. Calcium, phosphorous, and magnesium
   c. Sodium and bicarbonate
   d. All of the above
181. The order of the viral replication cycle is *(7)*
   a. Attachment, penetration, uncoating, assembly, and release
   b. Attachment, penetration, assembly, uncoating, and release
   c. Attachment, assembly, and release
   d. Attachment, penetration, assembly, release, and uncoating
182. Atopy is a genetically based condition where the patient *(8)*
   a. Does not possess IgE antibody
   b. Has an overreactive innate system
   c. Produces an excess of IgE antibody
   d. Is cell-mediated immunity deficient
183. What is the sheep's main means of defense? *(9)*
   a. Speed and flocking instinct
   b. Hooves and head
   c. Teeth and hooves
   d. Speed and head
184. Which of the following disinfectants is inactivated by the presence of organic debris? *(10)*
   a. Aldehydes
   b. Chlorine
   c. Phenols
   d. Biguanides
185. As the contrast of a radiograph decreases, you will have a *(11)*
   a. Brighter radiograph with few steps but greater differences between each step
   b. Brighter radiograph with many steps but little differences between each step
   c. Grayer radiograph with few steps but greater differences between each step
   d. Grayer radiograph with many steps but little differences between each step
186. A structure that contains cystic and solid lesions is *(12)*
   a. Hypoechoic
   b. Anechoic
   c. Complex
   d. Sonolucent
187. On a pedigree chart, what symbol represents unknown sex? *(13)*
   a. Half solid symbol
   b. Diamond
   c. Square
   d. Open symbol
188. Which statement is the best advice for cat owners who do not want to declaw their cat? *(14)*
   a. Buy leather furniture instead of fabric furniture
   b. Allow cat outdoors
   c. Rub the furniture with mothballs
   d. Get a second cat to entertain the first one
189. What is the most essential nutrient required for survival? *(15)*
   a. Water
   b. Protein
   c. Fat
   d. Carbohydrate

190. A nutritional disease of equines associated with acute overconsumption of grain, lush pasture, or water is *(16)*
   a. Heaves
   b. Rickets
   c. Laminitis
   d. Water belly
191. Which species has two pair of upper incisors (peg teeth)? *(17)*
   a. Degu
   b. Gerbil
   c. Hamster
   d. Rabbit
192. Autonomy in exotic medicine is the *(18)*
   a. Study of the parts of the body
   b. Slow movement of a turtle
   c. Ability of a lizard to shed its tail when captured
   d. Shedding of the skin in reptiles
193. Paradoxical breathing is characterized as which of the following? *(19)*
   a. Holding of breath on inspiration
   b. Increased respiration rate
   c. Abdomen rising and chest falling during an inspiration
   d. Increased tidal volume
194. Chemotherapeutic drugs require specific precautions for safe handling to prevent occupational exposure because they *(20)*
   a. Can cause a miscarriage
   b. Can affect rapidly growing cells in humans
   c. Will cause an allergic reaction in humans
   d. Are toxic to the skin and mucous membranes
195. The veterinarian gives you the following prescription to fill. "Levothyroxin sodium tablets 0.1 mg/10 pounds, SID for 4 weeks." The canine patient weighs 27 kg. The available tablet sizes are 0.1, 0.2, 0.3, 0.5, and 0.8 mg tablets. What should be written on the prescription label? *(21)*
   a. Give ¾ tablet each day for 28 days (0.8 mg tablet, quantity 21 tabs)
   b. Give 1 tablet each day for 28 days (0.2 mg tablet, quantity 28 tabs)
   c. Give 1 tablet each day for 4 weeks (0.2 mg tablet, quantity 28 tabs)
   d. Give 1 tablet twice a day for 28 days (0.1 mg tablet, quantity 28 tabs)
196. Which of the following is not a duty of a sterile assistant? *(22)*
   a. Provide hemostasis
   b. Touching the instruments with the bare hands
   c. Provide retraction of tissues
   d. Keep count of gauze squares
197. A Foley catheter is inserted in *(23)*
   a. The jugular vein for extended periods of time
   b. Only the female dog for collection of urine
   c. The male dog to facilitate a sterile collection of blood
   d. A dog's urethra for long periods of catheterization
198. In horses, there is a vaccine available for *(24)*
   a. Equine protozoal myeloencephalitis
   b. Equine infectious anemia
   c. Sleeping sickness
   d. Hyperkalemic periodic paralysis
199. Intramuscular injections, in animals entering the food chain, should be given in the *(25)*
   a. Gluteal muscles
   b. Semimembranosis muscles
   c. Semitendenosis muscles
   d. Lateral cervical muscles
200. With the triadan numbering system, the lower left fourth premolar is tooth number *(26)*
   a. 108
   b. 208
   c. 308
   d. 408
201. What statement best describes paradoxical respirations? *(27)*
   a. Labored inspiration
   b. Cheyne-Stokes
   c. Abdominal wall and chest wall does not move synchronously
   d. Labored expiration
202. *Toxocara* larva (in humans) typically does not migrate through which organs? *(28)*
   a. Viscera, somatic tissues
   b. Eyes
   c. Intestines
   d. Ears
203. All of the following are true about stress, *except* that it *(29)*
   a. Creates a feeling of tension and pressure
   b. Is never healthy
   c. Causes physical as well as mental symptoms
   d. Is created by lack of control over one's life
204. Which of the following is not a function of the autonomic nervous system? *(1)*
   a. Causing muscles of the foreleg to contract
   b. Contracting and dilating blood vessels
   c. Causing changes in heart rate
   d. Causing muscles of the intestine to contract
205. Which of the following is considered the least reliable method of determining urine specific gravity? *(2)*
   a. Reagent test strips
   b. Refractometer
   c. Urinometer
   d. All are unreliable
206. A sample that contains macrophages and 65% neutrophils is classified as *(3)*
   a. Purulent
   b. Granulomatous
   c. Suppurative
   d. Pyogranulomatous
207. All of the following are true of Trematodes *except* that they *(4)*
   a. Are hermaphroditic
   b. Have two suckers (oral and ventral)
   c. Are all host specific
   d. Require an intermediate host
208. *Campylobacter* sp. are bacteria that *(5)*
   a. Do not grow well on usual microbiology media
   b. Can be presumptively identified on a gram stain by their shape
   c. Are anaerobic
   d. Both a and b

209. If the exocrine function of the pancreas is abnormal, one would expect to find *(6)*
   a. Chronic or acute pancreatitis
   b. Hyperglycemia or hypoglycemia
   c. Normal blood lipase or amylase
   d. Abnormal blood or urine glucose
210. Which of the following is *not* a virology test that is commonly performed in veterinary clinics? *(7)*
   a. FA
   b. ELISA
   c. EM
   d. LA
211. Characteristics of killed or inactivated vaccines are that they *(8)*
   a. Usually require repeated administrations to produce a healthy level of immunity
   b. May cause a mild form of the disease in some patients
   c. Do not store well
   d. Cause abortions in pregnant patients
212. What method works best to move a pig from one place to another? *(9)*
   a. Yelling and shouting
   b. Get a large group of people to herd the pigs
   c. Use a dog to chase the pigs
   d. Use a hurdle or plastic pipe
213. Items sterilized in an ethylene oxide chamber must be ventilated for at least ___ hours to remove residual ethylene oxide. *(10)*
   a. 24
   b. 18
   c. 12
   d. 2
214. If you do not follow proper safelight procedures in the x-ray dark room, you will cause *(11)*
   a. Fogging of the film
   b. Underexposure of the film
   c. Clearing of the film when it is developed and fixed
   d. A dark border around the edges of the film
215. Lateral resolution depends on beam *(12)*
   a. Bandwidth
   b. Frequency
   c. Wavelength
   d. Width
216. Lordosis is *(13)*
   a. Vocalization
   b. Tail deflection
   c. Crouching and rolling on the floor
   d. A clear discharge from the vulva
217. For which of these behavior problems is drug therapy not a solution? *(14)*
   a. Obsessive/compulsive disorder
   b. Running away/escaping
   c. Separation anxiety
   d. Aggression
218. Ideal weight loss per week for a cat is *(15)*
   a. 0.25 lb (0.11 kg)
   b. 0.5 lb (0.22 kg)
   c. 1.0 lb (0.45 kg)
   d. 1.5 lb (0.68 kg)
219. Two animals that benefit nutritionally from consuming browse are *(16)*
   a. Pig and sheep
   b. Goat and llama
   c. Horse and cattle
   d. Horse and sheep
220. The most common health condition to affect workers in a laboratory animal facility is *(17)*
   a. Salmonellosis
   b. Giardiasis
   c. Laboratory animal allergens
   d. Pasteurellosis
221. The normal CaP ratio in a bird is *(18)*
   a. 51
   b. 1.51
   c. 15
   d. 101
222. Which of the following is an indication of hypoventilation? *(19)*
   a. Respiratory acidosis
   b. Respiratory alkalosis
   c. Metabolic acidosis
   d. Metabolic alkalosis
223. An otic drug may not be effective if ___________ and may cause toxicity if ___________. *(20)*
   a. The ear canal is dirty/the eardrum is ruptured
   b. The ear is infected/the eardrum is covered with wax
   c. The bacteria are not correctly identified/the patient has kidney or liver disease
   d. Parasites are present in the ear canal/parasites are present in the middle ear
224. What is the dose range in mg and mL for a 13-kg dog for atropine sulfate (0.5 mg/mL) at dosage of 0.02 to 0.04 mg/kg? *(21)*
   a. 2.6 to 6.5 mg/5.2 to 13 mL
   b. 0.26 to 0.52 mg/0.052 to 0.104 mL
   c. 0.26 to 0.52 mg/0.52 to 1.04 mL
   d. 0.26 to 0.26 mg/kg/0.052 to 1.04 mL/kg
225. What size surgical blade attaches to a no. 4 Bard Parker scalpel handle? *(22)*
   a. 20
   b. 15
   c. 11
   d. 10
226. A squamous cell carcinoma may be located in *(23)*
   a. The nasal cavity of a white cat and is malignant
   b. Mammary tissue and is benign
   c. Axillary lymph tissue and is cancerous
   d. Fibrous tissue and is metastatic
227. How are horses infected with equine protozoal myeloencephalitis? *(24)*
   a. Fomites
   b. Opossum feces
   c. Arthropods
   d. Aerosol
228. Which of the following is considered a quick release knot *(25)*
   a. Tom fool
   b. Square knot
   c. Bowline
   d. Slipknot

229. The surface of the incisor tooth facing the roof of the mouth is *(26)*
   a. Lingual
   b. Buccal
   c. Palatal
   d. Labial
230. What is the antidote for organophosphate toxicity? *(27)*
   a. Vitamin K_1
   b. Ethanol
   c. 2-PAM (pralidoxime)
   d. Methylpyrazole
231. Which group of animals is most likely to be a vector for human herpes B infection? *(28)*
   a. Reptiles
   b. Primates
   c. Canids
   d. Felids
232. A symptom of burnout is *(29)*
   a. Euphoria
   b. Exhaustion
   c. Mania
   d. Going to the movies
233. In glomerular filtration, metabolic waste from the plasma would *(1)*
   a. Pass into the distal convoluted tubule
   b. Remain in the plasma
   c. Pass into peritubular capillaries
   d. Pass into Bowman's capsule
234. Which of the following is not a granulocyte precursor? *(2)*
   a. Prorubricyte
   b. Myeloblast
   c. Band
   d. Metamyelocyte
235. A sample that contains few macrophages and greater than 70% neutrophils is classified as *(3)*
   a. Purulent
   b. Granulomatous
   c. Suppurative
   d. Pyogranulomatous
236. Examples of parasites in ruminant hosts that produce GIN-type eggs are *(4)*
   a. *Cooperia, Moniezia, Ostertagia*
   b. *Cooperia, Trichuris, Haemonchus*
   c. *Cooperia, Eimeria, Ostertagia*
   d. *Cooperia, Ostertagia, Haemonchus*
237. A lactose fermenting bacterial colony is what color on MacConkey agar? *(5)*
   a. Black
   b. Clear
   c. Dark pink or purple
   d. White
238. The following is true of hyperglycemia *except* that it *(6)*
   a. May be induced by stress
   b. Must be accompanied by glycosuria to confirm a diagnosis of diabetes mellitus
   c. Often accompanies pancreatitis
   d. Always leads to a diagnosis of diabetes mellitus
239. Which of the following is true regarding the analysis of viral samples? *(7)*
   a. It is usually performed to determine a course of treatment
   b. It is always performed in a clinic
   c. The virus is most easily cultured from animals just prior to and just after the onset of clinical signs
   d. Previous history is not needed
240. Once a vaccine is administered to a healthy patient, it is known that the patient is immune to the disease for which it was vaccinated. *(8)*
   a. True
   b. False
241. A hog snare has an optimum effect of *(9)*
   a. 3 to 5 minutes
   b. 8 to 10 minutes
   c. 15 to 20 minutes
   d. 25 minutes
242. The recommended method of quality control for autoclave sterilization in the veterinary clinic is *(10)*
   a. Bowie Dick Test
   b. Surface sampling
   c. Biological testing
   d. Thermocouple
243. When you increase the object-film distance, you will have a *(11)*
   a. Sharper image that is smaller
   b. Sharper image that is larger
   c. Fuzzier image that is smaller
   d. Fuzzier image that is larger
244. In ultrasonography, which organ is the most echogenic? *(12)*
   a. Bladder
   b. Liver
   c. Kidney
   d. Spleen
245. A gene that has been altered by the addition of exogenous DNA is called a(an) *(13)*
   a. Transgenic gene
   b. Independent allele
   c. Hybrid vigor
   d. Karyotype
246. Which of the following is not an example of olfactory communication in cats? *(14)*
   a. Urine spraying
   b. Feces in obvious locations
   c. Meowing
   d. Rubbing
247. An ingredient panel lists ingredients in *(15)*
   a. Alphabetical order
   b. Ascending order
   c. Descending order
   d. No order
248. Copper *(16)*
   a. Toxicity is a serious issue in cattle and sheep
   b. Is not needed for iron absorption
   c. Deficiency leads to reproductive failure
   d. Is a macromineral

249. Ringworm, a common zoonotic disease carried by rodents, guineas pigs, rabbits, etc, is caused by a *(17)*
    a. Parasite
    b. Bacterium
    c. Fungus
    d. Virus
250. A turtle's respiration is controlled by *(18)*
    a. The diaphragm
    b. The intercostal muscles
    c. Water depth during swimming
    d. Alternating body cavity pressure during locomotion and pharyngeal pumping
251. Replacement crystalloids during anesthesia are administered at which of the following rates? *(19)*
    a. Up to 5 mL/kg/hr
    b. 5 to 10 mL/kg/hr
    c. 10 to 15 mL/kg/hr
    d. 15 to 20 mL/kg/hr
252. Ophthalmic steroidal anti-inflammatory drugs are contraindicated when *(20)*
    a. There is a defect in the cornea
    b. There is an infection in the cornea
    c. The patient is also receiving an antiviral drug
    d. The patient is also receiving a miotic drug
253. Meloxicam at 1.5 mg/mL is prescribed for an arthritic 45-kg Irish wolfhound. On the first day of treatment the patient should receive 0.2 mg/kg SID PO AC. The maintenance dosage is 0.1 mg/kg body weight every other day. How much meloxicam should be prescribed for a 2-week period? *(21)*
    a. 8 mL
    b. 16 mL
    c. 15 mL
    d. 24 mL
254. What type of forceps has fine intermeshing teeth on the edges of the tips? *(22)*
    a. Brown-Adson
    b. Dressing
    c. Russian thumb
    d. Halstead mosquito
255. The following cancer therapy is not usually used to cure a patient *(23)*
    a. Cryosurgery
    b. Surgery
    c. Histopathology
    d. Antineoplastic antibiotics
256. The term "floating teeth" in reference to horses refers to *(24)*
    a. When a horse chews side to side
    b. Rasping down the sharp edges of teeth
    c. The removal of wolf teeth
    d. When a horse reacts to the bit
257. Tail bleeding is most commonly performed in which species *(25)*
    a. Cattle
    b. Goat
    c. Sheep
    d. Pig
258. The number of permanent teeth in cats is *(26)*
    a. 26
    b. 30
    c. 35
    d. 42
259. The most common occurring electrolyte imbalances associated with Addison's disease are *(27)*
    a. Hyperchloremia and hyperkalemia
    b. Hypernatremia and hypokalemia
    c. Hypokalemia and hypernatremia
    d. Hyponatremia and hyperkalemia
260. Newcastle disease causes which of the following symptoms in domestic poultry? *(28)*
    a. Watery, green diarrhea; tracheal exudate; facial edema; intestinal mucosa necrosis
    b. Gasping, coughing
    c. Twisted neck; paralysis; drooping wings; anorexia
    d. All of the above
261. When dealing with conflict, make sure you do all *except* *(29)*
    a. Separate the person from the problem
    b. Always walk away from the source of the conflict
    c. Identify options for possible solutions
    d. Focus on the interest, not the position
262. The part of a synovial joint that encloses the joint in a strong fibrous covering is *(1)*
    a. Synovial membrane
    b. Articular cartilage
    c. Joint capsule
    d. Synovial ligaments
263. The term for a variation in the size of erythrocytes is *(2)*
    a. Poikilocytosis
    b. Stomatocytosis
    c. Crenation
    d. Anisocytosis
264. A transudate would be expected to have a total protein concentration of *(3)*
    a. >7.5
    b. 7.5
    c. <7.5
    d. <3
265. A technician notes that during a patient's bath, the rinse water turned a red color. This could be an indication of an infestation of *(4)*
    a. *Ctenocephalides canis*
    b. *Ancylostoma caninum*
    c. *Strongylus vulgaris*
    d. *Oxyuris equi*
266. A bacterium that only grows on the TSA/blood agar plate is *(5)*
    a. An anaerobic bacteria
    b. Probably *Mycobacterium* sp.
    c. A fastidious organism
    d. All of the above

267. TLI (trypsin-like immunoreactivity) *(6)*
   a. Is highly specific for canine exocrine pancreatic insufficiency
   b. Uses EDTA anticoagulant
   c. Is completed on nonfasting animals
   d. Is used to determine if an animal has endocrine pancreatic insufficiency
268. What information is not needed when submitting virology samples for diagnosis? *(7)*
   a. The number of animals affected
   b. The clinical signs and treatment administered to date
   c. The veterinarian's tentative disease diagnosis
   d. Animal eye color
269. Which of the following is false with regard to maternal antibodies? *(8)*
   a. They are obtained by the neonates of all species via colostrum
   b. The antibodies do not prevent neonatal diarrhea
   c. They may block the effectiveness of vaccines when given too early in the neonate's life
   d. They convey short-lived immunity to the neonate
270. What does the standing part of the rope refer to? *(9)*
   a. The part of the rope that is attached to the animal
   b. The shortest part of the rope when tying a knot
   c. The part of the rope attached to an inanimate object
   d. The middle part of the rope
271. The recommended method of quality control for disinfection of the surgical suite in the veterinary clinic is *(10)*
   a. Bowie Dick test
   b. Surface sampling
   c. Biological testing
   d. Thermocouple
272. A black mark on a radiographic film could be caused by all of the following *except* for *(11)*
   a. Debris in the intensifying screen
   b. Static electricity
   c. Light leak
   d. Linear lines due to grid cutoff
273. Hertz refers to *(12)*
   a. Velocity
   b. Density
   c. Cycles per second
   d. Wavelength
274. In mares, the incidence of dystocia is *(13)*
   a. <1%
   b. <3%
   c. <5%
   d. <6%
275. Which factor is least important to consider when selecting a pet? *(14)*
   a. Exercise requirement
   b. Grooming requirement
   c. Financial resources
   d. Child's preferences
276. Food allergy/intolerance in pets may manifest themselves as *(15)*
   a. Gastrointestinal or dermatological signs
   b. Gastrointestinal or renal signs
   c. Hepatic or renal signs
   d. Cardiac or hepatic signs
277. The most critical nutritional requirement for newborns is *(16)*
   a. Water intake
   b. Carbohydrate intake
   c. Protein intake
   d. Colostrum intake
278. You have been asked to give a dehydrated adult mouse intraperitoneal fluid therapy. What would be the absolute maximum that you could safely give? *(17)*
   a. 1 mL
   b. 2 mL
   c. 3 mL
   d. 4 mL
279. In housing reptiles, the term "POT" refers to *(18)*
   a. Preferred outdoor tank
   b. Plastic outdoor tank
   c. Plastic oblong tank
   d. Preferred optimal temperature
280. If the patient's total protein is 3.5 g/dL, which of the following is not considered a suitable choice for intravenous fluids during anesthesia? *(19)*
   a. Plasma
   b. Crystalloids
   c. Dextran
   d. 15 to 20 mL/kg/hr
281. Analgesics that may be toxic to cats include *(20)*
   a. Narcotic analgesics
   b. Local anesthetics
   c. Nonsteroidal anti-inflammatory drugs
   d. Steroids
282. What volume of fluids did a patient receive if the drip rate was approximately 45 drops/min using a 20 drops/mL administration set, the IV line was in place at 800 mL, and the patient removed it at 1500 mL? *(21)*
   a. 945 mL
   b. Approximately 2 L
   c. 5.67 L
   d. 260 mL
283. When labeling sterile packs, what information is *not* necessary? *(22)*
   a. Content
   b. Date of sterilization
   c. Initial of the person who prepared the pack
   d. Intended patient
284. When performing wound lavage the most effective treatment is rinsing the wound with *(23)*
   a. Hydrogen peroxide using a Water Pik
   b. Normal saline in a 3-mL syringe using an 18-gauge needle
   c. Chlorhexidine diacetate solution in a spray bottle
   d. Povidine-iodine solution (10%) with a 60-mL syringe and 18-gauge needle
285. A major postoperative concern for the horse is *(24)*
   a. PCV and TP
   b. Moving the horse back to its stall as quickly as possible
   c. Proper grooming and shoe removal
   d. Ileus

286. When performing a tuberculin test, the tuberculin is injected *(25)*
    a. Intramuscularly
    b. Subcutaneously
    c. Intradermally
    d. Intravenously
287. The instrument used to scale the root of the tooth is a(an) *(26)*
    a. Sickle
    b. Explorer
    c. Probe
    d. Curet
288. What does SpO_2 measure? *(27)*
    a. Hemoglobin saturation
    b. PaO_2
    c. $PaCO_2$
    d. Lung sounds
289. Hookworm disease is not likely to be transmitted to humans via *(28)*
    a. Mosquitoes
    b. Walking barefoot where animals have defecated
    c. Fecal-oral route
    d. Poor sanitation and hygiene
290. When setting up a budget, you should *(29)*
    a. Just list household expenses
    b. List all expenses and income
    c. Include only your salary as income
    d. Make sure you have more expenses than income

1. b	30. c	59. a	88. d	117. b	146. d
2. c	31. b	60. d	89. c	118. c	147. b
3. d	32. c	61. d	90. b	119. b	148. a
4. b	33. a	62. c	91. c	120. c	149. a
5. a	34. a	63. b	92. a	121. d	150. b
6. b	35. d	64. c	93. a	122. d	151. a
7. a	36. c	65. a	94. b	123. c	152. b
8. a	37. b	66. c	95. b	124. d	153. c
9. c	38. a	67. d	96. a	125. a	154. b
10. b	39. c	68. b	97. a	126. b	155. c
11. c	40. a	69. c	98. c	127. a	156. c
12. a	41. d	70. c	99. d	128. c	157. b
13. d	42. d	71. c	100. a	129. b	158. c
14. b	43. c	72. d	101. c	130. a	159. d
15. b	44. b	73. b	102. b	131. a	160. b
16. c	45. a	74. c	103. a	132. b	161. d
17. b	46. c	75. a	104. b	133. a	162. c
18. b	47. c	76. a	105. a	134. b	163. a
19. c	48. b	77. b	106. a	135. a	164. a
20. d	49. c	78. a	107. c	136. b	165. d
21. b	50. d	79. b	108. b	137. d	166. c
22. c	51. a	80. b	109. d	138. c	167. c
23. a	52. d	81. d	110. b	139. d	168. a
24. c	53. a	82. a	111. c	140. d	169. c
25. d	54. c	83. d	112. c	141. b	170. d
26. d	55. b	84. c	113. a	142. d	171. b
27. c	56. d	85. b	114. c	143. d	172. a
28. a	57. d	86. b	115. a	144. c	173. b
29. c	58. c	87. c	116. c	145. c	174. a

175. c
176. d
177. c
178. b
179. b
180. d
181. a
182. c
183. a
184. b
185. d
186. c
187. b
188. b
189. a
190. c
191. d
192. c
193. c
194. b
195. a
196. b
197. d
198. c
199. d
200. c
201. c
202. d
203. b
204. a
205. a
206. d
207. c
208. d
209. a
210. c
211. a
212. d
213. a
214. a
215. d
216. c
217. b
218. a
219. b
220. c
221. b
222. a
223. a
224. c
225. a
226. a
227. b
228. d
229. c
230. c
231. b
232. b
233. d
234. a
235. a
236. d
237. c
238. d
239. c
240. b
241. c
242. c
243. d
244. d
245. a
246. c
247. c
248. a
249. c
250. d
251. b
252. b
253. d
254. a
255. d
256. b
257. a
258. b
259. d
260. d
261. b
262. c
263. d
264. d
265. a
266. c
267. a
268. d
269. a
270. d
271. b
272. a
273. c
274. a
275. d
276. a
277. d
278. c
279. d
280. b
281. c
282. a
283. d
284. c
285. d
286. c
287. d
288. a
289. a
290. b

APPENDIX H

Answer Key to Chapter Study Questions

Chapter 1
1. a
2. a
3. d
4. b
5. d
6. b
7. b
8. c
9. d
10. d

Chapter 2
1. b
2. c
3. d
4. b
5. a
6. b
7. a
8. c
9. b
10. c

Chapter 3
1. c
2. b
3. a
4. d
5. c
6. a
7. b
8. c
9. b
10. a

Chapter 4
1. b
2. a
3. a
4. c
5. b
6. b
7. a
8. d
9. d
10. d

Chapter 5
1. d
2. b
3. c
4. a
5. d
6. c
7. c
8. a
9. b
10. a

Chapter 6
1. c
2. c
3. b
4. c
5. b
6. b
7. a
8. a
9. b
10. d

Chapter 7
1. c
2. c
3. a
4. d
5. a
6. b
7. d
8. c
9. d
10. a

Chapter 8
1. d
2. d
3. d
4. c
5. d
6. b
7. a
8. b
9. a
10. a

Chapter 9
1. a
2. d
3. a
4. d
5. d
6. c
7. a
8. d
9. b
10. b

Chapter 10
1. c
2. b
3. c
4. a
5. d
6. c
7. d
8. b
9. d
10. c

Chapter 11
1. c
2. b
3. d
4. b
5. c
6. c
7. a
8. b
9. d
10. a

Chapter 12
1. a
2. b
3. c
4. c
5. d
6. a
7. d
8. b
9. c
10. d

Chapter 13
1. a
2. b
3. b
4. c
5. c
6. a
7. d
8. d
9. b
10. c

Chapter 14
1. a
2. a
3. d
4. b
5. a
6. a
7. c
8. b
9. c
10. c

Chapter 15
1. b
2. c
3. d
4. a
5. c
6. d
7. c
8. b
9. c
10. d

Chapter 16
1. d
2. c
3. c
4. a
5. a
6. c
7. c
8. a
9. b
10. b

Chapter 17

1. b
2. a
3. c
4. a
5. b
6. a
7. b
8. c
9. b
10. c

Chapter 18

1. b
2. c
3. b
4. a
5. a
6. a
7. b
8. b
9. b
10. d

Chapter 19

1. b
2. c
3. a
4. d
5. d
6. c
7. c
8. a
9. b
10. c

Chapter 20

1. c
2. b
3. a
4. a
5. c
6. a
7. c
8. c
9. d
10. b

Chapter 21

1. a
2. b
3. c
4. d
5. a
6. d
7. a
8. a
9. c
10. c

Chapter 22

1. b
2. b
3. d
4. a
5. d
6. a
7. c
8. b
9. c
10. a

Chapter 23

1. c
2. c
3. b
4. b
5. c
6. c
7. c
8. b
9. a
10. b

Chapter 24

1. c
2. d
3. a
4. a
5. d
6. b
7. a
8. b
9. c
10. b

Chapter 25

1. b
2. c
3. b
4. b
5. a
6. b
7. c
8. d
9. c
10. a

Chapter 26

1. c
2. c
3. d
4. b
5. a
6. b
7. a
8. d
9. b
10. c

Chapter 27

1. d
2. c
3. c
4. d
5. d
6. a
7. d
8. b
9. a
10. c

Chapter 28

1. c
2. c
3. c
4. b
5. d
6. d
7. d
8. a
9. b
10. d

Chapter 29

1. c
2. d
3. b
4. b
5. b
6. c
7. c
8. c
9. d
10. c

Index

Page numbers followed by f indicate figures; t, tables; b, boxes.

D

O

Q

R

S